BOVINE MASTITIS

BOVINE MASTITIS

Authors

NEELESH SHARMA
Assistant Professor
Division of Veterinary Clinical Medicine & Jurisprudence
Faculty of Veterinary Science & Animal Husbandry
Sher-e-Kashmir University of Agricultural Sciences & Technology of Jammu
R.S. Pura, Jammu- 181 102 (J&K), India

ANIL KUMAR SRIVASTAVA
Director and Vice-Chancellor
National Dairy Research Institute (Deemed University)
Karnal (Haryana), INDIA

GORAN BACIC
Reproduction and Theriogenelogy Clinic, Head of Ambulatory and
Herd Health Clinic Veterinary College
Zagreb University, 55 Heinzelova Av. 10000 Zagreb, Croatia, Europe

DONG KEE JEONG
Associate Professor
Animal Genetic Engineering and Stem Cell Biology Lab
Department of Biotechnology, College of Applied Life Sciences,
Jeju National University, Jeju, South Korea

RAJESH KUMAR SHARMA
Associate Professor
Department of Veterinary Pharmacology and Toxicology
College of Veterinary Science, M.P. Pashu Chikitsa Vigyan Vishwavidyalaya
Jabalpur (M.P.), INDIA

2012

SSPH

SATISH SERIAL PUBLISHING HOUSE
403, Express Tower, Commercial Complex, Azadpur, Delhi-110033 (India)
Phone : 011-27672852, Fax : 91-11-27672046
E-mail :info@satishserial.com, hkjain1975@yahoo.com Website : www.satishserial.com

Published by :

SATISH SERIAL PUBLISHING HOUSE

403, Express Tower, Commercial Complex, Azadpur, Delhi-110033 (INDIA)
Phone : 011-27672852 Fax : 91-11-27672046
E-mail : info@satishserial.com, hkjain1975@yahoo.com

ISBN 978-93-81226-03-2

Typeset at: Harminder *for* Laxmi Art Creation
Printed at: Salasar Imaging Systems, Delhi-110035

Dedicated to

DEAR READERS OF THIS BOOK

"It is important to cure diseased animals but even more important is, through skilled management and correct use, to prevent disease".

Erik Viborg, 1795
Danish Veterinarian

Preface

"Times are changing and so is veterinary medicine"

In all parts of the world milk production has been suffering from all kind of economic pressure and losses. This makes it imperative that producers become increasingly efficient in farm management. In particular it means that the milking cows used for milk production must be kept as productive and healthy as possible. There is a very thin line between healthy, high yielding dairy cow and sick, low producing animal on her exit to the slaughter house.

The food requirements and the resources to meet a projected human population of 8 billion people in the decade 2030–2040 appear to be unattainable. With grain yields increasing at 1.1% per annum and the world's population growing at 1.2% per annum the ability to satisfy food needs are gravely threatened. To reduce poverty, fight hunger and ensure global food security, there is an urgent need to increase livestock production in sustainable ways.

India is the largest milk producing country in the World. Dairying, by playing a significant role in strengthening rural economy, has brought about socio-economic transformation in India. Small farmers, marginal farmers and downtrodden constitute majority of milk producers. Dairying has vast potential to generate employment and has helped in poverty alleviation in the rural belt. Dairying provides definite and regular income and employment to millions of rural families throughout the year, especially to women thereby improving the quality of their life.

According to the 2003 livestock census, India possesses 185.2 million cattle and 97.9 million buffaloes, which is about 13.7% of the total cattle and 57.5% of the total buffalo population of the world. The dairy industry in India has made significant progress in the last few decades. Today, India is the largest producer of milk in the world. Milk production rose to about 117 million tonnes in 2010 from 17.0 million tonnes in 1950–1951. In India, although the proportion of buffaloes to cattle is 1:2, buffaloes contribute around 57% of the total milk obtained from cattle and buffaloes.

Technological and genetic developments in dairy farming have been tremendous over the last decades. These developments have resulted in more cows handled per man and per unit of space, have increased productivity, making dairy farming more intensified and larger scaled. Modern production and preventive medicine may be is not exciting as treating disease, does not involve the latest surgery techniques or molecular biology achievements; but it is the fundamental basis for welfare and health of dairy cows. It will become more and more important over the future years as more and more pressures are placed on the prevention before the treatment. At the same time markets became more competitive which resulted in smaller profit margin per cow. Today' s markets are also consumer driven which includes higher demands on animal welfare and product quality.

Mastitis (defined as an inflammatory reaction of the mammary gland) is one of the most important production diseases of dairy animals. Bovine mastitis is a complex disease in view of the complexity of its causes, pathogenesis, intensity, duration, residual effects, immunity, therapy and eradication. Although several strategies such as improved herd sanitation, antibiotic therapy, and vaccination have been developed to reduce the occurrence of mastitis, they are not effective in preventing or eliminating infections. The application of molecular or DNA-based methods in mastitis research and diagnostics has contributed to an increased understanding of mastitis epidemiology and control options. As well as the financial implications of mastitis, the importance of mastitis in public health should not be overlooked. The extensive use of antibiotics in the treatment and control of mastitis has possible implications for human health through an increased risk of antibiotic resistant strains of bacteria emerging that may then enter the food chain.

We place on record our sincere thanks to all authors whose work we have included in *Bovine mastitis.* Although nearly all the work presented in the book can be found in scientific literature but that is scattered in a lot of books, journals, reviews and symposia.

"Mastitis control is a never-ending battle for dairymen with many individual and interacting factors involved in causing problems"

Authors

Acknowledgement

At the onset, I pray with devotion before supreme 'Almighty' whose eternal blessing and inspiration enabled and emboldened me to complete this assignment.

I extend my respect and gratitude to Dr. B. Mishra, Honorable Vice Chancellor, Sher-e-Kashmir University of Agricultural Sciences and Technology, Jammu (J&K), India.

I am grateful to express my sincere thanks to Dr. A.R. Nazki, Dean, and Dr. M.S. Bhadwal, Associate Dean, Faculty of Veterinary Science, SKUAST-J, R.S. Pura, Jammu for meticulous guidance, constructive criticism and constant encouragement with relevant suggestions during entire period, in the preparation of this manuscript. I am also thankful to Dr. A.B. Srivastava, Dean, College of Veterinary Science, Jabalpur (M.P.) for constant encouragement and valuable suggestions. I sincerely thank to Dr. S.K. Gupta, Dr. Kafil Hussain and Dr. S.R. Upadhyay, F.V.Sc. & A.H., Jammu for their constant encouragement.

I feel very grateful to thank Dr. S.K. Maiti and Dr. S.L. Ali, College of Veterinary Science & A.H., Anjora, Durg (C.G.) for his awe-inspiring support, constant encouragement and charming loom since my M.V.Sc. programme. Words are not enough to express my special thanks to Dr. Varsha Sharma, College of Veterinary Science, Jabalpur (M.P.), who serves as a source of motivation to work hard without weary and remain pleasured even in odd circumstances and for their unreserved help, continuous motivation and well wishes for me as parents.

I extend sincere thanks to my senior colleagues Dr. Sunil Nayak, College of Veterinary Science, Jabalpur (M.P.), and Dr. K.V. Sharma, Dr. R.K. Tiwari and Dr. A.B. Sharma, for their even willing help, edifying, criticism and conductive advice during my normal life.

I am grateful to Dr. Vikash Vohra, Senior Scientist, NBAGR, Karnal for constant inspiration. It is my pleasure to thanks to my near and dear friend Dr. Vijay Pandey, College of Veterinary Science, Mathura, U.P., India. I am also thanks to Mrs. Melita Mesaric, Zegrab, Croatia for her moral support and positive criticism.

Last but not the least I would like to put across my heartiest and inexplicable gratitude to my beloved elder brother's (Mr. Virendra Sharma and Mr. Krishan Swaroop Sharma), their love brought me up to this stage.

Finally, but no my means least, I would like to thank my wife Satyabhama Sharma and Childrens Saloni (Daughter) and Vidip (Son), who have always been cooperative and helpful during the preparation of this book. I also express my love and affection to Tanu and Vedant.

I also equally thanks to Mr. Hemant Jain, and his team, Satish Serial Publishing House, Delhi for his keen interest in the publication of this book.

Neelesh Sharma

Abbreviations

µg	Microgram
AA	Arachidonic acid
ACTH	Adrenocorticotropic hormone
AI	Artificial insemination
AM	Apical plasma membrane
ATP	Adenosine triphosphate
b. wt.	Body weight
BAEC	Bovine aortic endothelial cells
BaM	Basement membrane
BC	β-carotene
BCP	Bromocresol purple
BHB	β-hydroxy butyrate
BHV	Bovine herpes virus
BID	Bis in a day
BIV	Bovine immunodeficiency virus
BLV	Bovine leukaemia virus
BM	Basal plasma membrane
BMSCC	Bulk milk somatic cell count
BoLA	Bovine lymphocyte antigens
bST	bovine somatotropin
BTB	Bromothymol blue
BUN	Blood urea nitrogen
BVDV	Bovine virus diarrhoea virus
CFU	Colony forming units
cm	Centimeter
CM	Clinical mastitis
CMIR	Cell mediated immune response
CMT	California mastitis test

CNS	Coagulase negative staphylococci
Co	Cobalt
COX	Cyclooxygenase
CR	Conception rate
CSF	Colony stimulating factors
Cu	Copper
DCP	Dry cow therapy
DHI	Dairy herd investigation
dl	Deciliter
DM	Dry mater
DMI	Dry mater intake
DNA	Deoxyribonucleic acid
E2	Estradiol
EC	Electrical conductivity
ECM	Extracellular membrane
FA	Fatty acid
Fe	Iron
FIL	Feedback inhibitor of lactation
FMD	Foot and mouth disease
FSH	Follicle-stimulating hormone
GA	Golgi apparatus
G-CSF	Granulocyte-colony stimulating factor
GH	Growth hormone
GJ	Gape junction
GM-CSF	Granulocyte-maccrophage colony stimulating factor
GnRH	Gonadotropin releasing hormone
GSHPx	Glutathione peroxidase
H_2O_2	Hydrogen peroxide
HETEs	Hydroxyeicosatetraenoic acids
HF	Holstein Frisian
HOCl	Hypochlorous acid
Hp	Haptoglobin
HUS	Hemolytic uremic syndrome
IDF	International dairy federation

IGF-I	Insulin-like growth factor-I
IL	Interleukin
IM	Intramuscular
IMI	Intramammary infection
IMM	Intramammary
INF	Interferon
INR	Indian rupee
IU	International unit
IV	Intravenous
kg	Kilogram
LBP	LPS-binding protein
LD	Lipid droplet
LF	Left fore
LH	Left hind
LH	Luteinizing hormone
LPS	lipopolysaccharide endotoxin
LS	Linear score
LSCC	Linear somatic cell count
MAMP	Modified Aulendorfer Mastitis Probe
MBC	Minimum bactericidal concentration
mcg	Microgram
MCMT	Modified California mastitis test
MCP	Myoepithelial cell process
MEC	Mammary epithelial cells
MEC	Minimum effective concentration
MFG	Milk fat globule
MFGM	Milk fat globule membrane
Mg	Magnesium
mg	Milligram
MGN	Mammary gland neutrophils
MHC	Major histocompatibility complex
MIC	Minimum inhibitory concentration
ml	Milliliter
MMPs	Matrix metalloproteinases

Mn	Manganese
MPO	Myeloperoxidase
mRNA	Messenger ribonucleic acid
MV	Microvillus
MWST	Modified Whiteside test
NAGase	N-acetyl-β-D-glucosaminidase
NEFA	Non-esterified fatty acids
NIRD	National Institute for Research into Dairying
NK	Natural killer
NMC	National Mastitis Council
NO	Nitric oxide
NPN	Non protein nitrogen
NS	Normal saline
NSAIDs	Non-steroidal anti-inflammatory drugs
OD	Once in a day
$OH^{\cdot}$	Hydroxyl radical
P_4	Progesterone
PAMPs	Pathogen-associated molecular patterns
PCR	Polymerase chain reaction
PG $F_2\alpha$	Prostaglandin $F_2\alpha$
PH-GSHPx	Phospholipid hydroperoxide glutathione peroxidase
PL	Phospholipids
PMN	Polymorphonuclear
ppm	Part per million
PRL	Prolactin
PRRs	pattern recognition receptors
PUFA	Polyunsaturated fatty acid
PVN	Paraventricular nuclei
RER	Rough endoplasmic reticulum
RF	Right fore
RH	Right hind
ROS	Reactive oxygen species
rRNA	Ribosomal ribonucleic acid
RUP	Ruminally undegredable protein

SAA	Serum amyloid-A
SC	Subcutaneous
SCC	Somatic cell count
SCM	Sub-clinical mastitis
SCS	Somatic cell score
Se	Selenium
SER	Smooth endoplasmic reticulum
SEs	Staphylococcal enterotoxins
SFMT	Surf field mastitis test
SLB	Swedish friesian breed
SLST	Sodium lauryl sulphate
SNF	Solid not fat
SOD	Superoxide dismutase
SON	Supraoptic nuclei
SRB	Swedish red and white breed
SV	Secretory vesicle
SVC	Small colony variants
TEC	Teat end callosity
TECT	Teat end callocity thickness
TJ	Tight junction
TLR	Toll-like receptors
TNF	Tumor necrosis factor
TSH	Thyroid-stimulating hormone
TSST	Toxic shock syndrome toxin
VERS	V*itamin E regeneration system*
VFAs	Volatile fatty acids
Vsps	Variable surface lipoproteins
WST	White side test
Zn	Zinc

Contents

CHAPTER

1

Introduction

History

As was so eloquently expressed in 1532 by Niccolo Machiavelli in *The Prince* (Machiavelli 1984), *"There is nothing more difficult to take in hand, more perilous to conduct, or more uncertain in its success, than to take the lead in the introduction of a new order of things."*

Mastitis must have been one of the first observed didease of farm animals when cattle were domesticated over 5000 years ago. Since then it will have been an ever present problem for all those who kept and milked dairy cattle. In first books published regarding mastitis problems (17th century) its importance was stressed and its association with poor cattle management and particularly with leaving cows half milked. From 19th century there has been constant stream of scientific and professional papaers in veterinary and animal science literature on mastitis causes and control. Scientific research followed Pasteur's demonstration of the „germ theory of disease" in 1860 and by 1900 it was established that most types of mastitis followed microbial infection. There were several common pathogens causing mastitis and therefore it was not a single disease. The clinical cases was readily detected by herdsman or milkers during milking but this was only the tip of the iceberg. Sub-clinical infections were much more common and caused bigger economic loses. Little or no progress had been made in reducing the infection level on dairy farms. In fact it was probably impossible at this time to devise control because there was no means of eliminating mastitis other than culling cows with cases of mastitis. A milestone was set in 1945 with the penicillin introduction for mastitis therapy so it it was possible to eliminate the most common mastitis pathogen (*S. agalactiae*) from infected udders. From that point it took another quarter of the century before an effective economic control was advised based on therapy but also on prevention, improved hygene and dairy cows herd management.

Main aim and objectives of book

The basic aim of our book is to describe and explain numerous factors which lead to poor milk quality and mastitis. If we all knows the way in which mastitis develops and occurs than we will be in better position for fight against it. We will be able to understand and implement required control measures for mastitis control despite the well known fact that mastitis can never be eradicated from our dairy herds". Environmental bacteria (such as *E. coli, Klebsiella* etc.) will always be present in cow environment. Also, it is hard to belive that some kind of magic mastitis vaccine" against all mastitis microbial causes will be find in the future.

Therefore, complete understanding of the basic mastitis principles will result in mastitis control program based on dairy herd management.

We, as authors will be very pleased and proud if mastitis incidence will be lower after reading this book and understanding of mastitis as multicausal dairy cattle health problem number one. We also expect economic benefits for dairy farming as well as cow welfare which will be the main objective of this book.

What mastitis means?

This is simply „udder inflamation". Most dairy farmers associate mastitis with inflamed quarter or udder resulting in change in the milk appearance. This changes are due to cow's inflammatory response to udder infection. Mastitis can also occur in sub-clinical form when there are no visible external changes on the udder despite the infection is present. As we previously mentioned majority of the information needed to reduce the mastitis incidence has been available for last 25-30 years. Research work carried out at National Institute for Research into Dairying (NIRD) in the UK and by National Mastitis Council (NMC) in the US in the 1960s formed the basis of the important mastitis control measures used today including the legendary „5 Point Plan" which recommended:

1. Recording and treating all clinical mastitis cases
2. Postdipping teats in disinfectant after each milking
3. Dry cow therapy all cows at the end of lactation
4. Culling all chronical cases of mastitis
5. Milking machine maintenance on regular basis

Over the past 50 years great progress has been made in reducing somatic cell counts (SCC) due to acceptance of the "5 Point Plan" by dairy farmers all over the World. Only in the UK, the clinical mastitis incidence has reduced from 121 cases per 100 cows per year in 1968, to between 40 to 50 in 2009 (one case is one quarter affected once).

Two, the most common types are environmental and contagious mastitis based on epidemiology of microorganisms which are responsible for the infection. The greatest progress has been made in reducing the incidence of contagious mastitis. Somatic cell counts relate to the severity of contagious infection. General decrease in average SCC all over the World can be seen as result of that progress. National SCC for UK decrese from almost 600.000 in 1970 to around 240.000 in 2009 (almost three times less than 40 years ago).

These days the aim is further reduction of contagious mastitis and SCC but main target is to reduce environmental infections. The incidence of environmental mastitis has remained more or less the same since 1960s, mostly due to increased milk yield and increased herd size. Flow rates have doubled over past 40 years and as we know milk yield is correlated to the milking speed. Over the same time faster milking speeds have led to twelve fold increase in mastitis susceptibility. Farm owners deserved big credit that they have improved the milking cow hygene and environment sufficiently to have prevented an increase in the clinical mastitis incidence over this period. Milk production are likely to increase in the future so at the same time the risk for new infections will also continue to rise.

Main target of modern dairy farmer is to produce large amount of high quality milk, not only the large quantity but high quality milk components such as milk proteins (casein), milk fat and lactose. Mastitis leads to a reduction in the useful milk components and increases the level of undesirable elements. Mastitis generally results in a less acceptable and lower quality product and of course the value of that low quality milk is greatly reduced.

Mastitis impact on economics

Mastitis is probably the most important health disorder and cause of highest economic loss on dairy farms. This is caused by a high incidence of clinical mastitis and a high prevalence of sub-clinical mastitis. Milk production loss in combination with treatment costs and culling due to mastitis problems constitute the major mastitis costs (Dijkhuizen, 1977). Mastitis affects the dairy farm economics in two main ways: through direct and indirect costs. Direct costs are discarded milk and drug and veterinary costs. Indirect costs are more complex and consisted of:

1. Penalties because of increased cell count.
2. Decreased milk yield during remainder of lactation due to udder damage and/or sub-clinical infection.
3. Extra labour requirements for treating and nursing.
4. Higher culling and replacement rates, leading to loss of genetic potential.
5. Deaths.

It is estimated that mastitis infections affected 30% of dairy cattle and cost the EU dairy industry about €1.55 billion in 2005 (Hillerton & Berry, 2005) and the US industry US$2 billion (Losinger, 2005). Costs of a clinical mastitis case in UK in 2009 was estimated between £100 and £200 (average cost of £125 is well accepted figure for 2009). In the US estimated cost are around US$185. This is assumed that there were 3 mastitis categories: mild, severe and fatal. The most common type of mastitis is the mild case which responds quickly to treatment. Discarded milk, intramammary tubes and reduced milk production for the remain of the lactation are main costs in mild mastitis case. Severe cases required additional veterinary treatment costs plus high risk of antibiotic residues in milk. In case of fatal outcome cost is the highest and cow will never return back to herd. The majority of economic losses in high SCC herds are from sub-clinical mastitis resulting in depressed milk production and reduced yield of casein, butterfat and lactose. SCC of 200000 is generally accepted as cutoff point for sub-clinical mastitis. For each SCC 100000 increase above that point there will be 2.5% yield reduction. If we add financial penalties for a low quality milk quite impressive financial loss will be generated.

For future prospects, we need to focus our efforts on improving environmental management, perhaps through the employment of novel bedding systems such as sand. Also to approach the management of mastitis in a more holistic manner by ensuring optimal nutrition, minimizing stress and encouraging farmers to pay attention to detail.

Conclusion

With good herd management it is possible to have an incidence of clinical mastitis below 30 cases per 100 cows per year, a herd SCC under 150,000 and bacterial counts under 20,000/ml. For "problem" herds this may take several years to achieve. Meeting these goals will improve profitability while ensuring a healthy future for both the dairy farmer and his cows. The farmers are therefore encouraged to keep reducing the herd SCC and bacterial count, and in so doing will ensure that they receive the premium price for their milk. This also benefits the consumer and the dairy industry, which will have a quality product with a good shelf life, suitable for manufacturing.

References

Dijkhuizen, A.A. (1977). Economic aspects of disease and disease eradication with special regards to mastitis (in Dutch). In: Publication 2, Department of Agricultural Economics, College of Veterinary Medicine, p. 87.

Hillerton, J.E. and Berry, E.A. (2005). J. Appl. Microbiol., 98: 1250-1255.

Losinger, W.C. (2005). J. Am. Vet. Med. Assoc., 226: 1652-1658.

Machiavelli, N. (1984). The prince. New York: Bantam Classics, Bantam Doubleday Dell Publishing Group (ISBN 0-553-21278-8); 1984. [Donno, D (Trans., editor; original work published 1532.]

CHAPTER

2

Mastitis Economics

Bovine mastitis, a condition recognized as long ago as the early 19th century, still presents a major challenge to the farmers, veterinary surgeons and research scientists in the new millennium. It is a most important production disease of dairy animals and is of considerable interest because of its high incidence and the extensive costs associated with the mastitis. Economics, as a science, primarily deals with the allocation of scarce resources (land, labour, and money) and as such deals with decision making, in which money is only one of the elements. Animal health economics, therefore, can be described as the discipline that aims to provide a framework of concepts, procedures, and data to support the decision making process in optimizing animal health management (Dijkhuizen, 1992). Improving udder health can play a major role in achieving efficient and economically rewarding milk production.

Mastitis is the most costly disease in dairy herds around the world. The effects of both clinical and sub-clinical mastitis on milk yield, and milk quality, in terms of fat, protein and somatic cell count (SCC) are significant. Mastitis has probably been observed since the cow first domesticated and remains the single health factor that is most influential in affecting milk production and causing enormous financial losses. Mastitis is great economic importance to milk producers, because the disease has negative impact on several important aspects of cow and herd performance. The economic losses associated with mastitis are due to loss of milk production, discarded milk, milk and milk product quality, veterinary services, treatment cost, extra labour cost and culling cost (Figure 2.1).

Incurred costs are of both direct and indirect nature (Kossaibati and Esslemont, 1997). ***Direct costs*** include veterinary costs, increased labour requirement, discarded milk, and reduced milk yield and quality. ***Indirect costs*** are those that are not always obvious to the milk producer, and are therefore referred to as *hidden costs*. They include increased risk of subsequent disorders, reduced fertility (extra services per conception and, as a result of this, an extended calving interval), increased risk of culling, and occasionally mortality (Nielsen, 2009). The total cost of mastitis can consequently be much higher than the direct cost (Kossabati and Esslemount, 1997).

Mastitis economic calculations vary between countries and even between regions within a country. In general, mastitis will cost farmers money, hence most farmers want to reduce the incidence of mastitis. In India most of farmers do not know about the most dangerous form i.e. sub-clinical mastitis and its consequences. Hence, there is a need of extensive awareness programmes to awake the dairy farmers regarding details of mastitis and economic losses due to this disease. Mastitis control is of paramount importance. The incidence of mastitis can be reduced by implementation of cost effective preventive measures. Mastitis prevention contributed to 48% of the total costs of disease prevention. As mastitis is generally a preventable disease, in many instances financial costs could be reduced, relatively easily, through implementation of current control programmes or the development of improved programmes at the farm level. Technology transfer is currently an important aspect of ensuring current knowledge is applied on farms and methods to implement this are required urgently.

The control and preventive measures are, however, associated with extra costs for the farmers in terms of investments and labour and interventions will only be made if the resulting increase in revenue can be expected to offset the incurred costs (Nielsen, 2009). Information about the economic loss associated with mastitis is, therefore, crucial when evaluating the viability of different preventive measures. The economic loss incurred by mastitis is also an essential part of other management decisions, such as treating infected udder quarters, culling mastitis cows, and discarding milk with high SCC in order to obtain a higher milk price. The contribution of individual component of economics in the total economic losses are as- reduced milk yield- 66%, discarded milk- 5.7%, replacement cost- 22.6%, extra labour- 0.1%, treatment cost- 4.1% and veterinary service- 1.5% of total losses (National Mastitis Council, 1996). Mastitis accounts for 38% of the total direct cost of all production diseases. Milk SCC is widely used as an indicator of udder health status, a high SCC is associated with sub-clinical intramammary infection (Figure 2.1). There is a negative relationship between milk yield and SCC (Jones and Herald, 1982), which is used to estimate the economic loss due to mastitis. These estimates are important in determining cost effective measures for mastitis control and prevention strategies.

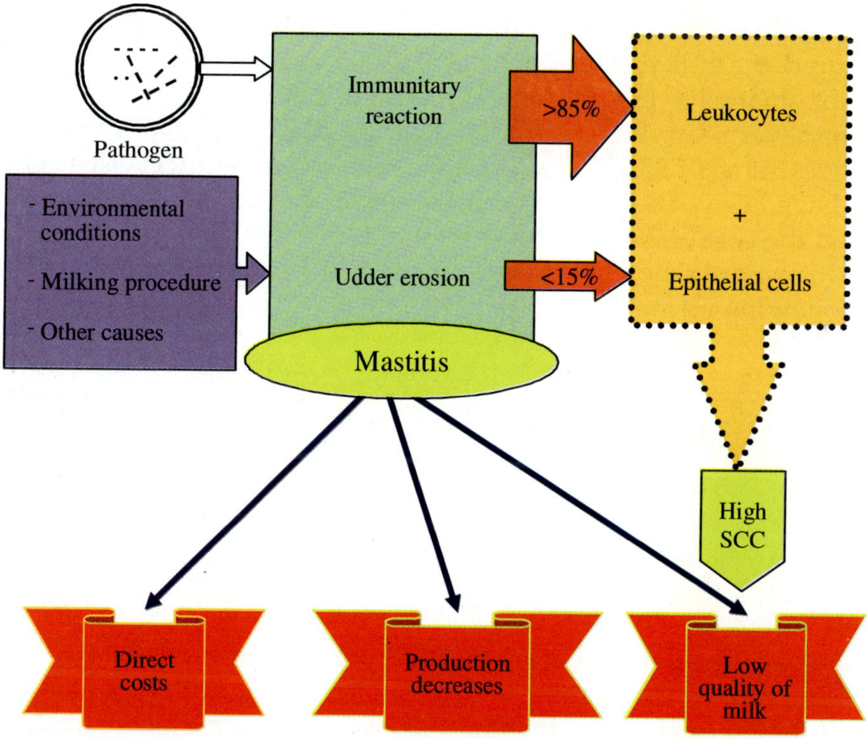

Figure 2.1 : Schematic demonstration of economic losses due to mastitis.

Many dairyman do not recognize fully the tremendous losses sustained through unrealized milk production. At the sub-clinical level dairymen could be unaware of the problem. Identifiable mastitis losses are not dramatic. Dairy farmers are more likely to become concerned about diseases that obviously affect the cow's health, even though such diseases may be of short duration and have less effect than mastitis on income from the herd (Blosser, 1979). The reduction or impairment of profitability caused by mastitis is hard to asses due to the impact of the many factors involved in the calculation, which are connected directly or indirectly to the dairy industry. Estimating economic losses resulting from mastitis becomes an extremely difficult task because of the many levels of infection and other factors. Therefore, a well-documented continued research and educational effort is necessary to increase producers awareness of cost of mastitis to the dairy enterprise.

The factors associated with economics of mastitis are explained below-

1. Milk Production Losses

The extent of yield loss depends on severity, causative pathogen, parity and the stage of lactation at which mastitis develops. In both clinical and subclinical mastitis, there is substantial loss in milk production. The loss in milk production does not only occur during the case itself, even after the mastitis case is cured, the milk production level of the cow stays lower. Milk production loss is not obvious to the producer, because this is milk never produced, and therefore never seen. Losses in total milk production range from 5 to 25%, with one extreme of 83.90%. In terms of milk losses per quarter per day, 9 to 43.30% have been observed (Janzen, 1970). Kossaibati and Esslemont (2000) estimated the cost of a mild, severe and fatal case of mastitis to be £145, £436 and £1418 respectively. The cost of reduced milk production can be calculated by the following formula :

Cost of reduced milk production per animal	=	Average milk losses due to clinical mastitis	x	Avg. daily milk yield of animal	x	Avg. price of milk	x	Avg. duration of mastitis case

OR

Cost of milk production loss per year	=	quarters	x	No. of production /CMT grade	x	Milk per litre loss/CMT grade		Milk price

The economic damage of lower milk production per cow also depends on the structure of the farming business. First of all, milk payment systems (payment based on amount of fluid milk or based on milk constituents such as fat and protein) may differ from state to state or country to country. Secondly, the calculation of the economic damage of decreased milk production differs between a quota system (e.g. EU, Norway or Canada) or a non-quota system. In India, the milk payment system is mainly based on milk components particularly milk fat. Moreover, the calculations of economic damage due to decreased milk production differ between a quota system (Halasa *et al.*, 2007). In a dairy system where farmers do not face a milk quota, the production potential of a farm is the number of dairy cows present on that farm. While in a quota system, calculation of economic damage for a decrease in milk production becomes much more complicated (Halasa *et al.*, 2007). The cows suffering from clinical mastitis causes an immediate drop in milk production and not regain production upto 60 days following clinical onset (Bartlett *et al.*, 1991). Steen (1978) recorded about 12.85% less milk yield in cows affected by mastitis as compared to the healthy cows and in India this report is about 10% less milk yield in clinical mastitic cow than before treatment (Sarma *et al.*, 1987). Clinical mastitis is associated with higher milk loss than sub-clinical mastitis (Hagnestam *et al.*, 2007; Hagnestam-Neilsen and Ostergaard, 2009). Because clinical mastitis is more severe form of mastitis and is associated with a larger amount of affected udder tissue, which results in more severe udder damage with decreased synthetic capacity of the mammary gland as a consequence. Udder tissue damage and case of clinical mastitis in early lactation will thus suppress milk yield throughout lactation. Also it is speculated that clinical mastitis in early lactation obstructs the differentiation of secretory cells, which takes place in this period and is responsible for the increase in milk yield until peak lactation (Capuco *et al.*, 2001). DeGraves and Fetrow (1993) estimated that 2.5 - 6.5% of expected annual yield is lost due to sub-clinical mastitis, whilst acute clinical cases caused a 6-11% reduction (Wood and Booth, 1983), and per-acute cases resulted in a 20-30% reduction in annual yield.

Multiparous cows loss approximately twice as much milk as first lactation cows. Cows with mastitis occurring before 150 days in lactation loss 1.4 times more milk compared with other cows (Bartlett *et al.*, 1991).

In primiparous cows, milk production loss is most severe when clinical mastitis is caused by *Staphylococcus aureus*, *E. coli* and *Klebsiella* spp., whereas, in multiparous cows, *Streptococcus* spp., *Staphylococcus aureus*, *E. coli*, *Klebsiella* spp. and *A. pyogenes* are responsible for the largest milk production loss (Grohn *et al.*, 2004). The lactational yield loss of 300 to 400 kg (4 to 6%) in multiparous cows and 200 to 300 kg in primiparous cows (Hortet and Seegers, 1998b). Lucey and Rowlands (1984) reported that a clinical case of mastitis would results in 6.4% drop in milk yield. Daily milk yield tended to decline 2 to 4 weeks prior to clinical mastitis, milk yield suppressed throughout lactation (Hagnestam *et al.*, 2007). As most researchers use the milk yield level of non-mastitic cows as reference for yield in healthy cows, the reported losses probably under estimate the true yield loss associated with clinical mastitis.

In addition to clinical mastitis, sub-clinical mastitis also has an important economic impact on dairying. It is generally agreed that 70 to 80% of the estimated loss from mastitis is associated with reduced milk production due to non-symptomatic i.e. sub-clinical mastitis. For every case of clinical mastitis in the herd, there are between 15 to 40 sub-clinical cases. Sub-clinical mastitis should be taken seriously and be thoroughly investigated because it can for example cause considerable losses in decreased milking capacity. Most commonly at the beginning, the infection does not appear as a clinical case but could gradually develop into one and thereby can cause even more damage. The milk production does not improve after complete recovery of sub-clinical mastitis (St. Rose *et al.*, 2003). Thus the assumed log-linear relationship might under estimate production losses due to sub-clinical mastitis (Halasa *et al.*,

2007). Dhakal and Thapa (2002) reported that about 68% of the total losses resulted from drop in milk production in buffaloes in Nepal.

Investigators have attempted to quantify these milk production losses by establishing the relationship between milk production of cows and concurrently measuring the somatic cell count (SCC) of milk. Milk SCC is widely used as an indicator of udder health status (Kirk, 1984), a high SCC is associated with sub-clinical mastitis (Table 2.1) and used to estimate economic loss due to mastitis. These estimates are important in determining cost-effective measures for mastitis control and prevention strategies. The SCC for an individual cow is a better indicator of milk loss than bulk tank SCC (Gill *et al.*, 1990). Sub-clinical mastitis (defined as cow with an increased SCC) causes economic losses because of production losses. The reduction in milk yield associated with sub-clinical mastitis (SCM) has been summarized as 80 kg (1.3%) and 120 kg (1.7%) per two fold increase in SCC above 50,000 cells/ml in primiparous and multiparous cows, respectively (Hortet and Seegers, 1998a). The greater the SCC increases 1,00,000 cells/ml, the greater the production losses. Primiparous cows are predicted to lose 0.31 (0.25 - 0.62) and 0.28 (0.20 - 0.35) kg of milk/day at an SCC of 200,000 cells/ml, for unadjusted and adjusted below SCC, respectively, while in multiparous cows 0.58 (0.54 – 0.62) and 0.50 (0.44 – 0.56) kg of milk/day respectively (Halasa *et al.*, 2009). The losses in milk yield due to mastitis are summarized in table 2.1, 2.2 and 2.3.

Table 2.1: Relationship between CMT, SCC and milk loss.

California Mastitis Test (CMT)	Somatic Cell Count (SCC)	Milk loss (%)	Milk loss (lb/cow/day)
Negative	1,00,000	0	0
T (trace)	3,00,000	3-6	5
1	9,00,000	10-12	7
2	2.7 million	16-28	8
3	8.1 million	25-46	10

Table 2.2 : Losses in milk production attributed to mastitis at world level.

Investigator	Loss in milk yield
Gayle and Moody (1959)	10-28 lb/cow/day
Gray and Schalm (1962)	6-24.5%
Forster (1964)	0.76-5.86 lb/quarter/day
Car (1964)	991.5-1500 kg/cow/lactation
Appleman *et al.* (1965)	0.9-6.8 lb/cow/day

Daniel *et al.* (1966)	49 lb/cow/month/unit CMT
Forster *et al.* (1967)	9.4-43.3/quarter/day
Philpot (1967)	2.8, 11.4, 25.6 and 45.5% in quarters with CMT scores of T, 1+, 2+ and 3+ respectively
Bishop and Compaan (1968)	30.5 lb/infection (28 day period)
Ward and Shultz (1972)	15% from quarters with SCC of 2 million/ml of milk
Fetrow *et al.* (1990)	25% from quarters with SCC of 4 million/ml of milk 200 kg/lactation
Schepers and Dijkhuizen (1991)	5-7%
Houben *et al.* (1993)	8.1%
Dhakal and Thapa (2002)	214.35 litre/lactation/buffalo
Shim *et al.* (2004)	0.36 kg (before clinical mastitis) 4.16 kg (during clinical mastitis) -0.03 kg (after clinical mastitis)
Wilson *et al.* (2004)	700 kg (in first lactation) 1200 kg (in second lactation)
Mungube *et al.* (2005)	1.2, 6.3 and 33% in quarters with CMT scores 1+, 2+ and 3+ respectively.
Hagnestam-Nielsen and Ostergaard (2008)	797 kg
Nielsen (2009)	*During clinical mastitis-* 0-9% (In primiparous cows) 0-11% (In multiparous cows) *During sub-clinical mastitis-* 2% (In primiparous cows) 5% (In multiparous cows)
Tesfaye *et al.* (2010)	6.8%

Table 2.3 : Losses in milk production attributed to mastitis in India.

Investigator	**Loss in milk yield**
Sarma *et al.* (1987)	2.35 litres/day in cross bred dairy cattle.
Singh *et al.* (1982)	0.35 litre/day/buffalo due to sub-clinical mastitis.
Singh *et al.* (1992)	50%
Dua (2001)	17.5%
Patel and Rao (2001)	11.76% (In cows due to SCM)
Sasidhar *et al.* (2002)	12.26%

The milk production loss during the period under treatment is calculated by the difference between the average milk yield potential of the animal and the average milk yield in unaffected quarters during treatment period. The milk yield potential of an animal is taken as the average of milk yield one week before and a week after treatment.

2. Discarded Milk Losses

When a cow suffering with mastitis, the affected cow is treated with various drugs including antibiotic. The milk of that cow must be withheld from the market until it is antibiotic free or for a certain period of time. The withdrawal period includes the days when a cow actually receives drug and a waiting time, usually consisting of some additional days, when there is a risk of antibiotic residues in the milk. The length of the withdrawal period depends on the production system (i.e. conventional or organic), and the drug used. The number of days the milk has to be discarded is usually around 8 days (Osteras, 2000). While in India, on an average 50% of the daily milk produced is discarded for 3 days. Half of the period of discarded milk is due to therapy and half is due to risk of therapeutic residues in milk. In addition, some milk is discarded because of altered composition prior to treatment.

Economic damage due to discarded milk is comparable with the damage of decreased milk production, but with one important difference: discarded milk is produced by the cow and is therefore associated with feed cost. This means that feeding costs for that amount of milk have to be taken into account in the calculations. The cost per unit of discarded milk is thus higher than the corresponding cost of milk not produced i.e. the economic damage of 100 kg discarded milk is therefore larger than for 100 kg decreased production. To calculate the economic loss due to discarded milk during this period has to be multiplied with the milk price, the farmer gets. The approximate cost of discarded milk can be calculated by the following formula :

Cost of discard milk = Average amount of discard milk per day x Number of days milk discarded x Avg. price of milk

OR

Cost of discard milk = 0.05 x Avg. daily milk yield of milk x Avg. price of milk x No.of days milk is discarded

OR

Cost milk discarded per year = Avg. lit of milk discarded animal milking x No. of cows having mastitis/year x Avg. duration of disease x Avg. price of milk per lit.

The cost of milk discarded in cows and buffaloes in India is Rs.26.52 and Rs.53.13 respectively (Dua, 2001) and Patel and Rao (2001) found that loss due to discarded milk or down graded contribute 4.44% of total loss per year. Natzke (1976) estimated discarded milk losses as 27 kg/day for 5 days for each clinical case. Another study estimated the losses from discarded milk as 34 kg/cow/year (Dobbins, 1977). Morse *et al.* (1987) reported the cost associated with discarded milk ranged from $29.72 to $166.18 per treated lactation and estimated average cost of discarded milk for parities 1, 2, 3, 4 and 5 ranged from $29.73 to $223.98 per lactation. Now days antibiotics are frequently and unnecessary using in the treatment of clinical mastitis, inspite of availability of other substitutive therapy. Administration of antibiotics usually requires a withdrawal time, during which milk is unusable, unmarketable and must be discarded or fed to calves (Shim *et al.*, 2004). This cost can be substantial and is used as justification for avoiding antibiotic use.

3. Veterinary Services

The cost of veterinary services render for each case is computed on the basis of time spent by each employee, his emoluments per day and the number of days taken for successful treatment of each mastitis case. The economic loss due to veterinary services includes the consultation charges or home visit of veterinarian. The veterinarian spends the time in the complete diagnosis and treatment of a case of mastitis. On an average a veterinary doctor spends 5 minutes for examining and suggesting the treatment, a compounder takes about 5 min to administer the medicine and an attendant needs 10 min for retraining the animal during examination and treatment (Sasidhar *et al.*, 2002). But in case of private practice, a veterinarian on an average spends 20 to 25 minutes in the complete diagnosis and treatment of a mastitis (clinical) case and they pays minimum 2 visits to treat a case of clinical mastitis. Average consultation charges of veterinarian are Rs.100 per visit and for two visits, it is Rs.200 in India. The consultation charges of veterinarian vary between state to state and country to country.

4. Cost of Drugs and Treatment

The immediate treatment of clinical mastitis in acute case is required new generation antibiotics with supportive therapy. The cost of medicine is a direct cause of economic damage to the farmers i.e. this is a straightforward economic damage. The cost of medicines varies between countries depending on the legislation and the infrastructure in a country. The total cost of treatment of a clinical case varies from veterinarian to veterinarian because it depends on the type of prescription (number and cost of medicines), which varies from individual to individual (veterinarian). In India, the common treatment protocol of a clinical mastitis with an average cost of drugs is given below-

Name of drug	Average cost of drug (Rs.)	Average total number of shots	Total cost (Rs.)
1. Antibiotic	63/shot	3	189
2. Intramammary tube	67/tube	6	402
3. Anti-inflammatory (Meloxicam)	30/shot	6	180
4. Fluid	720/shot	1	720
TOTAL (Rs.)	1491		

Note

1. Average cost of antibiotic is calculated from the recent price (2009-10) of four commonly used antibiotics e.g. Enrofloxacin, Ceftriaxone, Gentamycin, penicillin and tetracycline.
2. Average cost of intramammary tube is also calculated an average cost of 5 commonly used intramammary tubes in India e.g. Pendistrin SH, Mammal, Mammitel, Mastiwok, Tilox.
3. Average fluid cost is calculated from average cost of 3 fluids e.g. Ringers lactate, Calcium (Mifex) and Normal saline (NS).
4. The dose of drugs is calculated for 400kg b. wt. animal.

Dua (2001) calculated the cost of mastitis treatment in India, only on the basis of cost of intramammary tubes (as in formula-1). But this formula is not sufficient to represent the total cost of all medicines used in the treatment of a case of clinical mastitis. Here, authors are included the average cost of all commonly used drugs for the treatment of a case of mastitis in the formula.

Formula-1

Medicine cost = Cost of three tubes X Number of quarter affected per animal

Formula-2

Medicine cost = Average cost of drugs used/day/animal x Average number of days of treatment

OR

[A] Cost of parenteral antibiotics = Cost of antibiotic per shot x Avg. number of shots per day x Avg. number of days of treatment

[B] Cost of intramammary antibiotics = Avg. number of quarter affected x Cost of one tube

[C] Cost of supportive drugs = Avg. cost of supportive drugs x Avg. number of shots per day x Avg. number of days of treatment

[D] Total cost of medicine per animal (case) = [A] + [B] + [C]

The total veterinary costs are easily identified, and are often perceived by farmers as the full cost of mastitis. The cost of treatment constitute only part of the total cost of mastitis and that most costs are hidden. Therefore, suggested that treatment cost should be regarded as an investment to decrease the hidden costs (Osteras, 2000). Dua (2001) reported the cost of medicine Rs.138.60 and Rs.62.37 in cows and buffaloes respectively.

Esslemont (2002) has estimated the direct cost of a mild, severe and fatal case of clinical mastitis €13.58, €134.25 and €501.25 respectively for farmers in the UK. Natzke (1976) stated that antibiotic used to treat mastitis in a 200 cow herd cost the owner $500/year or $2.5/cow/year. Dubbins (1977) found a cost of $2.16/cow/year. The average cost of medicine and veterinary fee were NRs.872 ($13) and NRs.420 ($6) respectively in Nepal (Dhakal and Thapa, 2002).

5. Labour Cost

The extra labour is required for the management of mastitis case. The extra work included change of milking units, handling of cow, washing of extra equipment used in the treatment, diagnosis and discarding milk, treating cows, discarding milk and extra management practices.

The cost of labour is not easy to calculate. Opportunity costs of labour may differ from farm to farm. If the labour is separate or external used for the management of mastitis case, then the cost of labour for the time that has been used to prevent and treat the mastitis is quite easy to calculate (Formula). If the labour comes from the farmers free time, the opportunity costs are zero (Halasa *et al.*, 2007).

Labour cost = (Number of hours taken) X (wages per hour)

Each episode of clinical mastitis requires significant time for treatment and management. Fetrow (2001) estimated the time spent on a cow with severe clinical mastitis to be 4 hours with additional tasks consisting treatment, care, segregation and milking. The milking time to increase by 10 seconds per cow and milking, due to mastitis (Emanuelson and Hallen Sandgren, 1994). Dhakal and Thapa (2002) estimated NRs.750 ($11) as extra labour cost due to mastitis problem.

National mastitis advisory committee, England (Dairy insight research final report, 2005/2006) has made some assumptions for each episode of clinical mastitis-

- Five minutes required per milking during the treatment phase.
- Two minutes required per milking during the withholding period.
- Thirty minutes required per day for management of mastitis herd.

6. Losses Due to Change in Quality of Milk and Milk Products

The both clinical and sub-clinical mastitis affect the milk yield and its quality, in terms of fat, protein, total solids and SCC are significant (Sharma and Singh, 2005). Mastitis decreases the synthetic capacity of the mammary gland, which leads to decreased concentration of fat and caseins in the milk. The absolute fat yield loss due to clinical mastitis varies between 3 and 22 kg (1.5 - 7.5) (Hortet and Seegers, 1998a, 1998b). They also found that increase in protein content in milk produced by mastitic cows. This is due to a higher content of inflammatory non-coagulating proteins and whey proteins, but at the same time decreased proportion of casein, because casein is synthesized in the mammary gland (Sharma *et al.*, 2004).

It is well known that milk SCC increases during intramammary infection because they are first line of defense and helps in killing of infecting bacteria. When the somatic cells (phagocytic cells) destroy bacteria, enzymes that have been involved in the process are left behind. These enzymes are often resistant to pasteurization and attack on the milk fat and protein, which can result in serious off-flavours in dairy products. It may also significantly reduce shelf life, quality and yield of dairy products even when kept properly refrigerated (Ingalls, 1998). Increased SCC level is associated with decline in the milk constituents such as lactose (0.1 to 0.77%), solids not fat (0.1 to 0.57%), total solids (1.07%), fat (0.1 to 0.45%), total protein, casein, calcium, phosphorus and potassium (Janzen, 1970). Increased SCC also reduces the cheese yield. Rennet clotting time (RCT) in cheddar cheese making increased and cheese yield decreased to approximately 11.46% when sub-clinical mastitis milk was added to normal milk (Sirohi and Sirohi, 1995). The texture of cheese samples deteriorated as the mixing ratio of sub-clinical mastitis milk to normal milk increased (Le *et al.*, 1991). Some of these changes cause less efficient processing of milk and might result in products with less valuable properties (Santos *et al.*, 2003). The associated economic damage is difficult to calculate and the direct effect of this economic damage for the individual dairy farmer is even more difficult to estimate (Halasa *et al.*, 2007). Milk composition changes caused by mastitis can be neglected in economic calculations (Seegers *et al.*, 2003), because milk produced in connection with diagnosis is discarded due to treatment and later losses are proportional to the milk loss. The only changes in milk composition that are of economic importance to the dairy producer are those that affect the milk price, i.e. components that are part of milk payment scheme like milk fat, SCC etc.

7. Replacement or Culling Cost

Besides low production and reproduction, mastitis is one of the three major reasons why cows are removed from the herd (Young, 2000). The animals, which became non-productive as a sequel to mastitis, are normally discarded and to make up the loss in milk yield replacement with other animal is usually made (Dua, 2001). Clinical mastitis increases the risk of culling as well as mortality. The extent to which clinical mastitis affects the risk of culling depends on lactation stage at clinical onset. The culling is always a decision of the dairy farmer.

The cost of a culled cow is most simply defined as the *"cost of the replacement cow"* minus the *"value of the culled cow"*. Osteras (2000) defined the replacement cost at culling as the *"value of a pregnant heifer"* minus the *"value of the slaughter cow"* that was replaced.

Replacement cost = (Cost of a replacement cow or pregnant heifer) - (Cost of culled cow)

The economic losses to the farmer due to culling of animals can also be calculated by the following formula's (Dua, 2001).

[A]	Loss to the farmer by culling a mastitic animal	x	Avg. price of lactating animal	-	Price received for culled animal
[B]	Replacement value of new animal	x	Avg. price of lactating animal	+	Loss incurred for culling a mastitis animal

[C] Number of animals culled for mastitis = (Percent culling rate) - (Milch animal population)

[D] Total loss due to culling mastitic animals along their replacement = [B] - [C]

The cost due to premature replacement of animals due to mastitis is probably one of the largest areas of economic loss. However, it is very difficult to calculate precisely and it is also a hidden cost (Hogeveen, 2005). The both direct and indirect costs are involved in the culling cost. The *direct costs* that are the costs of rearing or buying a replacement animal (mostly heifers), while the *indirect costs* are a decreased efficiency of milk production by the replacement animals, because the milk yield of multiparous cows is higher than that of primiparous cows. Economic cost also arises as cows culled due to mastitis do not reach their full production potential (Osteras, 2005). Mastitis depreciated the market value of animal, when epithelial tissue of the udder is grossly damaged resulting in the loss of one or more quarters. Hence, the market value of the animal goes down considerably or may be completely lost if all the quarters get involved. It has reported that an average production life of a dairy cow being only three or four lactations (Young *et al.*, 1983).

Singh (1991) reported that the average culling rate due to mastitis in Punjab state of India is 2% and in India, it is 1%. Dua (2001) has been reported total economic losses due to culling of mastitic cows and buffaloes Rs.173.40

crores in Punjab state and Rs.1514.05 crores in India. Of these Rs.43.2 crores and Rs.130.2 crores losses due to culling of mastitic cows and buffaloes respectively in Punjab, and Rs.861.30 crores and Rs.652.75 crores respectively in India.

Seegers *et al.* (2003) reported that 5 to 17% of all culling was related to udder disorders and that the proportion reached 28.5%, when high SCC and teat injury were included. Roenfeldt (2000) reported that within 60 days of a severe clinical mastitis event, 13% of animals are culled and another 8% are dried off early. Furthermore, for clinical coliform mastitis, 23% of cows are either culled or die without completing their lactations. In U.K., it is assumed that, on average 10% of cows with mild mastitis are culled. In severe cases, the risk of culling is assumed to be at least 20%. A cull cow is assumed to cost £420 per cull, and the cost of a fatality is £1251 (Kossaibati and Esslemont, 2000).

Somatic cell counts above 3,00,000 cells/ml has been reported to increase the risk of culling in primiparous cows (Beaudeau *et al.*, 1995) and, in late lactation, sub-clinical mastitis is the most important disease influencing culling decisions regardless of parity of cow. Cows are culled when replacement is judged to the economically optimal alternative. Decisions can be taken at three levels- quarter/cow level, farm level and region/country level. Quarter or cow level decisions are those that are related to an individual cow and are mainly treatment of clinical or sub-clinical mastitis or culling (Halasa *et al.*, 2007).

8. Diagnosis Cost

The early diagnosis of mastitis particularly specific causal agent and their sensitivity to antibiotic have paramount importance in the successful treatment of clinical mastitis and it reduces the cost of treatment, because after receiving the antibiotic sensitivity report, a specific antibiotic (rational treatment) is used to treat the case. The diagnosis of mastitis is done by different techniques i.e. direct or indirect methods, but the cultural isolation and characterization is most accurate method to confirm the diagnosis. The diagnostic costs that are relevant to mastitis must be considered in the calculation of economics, for example cost of technical, chemical, reagents, diagnostic kits and culture media. Dutta *et al.* (1995) reported that the cost of testing milk with the help of the Modified Aulendorfer Mastitis Probe (MAMP) is very negligible. It amounted to a mere one Indian rupee (INR) per quarter per test.

After considering all individual factors in the calculation of mastitis economics, total losses due clinical and sub-clinical mastitis can be calculated by the following formula-

Total Economic Losses Due to Clinical Mastitis

Number of animals affected with clinical mastitis x Avg. incidence of clinical mastitis x Milch animal population

Total loss due to clinical mastitis = Total loss incurred on one animal x Number of animals affected with clinical mastitis x Total loss due to culling mastitic animals along with their replacement

Total Economic Losses Due to Sub-clinical Mastitis (SCM)

[A] Milk loss in one lactation due to SCM = % loss in milk yield x Avg. lactation yield x Avg. milk price

[B] Number of animals affected with SCM x Avg. incidence of SCM x Milch animal population

[C] Total loss due to SCM = [A] + [B]

Vast worldwide research on mastitis is going on for last several decades has not changed the situation significantly and the efforts have been aiming at early detection of the diseases rather than remedial measures about which there is no remarkable progress except knowing the list of large number of causative organisms and the results of their resistance to antibiotics and, prevalence reports from different regions.

Economic Losses due to Mastitis in India

The economic losses due to mastitis are enormous in India as well as in developed countries (Dhanda and Sethi, 1962; Dua, 2001; Sarma *et al.*, 1987; Irving, 1965; Hillerton *et al.*, 1992). Mastitis is the most important disease of dairy cattle and buffaloes and probably the most derelict in Indian field conditions where the veterinarians are required to treat so many clinical cases wherein the gland becomes very hard, fibrosed, losses milk producing capacity of the delicate gland cells and purulent and mixed watery secretion instead of milk. In such a case there is hardly anything that can be done to restore the normal functioning and the milk production from the udder, the intramammary antibiotics will at the best get rid of the infection but the glandular tissue is lost for ever and animal remains as a liability for the owner causing considerable loss to the country. It is estimated that a cow showing reaction as "trace" to California mastitis test records a total loss of 6% milk in a lactation against 24% milk loss in a cow showing strongly positive reaction to CMT.

In India, financial loss due to the incidence of 'blind teats' (that is, teats which become functionless as a result of mastitis) and milk loss from clinical mastitis. In 1962, it was calculated by Dhanda and Sethi that the annual loss due to mastitis in India was Rs.52.90 crores. Again in 1969, it was reported that the total economical damage due to mastitis in India was estimated to be around Rs.105.8 crores (Sinha and Prasad, 1969), which is nearly double than the losses in 1962.

In 1987, total economic loss to the owner was about Rs.170.40 per mastitis cow which included loss of milk (Rs.27.61) and the treatment cost (Rs.142.79) (Sarma *et al.*, 1987). This is equivalent to about 60 litres of milk or a week's milk yield of a cow producing about 9-10 (range 1.2 to 37.4 litres) litres per day.

In 1991, it was calculated that the total annual economic loss due to mastitis in India was Rs.1607.2 crores, which included Rs.889.51 crores for cows and Rs.717.69 crores for buffaloes (Singh, 1991).

In 1994, estimated Indian economic losses due to mastitis were Rs.1607 crores (Singh and Singh, 1994). Sirohi and Sirohi (2001) estimated economic losses in India due to mastitis Rs.2809.32 crores at 1994 prices, of these losses 76.55% losses were attributable to sub-clinical mastitis.

In 1995, reported total milk loss 38.13 litres during treatment including holding period, and economic damage Rs.305 due to milk loss (Dutta *et al.*, 1995).

In 1998, these total financial losses due to mastitis was Rs.1940 crores annually (Manickam, 1998).

In 2001, economic losses due to mastitis in India about Rs.6053.21 crores per annum (Dua, 2001). The details of economic losses during the year 2001 is given in table 2.4.

In 2001, Patel and Rao also carried out a study in 112 Kankrej cows and reported that mastitis caused an average economic loss of Rs.443.00 per cow per year which was 5.15% of the revenue from the sale of average lactation yield. Mean cost associated per clinical mastitis cow was Rs.1164.00 which was 13.50% of the revenue from the sale of lactation milk yield. Maximum economic loss were associated with reduced milk production (74.03%) followed by treatment cost (12.29%), veterinary expenses (8.59%), discarded milk (4.44%) and extra man-power expenses (0.64%). During this study, culling rate was reported about 11.76% due to mastitis. Sub-clinical mastitis caused the losses of Rs.33,545.00 with an average of Rs.1016.00 per sub-clinical mastitis case.

In 2002, calculated the total monetary loss to the dairy farmer about Rs.325.64 per mastitis cow which included loss of milk (Rs.106.80) and the treatment cost (Rs.218.84) only (Sasidhar *et al.*, 2002). This is near about double than the economic losses (Rs.170.40) during 1987.

Table 2.4: Estimated total economic loss (in Rs.) due to mastitis in bovines in India.

Parameter	Clinical mastitis		Sub-clinical mastitis	
	Cows	Buffaloes	Cows	Buffaloes
Cost of reduced milk production (Rs.)	44.20	88.55	945	1893.76
Cost of discarded milk (Rs)	26.52	53.13	-	-
Cost of Veterinary consultation (Rs)	100	100	-	-
Cost of drugs (Rs)	138.60	62.37	-	-
Total cost of one mastitic animal (Rs)	309.32	304.05	-	-
Economic loss due to culling/discarding one mastitic animal (Rs)	6000	7500	-	-
Economic loss due to replacement of one mastitic animal (Rs)	13500	17500	-	-
Total economic loss due to culling/discarding and replacement (crores)	861.30	652.75	-	-
Total economic loss due to mastitis (crores)	987.60	696.29	2646	1723.32
Total loss (crores)	**1683.89**		**4369.32**	
Grand total (crores)	**6053.21**			

Source: Dua (2001).

Rao and Patel (2003) estimated an economic losses due to mastitis at Holstein Friesian X Kankrej herd (27 cows), an average loss of Rs.1629 per cow/year which has been estimated 7.64% of the revenue from the sale of average lactation yield. Mean cost associated per clinical mastitis cows was Rs.2369. Maximum economic losses were in terms of reduced milk production (89.99%), followed by veterinary expenses (4.22%), discarded milk (3.03%), treatment cost (2.53%) and extra man power expense (0.21%). It was also estimated that the losses of Rs.20881 with an average of Rs.2320 per cow suffering from sub-clinical mastitis.

The lots of papers have been published on prevalence/incidence, etiology, antibiogram, diagnosis and treatment of mastitis from all over the India for the past several decades when the first record of the disease was made by Land in 1926, but there is a lack of systemic work on mastitis economics due to poor data recording system. However, no single author consider all factors (as described in a review article of Halasa *et al.*, 2007) in the calculation of economic losses due to mastitis in India. Hence, present (available) data of mastitis economic losses are not true representative of actual economic losses due to mastitis i.e. underestimated in India. The dramatic increase (approximately 115 times) in the economic losses from 1962 (Rs.52.80 crores/annum) to 2001 (Rs.6053.21 crores/annum) due to mastitis in India, divert the mind of researchers, policy makers and dairy farmers toward this costliest disease to control it. However, all these reports on the economic losses in India are not undertaken all the factors involved in the losses in the mastitis economics calculation. Hence, there is ardent need for a systemic study to produce the precise and unbiased data on mastitis economics. These precise and complete data will help in awaking the dairy farmers to control this disease with keeping in mind economically effective principles.

Economic Losses due to Mastitis Globally

Mastitis is known as a disease that causes the greatest economic losses to milk producers and to the dairy industry world wide. The majority of milk producers are unable to asses the damage caused by this disease. The main component of the financial loss is reduced production levels in affected cows. The economic losses due to mastitis from most of the countries/states are summarized in table 2.5.

Table 2.5 : Estimates of total economic losses due to mastitis from different countries.

Country/State	Total annual economic loss	Reference
USA	$411 million	Irving (1965)
USA	$400-500 million	Janzen (1970)
USA	$179/cow	Bar *et al.* (2008)
France	Fancs 644 - 1244 million	Plomet and leLouedee (1972)
Denmark	$21-26 million	Ellis and Asby (1975)
German Federal	DM 370-450 million	Hamann (1975)
Netherland	Guilders 150 million	Jaartsveld (1975)
Netherlands	Dfl 136/cow	Schakenraad and Dijkhvizen (1990)
Georgia	$90-250/cow	Dubbins (1977)
Pakistan	Rs.240 million	Chaudhry and Khan (1978)
Norway	Kroner235 million	Waage (1989)
Egypt	£ 177.16/cow	Badran and Ebeid (1990)
U.K.	£ 6.22 million	Hillerton *et al.* (1992)
U.S.	$185/cow	Costello (2004)
Brazil	US$126/cow	Holanda Junior *et al.* (2005)
Sweden	€97/cow	Hangnestam-Nielsen and Ostergaard (2008)

The effects of sub-clinical mastitis in developing countries may be similar to its effects in developed countries, that is, a reduction in the yield and quality of milk, and an increase in the risk of clinical mastitis. In Costa Rica, for example, the reduction in milk yield due to sub-clinical mastitis, as defined by the California mastitis test, was estimated to be 1.56 kg of milk per day, and 17.6% of total daily yield, compared with normal cows and normal quarters, respectively (deGraaf and Dwinger 1996).

Mungube (2001) had been reported the total economic losses due to mastitis Birr115,526.34 per year. The maximum losses (66.20%) were due to culling of animals followed by reduced milk production (25.40%), treatment cost (6.20%) and losses due to withdrawal of milk (2.2%).

In Norway, mastitis causing loss is estimated to have cost approximately 190 million NOK (approximately 23.5 million €) in a population of 270,000 dairy cows, or 0.13 NOK (€ 0.016) per liter of milk produced in 2003 and 2004 (Osteras, 2006). The loss corresponds to 4% of the market value of milk at farm level.

In Sweden, Hangnestam-Nielsen and Ostergaard (2008) estimated yearly cost of clinical mastitis at herd (150 cows) level was about €14,504, corresponding to 6.9% of the net return given the initial incidence of clinical mastitis. They expressed per cow/year, the cost of clinical mastitis was €97. Therefore, the cost of clinical mastitis in Sweden today is thus €427.

Mastitis costs the U.S. dairy industry about $1.7-2 billion annually or 11% of total U.S. milk production. Much of this cost is attributed to reduced milk production, discarded milk, and replacements which are estimated at $102, $24, and $33 per cow per year. The obvious costs for treatment medication, labor, and veterinary services are low, estimated to total $13 per cow. It must be recognized that mastitis cannot be eliminated from a herd. However, the total cost of mastitis in the average herd enrolled in dairy herd investigation (DHI) is approximately $171 per cow, which amounts to $18.6 million cost to the Virginia dairy industry annually. If the goal for each herd was to have an average DHI SCC score of 2.0 and no more than 3 cases of clinical mastitis per 100 cows per month, the average herd of 128 cows could increase annual net income by $57 per cow or $7,296. Blosser (1979) estimated that mastitis costs $117.35 annually for each cow in the United States. Yearly costs per cow were 386 kg of discarded milk, veterinary costs $1.97, drugs $3.86, labor $2.28, and decreased sale value per cow $5.72. Jasper *et al.* (1982) calculated that losses directly from mastitis averaged $182 per cow or in excess of 2 billion dollars annually in the United States. In the U.K., the annual mortality rate from mastitis in dairy cows has been estimated at 0.2% (Wilesmith *et al.*, 1986; Menzies *et al.*, 1995), the majority of these being due to coliform infections. Additionally, it has been estimated that coliform infection of the udder incurs an annual total cost to the average farmer of over Stg£30 per cow (Hogan *et al.*, 1989; Anon., 1996).

A recent study of Huijps *et al.* (2008) in the Netherlands, reported the economic losses of a clinical case in a default situation were calculated as €210, varying from €164 to €235 depending on the month of lactation. The total economic losses of mastitis (sub-clinical and clinical) per cow present in a default situation varied between €65 and €182 per cow per year depending on the bulk tank somatic cell count. In another recent study, Halasa *et al.* (2009) developed a stochastic bio-economic model to calculate the costs of bovine intramammary infections. They found that the cost of a clinical case of mastitis was €185, varying between €124 and €331 per case. The average net cost of a sub-clinical mastitis case was €96 (€10 to €265).

The cost of mastitis under an optimal policy in California, vary between $142 to $225 per cow per 305-d lactation, and depend strongly on mastitis prevalence, SCC threshold, milk price, milk production level of cow, and parity. Bar *et al.* (2008) reported the average cost of a clinical mastitis case was $179. It was composed of $115 due to milk yield losses, $14 because of increased mortality, and $50 because of treatment-associated costs.

Tesfaye *et al.* (2010) carried out a study on mastitis economics in Ethiopia. Milk yield losses for CMT positive quarters were estimated by comparing production of quarters with CMT score 0 and quarter milk production was measured over a period of 8 days. Mean milk yield for uninfected healthy quarters was 1.66 kg per milking and the rate of milk reduction for quarters with CMT scores of 1+, 2+, and 3+ was 25%, 33%, and 48%, respectively. Economic losses at different farm-size levels were calculated by multiplying the prevalence of CMT scores with milk yield losses associated with respective CMT scores. In Debre Ziet dairy herds, a quarter with SCM due to *Staph. aureus* lost an average of 34.5% of its potential milk production while the total milk yield loss per cow was estimated at 6.8%. Losses were highest in large-scale (13%) farms and lowest (3.7%) in small-scale. Based on the prevalence, the overall financial loss for each cow per lactation was 984.64 Eth Birr (US$78.65) and losses in large farms (1,882.40 Eth Birr or US$150.35) were over 3.5 times the loss in small-size farms.

References

Anon. (1996). Mastitis - technical bulletin. Information leaflet produced by Schering-Plough Animal Health. Welwyn Garden City: Schering-Plough Ltd., p. 2.

Appleman, R.D., Rowe, G.A. and Forker, O.D. (1965). J. Dairy Sci., 48: 829.

Badran, A.E. and Ebeid, A.B. (1990). Indian Vet. J., 67(1): 43-46.

Bar, D., Tauer, L.W., Bennett, G., Gonzalez, R.N., Hertl, J.A., Schukken, Y.H., Schulte, H.F., Welcome, F.L. and Grohn, Y.T. (2008). J. Dairy Sci., 91: 2205-2214.

Bartlett, P.C., Wijk, J.V., Wilson, D.J., Green, C.D., Miller, G.Y., Majewski, G.A. and Heider, L.E. (1991). J. Dairy Sci., 74: 1561-1572.

Beaudeau, F., Ducrocq, V., Fourichon, C. and Seegers, H. (1995). J. Dairy Sci., 78(1): 103-117.

Bennedsgaard, T.W., Enevoldsen, C., Thamsborg, S.M. and Vaarst, M. (2003). J. Dairy Sci., 86(10): 3174-3183.

Bhardwaj, A., Dixit, V.B. and Sehi, R.K. (2006). Indian J. Dairy Sci., 59(5): 322-327.

Bishop, E.J.B. and Compaau, J.P. (1968). Farming in South Africa 44(11): 17, 19, 21. [Dairy Sci. Abstr., 31:2253.]

Blosser, T.H. (1979). J. Dairy Sci., 62: 119-127.

Blosser, T.H. (1979). J. Dairy Sci., 62: 119.

Cabrera, E., Pantoja, J., Ruegg, P. and Shook, G. (2009). Decision-making for early postpartum sub-clinical mastitis. V., J. Anim. Sci. Vol. 87, E-Suppl. 2/J. Dairy Sci. Vol. 92, E-Suppl. 1 (Abstract). pp.201-202.

Capuco, A.V., Wood, D.L., Baldwin, R., Mcleod, K. and Paape, M.J. (2001). J. Dairy Sci., 84(10): 2177-2187.

Car, M. (1964). Dairy Sci. Abstr., 26: 3308.

Chaudhry, N.A. and Khan, B.B. (1978). Estimation of economic losses due to animal diseases in Punjab (Final Report of Research Project). Univ. of Agri. Faisalabad, Pakistan.

Costello, S. (2004). Consultants guide to economics of mastitis. Extension Letter of Penn State University.

D. Bar, L.W. Tauer, G. Bennett, R.N. González, J.A. Hertl, Y.H. Schukken, H.F. Schulte, F.L. Welcome and Y.T. Gröhn (2008). J. Dairy Sci., 91: 2205-2214.

Daniel, R.C.W., Biggs, D.A. and Barnum, D.A. (1966). Canadian Vet. J., 7: 99. [Dairy Sci. Abstr., 28: 2526]

Degraaf, T. and Dwinger, R.H. (1996). Prev. Vet. Med., 26: 215-222.

DeGraves, F. J. and Fetrow, J. (1993). Vet. Clin. North Am., 9: 421-434.

Deluyker, H.A., Roldan, P., Carleos, C., Grillo, G.J. and Perez, M.A. (2005). J. Dairy Sci., 72: 93-100.

Dhakal, I.P. and Thapa, B.B. (2002). Buffalo J., 2: 225-234.

Dhanda, M.R. and Sethi, M.S. (1962). Investigation of mastitis in India. ICAR series No. 35, Indian Council of Agricultural Research, New Delhi.

Dijkhuizen, A. A. (1992). Modelling animal health economics. Inaugural speech, Wageningen University and Research Centre, Wageningen. p. 28.

Dobbins, C.N.Jr. (1977). J. Am. Vet. Med. Ass., 170(10, 11): 1129-1132.

Dua, K. (2001). Indian Dairyman, 53(10): 41- 48.

Dutta, G.N., Saxena, R.K. and Buragohain, J. (1995). Indian Vet. J., 72(4): 420-422.

Ellis, P.R. and Asby, C.B. (1975). The economics of mastitis control. In: Proc. IDE. Seminar of mastitis control, Reading University. Pp.453.

Emanuelson, U. and Hallén Sandgren, C. (1994). Ekonomiskt effektiv mjölkproduktion, hög mjölkmängd och/eller god hälsa? Djurhälsoavdelningen, SHS. Summary of lecture at Gällöfsta (November 1994), pp. 17.

Esslemont, D. (2002). Dairy farmer, December, pp 30-31.

Fetrow, J., Mann, D., Butcher, K. and McDaniel, B. (1990). J. Dairy Sci., 74: 833-839.

Forster, T. L. (1964). J. Dairy Sci., 47: 696.

Forster, T.L., Ashworth, U.S. and Luedecke L.O. (1967). J. Dairy Sci., 50(5): 675-682.

Gayle, Gilda, and Moody. E.G. (1959). J. Dairy Sci., 42: 1740.

Gill, R., Howard, W.H., Leslie, K.E. and Lissemore, K. (1990). J. Dairy Sci., 73: 3340-3348.

Gray, D.M. and Sehalm, O.W. (1962). Am. J. Vet. Res., 23: 541.

Gröhn, Y.T., Wilson, D.J., Gonzalez, R.N., Hertl, J.A., Schulte, H., Bennett, G. and Schukken, Y.H. (2004). J. Dairy Sci., 87(10): 3358-3374.

Hagnestam, C., Emanuelson, U. and Berglund, B. (2007). J. Dairy Sci., 90(5): 2260-2270.

Hagnestam-Nielsen, C. and Ostergaard, S. (2008). Economic impact of clinical mastitis in a dairy herd assessed by stochastic simulation. In: Mastitis Control from science to practice, edited by Lam, T.J.G.M., 1 edn., Wageningen Academic publisher, The Netherlands. Pp. 423-429.

Hagnestam-Nielsen, C. and Østergaard, S. (2009). Animal 3(2): 315-328.

Halasa, T., Nielen, M., DeRoos, A.P.W., Van Hoorne, R., deJong, G., Lam, T.J.G.M., van Werven, T. and Hogeveen, H. (2009). J. Dairy Sci., 92: 599-606.

Halasa, T., Nielen, M., Huirne, R.B.M. and Hogeveen, H. (2009). Livest. Sci., (124): 295 - 305.

Hamann, J. (1975). Tierzuchter, 27: 237-238.

Hillerton, J.E., West J.G.H. and Sheran M.F.H. (1992). Vet. Rec., 131(14): 315-317.

Hogan, J.S., Smith, K.L., Hoblet, K.H., Schoenberger, P.S., Todhunter, D.A., Hueston, W.D., Pritchard, D.E., Bowman, G.L., Heider, L.E., Brockett, B.L. and Conrad, H.R. (1989a). J. Dairy Sci., 72: 1547-1556.

Hogeveen, H. (2005). In: Proc. British mastitis conf., Stoneleigh, pp. 1-13.

Hogeveen, H. and Østerås, O. (2005). Mastitis management in an economic framework. In: Hogeveen, H. (Ed.) Proceedings of 4th IDF International Dairy Conference: Mastitis in dairy production - Current knowledge and future solutions. Wageningen: Wageningen Academic Publishers. pp. 41-52.

Holanda Junior1, E.V., Madalena, F.E., Holanda, E.D., Miranda, W.M. and Souza, M.R. (2005). Prod. Anim., 13(2): 63-69.

Hortet, P. and Seegers, H. (1998). Prev. Vet. Med., 37(1-4): 1-20.

Hortet, P. and Seegers, H. (1998a). Vet. Res., 29(6): 497-510.

Hortet, P. and Seegers, H. (1998b). Prev. Vet. Med., 37(1-4): 1-20.

Houben, E.H.P., Dijkhuizen, A.A., Arendonk, J.A.M.V. and Huirne, R.B.M. (1993). J. Dairy Sci., 76: 2561-2578.

Huijps, K., Lam, T.J.G.M. and Hogeveen, H. (2008). J. Dairy Res., 75: 113-120.

Ingalls, W. (1998). Somatic cells, mastitis and milk quality. http://www.southdairyextension.org/milk_mgmt_economics.asp

Irving, G.W.Jr. (1965). Losses in agriculture. USDA, ARS, Agr. Handbook 291: 73.

Jaartsveld, F.H.J. (1975). Tijdschroft voor Diergenerskune, 100(23): 2173-2174.

Janzen, J.J. (1970). J. Dairy Sci., 53(9): 1151-1160.

Jasper, D.E., S. McDonald, J., Mochrie, R.D., Philpot, W.N., Farnsworth, R.J. and Spencer, S.B. (1982). In: Proc. Annu. Mtg. Natl. Mastitis Counc., p. 184.

Jones, G.M. and Herald, C.W. (1982). Milk loss, somatic cell counts and udder infections in Virginia herds. In: Proc. Annu. Mtg. Natl. Mastitis Conc., Arlington, VA.

Jones, G.M., Pemson, R.E., Clasgaugh, G.A. and Heald, C.W. (1984). J. Dairy Sci., 67: 182.

Kirk, J.H. (1984). Somatic cells in millk: current con-cepts. Comp. Contin. Educ. 6237.

Kossaibati, M.A. and Esslemont, R.J. (2000). The Cost of clinical mastitis in UK Dairy Herds. In : Proc. of MDC meeting on mastitis, Honiley Court, Warwick. 2000. 7-3-2000.

Kossaibati, M.A. and Esslemont, R.J. (2000). The cost of clinical mastitis in UK dairy herds. Abstract for MDC meeting on mastitis, Honiley Court, Warwick, March 7th, 2000.

Le, S.C., Yu, J.H., Jeong, C.L.; Back, Y.J. and Yoon, Y.C. (1991). Korean J. Dairy Sci., 13: 217-223.

Lucey, S. and Rowlands, G.J (1984). Anim. Prod., 39(2): 165-175.

Manickam, R. (1998). Milcow, 3: 21-25.

Menzies, F.D., Bryson, D.G., McCallion, T. and Matthews, D.A. (1995). Vet. Rec., 137: 531-536.

Morse, D., DeLorenzo, M.A., Natzke, R.P. and Bray, D.R. (1987). J. Dairy Sci., 70: 2411-2418.

Mungube, E.O. (2001). Management and economics of dairy cow mastitis in the urban and periurban areas of Addis Ababa. Free University of Berlin and Addis Ababa University, MSc thesis.

Mungube, E.O., Tenhagen, B.A., Regassa, F., Kyule, M.N., Shiferaw, Y., Kassa, T. and Baumann, M.P. (2005). Trop. Anim. Hlth. Prod., 37(6): 503-512.

National Mastitis Council (1996). Current concepts of Bovine Mastitis, 4th ed., Arlington, VA.

Natzke, R.P. (1976). The economics of mastitis control. In: Proc. large herd management symposium, University of Florida, January, 1976.

Nielsen, C. (2009). Economic impact of mastitis in dairy cows. PhD thesis, Swedish University of Agricultural Sciences. Uppasala, Sweden.

Østerås, O. (2000). In: Proc. of the British Mastitis Conf - 2000, Shepton Mallet, U.K. pp. 67-77.

Østerås, O. (2000). In: Proc. Brit. Mastitis Conf., pp. 67-77.

Østerås, O. (2005). Bulletin of the International Dairy Federation. 394: 1-25.

Osteras, O. (2006). Mastitis epidemiology practical approaches and applications. In: Proc. of XXIV World Buiatrics Congress, Nice, France.

Patel, P.R. and Rao, N. (2001). In: Proc. 2nd Round table conference on mastitis, Ludhiana, (Pb), India, 22-23 Feb., pp. 99-103.

Philpot, W.N. (1967). J. Dairy Sci., 50: 978.

Plommet, M. and leLoudee, C. (1972). Dairy Sci., 35(1): 84.

Rao, N. and Patel, R.R. (2003). In: Proc. Natl. Symp. XXI ISVM convention. P. 245.

Ruegg, P.L. (2004). Treatment of clinical mastitis. http://www.uwex.edu/milkquality/PDF/treatment_clinical_mastitis.pdf

Salskg, E., Meek, A.H. and Martin, S.W. (1984). Can. J. Comp. Med., 48: 251.

Sarma, P.V., Rao, S.V.N. and Sampath, S.R. (1987). Indian Dairyman, 39(10): 477-479.

Sasidhar, P.V.K., Reddy, Y.R. and Rao, B.S. (2002). Indian J. Anim. Sci., 72(6): 439-440.

Schakenraad, M.H.W. and Dijkhuizen, A.A. (1990). Netherlands J. Agric. Sci., 38(1): 89-92.

Schepers, J.A. and Dijkhuizen, A.A. (1991). Prev. Vet. Med., 10: 213-224.

Schneider, M.P., Strandberg, E., Emanuelson, U., Grandinson, K. and Roth, A. (2007). Prev. Vet. Med., 80(2-3): 179-192.

Schroeder, J.W. (1997). Mastitis control programmes: Bovine mastitis and milking management. Extension publication, North Dakota State University Extension Service, April, 1997 (AS-1129).

Seegers, H., Fourichon, C. and Beaudeau, F. (2003). Vet. Res., 34: 475-491.

Seegers, H., Fourichon, C. and Beaudeau, F. (2003). Vet. Res., 34(5): 475-491.

Sharma, N. and Singh, R. (2005). Indian Dairyman. 57(7): 43-47.

Sharma, N., Maiti, S.K. and Singh, R. (2004). Dairy Planner. 1(1):40-41.

Shim, E.H., Shanks, R.D. and Morin, D.E. (2004). J. Dairy Sci., 87: 2702-2708.

Singh, N., Sharma, V.K., Rajani, H.B. and Sinha, Y.R. (1982). Indian Vet. J., 59: 693-696.

Singh, P.J. (1991). Studies on mastitis in cattle at machine milked farms in Punjab. MVSc. Thesis, Punjab Agricultural University, Ludhiana, India.

Singh, P.J. (1991). Studies on mastitis in cattle at machine milked farms in Punjab. M.V.Sc. thesis submitted to PAU, Ludhiana, India.

Singh, P.J. and Singh, K.B. (1994). Indian J. Dairy Sci., 47: 265-272.

Singh, P.J. and Singh, K.B. (1994). Indian J. Dairy Sci., 47: 265-272.

Singh, P.J., Singh, K.B., Nauriyal, D.C., Dhingra, P.N. and Bansal, B.K. (1992). Journal of Research, PAU, 29: 525-534.

Sinha, M.N. and Prasad, L.B.M. (1969). Indian J. Anim. Hlth., 8: 71.

Sirohi, Smita and Sirohi, S.K. (1995). Agri. Review 16(2): 81-87.

Steen, G.U. (1978). Dairy Sci. Abstr., 43: 7077.

Tesfaye, G.Y., Regassa, F.G. and Kelay, B. (2010). Trop. Anim. Hlth Prod., 42(5): 925-931.

Waage, S. (1989). Nork-Veterinaertidsskrift, 101(2): 93-100.

Ward, G.E., and Schultz, L.H. (1972). J. Dairy Sci., 55: 1428.

Watts, J.L. (1990) Bovine Mastitis. In: Diagnostic procedures in veterinary bacteriology and mycology, 5th edn. (eds. Carter G. R., Cole J. R.). Academic Press: London, 469-478.

Wilesmith, J.W., Francis, P.G. and Wilson, C.D. (1986). Vet. Rec., 118: 199-204.

Wilson, D.J., González, R.N., Hertl, J., Schulte, H.F, Bennett, G.J., Schukken, Y.H and Gröhn, Y.T. (2004). J. Dairy Sci., 87: 2073-2084.

Wood, P.D.P. and Booth, J.M. (1983). Anim. Prod., 36: 335-339.

Young, A. (2000). Can mastitis have an effect on reproduction? http://extension.usu.edu/files/agpubs/mastrepr.htm

Young, G.B., Lee, G.J., Waddington, D., Sales, D.I., Bradley, J.S. and Spooner, R.L. (1983). Vet. Rec., 113: 107-111.

□□□

CHAPTER

3

Bang of Mastitis of Milk Quality and Production

Bang on milk quality and yield

Mastitis influences the total milk output and modifies its composition and technological usability. The effects of both clinical and subclinical mastitis on milk yield, and milk quality, in terms of fat, protein and somatic cell count (SCC) are significant. Mastitis is always related to low milk production (Harmon, 1994), changes to milk consistency (density), reduced possibility of adequate milk processing, low protein and high risk for milk hygiene which may even contain pathogenic organisms. Subclinical mastitis also alters the composition of the milk in addition to suppressing milk yield (Harmon, 1994). It is well known that mastitis causes a decrease in the concentration of milk lactose (Nguyen and Neville, 1998), which may be due to leakage of lactose into the extracellular fluid and blood after the destruction of the normal lactose barrier (Mielke, 1975). Ogola *et al.* (2007) investigated the impact of mastitis infection on the quality of milk composition in small-scale dairy bovine herds. They found that in infected quarters milk, the concentrations of non-casein fractions, sodium, chloride, and free fatty acid were higher, while the casein content, lactose, casein-to-total protein, potassium, and calcium were lower compared to normal quarters.

Streptococcus agalactiae infection in dairy cattle plays an important role in reducing the production of quality milk and milk products. Variations in the composition of whole milk affect the properties of many other dairy products. Changes in milk composition result in reduced nutritional value of milk, increased processing problems, and off flavors. The shelf life of fluid milk products is also decreased, due to augmentation of the growth of spoilage bacteria.

During the inflammatory process (mastitis), three mechanisms are involved in milk composition change: a decrease in synthesis, an increase in the permeability of the milk barrier and an increase in the proteolytic activities in milk (Roux *et al.*, 2003). The impact of mastitis on milk composition is also discussed in detail in chapter 5 (Physiology of synthesis and secretion of milk). The concentrations of many minerals are altered during mastitis, and these changes can play significant roles in determining the manufacturing quality of the milk and diagnosis of sub-clinical mastitis. Certain nutritionally important minerals (Ca, P, Na, K, Cu, Mn, Fe and Zn) in skim milk or in the whey may undergo significant change as a consequence of secretory disorders in the mammary glands and increased permeability of blood capillaries (Singh and Mathur, 1990; Middleton *et al.*, 2004). The main mastitis effects on milk components are visible in table 3.1.

Table 3.1: The effect of mastitis on milk components (from Philpot and Nickerson, 1991).

	Components	Subclinical mastitis effects
Desirable	Total proteins	Decreased slightly
	Casein	Decreased between 6 and 20%
	Lactose	Decreased between 5 and 20%
	Solids non fat (SNF)	Decreased by up to 8%
	Butterfat	Decreased between 4 and 12%
	Calcium	Decreased
	Phosphorus	Decreased
	Potassium	Decreased
	Stability and keeping quality	Decreased
	Taste	Deteriorates and becomes bitter
	Yogurt starter cultures	Inhibited
Undesirable	Plasmin (degrades casein)	Increased
	Lipase (breaks down fat)	Increased
	Immunoglobulins	Increased
	Sodium	Increased – hence the "bitter" taste

The relationship between the raw milk somatic cell count and milk components has been well documented (Ma *et al.*, 2000; Schallibaum, 2001) (Table 3.2). According to Harmon (1994), the mastitis or elevated SCC is associated with a decrease in lactose, α-lactalbumin, and fat in milk because of reduced synthetic activity in the mammary tissue. The largest negative consequences of the presence of SCC are related to shorter shelf time and less sensory content or un-desirable organo-leptic characteristics of the final product, due to enzymatic activities from somatic cells (Topel, 2004). The higher levels of free fatty acids in high cell count milk may produce a *rancid* flavor. Milk from cows with sub-clinical mastitis decreases the quality of cheese and other manufactured milk products. Cheese from high cell count milk has been reported to be lower than it is from low cell count milk (Everson, 1980) and it may be due to the degradation of casein by the plasmin. As the SCC continues to increase with more severe and chronic cases of mastitis, the impact on casein becomes more intense. In addition to the yield losses, there is also reduced curd firmness, increased fat and casein loss in the whey and compromised sensory quality. Each of these affects the bottom-line of the cheese industry along with consumer acceptance. Decreasing SCC from 340000 cells/ml to 24,0000 cells/ml increased cheese yield 1% and decreasing SCC from 640000 cells/ml to 240000 cells/ml increased cheese yield 3.3%. The high presence of SCC in milk affects the activity of yogurt fermentation (Tamime and Robinson, 1999) and can even stop this process. Fernandes *et al.* (2007) studied the effect of SCC in raw milk on the chemical and physical properties of yogurt. He concluded that an increase in SCC causes an increase in fatty acids in yogurt during the preservation period and thus shortens the time of preservation of this product. The reduced heat stability of high SCC

Table 3.2 : Changes in milk constituents with elevated SCC.

Milk constituent	SCC (X 10^3 cells/ml)				Reason of changes
	<100	<250	500-1000	>1000	
Decrease (in g/100 ml)					
Lactose	4.90	4.74	4.60	4.21	
Casein	2.81	2.79	2.65	2.25	Reduced synthesis
Fat	3.74	3.69	3.51	3.13	
Increase (in g/100 ml)					
Whey proteins (Total)	0.81	0.82	1.10	1.31	
Serum albumins	0.02	0.15	0.23	0.35	
Immunoglobulins	0.12	0.14	0.26	0.51	Leakage from blood
Chloride	0.091	0.096	0.121	0.147	
Sodium	0.057	0.062	0.091	0.105	
Potassium	0.173	0.180	0.135	0.157	
pH	6.6	06.6	6.8	6.9	

Source: Schallibaum, Melchior. (2001). National Mastitis Council, Inc. 40th Annual Meeting Proceedings. 2001

milk causes flocculation during heat treatment processes such as pasteurization and evaporation (Sharma *et al.*, 2011). Milk SCC is widely used as an indicator of udder health status, a high SCC is associated with subclinical intramammary infection. There is a negative relationship between milk yield and SCC (Jones and Herald, 1982), which has been used to estimate the economic loss due to mastitis. These estimates are important in determining cost effective measures for mastitis control and prevention strategies.

In both clinical and subclinical mastitis, there is substantial loss in milk production. It is generally accepted that 70 to 80% of the estimated loss from mastitis is associated with reduced milk production due to subclinical mastitis. The extent of yield loss depends on severity, causative pathogen, parity and the stage of lactation at which mastitis develops. DeGraves and Fetrow (1993) estimated that 2.5-6.5% of expected annual yield is lost due to subclinical mastitis, whilst acute clinical cases caused a 6 - 11% reduction (Wood and Booth, 1983), and per-acute cases resulted in a 20 - 30% reduction in annual yield. The lactational yield loss of 300 to 400 kg (4 to 6%) in multiparous cows and 200 to 300 kg in primiparous cows (Hortet and Seegers, 1998). The loss in milk production does not only occur during the case itself, even after the mastitis case is cured, the milk production level of the cow stays lower. Losses in total milk production range from 5 to 25%, with one extreme of 83.90%. In terms of milk losses per quarter per day, 9 to 43.30% have been observed (Janzen, 1970). The cows are suffering from clinical mastitis causes an immediate drop in milk production and not regain production upto 60 days following clinical onset (Bartlett *et al.*, 1991). Steen (1978) recorded about 12.85% less milk yield in cows affected by mastitis as compared to the healthy cows and in India this report is about 10% less milk yield in clinical mastitic cow than before treatment (Sarma *et al.*, 1987). Clinical mastitis is associated with higher milk loss than subclinical mastitis (Hagnestam *et al.*, 2007; Hagnestam-Neilsen and Ostergaard, 2009). Because clinical mastitis is more severe form of mastitis and is associated with a larger amount of affected udder tissue, which results in more severe udder damage with decreased synthetic capacity of the mammary gland as a consequence.

Bang on reproduction

Udder health, production and reproduction are closely interacting factors in a dairy operation. The lifetime productivity of a dairy cow depends on the number of calves born and the amount of milk produced during its active reproductive phase. Efficient reproduction requires that calving intervals are optimized and there is adequate nutrition to support milk production and calf growth to reach puberty early in life. Mastitis is the most common and costliest disease in dairy cattle with the second most common disorder being reproductive disorders, including abortions and breeding problems. The total cost of mastitis and reproductive disorders to the dairy industry is difficult to predict, but it is known that these two conditions account for the overwhelming majority of disease costs to the dairy farmer. Mastitis has been reported to have a negative effect on both production and reproduction in dairy cattle. The negative effect is greatest on those cows having mastitis early in lactation (Kirk, 2004). Cows suffering from clinical and sub-clinical mastitis are at increased risk for reduced conception rate and increased fetal loss, regardless of clinical case being caused by either Gram- positive or Gram-negative bacteria (Santos *et al.*, 2004; Barker *et al.*, 1998; Schrick *et al.*, 2001). All types of mastitis, both Gram-positive (contagious pathogens) and Gram-negative bacteria (environmental pathogens), decreased reproductive performance in a similar manner. Previously, it was thought that only Gram-negative, environmental infections caused by coliform bacteria had an effect on reproductive performance.

Among the associations between mastitis and impaired reproductive function was an increase in services per conception (a term to describe the number of inseminations required to achieve a confirmed pregnancy) for cows diagnosed with clinical mastitis between first insemination and confirmed pregnancy when compared with cows that were diagnosed with mastitis at other times or to cows without clinical mastitis (Barker *et al.*, 1998) (Table 3.3). The greatest increase in services per conception is observed when cows experienced sub-clinical mastitis that progressed to clinical mastitis (Schrick *et al.*, 2001). The increase in services per conception caused by mastitis in these studies suggests that mastitis is associated with either anovulation at estrus, fertilization failure, or embryonic mortality. One cannot rule out the

Table 3.3: The effect of mastitis on reproduction performance in early lactation cows.

Parameter	Mastitis	Uninfected	Reference
Conception rate$	48%	63%	Frago *et al.*, 2004*
Days open	107±5	88±2	
Service per conception	2.1±0.1	1.6±0.1	
Days to first service	77.3±2.7	67.8±2.2	Shrick *et al.*, 2001**
Days open	110±6.9	85.4±5.8	
Service per conception	2.1±0.2	1.6±0.2	
Conception rate	48%	63%	
Conception rate	38%	46%	Kelton *et al.*, 2001***

*Based on clinical mastitis cases

**Based on clinical mastitis before first service

***Based on clinical mastitis event within 30 days post insemination

$ Conception Rate = Pregnancies/Services (Inverse of Services/Conception rom trial data)

possibility that the association between mastitis and services per conception occurs because cows that are pre-disposed to developing mastitis (for example, because they are experiencing some form of stress) are also predisposed to reproductive problems (Hansen *et al.*, 2004). Mastitis also affects the interval from calving to first service (Barker *et al.*, 1998; Schrick *et al.*, 2001). A mastitis event at or shortly after breeding may have a negative impact on the establishment and/or maintenance of pregnancy through either the hypothalamo-pituitary-ovarian axis, the uterine-ovarian axis or a nutritional effect on hormone levels (Hockett *et al.*, 1997; Jackson *et al.*, 1990).

Chebel *et al.* (2004) evaluated factors that affect conception rates (CR) and pregnancy loss in lactating Holstein cows from three different dairy herds in the Central Valley of California. In this study a total of 7,633 artificial insemination (AI) were used for evaluation of factors affecting CR and 1,465 cows diagnosed pregnant by ultrasonography at 31 day after AI and re-examined 14 d later were used for evaluation of factors affecting pregnancy loss. Among the factors evaluated was occurrence of mastitis between AI and pregnancy confirmation at approximately 45 day after AI. Cows that experienced mastitis during this interval had similar conception rates (24.0%) compared with those cows that did not experience mastitis (25.5%). However, when cows had mastitis between AI and pregnancy confirmation they were 2.8 times more likely to experience pregnancy loss between 31 and 45 d after AI compared with those cows that did not have mastitis. In a subsequent study, the same group evaluated the correlation between subclinical mastitis and pregnancy maintenance (Moore *et al.*, 2005). Cows were classified as experiencing subclinical mastitis when they had linear somatic cell count (LSCC) > 4.5 in the test day immediately prior to the AI but had no clinical signs of mastitis. Pregnancy was diagnosed at 28 day after AI by ultrasonography and at 35 d after AI by palpation per rectum. Cows classified as experiencing subclinical mastitis immediately prior to AI were 2.40 times more likely to lose the pregnancy between 28 and 35 day after AI compared with those cows that had LSCC < 4.5 (Moore *et al.*, 2005).

The stronger effect of clinical mastitis from Gram-negative bacteria on reproduction had been confirmed by a recent study (Hertl *et al.*, 2010). They reported that clinical mastitis occurring any time between 14 days before until 35 days after an A.I. was associated with lower probability of conception. The greatest effect was an 80% reduction associated with Gram-negative clinical mastitis occurring in the week after AI. Also, clinical mastitis due to Gram-negative bacteria had a more detrimental effect on probability of conception than did clinical mastitis caused by Gram-positive bacteria or other organisms.

Mechanisms by which mastitis may affect fertility

There are plenty of possible mechanisms/hypothesis by which mastitis could negatively affect fertility. There are some interesting speculation regarding the mechanisms by which mastitis, especially mastitis contracted between conception and approximately 40 days later, might cause loss of embryos. These possibly include fever, endotoxins from mastitis bacteria, production of cytokines as part of the cow's immune response and prostaglandins in the blood of the infected cows. However, there has not been conclusive evidence of exactly how mastitis affects reproduction? Most commonly accepted theories in the support of mechanisms by which mastitis may affect fertility.

1. Pyrexia/fever as a cause of reduced pregnancy

Pyrexia may result from both Gram-positive and Gram-negative infections of the mammary gland (Wenz *et al.*, 2001). In cattle, for example, heat stress during the period of oocyte maturation (Putney *et al.*, 1988) or early embryonic development (Putney *et al.*, 1988; Ealy *et al.*, 1993) leads to reduced embryonic survival. At least some of the effect of heat stress on embryonic survival is because of the direct effects of elevated temperature on oocyte and embryo function as culture of maturing oocytes (Edwards and Hansen, 1997) or pre-implantation embryos (Edwards and Hansen, 1997; Krininger *et al.*, 2002) reduced development to the blastocyst stage. It also appears that oocyte competence can be compromised by heat stress during follicular development (Hansen *et al.*, 2004). Furthermore, when lactating dairy cows and dairy heifers were exposed to heat stress, the fertilization rate and the proportion of excellent/good quality embryos were dramatically smaller for lactating dairy cows compared to heifers (Sartori *et al.*, 2002). This indicates that exposure of oocytes and embryos to heat stress compromises fertilization and development. Aside the direct effect of elevated body temperature on oocyte and embryo quality and development, fever can indirectly affect reproductive performance because cows that experience it have decreased feed intake and body condition (Maltz *et al.*, 1997). Therefore, if a cow develops mastitis and fever during early postpartum, a period of the lactation in which cows are already predisposed to reduced feed intake, greater loss of body condition and more pronounced negative energy balance may occur, which could delay resumption of ovarian cyclicity (Buttler, 2000; Chebel, 2007).

2. Inflammatory mediators may disrupts the oocyte maturation, embryonic development and uterine changes-

In Gram negative mastitis, endotoxin is released from Gram negative bacterial cell walls, which stimulate the body cellular response like polymorphonuclear cells (PMN) and other phagocytic cells. In the response of endotoxin these cells start produce a number of inflammatory mediators. Among them interleukin (IL)-1α, IL-1β, IL-6, IL-10, IL-12, and tumor necrosis factor-α (TNF-α) have been isolated from milk-derived cells from infected mammary glands (Riollet *et al.*, 2001). Prostaglandin $F_2\alpha$ (PGF2α) produced by the endometrium (one of the layers of the uterine wall) is also responsible for luteolysis, which occurs at the end of the estrous cycle if an embryo is not present. Mastitis and endotoxin treatment increased concentrations of nitric oxide (NO) in milk and intramammary infusion of *E. coli* endotoxin resulted in increased milk concentrations of PGF2α. It has been demonstrated that production of $PGF_2\alpha$ can be stimulated by cytokines such as TNF-β and IL-1c (Skarzynski *et al.*, 2000). Therefore, mastitis can lead to an increase in secretion of $PGF_2\alpha$ and consequently premature luteolysis, which could result in embryonic/fetal death. Of these molecules, TNF-α, NO, and $PGF_{2\alpha}$ can affect embryonic development by acting either on the oocyte or on the developing embryo (Figure 3.1). Elevated concentrations of NO have also been associated with early embryonic death. Culture with sodium nitroprusside dihydrate, a NO donor, inhibited development to the blastocyst stage of bovine (Soto *et al.*, 2003; Lim and Hansel, 1998) and mouse embryos (Sengoku *et al.*, 2001; Chen *et al.*, 2001). The toxic effects of NO may occur through interaction between NO and O_2^- to form the oxidant peroxynitrite (Hobbs *et al.*, 1999). It is not known whether mastitis is associated with increased synthesis of PGF2a and NO in the reproductive tract but this is possible because synthesis of both molecules is under cytokine regulation.

Maturation of bovine oocytes in the presence of TNF-α resulted in reduced proportion of fertilized oocytes developing to the blastocyst stage (Soto *et al.*, 2003). Furthermore, embryos cultured in the presence of TNF-α, PGF2α, or NO had either increased number of apoptotic cells (dead cells) or compromised development to the blastocyst stage (Wuu *et al.*, 1999; Chen *et al.*, 2001). Cullor (1990) indicated that endotoxins from the cell wall of Gram-negative bacteria, induced luteolysis and influenced conception and early embryonic survival apparently via the release of inflammatory mediators such as PGF2α. Intrauterine infusion of live *E. coli* into heifers on days 7-9 of the estrous cycle caused luteal regression and shortened estrous cycles (Gilbert *et al.*, 1990). Cytokines could also exert other effects on endometrial or oviductal tissue that impede embryonic development. IL-1β, for example, reduced proliferation of endometrial stromal cells and IFN-α reduced proliferation of oviductal epithelial cells (Kamwanja and Hansen, 1993).

Endotoxin absorbed from the uterine cavity has been reported to suppress the formation of preovulatory luteinizing hormone (LH) peak and to induce the cystic degeneration of dominant follicles in post-parturient cows (Peter *et al.*, 1989; Lopez-Diaz and Bosu, 1992). Therefore, although all details of the neuroendocrine regulation have not been fully known yet, endotoxin appears to disrupt the progression of the proestrous phase in ruminants and interrupt the preovulatory 17β-estradiol (E2) rise thus delaying or blocking the LH surge and the subsequent ovulation.

3. Changes in Hypothalamic-Pituitary-Ovarian Axis

Hypothelamic-pituitary-ovarian axis play important role in the reproductive cycle of cows. Reproductive cycles in cows are regulated by hormones produced in the hypothalamus (GnRH = gonadotropin releasing hormone) and pituitary (FSH = follicle stimulating hormone and LH = luteinizing hormone), which are glands located in the brain, and ovaries (E2 = estradiol and P4 = progesterone). Briefly, GnRH is responsible for stimulating the secretion of FSH and LH. Follicle stimulating hormone is responsible for stimulating initial growth of follicles in the ovaries, while LH is responsible for maturation of follicles and ovulation and also for stimulation of P4 secretion by the corpus luteum. Estradiol, produced by the follicles, is responsible for nstimulating the peak of LH that causes ovulation, while P4 is responsible for stimulating embryo growth and maintenance of pregnancy. Therefore, it is clear that the disruption of production or secretion of one of these hormones may dramatically affect the fertility of dairy cows (Chebel, 2007).

Another possible reason for increased number of services per conception in cows with mastitis is inhibition of gonadotropin secretion leading to reduced gonadotropin support for ovulation, oocyte maturation, folliculogenesis and luteal function. It has been demonstrated that cytokines can decrease LH release (McCann *et al.*, 2000). In cattle, for example, IFN-α has been shown to have such an action (Hansen *et al.*, 2004). Furthermore, mastitis and exposure of cows to endotoxins secreted by gram-negative bacteria result in increased blood concentrations of cortisol, a hormone that blocks the release and the peak of LH (Li and Wagner, 1983; Padmanabhan *et al.*, 1983). The decrease or lack of LH secretion may result in compromised follicle and oocyte development, lack of ovulation, and suboptimal luteal function. The whole mechanism in brief is mentioned in figure 3.1.

Cytokines released during mastitis can also have direct effects on the ovary. IL-6 blocks follicle stimulating hormone-induced estradiol secretion from bovine granulosa cells, especially from cells isolated from small follicles (Alpizar and Spicer, 1994). Both TNF-α and IFN-γ are cytotoxic to bovine luteal cells (Fairchild and Pate, 1991; Petroff *et al.*, 2001).

Therefore, preventing mastitis in early lactation animals improves reproductive efficiency. Beyond the udder health benefits, there are dramatic improvements in days to first service, days to conception, and services per conception in cows that are infection-free at first service compared to those herd mates infected near first service.

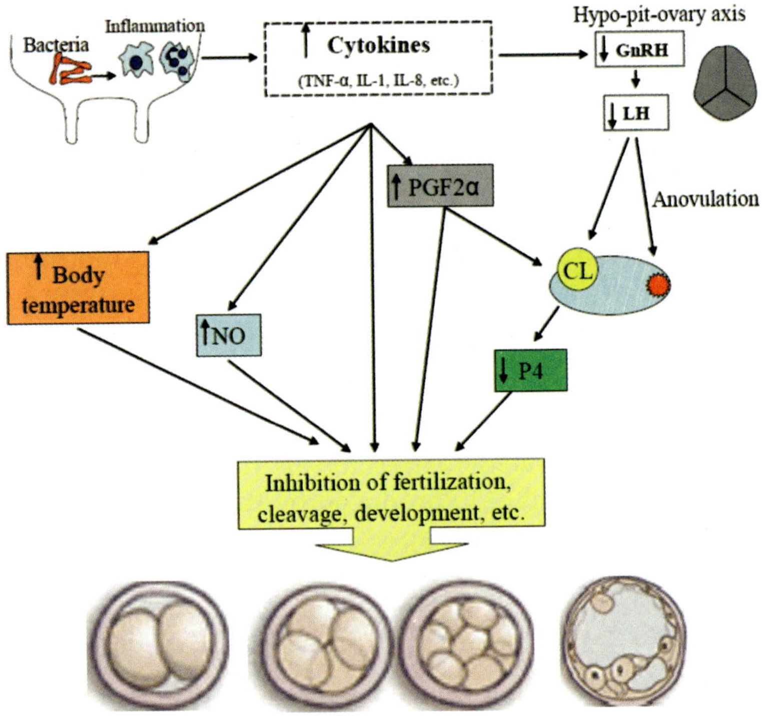

Figure 3.1: Hypothetical model by which mastitis affects fertility in lactating dairy cows. Modified and adapted from Chebel (2007).

Bang on animal welfare

Animal welfare is a sensitive issue for many consumers. Standards in which animals are kept vary from farm-to-farm and country to country. For example, on conventional dairy farms, cows do not have to be given bedding or much room to move. Some farms never allow their cows to graze outside, restricting them to indoor stalls. Calves may be kept isolated from their mothers and experience great distress. Farm animal welfare is an increasingly important consideration for çonsumers, farmers, the veterinary profession and government, as a criterion for ensuring acceptable standards and conditions of food production (Hristov *et al.*, 2008). There are many definitions of animal welfare. The most generally accepted single definition of animal welfare has been defined "*as its state at it seeks to cope with* its environment" (Fraser and Broom, 1990). It is well known the health is an important component of dairy cow welfare. The incidence and duration of an illness considerable affects the health of the animal (Webster, 2005; Vucinic, 2006). However, in terms of animal welfare, the intensity of pain and discomfort suffered from that disease are important. The welfare of farm animals is affected by the production system itself as well as the way the individual farmer applies the system.

The disorders, which have the greatest impact on welfare, are either acute disease processes, causing suffering or long-term progressive conditions involving chronic pain (Sorensen *et al.*, 2002). The mastitis is one of them. It is well noun that clinical mastitis causes severe pain and discomfort to animal and its current incidence and prevalence in the India and world over, still give cause for great concern. Mastitis is a serious animal welfare issue as the associated swelling and inflammation of the udder is very painful. Affected cows exhibit clear signs of discomfort, including abnormal posture, increased sensitivity, rapid breathing and heart rate, and a high temperature. Unfortunately, mastitis is not always easy to detect in its early stages, particularly when the redness and swelling of the udder is not obvious. If left untreated, severe mastitis may cause the death of the cow. It is more important aspect in regard to animal welfare. It is the most common disease and is a major reason for premature culling.

References

Alpizar, E. and Spicer, L.J. (1994). Biol. Reprod., 50: 38-43.

Barker, A.R., Schrick, F.N., Lewis, M.J., Dowlen, H.H. and Oliver, S.P. (1998). J. Dairy Sci., 81: 1285-1290.

Bartlett, P.C., Wijk, J.V., Wilson, D.J., Green, C.D., Miller, G.Y., Majewski, G.A. and Heider, L.E. (1991). J. Dairy Sci., 74: 1561-1572.

Buttler, W.R. (2000). Anim. Reprod. Sci., 60: 449.

Chebel, R.C. (2007). In: Proc Natl. Mastitis Counc. Reg. Meeting, pp. 43-55.

Chebel, R.C., Santos, J.E.P., Reynolds, J.P., Cerri, R.L.A., Juchem, S.O. and Overton, M. (2004). Anim. Reprod. Sci., 84: 239.

Chen, H.W., Jiang, W.S. and Tzeng, C.R. (2001). Fertil. Steril., 75: 1163-1171.

Cullor, J.S. (1990). In: Proc. International Symposium on Bovine Mastitis, Indianapolis, IN. pp. 176-180.

DeGraves, F. J. and Fetrow, J. (1993). Vet. Clin. North Am., 9: 421-434.

Ealy, A.D., Drost, M. and Hansen, P.J. (1993). J. Dairy Sci., 76: 2899-2905.

Edwards, J.L. and Hansen, P.J. (1997). Mol. Reprod. Dev., 46: 138-145.

Everson, T.C. (1980). In: Proc. Nat. Mast. Coun., pp. 153-166.

Fairchild, D.L. and Pate, J.L. (1991). Biol. Reprod., 44: 357-363.

Fernandes, A.M., Oliveira, A.F. and Lima, C.G. (2007). Intl. Dairy J., 17: 111-115.

Frago, F., Ahmadzadeh, A., Shafii, B., Dalton, J.C., McGuire, M.A. and Price, W.J. (2004). J. Dairy Sci., 87(1): 258.

Fraser, D. and Broom, D.B. (1990). Farm animal behaviour and welfare. CAB International, Wallingford, Oxon.

Gilbert, R.O., Bosu, W.T.K. and Peter, A.T. (1990). Theriogenology, 33: 645-651.

Hagnestam, C., Emanuelson, U. and Berglund, B. (2007). J. Dairy Sci., 90(5): 2260-2270.

Hagnestam-Nielsen, C. and Østergaard, S. (2009). Animal, 3(2): 315-328.

Hansen, P.J., Soto, P. and Natzke, R.P. (2004). Am. J. Reprod. Immunol., 51: 294-301.

Harmon, R.J. (1994). J. Dairy Sci., 77: 2103-2112.

Hertl, J.A., Gröhn, Y.T., Leach, J.D.G., Bar, D., Bennett, G.J., Gonzalez, R.N., Rauch, B.J., Welcome, F.L., Tauer, L.W. and Schukken, Y.H. (2010). J. Dairy Sci., 93: 1551-1560.

Hobbs, A.J., Higgs, A. and Moncada, S. (1999). Annu. Rev. Pharmacol. Toxicol., 39: 191-220.

Hockett, M., Oliver, S.P., Lewis, M.J., Hopkins, F.M. and Schrick, F.N. (1997). J. Dairy Sci. 80(Suppl. 1): 173.

Horted, P. and Seegers, H. (1998b). Prev. Vet. Med., 37(1-4): 1-20.

Hristov, S., Stankovic, B., Zlatanovic, Z., Joksimovic Todorovic, M. and Davidovic, V. (2008). Biotech. Anim. Husbandry, 24 (1-2): 25-35.

Jackson, J.A., Shuster, D.E., Silvia, W.J. and Harmon, R.J. (1990). J. Dairy Sci., 73: 627-632.

Janzen, J.J. (1970). J. Dairy Sci., 53(9): 1151-1160.

Jones, G.M. and Herald, C.W. (1982). In: Proc. Annu. Mtg. Natl. Mastitis Conc., Arlington, VA.

Kamwanja, L.A. and Hansen, P.J. (1993). Horm. Metab. Res., 25: 500-502.

Kelton, D., Petersson, C., Leslie and Hansen, D. (2001). In: Proc. 2nd International Symp. on Mastitis and Milk Quality. Pp. 200-202.

Kirk, J.H. (2004). Effect of mastitis on production and reproduction. Dairy Diary, University California Cooperative Extension. Pp. 3-4.

Krininger, C.E. III, Stephens, S.H. and Hansen, P.J. (2002). Mol. Reprod. Dev., 63: 335-340.

Li, P.S. and Wagner, W.C. (1983). Biol. Reprod., 29: 25.

Lim, J.M. and Hansel, W. (1998). Mol. Reprod. Dev., 50: 45-53.

Lopez-Diaz, M.C. and Bosu, W.T.K. (1992). Theriogenology 37: 1163-1183.

Ma, Y., Ryan, C., Barbano, D.M., Galton, D.M., Rudan, M.A. and Boor, K.J. (2000). J. Dairy Sci., 83: 264-274.

Maltz, E., Devir, S., Metz, J.H.M. and Hogeveen, H. (1997). Livest. Prod. Sci., 48: 175.

McCann, S.M., Kimura, M., Karanth, S., Yu, W.H., Mastronardi, C.A. and Rettori, V. (2000). Ann NY Acad Sci., 917: 4-18.

Middleton, J.R., Luby, C.D., Viera, L., Tyler, J.W. and Casteel, S. (2004). J. Dairy Sci., 87: 976-979.

Mielke, H. (1975). Veterinaermed., 30: 334.

Moore, D.A., Overton, M.W., Chebel, R.C., Truscott, M.L. and BonDurant, R.H. (2005). J. Am. Vet. Med. Assoc., 226: 1112.

Nguyen, D.-A.D. and Neville, M.C. (1998). J. Mammary Gland Biol. & Neoplacia., 3(3): 233-246.

Ogola, H., Shitandi, A. and Nanua, J. (2007). J. Vet. Sci., 8(3): 237-242.

Padmanabhan, V., Keech, C. and Convey, E.M. (1983). Endocrinology, 112: 1782.

Peter, A.T., Bosu, W.T.K. and DeDecker, R.J. (1989). Am. J. Vet. Res., 50: 368-373.

Petroff, M.G., Petroff, B.K. and Pate, J.L. (2001). Reproduction, 121: 753-760.

Philpot, W.N. and Nickerson, S.C. (1991). Mastitis: Counter Attack. Babson Bros. (Westfalia-Surge), Naperville, Illinois.

Putney, D.J., Drost, M. and Thatcher, W.W. (1988). Theriogenology, 30: 195-209.

Putney, D.J., Mullins, S., Thatcher, W.W., Drost, M. and Gross, T.S. (1988). Anim. Reprod. Sci., 19: 37-51.

Riollet, C., Rainard, P. and Poutrel, B. (2001). J. Dairy Sci., 84: 1077.

Roux, Y.L., Laurent, F. and Moussaoui, F. (2003). Vet. Res., 34: 629-645.

Santos, J.E.P., Cerri, R.L.A., Ballou, M.A., Higginbotham, G.E. and Kirk, J.E. (2004). Anim. Reprod. Sci., 80: 31-45.

Sarma, P.V., Rao, S.V.N. and Sampath, S.R. (1987). Indian Dairyman, 39(10): 477-479.

Sartori, R., Sartor-Bergfelt, R., Mertens, S.A., Guenther, J.N., Parrish, J.J. and Wiltbank, M.C. (2002). J. Dairy Sci., 85: 2803.

Schallibaum, M. (2001). In: Proc. Natnl. Mastitis Counc. Inc. 40th Annual Meeting. pp. 38-46.

Schrick, F.N., Hockett, M.E., Saxton, A.M., Lewis, M.J., Dowlen, H.H. and Oliver, S.P. (2001). J. Dairy Sci., 84: 1407-1412.

Sengoku, K., Takuma, N., Horikawa, M., Tsuchiya, K., Komori, H., Sharifa, D., Tamate, K. and Ishikawa, M. (2001). Mol. Reprod. Dev., 58: 262-268.

Sharma, Neelesh, Singh, N.K. and Bhadwal, M.S. (2011). Asian-Australasian J. Anim. Sci., 24(3): 429-438.

Singh, M.N. and Mathur, B.N. (1990). Indian J. Dairy Sci., 43: 95-98.

Skarzynski, D.J., Miyamoto, Y. and Okuda, K. (2000). Biol. Reprod., 62: 1116.

Sørensen, J.T., Hindhede, J., Rousing, T. and Fossing, C. (2002). In: Proc. First North American Conference on Robotic Milking - March 20-22, 2002. Pp. VI54-56.

Soto, P., Natzke, R.P. and Hansen, P.J. (2003). Am. J. Reprod. Immunol., 50: 380.

Steen, G.U. (1978). Dairy Sci. Abstr., 43: 7077.

Tamime, A.Y. and Robinson, R. (1999). Yoghurt Science and Technology. 2nd ed. Woodhead Publishing Ltd., Cambridge, UK.

Topel, A. (2004). Chemie und Physik der Milch. Behr's Verlag GmbH & Co. KG, Hamburg DE, 756, pp. 369-434.

Vucinic, M. (2006). Ponašanje, dobrobit i zastita zivotinja. Fakultet veterinarske medicine, Beograd.

Webster, J. (2005). Animal Welfare: Limping Towards Eden. Blackwell Publishing.

Wenz, J.R., Barrington, G.M., Garry, F.B., McSweeney, K.D., Dinsmore, R.P., Goodell, G. and Callan, R.J. (2001). J. Am. Vet. Med. Assoc., 219: 976.

Wood, P.D.P. and Booth, J.M. (1983). Anim. Prod., 36: 335-339.

Wuu, Y.D., Pampfer, S., Becquet, P., Vanderheyden, I., Lee, K.H. and De Hertogh, R. (1999). Biol. Reprod., 60: 479.

□□□

CHAPTER

4

Udder Anatomy

Mammary gland is a complex organ that proceeds through the early embryonic stages, into pregnancy, lactation and finally regression. To understand the etiology, pathogenesis and mastitis treatment, it is very important to know the anatomy of the mammary gland. Morphologically the mammary glands are *modified sweat (sudoriferous) exocrine glands.* The cow mammary gland is commonly named the *'udder'*. The udder consists of four separate functional mammary glands (quarters): *two fore* and *two rear quarters* (Figure 4.1A, B). The fore and rear quarters are separated by fine membrane. Each quarter is separate and no milk transfer occurs between quarters. Still antibiotics can be transferred from one quarter to the other through the extensive blood network throughout the udder. This is the reason why all milk should be discarded even if just one quarter was treated with antibiotics. Parenteral administration of antibiotics will also end up in the milk via the blood. Generally, the rear quarters are slightly more developed and produce more milk (60%) than the fore quarters (40%). Anatomical structure of each quarter is helpful in minimizing the spread of infection within the udder unless the infection become hematogenous. A prominent *median intermammary groove* (medial suspensory ligament) generally marks the division of the udder into right and left halves. Mammary glands are present in both male and female animals but normally develops only in female. The appearance of the udder varies greatly, depending on maturity and functional status as well as on individual and breed characteristics.

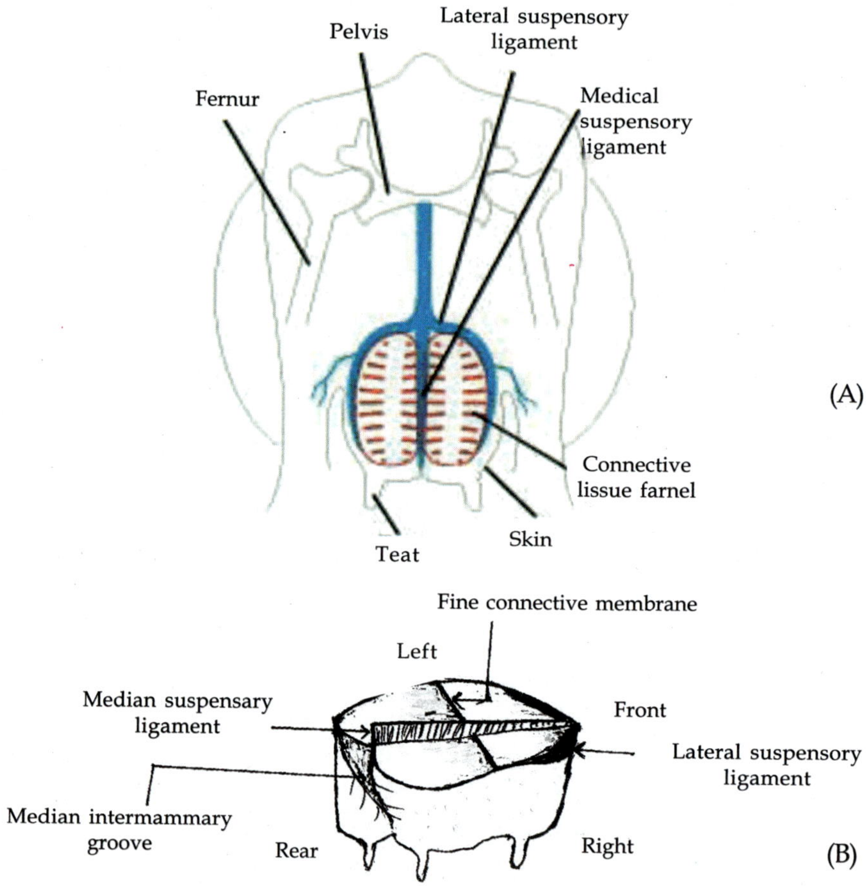

Figure 4.1 : Gross structure of the udder.

Certain features of conformation, particularly the size, shape and position of the teats, do have a practical importance in determining the suitability of the udder to milking and a particular size and shape of teats is more susceptible to the development of mastitis. Anatomical position of the udder probably disposes to many affections/infections resulting in loss of milk production and value of the animal is decreased (Singh and Varshney, 1999). The each udder half is almost completely independent, and has its own vascular system, nerve supply and suspensory apparatus.

Mammary Gland Development

Mammogenesis is the term used for development of mammary gland and refers to the development of mammary gland structures or it may defined as the growth and differentiation of the mammary gland to the stage prior to active secretion. This is most often assumed to occur during pregnancy, however mammary development begins when the animal is in early feta stagel and proceeds beyond begining of lactation. The mammary gland develops from the ectoderm as a single layered sheet of cuboidal cells, which differentiates it from the underlying mesenchyme (Figure 4.2). When first distinguished, it is known as *mammary band*. The mammary band is found at ~32 days after conception. A little later, when it becomes more localized, it is referred as the *mammary streak*. The mammary streak becomes further differentiated and form the *mammary line* by the 4-5th week of pregnancy. The ectodermal cells continue to grow into the mesenchymal layer, resulting

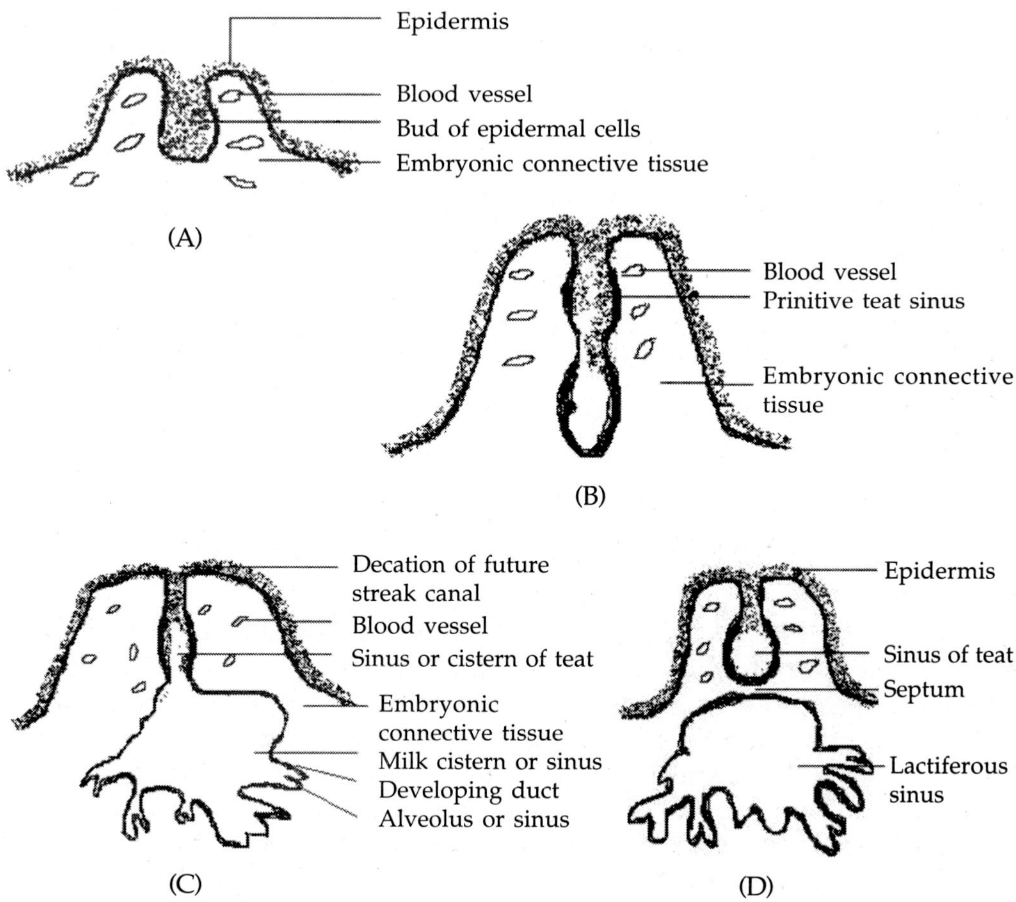

Figure 4.2: Schematic drawings of some stages in the embryonic development of the udder. a) Mammary bud extends into the cutis or dermis; b) mammary bud lengthened, showing some canalization for the teat canal and for the lactiferous sinus; c) further growth of the mammary bud with enlargement of the lactiferous sinus; d) Schema of the formation of septum (vail) between the lactiferous sinus and the teat sinus.

in formation of a spherical or globular structure known as *mammary bud.* In the bovine species by seventh week of gestation in fetuses 9 cm long, four primary mammary buds are usually present, two on each side and ultimately will give rise to the fore and rear quarters. Extra buds occasionally form and develop into supernumerary teats. The mammary bud formation is a critical stage in mammary development. After the bud formation finished several other important processes begin.

Active proliferation of mesenchymal cells around the mammary bud lifts the epidermis into a rudimentary teat by the 8-cm stage. Simultaneously, vigorous proliferation of cells near the inner end changes the mammary bud into a solid cellular column, which elongates vertically into the mesenchyme as the rudiment of the ductal system, the future single galactophore. Meanwhile, division among the epidermal cells below the original bud produces an epidermal cone at the base of the duct primordium. By the 19cm stage the growing duct primordium is longer than the teat and slightly swollen at the inner end. Here a cavity or lumen appears and soon spreads proximally towards the teat end. On reaching the epidermal cone the split remains narrow as the lumen of the future teat canal. Later this will open on the teat end and both teat canal and superficial epidermis will be lined by a common, thick, stratified squamous, keratinizing epithelium. By the 35-cm stage the growing duct rudiment has differentiated into three distinct regions-

1. An upper spheroid chamber distended with fluid represents the future gland sinus or milk reservoir.
2. A slightly longer mid-portion forms the more slender teat sinus.
3. A narrow teat canal within the epidermal cone, but still closed from the exterior by a plug of horny cells.

From the domed roof of the gland sinus several short solid epithelial cords, the secondary sprouts, project dorsally into the overlying pad of differentiating adipose tissue. When canalized these secondary sprouts represent the bases of the 10 or more major lactiferous ducts, which in the adult deliver milk into the gland sinus for storage. The teat sinus, gland sinus and duct bases are lined by a two layer cuboidal epithelium. As also in the terminal alveoli, which differentiate later in pregnancy, the inner cells are potentially secretory, while the outer differentiate into myoepithelial elements. In contrast the lowest and narrowest part of the axial lumen, forming the teat canal, is lined by thick, stratified squamous epithelium continuous with and identical to the glabrous epidermis of the teat. The latter is distinctly thicker, even in the fetus, than the epidermis above the teat where hair follicles differentiate from solid cellular ingrowths. The mesenchyme around and between the rudimentary epithelial ducts differentiates to provide blood vessels, lymphatics, small amounts of smooth muscle and an extensive fibroelastic stroma. One or more epidermal sprouts grow from the mammary bud into the connective tissue of the teat and begin to canalize at about the time of birth. Each sprout is destined to form a separate duct system with associated glandular tissue. When there is only one sprout (bovine), the mammary gland arising from it has a single duct system leading to single orifice at the teat end. The growth of the ducts and gland tissue is continued after puberty and especially during the first pregnancy. Tracts of denser white fibrous and elastic tissue form the suspensory ligaments and dorsally numerous lobules form in the pad of adipose tissue. Just before birth tertiary sprouts develop as short side branches from the secondary ducts, but thereafter the gland remains in an arrested state of development until puberty. Some extension to the ducts occurs during oestrous cycles, but full structural differentiation of the mammary gland is completed only during pregnancy under the influence of progesterone from the corpus luteum and other hormones. Most of the major developmental changes that will occur before birth have occurred by mid gestation. After birth, the bovine udder keeps pace with the normal growth of the animal, mostly by the deposition of fat, until puberty. The developmental changes in the udder at the time of birth are- teats are well developed, growth of the sprouts is limited to the area around the gland cistern. Only a few tertiary sprouts are present, non-secretory tissue is well formed (connective tissue, blood vessels and lymph vessels), and secretory or glandular parts are not developed at this time.

From the 4th or 5th month of pregnancy, the udder gradually enlarges owing to the formation of true alveoli. When the alveolar growth is complete, glandular activity is manifested a variable time before parturition by a tremendous increase in the size of the gland, frequently referred to as *"bagging up"* or *"making bag"*.

Growth of the pregnant Heifers udder

The udder tissue of 3 month pregnant heifer is similar to that of a non pregnant heifer (Kwong, 1940). No secretory tissue can be found. The ductules are at their height of proliferation. At the first month of pregnancy the connective bands are denser and more numerous in comparison with those in non pregnant heifer. While the secretory tissue has not developed by the end of the 3rd month of pregnancy, the elementary lobes and lobules can be treated by the groupings of the ductules. Between the 4th and 7th months of pregnancy, the secretory tissue is formed and begins to function. Individual or breed differences may account for the variation in the formation of the secretory tissue. Bizzozero and Vassale (1887) were the first to report the cellular changes of the mammary gland during pregnancy.

Benda (1894) found that in the resting stage of the mammary gland of the cow there is a layer of cells just outside of the alveolar epithelium continuing down along the ductules. During lactation this external layer disappears and is represented by myoepithelial layer that takes an active part in the mechanism of milk secretion. In the later part of the 4th to 7th month of pregnancy the alveoli are full of milk, which is a good indication of complete development. The interlobular spaces are filled with connective fibers, cellular elements, blood vessels, lymph spaces, and nerves.

During the 8th and 9th months of pregnancy, the alveoli are large and can be compared with those of lactating udders, and they are full of secretion. The interlobular and interlobar connective tissues are narrow, which indicates that the alveoli have fully developed and have occupied all the space available to them.

Role of hormones in the udder development

For the maintenance of pregnancy and the growth of the udder the two hormones of the ovary, *estrogen* and *progesterone are responsible*. When heifers reach sexual maturity and pass through estrus cycles, the hormone estrogen secreted (from the Graafian follicle) acts upon the pituitary gland and stimulates the secretion of a hormone called the *"mammogen-duct factor"*. Mammogen in turn acts upon the udder and stimulates the growth of the duct system and the cisterns. Each estrus cycle causes further growth, but the extent of this growth in non pregnant heifers is rather limited. When cows become pregnant, the progesterone (secreted from the corpus luteum) also acts upon the pituitary and stimulates the secretion of a second mammogenic hormone, the *lobule-alveolar factor* or *mammogen-lobule factor*, which causes the growth of the secretory parts of the udder at the ends and sides of the duct system. This part of the udder is called the lobule-alveolar system. Thus the growth of the udder is stimulated by the following hormones of the ovary acting upon the pituitary.

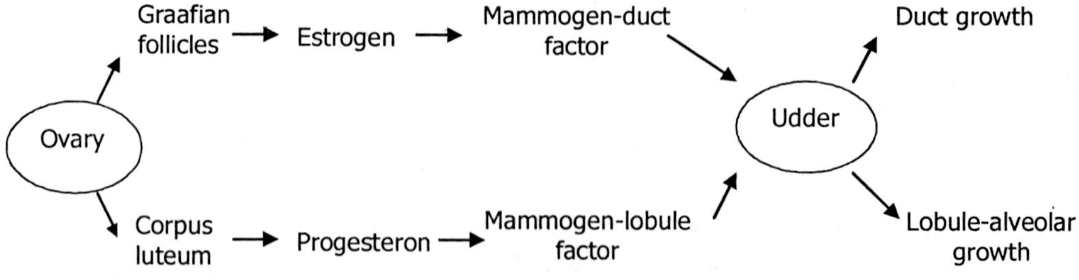

In addition, estrogen has a direct action on the tissues surrounding the mammary glands in each quarter of the udder, increasing the blood supply and the permeability of the capillaries and thus allowing the hormones in the blood to reach the tissues in increasing amounts and the blood to furnish the nutrients required for rapid growth of the udder.

Gross Structure of the Mammary Gland

The cow's udder comprises four quarters, each an individual gland drained by a teat. The four secretory glands are structurally separate and function independently, without milk flow between them. Receiving a large flow of blood and laden with stored milk, the lactating udder often weights 50–60 kg. A desirable udder should be strongly attached extending well forward with a rear attachment high and wide. The feature of the udder should be soft, pliable and elastic and well collapsed after milking.

The udder is attached to the body wall under the pelvis by strong lateral suspensory ligaments (suspensory apparatus) and skin. The main function of the skin appears to be assisting the support of the udder, especially anteriorly, and to prevent undue pendulum movement. It also provides the outward protection to the udder. The udder is attached to the skin by a *fine connective tissue* and a *course connective tissue* attaches the forequarters to the abdominal wall. The skin of the udder is thin, soft, pliable and freely movable and covered with a fine hair except at the teats and around the base of the teats, where hair is absent. The skin covering the teats may be smooth or wrinkled, depending on the degree of fullness. Bjorck (1963) classified the udder as *globular, trough shaped, bowl shaped* and *pendulous*; and teats as *conical, cylindrical, funnel* and *bottle shaped*. He also stated that pendulous udders are more prone to mastitis.

The Suspensory apparatus

A stronger udder supportive (suspensory) system is required to maintain proper attachments of the udder to the body. In dairy cows, the udder is very large can weight upto 60 kg. However, weight upto 100 kg have been reported (Little and Plastridge, 1946). Therefore, the udder has to be very well attached to the body (skeleton and muscles). The suspensory apparatus consists two major (suspensory) ligaments- *medial* and *lateral suspensory ligaments* (Figure 4.1A, B).

1. Medial suspensory ligaments

The medial suspensory ligament is the most important suspensory structure of the udder. It is formed by two lamellae of *yellow elastic* and *fibrous connective tissue,* originating from the abdominal tunic, which are reflected ventrally from the linea alba between the halves of the mammary glands. The lamellae of the medial suspensory ligament anastomose with the lateral suspensory ligaments of their respective sides on the ventral surface of each of the mammae in the formation of a sling. The elastic tissue of the medial suspensory ligament provides the necessary elasticity needed by the udder as it fills with milk to expand away from the body. The medial suspensory ligaments are attached to the pelvic bone and to tendon of the external oblique abdominal muscles. These ligaments run parallel to each other and pass ventraly between the two udder halves, forming an *intermammary groove* (Figure 4.1A, B). The ligaments then separate to cover the anterior, posterior and ventral portions of the glandular tissue on each udder half but terminate at the base of the teats (Nickerson, 1994). The median suspensory ligament has tensile strength. It is located at the center of gravity of udder to give it a balanced suspension. When the cow is viewed from behind, a distinct midline groove, marks the position of medial suspensory ligament.

2. Lateral suspensory ligaments

The lateral suspensory ligament of each udder half originates from the subpubic and prepubic tendons. Lateral suspensory ligaments contain more collagen (fibrous non-elastic strands) than elastin and thus provide support but not elasticity to the udder. The lateral suspensory ligaments continues to the ventral border of the gland, where it fuses with the medial suspensory ligament to form a *suspensory sling*. This fusion of the lateral suspensory ligaments with the medial suspensory ligaments usually extends onto the posterior and anterior borders of their respective glands. The lateral suspensory ligaments cover the lateral surface of the mammary glands. In young animals before the first lactation, the lateral suspensory ligaments are very difficult to differentiate from the facial layers.

Both the medial and lateral suspensory ligaments have lateral branches that are inserted into the glandular tissue and become continuous with the connective tissue stroma, supporting the parenchyma in a *cradle-like fashion* (Swett, 1942). In any condition when this suspensory apparatus becomes loose e.g. in high yielder cows, immediately after parturition when milking is not done regularly or in old ages, the udder becomes *pendulous*. It swings very fast while walking and may came in contact with various obstruction e.g. barb wires, bushes and walls. Thus pendulous udder is very easily affected with contusion, open wound, gangrene etc. which ultimately leads to mastitis (Pathak, 2003).

The Circulatory system

1. Arterial system

Milk production demands a lot of nutrients that are brought to the udder by the blood. The rate at which blood flow to the mammary gland is one of the key factors in determining milk synthetic rate. Approximately 400-500 liters of blood flowing the mammary gland to produce one liter of milk (Turner, 1981). For a cow with an average milk production level, this translates to about 20% of the entire output by the heart. Total udder blood volume for lactating cows is about 8% of total body blood volume, while for a non-lactating cow it is about 7.4%. There is a 2-6 fold increase in blood flow in the mammary gland during last 2-3 days prepartum. However, the decrease in milk production in later lactation is not due a reduction of blood flow to the mammary glands, rather it is due to the loss of secretory epithelial cells through a process programmed cell death (apoptosis). This is also suggests that the efficiency of extraction of milk precursors (e.g. glucose, amino acids, fatty acids) from the blood while it passes through the mammary glands is very important. In order to supply the udder, the blood is conducted from the left ventricle of the heart into the descending, or abdominal aorta. The abdominal aorta proceeds posteriorly, ventral to the thoracic and lumbal vertebrae until it reaches the fifth or sixth lumbal vertebra, where it divides into the right and left *external* and *internal iliac arteries* (Figure 4.3).

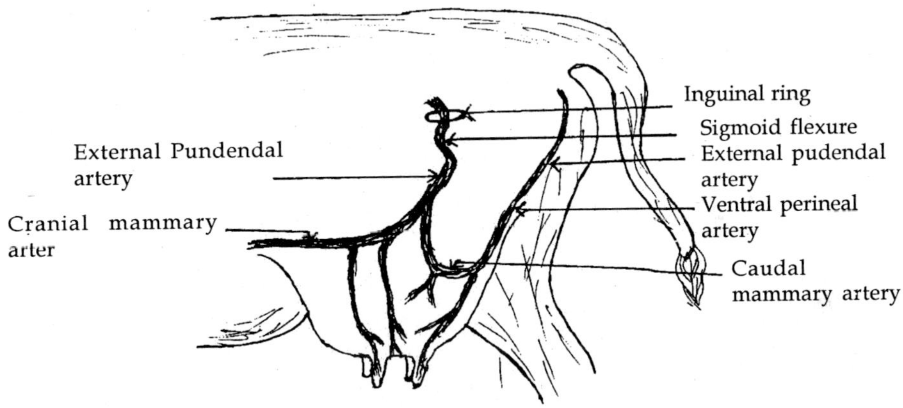

Figure 4.3 : The arterial system of the udder.

The external iliac artery proceeds posterolateral and slightly ventral along the side of the pelvic inlet and continued as the femoral artery. The internal iliac artery gives off the *prepubic artery*, which divides into *posterior abdominal* and *external pudic arteries*. The external pudic artery descends on the inguinal ligament through the medial part of the inguinal canal and emerges at the medial angle of the external inguinal ring deeply to the anterior border of the lateral suspensory ligament. Upon emerging from the inguinal canal, the mammary artery as well as the associated mammary vein, follow a tortuous route forming an *S-shaped curve (Sigmoid flexure)*. This allows for downward distention of the udder as it fills with milk, without stressing blood vessels.

The sigmoid flexure appears to be lacking in the young animal that has not reached the lactating stage. It probably occurs during the first lactation period and is very likely the result of a stretching of the vessels to supply the glands following the stimulus of the first pregnancy.

Just after leaving the external inguinal ring, the external pudic artery divides into the *subcutaneous abdominal artery* and the *mammary artery,* the later being about 1 cm in diameter. The mammary artery enters the glandular tissue, giving off a small branch posteriorly about 0.2 cm in diameter that ramifies in the supramammary lymph gland. The mammary artery soon divides into *posterior* or *posterior* and *anterior* or *anterior* mammary arteries, which usually supply in their respective quarters. The anterior mammary artery is about 0.5 cm in diameter and supplies the front side of the udder. The posterior mammary artery, soon after begins gives off a large anterior branch that describes a wide are anteriorly and is continued ventrally in the glandular tissue, giving off numerous small branches as it proceeds. This branch usually terminates in the lateral wall of the posterior teats as the papillary arteries. The larger papillary arteries usually occupy a lateral position of the teats. The main trunk of the posterior mammary artery proceeds ventrally and posteriorly giving off two large branches posteriorly and one anteriorly, itself ramifies in the *accessory teats,* if present, and the surrounding glandular tissue.

Variations occur in the arterial distribution to the mammary glands in different animals and even in the two halves of the same individual. Near the base of the udder, the arteries, veins, lymph vessels and nerves are widely dispersed, but as they proceed ventrally they usually become *satellites* of large milk collecting ducts.

2. Venous System

The blood from each half of the udder flows through two veins- the *external pudic veins* and the *subcutaneous abdominal veins (milk veins)* (Figure 4.4). The majority of the veins carrying blood from the teat to the

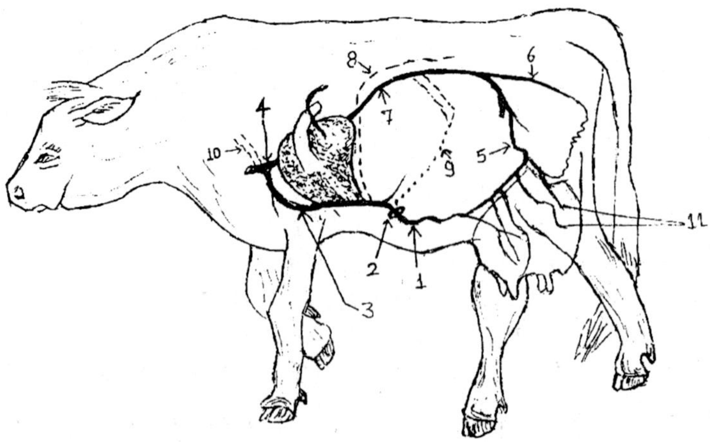

Figure 4.4: The venous system of the udder. 1. Milk vein 2. Milk "well" 3. Internal thoracic vein 4. Craniul vena cava 8. Diaphrogm 9. Costal arch 10. First rib 11. Venous tributories from gland parenchyma.

larger vessels at the base of the udder. They are usually superficial on the lateral surfaces of the udder.

Satellite veins of the arteries collect the blood from the parenchymatous tissue and the milk collecting duct and alveolar system and proceed dorsally into the glandular tissue commitant to the larger milk collecting ducts. Near the base of the udder these veins become almost twice the size of the arteries of which they are satellites, deviate from them, and join the vessels forming the venous circle at the base of the udder. A tortuous well developed *venous circle* is formed by anastomoses between anterior and posterior mammary veins infront of the mammary glands. It is generally regarded as the desirable character among the good milkers. The division between the anterior and posterior mammary veins is the point of origin at the base of the udder of the external pudic trunks almost directly dorsal to the posterior teats of their respective sides. Several veins leaves the anterior border of the base of the udder and become subcutaneous. The most lateral on each side is a continuation of the anterior veins and are termed the *subcutaneous abdominal vein (milk vein)* from this point anteriorly.

The external pudic veins

The external pudic vein arises from the venous circle at the base of the udder almost directly dorsal to the posterior teat. The diameter of this vessel is usually twice the diameter (2-3 cm) of the artery to which it is a satellite. It forms the *S-shaped curve* anterior to the artery and ventral to the external inguinal ring. Blood flows through this vein from the udder to the posterior vena cava. Emmerson (1928) opined that the external pudic vein is the most contant channel by which the blood returns to the heart from the udder. It is of sufficient size to backflow the blood from the udder, and it remain the most constant in size of the veins. Greaves (1916) ligated the mammary veins in two lactating cows and found that there was no appreciable variation in the amount of milk secreted after the ligation.

The subcutaneous abdominal veins

The subcutaneous abdominal veins also known as the *mammary* or *milk veins,* emerges from the anterior basal border of the mammary glands. These are the large veins that are visible under the skin of the cows abdomen. The largest veins emerging from the lateral parts of the anterior basal border of the udder are subcutaneous continuations of the anterior mammary vein of their respective sides also known as the subcutaneous abdominal veins.

The subcutaneous abdominal veins proceed anteriorly to a transverse plane through the xyphoid cartilage, receiving numerous smaller radicles draining the ventral and lower lateral abdominal wall, and enters the abdominal wall about a hand-breath on either side of the xyphoid cartilage via *"milk wells"* (Figure 4.4). These milk wells may occur at any point along the course of the subcutaneous abdominal veins between the umbilicus and the xyphoid cartilage. Within the abdominal cavity the subcutaneous abdominal veins pass forward beneath the insertion of the diaphragm to join the *internal thoracic veins.* The internal thoracic veins are converge with the brachial veins of their corresponding sides. The brachial veins, along with the common jugular form the anterior vena cava, which empties into the right atrium of the heart.

The another route of blood return to the heart is observed when occasionally a small venous radicle leaves the lateral surface of the udder to pass over the reflection of the skin from the lateral surface of the udder to the medial surface of the thigh to join the saphenous vein.

The exact route is probably dependent upon the position of the animal. When the cow is in the standing position, most of the blood returns to the heart via the milk veins. However, when the cow lies down and shuts off blood flow through the milk vein, milk production is not affected because of alternative way of blood flow.

The Lymphatic System

The interstitial fluid originating from capillaries that nourish the mammary parenchymal cells recirculating via the lymphatic system, which carries waste products away from the udder. Lymph originates as a filtrate of the blood serum and is similar in composition to it except that lymph has no red blood serum and about half the protein content.

Lymph flows from the udder (Supramammary lymph nodes) to the thoracic duct and is eventually discharged into the blood system via anterior vena cava (Figure 4.5). The rate of lymph flow through the mammary gland of lactating cow is 1300 ml/hour or 31,200 ml/day, and 1.6 units lymph leave udder for every unit milk produced. In response to infection (e.g. mastitis) lymph nodes increase the output of lymphocytes, which are transported to the udder to squash infection.

Very small afferent lymph vessels pass dorsally in the muscular part of the teat wall and beneath the mucous membrane to join the larger lymph ducts of the udder. These lymph ducts form a profuse network at the base of the teat. They proceed dorsally toward the supramammary lymph glands. Either they are equally distributed in the superficial fascia covering the lateral surfaces of the udder, or they may pass posteriorly and proceed dorsally in a group directly over the posterior teats. The majority of the lymph vessels of the teat join these superficial lymph ducts.

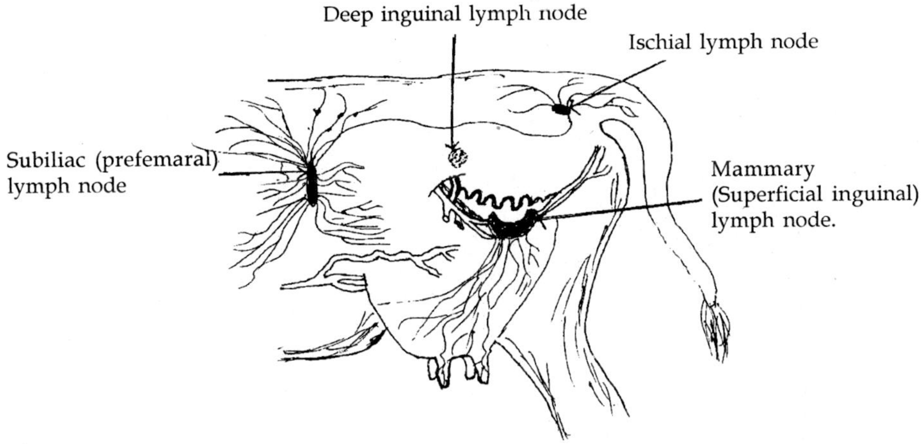

Figure 4.5 : Left lateral view of the mammary gland showing the lymphatic drainage.

The *superficial afferent lymph ducts* penetrate the lateral suspensory ligament on a horizontal plane drawn through the ventral border of the supramammary lymph glands. The course of these lymph ducts medial to the lateral suspensory ligament is toward the supramammary lymph glands, which they enter.

The *deep afferent lymph ducts* may receive small lymph vessels from the teat, as well as numerous vessels from the lymph spaces of the glandular tissue and the milk collecting ducts. The deep lymph ducts pass toward the base of the udder in company with the arteries, veins and nerves, which are all usually satellites of some large milk collecting duct.

The supramammary lymph glands are located just posterior to the inguinal vessels as the later emerge from the external inguinal ring and between the lateral suspensory ligaments on the posterodorsal surface of the udder (Figure 4.5), which serve as filters to remove foreign substances. They may vary greatly in number, size and shape. Two supramammary lymph glands are most frequently found, although three are not infrequent and as high as seven small glands have been recorded (Little and Plastridge, 1946). The large glands are usually 2 to 4 inches (about 6-10 cm) long, the smaller ones ¼ to ½ as large. The supramammary lymph glands are often kidney shaped and are compressed laterally. The right and left glands may lie in apposition to each other, or the glandular tissue of the udder and fat may be interposed between them. Occasionally, one finds the right and left lymph glands fused at their dorsal extremities. Supra-mammary lymph glands receive afferent vessels from the udder and teats, and from the medial side of the thigh.

The prefemoral lymph glands

The efferent ducts of the prefemoral lymph glands pass dorsally toward the tubercoxae, penetrate the abdominal wall a few centimeters below it, and usually become afferent ducts to the deep inguinal lymph glands, sometime to the iliac lymph glands. From the deep inguinal lymph glands and the external iliac lymph glands the lymph passes to the thoracic duct and hence into the *cisterna chyli.*

Around the time of parturition, the filtration of lymph out of the blood capillaries in the udder may exceed the drainage back into the blood, resulting accumulation of fluid in the intercellular tissue spaces and; the accumulation of milk within the udder compresses the lymphatics, causing the *udder edema.* This is more serious in first calf heifers and in older cows with pendulous udders. This situation can be remedied, in part by massaging the surface of the udder in a direction toward the supramammary lymph nodes to promote movement of lymph and reduce swelling. Sharma *et al.* (2005) had reported a case of post parturient of udder edema in Sahiwal cow.

The Nervous System

The innervation of the udder is sparse as compared with other tissue of the body. The major nerves of the udder are sensory (afferent) nerves that carry impulses from the quarters to the brain. The sensory nerves are involved in milk ejection and found in the teats and skin. Innervation of the udder is greatest in the dermis of the teats. Similar to other skin glands, *there is no parasympathetic innervation* to the mammary glands. There is no innervation of the secretory system (St. Clair, 1940). Myoepithelial cells of the alveoli, contract in response to blood borne hormone oxytocin and not response to direct innervation.

The nerve supply to the udder and teats of the cow is mainly from three sources:-

a) Inguinal nerve
b) Perineal nerve and
c) Sympathetic innervation of the udder.

a) Inguinal nerve

The inguinal nerve is formed by the ventral branches of the 2nd, 3rd and 4th lumbar spinal nerves. The third lumbar spinal nerve always supplies the inguinal nerve, but the second and fourth may not always contribute to it. Just before entering the internal inguinal ring, the nerves commonly unite to form a single inguinal nerve trunk. If a common inguinal trunk enters the internal inguinal ring, it immediately divides into *anterior* and *posterior inguinal nerves.*

The *anterior inguinal nerve* emerges from the extreme anterior part of the external inguinal ring. This nerve supplies the skin of the fold of the flank and the anterior part of the fore quarter and teat but it supplies the glandular tissue only slightly.

The *posterior inguinal nerve* always passes entirely through the inguinal canal. It usually passes over the dorsal part of the S-shaped curve of the vein, after traversing the inguinal canal anterior to the external pudic vein. Just outside the external inguinal ring it gives off one or two small anterior branches, which supply the glandular tissue somewhat but mainly innervate the skin of the lateral part of the anterior gland quarter as far posteriorly as the interquarter junction. These branches also supply the skin of the posterior part of the anterior teats. The posterior or main portion of the posterior inguinal nerve is the only part of the inguinal nerve that makes an S-shaped curve with the external pudic vessels. It also sends a small branch to the supramammary lymph node area.

b) Perineal nerve

It originating from the ventral branches of the third and fourth sacral nerves are the pudic and posterior hemorrhoidal nerves. The perineal nerve is a branch of the pudic nerve that passes over the ischial arch to descend in the perineum with the perineal vessels. It is small and superficial, supplying the skin of the escutcheon and posterior part of the udder as far as the posterior basal border of the rear teats.

c) Sympathetic innervation

The sympathetic innervation of the udder is accomplished through fibers incorporated in the nerve trunks of the inguinal nerves that originating from the posterior mesenteric plexus (Montane and Bourdelle, 1917). According to St. Clair (1940), the sympathetic nerve supply to the mammary gland is from the postganglionic fibers carried by the spinal nerves. The primary function of the sympathetic nerve fibers are- the control of the blood supply to the udder and innervation of the smooth muscle surrounding the milk collecting ducts and the sphincter muscles within the teat.

Since the third lumbar spinal nerve always supplies the inguinal nerve, whereas the second and fourth do not always contribute to it, the third is unquestionably the principal source of the sympathetic fibers to the inguinal nerves, thence to the nonstriated musculature of the udder and teats.

The nerves to the blood vessels of the udder and teat reach them through the spinal nerves. The sympathetic nerves to the udder are *motor to the smooth muscle* and *vasoconstrictor to the blood vessels*. Stimulation of the sympathetic nervous system causes a vasoconstriction of the blood vessels and this has an inhibiting effect on milk secretion.

The nerves to the glandular tissue pass through the connective tissue and are probably not secretory. The nerves of the sympathetic nervous system carry impulses to the smooth muscle bundles of teat, which undergo continuous rhythmic contractions between milkings. When these nerves are blocked, cows tend to leak milk because the rhythmic contractions can no longer take place (Emmerson, 1914). During milking, impulses from the brain and spinal cord cause the smooth muscle bundles surrounding the teat canal to relax, allowing the teat canal to dilate for the flow of milk (Nickerson, 1994).

Interior Structure of the Mammary Gland

Duct and milk secretory system

The udder is divided into two distinct, equal halves by the median suspensory ligament. Each half is composed of two mammary gland, that are characterized by the presence of a teat on their ventral surface. These parts or complex are popularly called *"quarters"* (Frei, 1926). Each of the four quarters functions as separate gland within the udder and has its own milk secretory tissues. The interior structure of the mammary gland consists of (Figure 4.6)

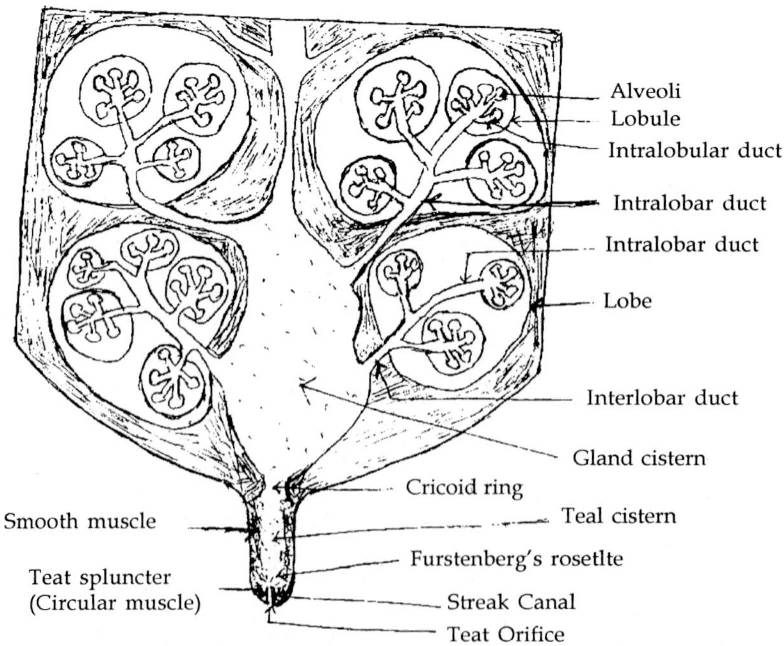

Fig. 4.6 : Longitudinal diagram of quarter illustrating the interior structure of the mammary gland.

1. Connective tissue
2. Secretory tissue
3. Ductular system

1. Connective Tissue

The function of the connective tissue is to support and protects the ductular and the secretory tissues. A desirable udder should contain a minimal amount of connective tissue and a maximal amount of secretory tissues. It is a common belief that a big udder is related to a high milk production. This is, however, not true in general, since a big udder might include a lot of connective and adipose tissue. Udders with a large proportion of connective tissue relative to secretory tissue lobules are referred as *"meaty"*.

2. Secretory Tissue

The secretory tissue consists of billions of alveoli. The alveoli are microscopic, spherical structures 50 to 250 mm in diameter, depending upon the volume of accumulated milk. Each alveolus is supplied with tiny capillaries, which lie outside the secretory cells (stroma). An alveolus is the sac like structure, where milk is synthesized and secreted, and therefore considered the *milk producing structural unit of the udder* (Figure 4.7). The word alveolus is

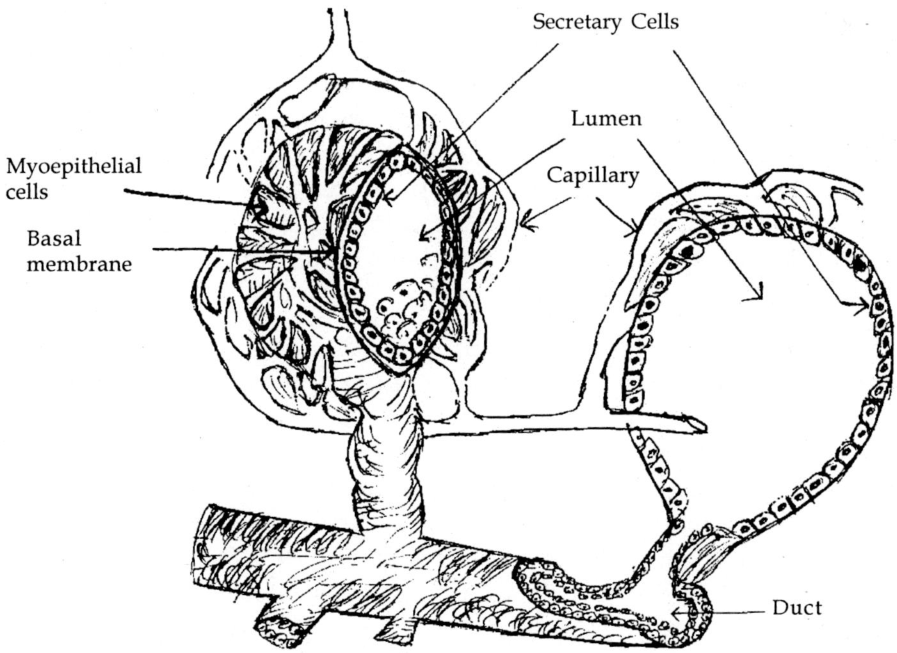

Figure 4.7 : Structure of the alveoli.

derived from the Latin word *"alveus"* meaning *"hollow"*. It is estimated to hold ~1/5 of a drop of milk. The lumen of the alveolus is lined by a single layer of *cuboidal* to *columnar shaped epithelial cells*. The epithelial lining is surrounded by contractile epithelial (muscle fiber) cells known as the *myoepithelial cells*. These smooth muscle cells also surround the small ducts, running in a lengthwise direction and these cells contract in response to the hormone *oxytocin*, resulting in the letdown of milk. Outside the myoepithelial cells, the alveolus is surrounded by a connective tissue *basement membrane*. A cluster of 150-250 alveoli encapsulated by connective tissue sheath and their ducts constitute a *lobule*. The structure of this area is very similar to the structure of the lung. A group of lobules are surrounded by a septum of connective tissue and form a *lobe*.

3. Ductular System

The ductular system of the mammary gland starts at the alveolus and ends at the streak canal. The milk collecting system consists of a network of collecting tubules and ducts. The duct systems of the four quarters are independent having no connection with each other. Despite this, infection may spread directly between the tissues of the quarters of the same side (Dycee *et al.*, 1996). The terminal ducts of alveoli unite successively to form *intralobular ducts*. The intralobular ducts found within the lobule and they unite to form large ducts i.e. *interlobular ducts*. Subsequently these ducts unite successively to form *intralobar* and *interlobar ducts*, they present within the lobe and between the lobes respectively. These various order of ducts eventually empty into a large basin, the *lactiferous sinus*. Reinder (1903) found that the number of large milk ducts entering the lactiferous sinus is usually 9 to 11, while Zwart (1911) found that 15 lactiferous ducts emptying into the lactiferous sinus. Lactiferous sinus is multilocular dilatation, because the openings of the large collecting ducts are overlapped and surrounded by connective tissue and smooth muscle fibers covered. The lactiferous sinus empty into a large cavity within the quarter proper, the *gland cistern*.

Gland cistern is the largest collecting point of milk (~400ml). According to Nickerson (1994) gland cistern can accommodate milk up to 2 liters. The gland cistern is opened into the *teat cistern*. The teat cistern holds the milk about 30 to 40 ml. The gland cistern and teat cistern is partially separated or demarcated by an annular fold known as *cricoid rings*. The teat cistern is continued with the exterior of teat trough a narrow tube (5 - 10 mm) known as *streak canal*. At the junction of teat cistern and streak canal, the lining of the teat is arranged in a group of radial folds called the *rosette of Furstenberg's* (Pathak, 2003). The rosette of Furstenberg's may fold over the canal opening due to pressure when the udder is full. It may be a major point of entry for leukocytes leaving the teat lining.

The teat is the external opening of the milk collecting system. An external opening, present at the ventral extremity of the teats, is known as the *teat orifice*. At the end of the teat is surrounded by sphincter composed of circular smooth muscle fibers which remains constricted and prevent leakage of milk until milking commence and entry of the organisms into the teat canal. The teat orifice is tightly closed in buffaloes due to well developed circular muscles. The teats are suspended in a perpendicular manner from the ventral part of each gland. Four teats normally are present on the ventral surface of the cow udder. These vary greatly in shape, length and diameter in the various breeds and in animals of the breed. The average length of the fore teats is 6.6 cm with an average diameter of 2.9 cm, while the rear teats 5.2 cm in length and 2.6 cm in diameter (Emmerson, 1928), while Sisson *et al.* (1975) states that the average length is 7 to 8 cm. Teat duct length was shown to be an important factor in mastitis susceptibility with intramammary infections increasing in probability with decreasing teat canal length (Lacy-Hulbert and Hillerton, 1995). The diameter of the teat duct has been shown to affect susceptibility to intramammary infection with wider diameters being associated with increased bacterial penetration (McDonald, 1975) resulting increased the chances of mastitis (Motomura *et al.*, 1994). The shape and length of teats are very important as too long teats are always prone to injuries and consequent infections (Khire and Kothekar, 2002). In 1960, Tomar and Tomar suggested that the size of teats had significant relationship with milk production. The short teats are more superior for level of production and had less chances of mastitis (Hickman, 1964). The mucous membrane is very thin and is closely adherent to the muscular coat. Between the mucous membrane and the muscular coat are interposed the papillary blood vessels.

About 50% of all cows have extra teats, referred to as *accessory* or *supernumerary teats*. Some of these extra teats open into a "normal" gland, but many do not. Generally they are removed before 1 yr of age. A pseudo-teat has no streak canal, and therefore, no connection to the internal structures of the gland. Emmerson (1928) studied that both dairy and beef cows had 44% accessory teats. Of these, 22.5% had one accessory teat, 19% had two accessory teats, and 2.5% had three accessory teats.

References

Benda (1894). Dermatol. Z., 1: 94.

Bizzozero, G. and Vassale, G. (1987). Virchow's Arch. Path. Anat., 40: 155-214.

Bjorck, G.R. (1963). Zhivotnovodstov mosk. 27 (15): 105-123.

Dyce, K.M., Sack, W.O. and Wensing, C.J.G. (1996). In Text book of Veterinary Anatomy. 2nd ed., W.B. Saunders Co., Philadelphia. pp. 727-736.

Emmerson, M.A. (1928). Studies on the macroscopic anatomy of the bovine udder and teat. M.S. thesis, Iowa State College Library, Ames, Iowa.

Emmerson, M.A. (1941). University of Penn. Vet. Ext. Qtrly. 41:80.

Frei, W. (1926). Joest's spezielle pathologische Anatomie der Haustiere, vol. IV, Verlagsbuchhandlung von Richard Schoetz, Berlin.

Greaves, R.R. (1916). Hoard's Dairyman, 52: 687.

Hickman, C.G. (1964). J. Dairy Sci., 45: 777.

Khire, D.M. and Kothekar, M.D. (2002). In compendium of IAAVR round table Conf. on mastitis., 4-5 Feb, 2002. Nagpur (MS), India. Pp. 126-129.

Kwong, F.J. (1894). Am. Vet. Med. Assoc., 94:36-40.

Lacy-Hulbert, S.J. and Hillerton, J.E. (1995). J. Dairy Sci., 62(3): 395-404.

Little, R.B. and Plastridge, W.N. (1946). Bovine mastitis. 1st edn., Mc Graw Hill book Comp. INC, New York. p. 42.

McDonald, J.S. (1975). Cornell. Vet., 65(4): 492-496.

Montane, L. and Bourdelle, E. (1917). Anatomie regionale des animaux domestiques. Vol. II, J.C. Bailliere et fils, Paris.

Motomura, Y., Yugi, H., Kamimura, S. and Hamana, K. (1994). J. Japan Vety. Med. Assoc., 47(6): 387-389.

Nickerson, S.C. (1994). Dairy Research Report., Hill Farm Research Station, Lousiana State University :274.

Pathak, A. (2003). In compendium of IAAVR round table Conf. on mastitis., 14-15 April, 2003. Palampur (H.P.), India. Pp. 74-78.

Reiderer (1903). Arch. Wiss. Prakt. Tierheilk. 29:593-625.

Sharma, Neelesh, Maiti, S.K., Mukherjee, K., Ghose, R.C. and Roy, S. (2005). 82(6): 103-104.

Singh, M. and Varshney, A.C. (1999). Himachal Vet. J., 3:64-66.

Sisson, S., Grossman, J.D. and Robert, G. (1975). The anatomy of the domestic animals. 5th ed., W. B. Saunders Company, Philadelphia.

St. Clair, L.E. (1940). The nerve supply to the bovine mammary gland. M.S. thesis, Iowa State College Library, Ames, Iowa.

Swett. W.W. (1924). J. Agric. Res., 65:19.

Tomar, M.S. and Tomar, S.P.S. (1960). Indian J. Dairy Sci., 26(1): 25.

Turner, C.W. (1981). In Harvesting Young Milk Crop. Babson Bros., Dairy Research and Educational Services, Oak Brook, II, USA.

Zwart, S.G. (1911). Beitrage zur Anatomie und Physiologie der Milchdrüse des Rindes. Inaugural Dissertation, Bern.

□□□

CHAPTER

5

Physiology of Synthesis and Secretion of Milk

As an introduction to the study of bovine mastitis, it is important to understand the physiology of the synthesis and secretion of milk and normal growth of the udder, the hormones regulating the initiation and maintenance of milk secretion, and the reactions occurring at the time of milk removal. Complete removal of milk is very important in the control of mastitis (Schalm and Mead, 1943). The mammary glands of the dairy cows are the largest glands of the body. There are an integral part of the reproductive system and designed to secret the milk to furnish nutrition to the new born calf. *Milk* is the normal product of mammary gland secretion. Milk is a complex, nutritious product that contains more than 100 substances that are either solution, suspension or emulsion in water. Milk provides energy in the form of lactose and fat, and amino acids in the form of protein. It is also a source of antibodies, vitamins, and minerals.

During the first-half to two-thirds of pregnancy, the secretory tissue of the cow's udder develops. The alveoli are the functional unit of the udder for the synthesis and secretion of milk. The functions of the alveoli are to remove nutrients from the blood and transform these nutrients into milk and, finally discharge the milk into the lumen. Following the formation of the cells lining the alveoli, they gradually enlarge with secretory products and eventually fill the lumen of the alveoli and the connecting ducts with secretion. This secretion is called *"colostrum"*. The alveolar epithelial cells, surrounded by a cell membrane, contain the machinery or organelles necessary to convert precursors absorbed from the blood into milk constituents. The *lactation* is the combined process of milk synthesis, secretion and its removal (milk ejection) from the mammary gland. Lactation completes in two processes- 1) milk secretion and, 2) milk ejection.

Milk secretion

Synthesis of milk by alveolar epithelial cells and its passage through the duct system is called *milk secretion*. The milk secretion involves both intracellular synthesis of milk and subsequent passage of milk from the cytoplasm of the epithelial cells into the alveolar lumen. This process has two phases-:

A) Lactogenesis (initiation of milk secretion)
B) Galactopoesis (maintenance of milk secretion).

A) Lactogenesis

Lactogenesis is a process of differentiation whereby the mammary alveolar cells acquire the ability to secrete milk. During pregnancy particularly in later months, more quantity of prolactin is secreted. But the activity of this hormone is suppressed by estrogen and progesterone secreted by placenta and lactation is prevented during pregnancy. Progesterone also decreases the ability of prolactin to induce secretion of α-lactalbumin, an enzyme moiety of lactose synthetase. Moreover, progesterone significantly reduces the synergism between estrogen and prolactin. Immediately after the delivery of calf and expulsion of placenta, there is sudden loss of estrogen and progesterone. Now the prolactin is free to exert its action on mammae and to promote lactogenesis.

B) Galactopoiesis

Galactopoiesis is the maintenance of lactation, once lactation has been established. Maintenance of lactation requires maintenance of alveolar cell numbers, synthetic activity per cell, and efficacy of the milk-ejection reflex. Two key interrelated components contribute to the maintenance of lactation like *galactopoietic hormones* and *removal of accumulated milk.* Any substance that is administered to a lactating animal and that results in increased milk production considered as *galactogogue*. Milk yield is dependent of the amount of secretory tissue and the rate of secretion (per unit of time). Secretion rate is affected by the accumulation of milk in the alveolar lumen. Secretion rate is affected by the accumulation of milk in the lumen increases the intra-mammary pressure. Once the intra-mammary pressure reaches a certain level, secretion rate declines. If the pressure increases enough (~70mm Hg), then the secretion stops and milk starts to be reabsorbed. In the dairy cow secretion rate reaches zero at about 35 hours after the last milking.

The interior of the cell is composed of cytoplasm in which organelles such as the nucleus, ribosome, lysosome rough endoplasmic reticulum, smooth endoplasmic reticulum, mitochondria and Golgi apparatus are dispersed. The initiation of secretory activity on the part of the udder epithelial cells in late pregnancy and post partum is due to the pituitary hormone called "prolactin". The galactopoietic hormones include prolactin, growth hormone, thyroid hormone and glucocorticoids, which are essential for continuous supply of milk precursors like glucose, amino acids, minerals and other substances which are essential for the production of milk.

It is well known that just before calving, estrogen, now produced by the placental membranes, increases in its rate of secretion and physiologically overrides the progesterone produced by corpus luteum. Estrogen causes an increase in uterine motility and acts upon the placental circulation, thus precipitating parturition. Estrogen also acts upon the pituitary, stimulating an increased secretion of prolactin, which in turn stimulates the milk secretion. Thus, at the time of parturition, when the calf becomes separated from its placental connections the secretion of milk is stimulated intensely by the rising secretion of the lactogenic hormone (Hurst and Tunner, 1942). While the presence of estrogen in increasing amounts just before parturition initiates the intense secretion of prolactin hormone, it is the stimulus of milking and the removal of milk that maintain the lactation process. It has been shown that, each time the teats are stimulated by milking, the lactogenic hormone accumulating in the pituitary during the interval between milking is gradually discharged into the blood stream and stimulates the secretion of milk during the interval between milking (Reece and Turner, 1937). Thus regular milking is necessary for the maintenance of the secretion of the prolactin (lactogenic hormone), which in turn is partly responsible for maintenance of milk secretion. The amount of prolactin secreted by the pituitary of the individual cow and the maintenance of the secretion rate during the progress of the lactation period undoubtedly play an important role in stimulating the cells of the udder to maximum milk secretion and persistency.

Role of prolactin in milk secretion

Prolactin is a polypeptide hormone which is secreted by the *mammotropes cells* of the anterior pituitary (adenohypophysis). The role of prolactin hormone is well established in maintenance of lactation (Tucker, 1994). The role of prolactin in cows is ambiguous. Prolactin is released at the time of milk removal, and it remains a key systemic modulator of milk secretion during lactation. Prolactin is considered the major galactopoietic hormone in ruminants. Inhibition of prolactin secretion or administration of prolactin to lactating cows has little effect on milk yields (Karg and Schalms, 1974; Plaut *et al.*, 1987). An inhibiting hormone termed *prolactin inhibiting factor (PIF)* regulates secretion of prolactin. PIF is probably the catecholamine, dopamine, that is an amine of low molecular weight synthesized from L-tyrosine. It is secreted from nerve terminals mostly in the arcuate nucleus located in the median eminence and transported through the hypophyseal portal system to the adenohypophysis.

Role of thyroid hormone in milk secretion

The lactogenic hormone is the only factor that will cause the cells of the udder to begin to secrete milk, but there are some other hormones that will increase established lactation. The most important of these hormones *thyroxin*, which is secreted by the thyroid gland. If the thyroid gland is removed from a milking cow, the milk yield may decline as much as 30 to 40%. On the other hand, if desiccated thyroid tissue is fed or if the pure thyroxin is injected into dairy cattle resulting increase in milk yield. The content of the milk is markedly increased as well (Herman *et al.*, 1938; Ralston *et al.*, 1940). The feeding of thyroprotein causes an increased need for nutrients, a loss of body weight, and increased heart rate, respiration rate and body temperature. Injection of thyroid hormone into dairy cows increases milk production for a short period of time (several weeks). Administration of thyroid hormone for more than 7 weeks have no effect on milk yield. Thyroprotein (iodinated casein) is a commercial product that increases milk yield in cows by about 10% in early lactation (first 100 days) and by 15-20% in whole lactation. It is to be expected that thyroprotein feeding will be particularly effective in cows tending to be slightly hypothyroid, in cows of advanced age in which the rate of thyroxin secretion tend to fall off, and during the summer months when the high environmental temperature normally depresses the thyroid. However, the positive effect only lasts for 2-4 months and subsequent yield is below normal. Therefore, generally there is no benefit in feeding thyroprotein over the entire lactation. Thyroid hormone influence milk synthesis as well as the intensity and duration of milk secretion. The thyroid hormones stimulate protein synthesis and milk yield (Nickerson, 1994).

It is not entirely clear that how thyroxin influences the rate of milk secretion. It is known that it increases the appetite of animals and aids in the absorption of food nutrients, particularly carbohydrates, from the digestive tract. Thus the feed consumption may be increased. Thyroxin also increases the rate of energy metabolism in proportion to the amount administered. The heart rate may increased by thyroxin and thus cause more blood to flow through the udder. As milk secretion is dependent upon the availability of precursors in the blood, the increased blood flow and the increased uptake of the various constituents of the blood by the more active cells of the udder may be responsible in part for the action of the thyroid hormone. The cows having an inheritance for high milk and fat production probably have also an inheritance for the secretion of optimum amounts of thyroxin.

Role of growth hormone in the milk secretion

Growth hormone (GH) is generally considered to be the predominant galactopoietic hormone in ruminants (Bauman, 1992). It has been known for many years that growth hormone has a dose dependent effect on stimulation of milk yield in dairy cows. Growth hormone does not produce its effects by direct stimulation of the mammary gland in bovines. It appears to exert its galactopoietic effect by change in body tissues and physiological processes that support increase in synthesis of lactose, protein and fat in mammary gland. Sakamoto *et al.* (2005) have been reported that GH acts on bovine mammary epithelial cells and indices the expression of both a-casein gene and protein because its receptors are present on the membrane as well as in the cytoplasm of bovine mammary epithelial cells. The bovine growth hormone is now commercially produced and available bovine somatotropin (bST). By the use of bST, 10 to 40% increase in milk yield has been reported. It increases the blood flow to the mammary gland which ultimately improves the efficiency of milk production (Singh *et al.*, 2007). Although bST has been banned in Europe. It is found that if the cows keep on bST for long duration (for two lactations) and after that those cows are mostly culled because of numerous problems (low milk production, low fertility, hoof problems, metabolic problems etc. Sometimes culling rate in bST herds are over 35-40% per year.

Role of other hormones in milk secretion

It has been demonstrated that the anterior pituitary secretes several hormones that may directly or indirectly influence the rate of milk secretion. It has been found that the use of crude pituitary extract stimulate a greater increase in milk yield than the equivalent amount of the lactogenic hormone. This can be explained most convincingly by the assumption of lactation stimulating action of other pituitary hormones (Table 5.1).

Adrenocorticotropic hormone (ACTH) plays a direct role in maintaining lactation by exerting its effects on maintenance of mammary cell numbers and metabolic activity. Cortisol is the prominent endogenous glucocorticoid in cattle whose major function at the mammary gland is to cause differentiation of the lobule-alveolar system (Tucker, 2000). *Oxytocin* is required for milk removal; where as several other hormones are essential for maintenance of intense milk synthesis and secretion. The administration of estrogen in very low doses is galactopoietic. However, higher doses have inhibitory effects. Estrogen initiates the lactation in the periparturient period. It acts in atleast two ways to initiate lactation: 1) it caused release of prolactin from the anterior pituitary gland into blood, which in turn, would initiate lactation; and 2) estrogen increased the number of prolactin receptors in mammary cells. A combination of estrogen and progesterone is more inhibitory than estrogen alone. Progesterone alone has no effect on galactopoiesis because there are no progesterone receptors in the mammary gland during lactation.

Table 5.1: Major hormones affecting mammary gland function.

Endocrine gland	Hormone secreted	Major function associated with mammary gland
Anterior pituitary	Follicle-stimulating hormone (FSH)	Estrogen secretion from ovarian follicles
	Luteinizing hormone (LH)	Progesteron secretion from corpus luteum
	Prolactin (PRL)	Mammary growth, initiation and maintenance of lactation.
	Growth hormone (GH)	Stimulates milk secretion
	Thyroid-stimulating hormone (TSH)	Stimulates thyroid gland to secrete thyroxin, triiodothyronin
	Adrenocorticotropic hormone (ACTH)	Stimulates adrenal gland to secrete glucocorticoids
Posterior pituitary	Oxytocin	Milk ejection
Hypothalamus		
	Growth hormone-releasing hormone	Stimulates GH release
	Somatostatin	Inhibit GH release
	Prolactin-inhibiting factor	Inhibits prolactin release
Thyroid	Thyroxin; triiodothyronine	Stimulates oxygen consumption, protein synthesis, and milk yield.
	Thyrocalcitonin	Calcium and phosphorus metabolism
Parathyroid	Parathyroid hormone	Calcium and phosphorus metabolism
Pancreas	Insulin	Glucose metabolism
Adrenal cortex	Glucocorticoids	Initiation and maintenance of lactation.
	Mineralocorticoids	Electrolyte and mineral metabolism
Adrenal medulla	Epinephrine and norepinephrine	Inihibition of milk ejection
Ovary	Estrdiol/estrogen	Mammary duct growth
	Progesteron	Mammary lobule-alveolar growth; inhibition of lactogenesis
Placenta	Estrdiol/estrogen	See ovary
	Progesteron	See ovary
	Placental lactogen	Mammary growth

Adopted from Tucker (1985). In Larsen, ed., Lactation, Iowa University Press, Ames, Iowa.

There is a critical role of some *local mammary factors* in maintenance of milk secretion. One such factor that plays a major role in regulating milk secretion is a *feedback inhibitor of lactation (FIL)* found in milk (Wilde *et al.*, 1995). FIL is thought to be produced by the mammary cells as they synthesize and secrete milk. A milk whey protein has been identified as FIL. Accumulation of FIL in the milk producing alveoli results in feed back inhibition of milk synthesis and secretion. Frequent removal of milk from the gland minimizes local inhibitory effects of FIL and increases milk secretion (Wilde *et al.*, 1987; Wilde and Knight, 1989; Wilde and Peaker, 1990).

Synthesis of milk

Anatomical study of the mammary gland in full lactation shows that the milk is secreted, by the epithelial cells lining the alveoli from the blood brought up by the blood stream. Some constituents of milk are present in the blood and are merely transferred to the milk (Fig 5.1). Other constituents of milk are not present in the blood and therefore must be built up, or synthesized from other constituents of the blood. For many years it was thought that about one-half of the milk present in the udder at milking time was formed in the udder during the interval between milking and the other half during the process of milking. It is now generally agreed that all the milk obtained at milking time is present preformed in the cows udder. Within the cells of mammary glands, the cycle of milk secretion includes, first a period of synthesis during which milk is formed within the cells, followed by the discharge of the milk into the cavity of the alveolus.

McManaman and Neville (2003) states that a lactating mammary gland is composed of a branching network of ducts formed of epithelial cells ending in extensive lobulo-alveolar clusters which are the sites of milk secretion. Linzell and Peaker (1971), there is only one type of secretory cell in the mammary gland. The cytoplasm of lactating mammary secretory epithelial cell is filled with a spherical nucleus, free ribosomes, rough endoplasmic reticulum (RER), mitochondria, Golgi apparatus and products of synthesis fat globules and protein granules (Figure 5.2) (McManaman and Neville, 2003). Synthesis of nucleic acid code and mRNA and rRNA occurs in the nucleus. The endoplasmic reticulum is the site of protein synthesis, esterification of fatty acids to glycerol to form triglycerides, phospholipids synthesis, and fatty acids desaturation. The mitochondrion is the production site of ATP, nonessential amino acid precursors, and fatty acid precursors. The Golgi apparatus is the site where lactose synthesis, glycoprotein synthesis, casein phosphorylation, and packaging of water occur. The secretory cells are connected to each other through an *apical junction complex* composed of adherens, and tight junctional elements that function to inhibit direct paracellular exchange of substances between vascular and milk compartments during lactation. *Tight junctions,* as described by Nguyen and Neville (1998), form a narrow, continuous seal that surrounds each endothelial and epithelial cell at the apical border, and act to regulate the movement of material between the cells. During lactation, the tight junctions of the alveolar epithelial cells are impermeable, allowing milk to be stored between milking periods while restricting the leakage of milk components from the lumen or leakage of interstitial fluid components into the milk.

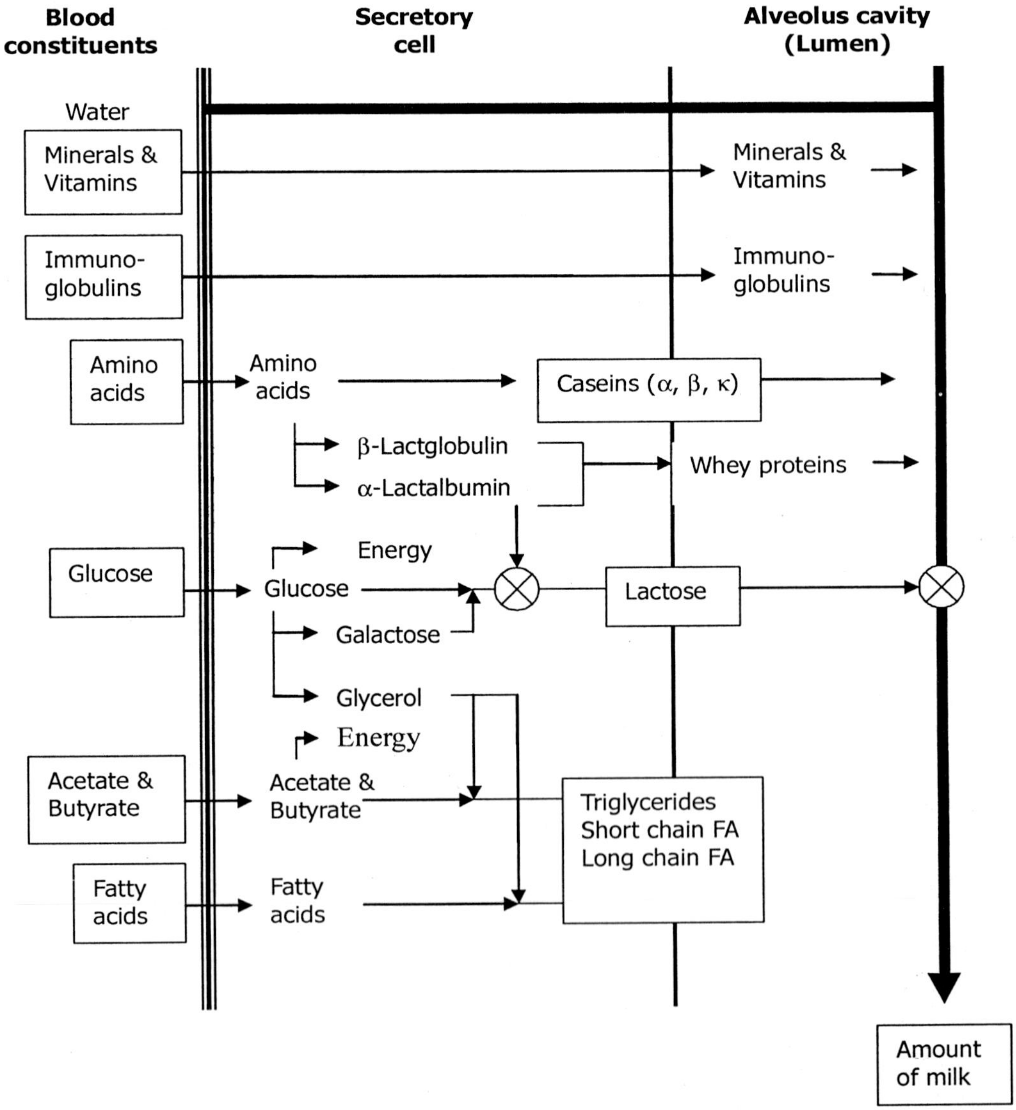

Figure 5.1: Overview of synthesis of milk constituents from respective precursors in the alveolar secretory cell (cross circles indicate key regulatory steps).

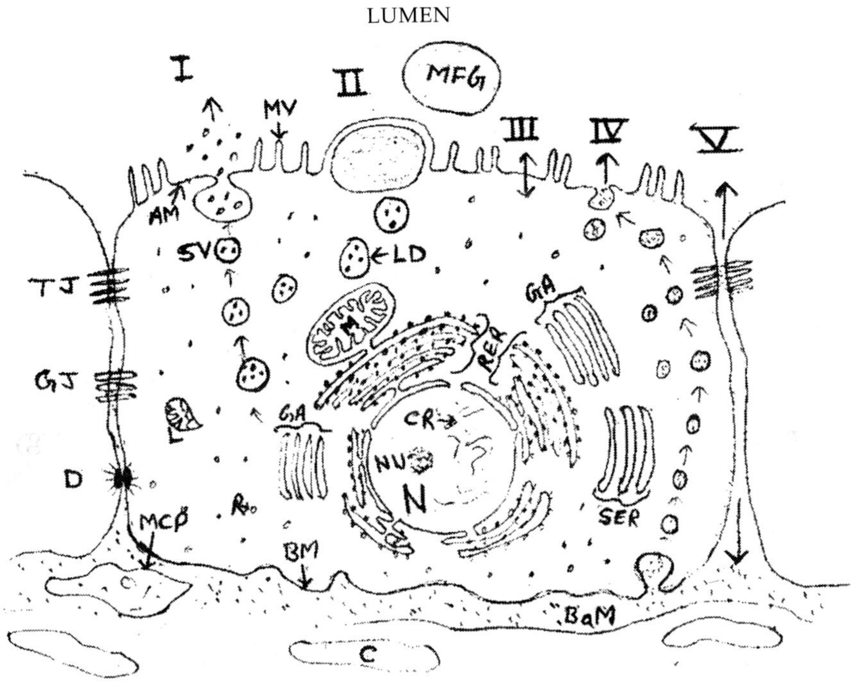

Figure 5.2. Diagram of secretory alveolar cell from lactating mammary gland.

MFG- Milk fat globule, MV-Microvillus, AM- Apical plasma membrane, SV- Secretory vesicle, LD- Lipid droplet, M-Mitochondria, RER- Rough endoplasmic reticulum, GA-Golgi apparatus, SER- Smooth endoplasmic reticulum, L- Lysosome, R- Ribosome, BM- basal plasma membrane, BaM- Basement membrane, MCP- Myoepithelial cell process, C-Capillary, N- Nucleus, NU- Nucleolus, CR- Chromosomes, TJ- Tight junction, GJ- Gape junction, D- Desmosome.

Secretory pathways- I (Exocytosis), II (Milk fat), III (Apical transport), IV (Transcytosis) and V (Paracellular pathway).

The Precursors of Milk

Although the site of milk synthesis is the tiny epithelial cells lining the alveoli, some milk components (e.g. vitamins, minerals, certain proteins) are not synthesized here. They are simply filtered out from the blood through the cells into the milk. Lactose, fat and proteins (mainly casein) are formed in the epithelial cells from substrates carried in the blood. Each epithelial cell is believed to do a complete milk producing job. That is, each secretory epithelial cell secretes the lactose, casein, fat and other complex constituents of milk together instead of there being groups of cells specialized in protein secretion, fat secretion, or carbohydrate secretion. Some milk constituents come preformed from the blood such as minerals, certain hormones and several proteins including some of the immunoglobulins passed unchanged into milk

(Figure 5.1). However, whether the individual constituents of milk come preformed from the blood or are synthesized into unique milk constituents from other constituents of the blood, the cells play a dynamic role in selecting from the blood plasma the amount required for the milk produced. The substrates are filtered from the blood and pass into each epithelial cell through the basal membrane is injured by some means as by the toxic products of pathologic organisms (e.g. mastitis), changed physiological conditions, or the introduction of foreign compounds or solutions. Then their ability selectively to absorb the precursors of the various constituents of milk from the blood is break down or altered, resulting abnormal milk may be produced. Some precursors of milk components are produced in the rumen and then reach the blood circulation. Digestion of fiber in the rumen produces the volatile fatty acids (VFAs), acetate and butyrate. Butyrate produces energy for the rumen wall, and much of it is converted to b-hydroxybutyrate in the rumen wall tissue. About half of the fat in milk is synthesized in the udder from acetate and b-hydroxybutyrate. The other half of milk fat is transported from the pool of fatty acids circulating in the blood. These can originate from body fat mobilization, absorption from the diet, or from fats metabolized in the liver.

Rumen microbes convert dietary protein into microbial protein, which is a primary source of essential amino acids for the cow. These amino acids are used by the mammary gland to synthesize milk proteins. Glucose is required to provide energy to support this protein synthesis. Glucose is either formed from the propionate in the liver, or absorbed directly from the small intestine. If too little propionate is absorbed from the rumen, the cow will have to break down amino acids and convert them to glucose (gluconeogenesis), this can reduce the supply of amino acids available to make milk protein.

Since the secretion of milk is dependent upon the passage through the udder of huge supplies of blood. It has been estimated that 400 to 500 liters of blood must pass through the cows udder to produce 1 liter of milk. It has been observed that it requires about 52 seconds for the blood to make a complete circuit from the udder to the heart and return through the udder in cows with an average pulse rate of 63 beats per minute. This is evidence indicating that the differences in the milk secreting ability of cows is more largely due to the differences in the total volume of blood passing through the cows udder than to differences in the rate of uptake of the precursors of milk from the blood. In fact, with increasing volume of blood flow, the uptake of milk precursors per unit of blood might decline, yet the total milk yield increases. The plasma like fluid that bathes the secreting cells of the udder contains many compounds. The amount of these compounds may vary to some extent due to the amount and quality of the feed supply, the rate and efficiency of absorption from the digestive tract, and the hormones that influence their metabolism and storage.

These blood constituents are in part transformed into new milk constituents by the cells enzyme systems. When a cell becomes filled with the newly secreted milk, it is ready to discharge the contents into the hollow central cavity of the alveolus called the ***"lumen"***. Many cycles of synthesis and secretion, then discharge of the preformed milk go on each cell during the interval between milkings.

Biosynthesis of various constituents of milk

Lactose

Lactose or milk sugar, is a disaccharide found exclusively in milk and formed by the union of two simple sugars, ***glucose*** and ***galactose***. The concentration of lactose in the milk is relatively constant and averages about 5% (4.8 to 5.2%). The molecules from which lactose is made are found in much lower concentrations in milk- glucose (14mg/100g) and galactose (12mg/100g). Much study has been devoted to the determination of the precursors of lactose. Each time the blood flows through the udder, almost 20% of the glucose is taken up (Blackwood and Stirling, 1932). However, some of the glucose taken up by the cells of the udder may be used as a source of energy for the formation of milk. This has been estimated as about 10% of the energy content of the milk. Although glucose in the diet is entirely fermented in the rumen in volatile fatty acids (acetic, propionic and butyric acids), it is needed in large amounts by the lactating udder. The liver transforms propionic acid back into glucose which is transported by the blood to the udder where it is taken up by the secretory cells. Glucose plays a central role in the metabolism of the mammary gland. Glucose can be used in one of three ways- 1) conversion to the galactose moiety of lactose, 2) formation of triose phosphate via the glycolytic pathway, and 3) conversion of 6-phosphogluconate via the pentose phosphate pathway. These pathways generate immediate precursors and co-factors for the synthesis of milk components. Enzymes for lactose synthesis are located in the Golgi apparatus. The a-lactalbumin moiety is glycosylated in transit through Golgi components where it combines with membrane bound galactosyltransferase to produce functional lactose.

The synthesis of lactose is controlled by a two-unit enzyme called lactose synthetase and the sub unit a-lactalbumin is found in the milk as a whey protein. In addition to *blood glucose*, there are several other blood constituents that may be used in part by the cells to form lactose. The *lactic acid*, a break down product of glucose, is taken up by the udder and may be used as lactose precursor (Graham, 1937). Another blood constituent is *glycoprotein*.

Glycoprotein consists of a sugar bound to a protein. This compound is taken up by the udder and may serve as a source both of protein and of sugar by the secreting cells. A fourth source of lactose is a rather unexpected one that is *amino acids*. When amino acids, the building blocks of the proteins, are themselves broken down, many form a carbohydrate fragment. The break down of amino acids normally occurs in the liver with the production of sugar and urea as a waste product. It has been discovered that urea is also formed in the udder and is discharged back into the blood. This report indicates that amino acids are being broken down by the udder cells to form an additional source of carbohydrates, with the elimination of urea as a by product. On the basis of blood glucose alone, there is a concentration of 80 times in the form of lactose in the milk. This indicates that glucose is very permeable to the secreting cells; yet only small amount pass through into milk unchanged.

Because lactose is the major osmotically active milk constituent, alteration of lactose synthesis has a marked influence on milk yield. Lactose secretion into the cavity of an alveolus increases the concentration of dissolved substances (osmotic pressure) relative to the other side of the secretory cells where the blood flows. As a result, the concentration of dissolved substances on each side of the secretory cells is balanced by drawing water from the blood and mixing with the other milk components found in the cavity of the alveolus. For normal milk, a balance is reached when there is 4.5 to 5% lactose in milk. Thus lactose production acts as a *"valve"* that regulates the amount of water drawn into the alveoli and therefore the volume of milk produced. Secretory vesicles that carry casein are the main vehicles for lactose transport into milk.

When the quarter becomes infected with mastitis causing organisms, the secretion of lactose is reduced. The pH of the normal milk is ranged from 6.45 to 6.7, and mastitis milk tend to be more alkaline, approaching the pH of blood (7.4) or >7.4. In a few cases of mastitis a very acid type of milk has been observed, but this may be owing to the presence of sugar fermenting organisms in the milk, which alter the milk after it is secreted.

Protein

The chief milk proteins are the caseins (α, β and k-casein) upto 80% of the total milk and 20% whey proteins (α-lactalbumin, β-lactglobulin and immunoglobulins). Lactoferrin and lysosomal enzymes are quantitatively important proteins in milk. Immunoglobulins and blood serum albumin enter the mammary cell as preformed proteins from the blood. The immunoglobulins are synthesized by the immune system, and these usually large proteins are drawn from the blood into the milk. IgG immunoglobulins are serum derived whereas IgA and IgM are synthesized in udder and pass into milk through mammary epithelium with IgG. The permeability of the secretory cells to immunoglobulins is high during the synthesis of colostrum, but decreases sharply with the onset of lactation. The concentration of protein varies with the breed of the cow and proportion to the amount of fat in the milk. There is a close relationship between the amount of fat and the amount of protein in milk- the higher the fat, and higher the protein. It is formerly considered that each animal protein is built up completely from the amino acids of the blood. It is generally accepted that amino acid nitrogen is the precursor of milk protein. It has been reported that the total uptake of amino acids is not sufficient to account for more than half the protein of milk. The availability of amino acids for protein synthesis is further reduced because some amino acids are broken down in the udder with the production of urea. Another blood protein that has been shown to be taken up by the active mammary gland is *glycoprotein*. The glycoprotein is believed to be composed of three sugars- mannose, galactose and glucosamine bound to globulin. The uptake of this compound would provide the udder with both sugar and protein. Several non protein nitrogen constituents of the blood have been investigated as sources of milk protein. Urea has been shown actually to pass from the active udder rather than to be taken up.

The casein is synthesized in alveolar epithelial cells from free amino acids absorbed from the blood stream. The site of casein synthesis is the *rough endoplasmic reticulum (RER)*, from where it is transported to the Golgi apparatus and eventually into the collecting spaces of lactating tissue. The mechanism of protein synthesis in the mammary gland appears to be comparable to those found in most other protein synthesizing cells of the body. Milk protein synthesis is controlled by hormonal regulation of gene transcription, the stability of mRNA and the rate of mRNA translation. In the presence of DNA-dependent RNA polymerase and appropriate nucleotide precursors, DNA is transcribed to mRNA. The mRNA carries the encoded message from the nucleus to the cytoplasmic ribosomes located on RER. Synthesis takes about 3 to 15 minutes. Individual casein proteins begin to aggregate into rudimentary casein micelles during packaging in secretory vesicles. Casein laden secretory vesicles originating from Golgi apparatus then proceed through the apical cytoplasm, fuse with the luminal plasma membrane, and release their contents. Changes in the relative amounts of the milk proteins are produced during the mastitis. Casein secretion is gradually reduced and, true lactalbumin as well.

Fat

Milk fat plays a central role in dairy products and farm efficiency. Fat is a major contributor to the energy density of whole milk and is essential to many of the physical properties, manufacturing qualities and organoleptic characteristics of dairy products. Fat is the most variable component of milk and is affected by many factors including genetics, physiological state and environment. Synthesis of milk fat requires the coordination of multiple biochemical processes and cellular events in the mammary epithelial cell (Figure 5.3). Milk fat consists mainly of triglycerides, which are synthesized from glyceroles and fatty acids. Ruminant milk fat is estimated to include over 400 individual fatty acids that differ primarily in chain length and number and orientation of unsaturated bonds (Jensen, 2002). Over 95% by mass of the fatty acid are esterified in triglycerides while the remaining are found in phospholipid, cholesterol ester, diglyceride, monoglyceride and free fatty acid fractions (Harvatine *et al.*, 2009). Long chain fatty acids are absorbed from the blood. The short chain fatty acids (C_4 – C_{12}) are synthesized in the udder epithelial cells since bovine blood is free of these fatty acids. The fatty acids, glycerol and other related intermediates are synthesized in the cytosol and

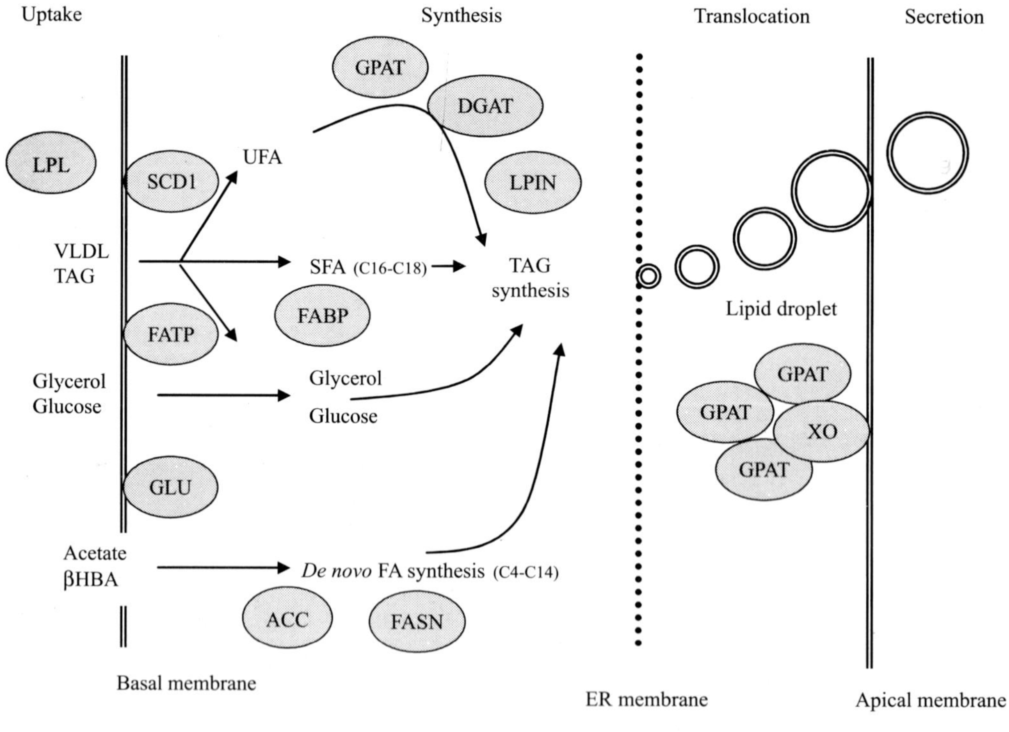

Figure 5.3 : Diagram representing activities and pathways coordinated during the synthesis and secretion of milk fat. Key proteins are shown in ovals: lipoprotein lipase (LPL); stearoyl-CoA desaturase (SCD); fatty acid transport proteins (FATP); glucose transporters (GLUT); glycerol phosphate acyltransferase (GPAT); diacylglycerol acyltransferase (DGAT); lipin (LPIN); fatty acid binding proteins (FABP); acetyl-CoA carboxylase (ACC); fatty acid synthase (FASN); mucin 1 (MUC1); butyrophilin (BTN1A1); xanthine oxidoreductase (XO) and adipophilin (ADPH). FA5fatty acid; UFA5unsaturated fatty acid; SFA5saturated fatty acid; VLDL5very low-density lipoprotein; TAG5triacylglycerol and bHBA5b-hydroxybutyrate. Adapted from McGuire and Bauman (2002).

biosynthesis of triglycerols takes place in or near the endoplasmic reticulum of the mammary epithelial cells. Undoubtedly, the natural fat and free fatty acids of the blood are the chief source of milk fat. Adipose tissue mobilization accounts for less than 10% of preformed fatty acids in milk fat, except during periods of negative energy balance when their proportion increases substantially. The fat is broken down into fatty acids and glycerine, and then reconstituted into the fats of varying carbon chain length characteristic milk fat. The milk fat is mainly contains long chain fatty acids and short chain fatty acids.

The long chain fatty acids are the either dietary or rumen microbial origin and are mainly palmitic (C_{16}) and, stearic, oleic and linoleic (C_{18}) acids. More than half of the fatty acids in cows milk are derived directly from the blood. The long chain fatty acids are not synthesized in the secretory cell of the udder. However, since the short chain fatty acids are not present in the blood, they must be formed by the secretory epithelial cells of the udder by one or more sources of precursors like-1) by the acetate and β-hydroxybutyric acid transported from the rumen. In cows, ketone bodies enter the blood as a result of rumen digestion and from the metabolism of fat. Acetate, via the melonyl Co-A pathway, contributes to all short chain (C_4- C_{14}) fatty acids, 2) by the break down of long chain fatty acids and, 3) by carbohydrates. The animal body can convert carbohydrates (blood glucose) into fat. This evidence that, dairy cows fed a low fat diet actually secretes more milk fat than they are fed. It has long been recognized that the liver is the site of conversion of excess sugar or glycogen into depot fat. Milk fat contains predominantly short chain fatty acids built from acetates derived from fermentation in the rumen. This is a unique feature of milk fat compared with other kinds of animal and plant fats.

After lipid synthesis is initiated, droplets are transported to the apical cytoplasm. The most widely accepted mechanism of lipid secretion from the mammary cell is progressive envelopment of the protruding droplet by the apical plasma membrane and release into the alveolar lumen (Nickerson, 1994). Lastly, due to the hydrophobic nature of esterified FA, milk fat is secreted from the mammary epithelial cell as a lipid droplet surrounded by a protein-rich polar lipid coat called the *"milk fat globule membrane"* (MFGM). Milk fat droplets also contain compounds such as phospholipids, sterols, carotenoids, and fat soluble vitamins. Lecithin is also considered to be an important precursor of milk fat. Lipids mobilized from body reserves in early lactation are another building block for milk fat synthesis.

Minerals and Vitamins

Although minerals in the milk are derived from the blood, it is not known conclusively whether they are absorbed in proportion to their concentration in blood or whether there are mechanism that allow selective uptake. It is probable that the passage of water and dissolved substances through the arterial capillary membrane to the secreting cells is due to the hydrostatic pressure of the blood. Arterial capillary pressure is about 32 mm. The hydrostatic pressure of the arterial capillary is the force causing the passage of water and milk precursors to the cells is indicated by the fact that milk secretion continues until an intraudder or milk pressure of about 30 mm is reached. The osmotic equilibrium of blood and milk is of great importance in regulating the composition of milk. The living normal milk secreting cell membrane selectively permits the passage of some constituents from the blood into milk more readily than others. When the cell membrane is injured as in mastitis, then its selectivity is injured and constituents of the blood pass through it more nearly in proportion to their presence in the blood. The unique constituents of milk (those secreted by the secretory epithelial cell) become reduce, and the milk more nearly approaches the composition of blood. The osmotic equilibrium of blood and milk provides a mechanism for the concentration of some constituents in greater amount in milk than in blood. Thus the glucose molecule in blood exerts twice as much osmotic pressure as does the lactose molecule in milk following its synthesis in the cell. Further, in the case of many inorganic constituents, following their passage into the secreting cell they are transformed into osmotically inactive compounds by their combination with protein or precipitation from solution. Milk is an excellent source of most of minerals required for the growth of the young (e.g. calcium, phosphorus and magnesium). Minerals contribute to the buffering capacity of milk, the maintenance of milk pH, the ionic strength of milk, and milk's osmotic pressure. The blood *calcium* is present in two forms. About two-third is soluble or diffusible and contributes to the osmotic pressure of the blood, and the remainder is firmly bound to the blood proteins. The Ca is 15 times more concentrated or higher in milk than in the blood. The blood inorganic *phosphorus* is combined as the phosphoric acid radical of Ca, Mg, Na and K. In milk these same compounds are present, but in addition new combinations are formed (e.g. phosphoprotein).

Much of the osmotic activity of blood serum is due to the presence of *sodium chloride*. However, the normal milk secreting cell has the ability of preventing this highly soluble ionizable compound from blood into the milk. *Iodine* is the only mineral constituent of the feed that when fed in increased amounts will cause an increased amount to be present in the blood and to pass in increased amounts into milk. Another mineral of interest in the milk is *iron*. The low iron concentration milk cannot meet the needs of the calf, but this low level turn out to have a positive aspect because it limits bacterial growth in milk (bactericidal)- iron is essential for the growth of many bacteria. Most of the *Vitamins* cannot be synthesized by the mammary gland, so vitamins present in milk come preformed from the blood. Milk contains considerable amounts of vitamin A, very small amounts of vitamin C and D, and traces of vitamins E and K. Milk is also a good source of all vitamins B.

Mechanism of secretion of milk constituents

There are five major pathways (Figure 5.2) utilized by the secretory mammary epithelium in the milk constituents secretion across the mammary secretory epithelium from the blood into the milk. These pathways operate in parallel to transform precursors derived from the blood or interstitial fluid into milk constituents. Four of these pathways are transcellular: I) Exocytosis or Golgi pathway, II) milk fat pathway, III) transmembrane pathway, and IV) transcytosis. The fifth is paracellular pathway that allows direct exchange of interstitial and milk components (Shennan and Peaker, 2000). The transport through these pathways is affected by the functional state of mammary gland and regulated by direct and indirect actions of hormones and growth factors (McManaman and Neville, 2003).

I) Exocytosis or Golgi pathway

Most of the components or secretory products of the aqueous phase of milk are transported to or sequestered by the Golgi apparatus and secreted into the lumen of the alveolus by exocytosis (Figure 5.2). The aqueous solutes including the major milk proteins, oligosaccharides (lactose), citrate, phosphate and calcium. Proteins synthesized on ribosomes are transferred to the lumen of the rough endoplasmic reticulum. From there it is transported to the Golgi apparatus where they are further processed by the addition of carbohydrate, phosphate or other groups and packaged into secretory vesicles. Secretory vesicles are thought to be the source of most of the constituents of the aqueous phase of the milk including citrate, nucleotides, calcium, phosphate and probably monovalent ions and glucose, and concentration of these substances may be adjusted by direct membrane transport. Secretory vesicles containing essentially non fat constituents, travel toward the apical surface of the mammary epithelial cell and fuse with the plasma membrane, where the vesicular contents are discharged into the lumen.

II) Milk fat pathway

The milk fat pathway is unique in the mammary secretory cells. Triglycerides, synthesized in the smooth endoplasmic reticulum of the mammary alveolar cells from precursor fatty acids and glycerol, coalesce into large droplets that are drawn to the apex of the cell (Figure 5.2). The fat droplets bulge against and gradually become enveloped in apical plasma membrane, finally separating from the cell as the milk fat globule and discharged into alveolar lumen.

III) Transmembrane pathway

In contrast to the other pathways for milk secretion, the pathways for the direct transport of substances across the apical membrane of the mammary alveolar cell are poorly understood. The sodium, potassium, chloride and certain monosaccharides as well as water directly permitted this membrane (Linzell and Peaker, 1971), but calcium, phosphate and citrate did not (Neville and Peaker, 1981). Linzell and Peaker (1975) states that chloride-bicarbonate exchange takes place at the apical membrane. The function of apical pathways is not clear, however, apical pathways are limited to a modest number of small molecules. Many drugs enter milk by direct transfer across both basolateral and apical membranes of the mammary alveolar cell. For this reason most therapeutic drugs are transferred efficiently into milk (Fleishaker and Mc Namara, 1988).

IV) Transcytosis

Intact proteins can cross the mammary epithelium from the interstitial fluid either by transcytosis or through the paracellular pathways. During lactation only the transcytotic pathway is available (Figure 5.2). By the transcytosis, there is secretion of macromolecular substances derived from serum or stromal cells, including serum proteins such as immunoglobulins, albumin and transferring; endocrine hormones such as insulin, prolactin and estrogen.

V) The paracellular pathway

Because of the tight junctions between epithelial cells, there is little or no "flow" of anything between the cells, except perhaps water and some ions. Anytime something passes between the cells through the tight junction, this is called the *paracellular pathway*. This pathway allows passage of substances between epithelial cells, rather than through them (Figure 5.2). The paracellular pathway provides a direct passage of interstitial fluid and serum components into milk between the cells via leaky tight junctions. Normally this pathway is closed in the fully lactating gland providing tight junctions between the milk and interstitial spaces. When the udder is inflamed, such as during mastitis or involution, or when oxytocin is causing milk ejection, the tight junctions open some or become *'leaky'*. This allows lactose and potassium to move from the lumen into the extracellular space, and for sodium and chlorine to move into the lumen from the extracellular space. This results in a change in electrical conductivity of the milk (as diagnostic indicator of mastitis). At the same time milk components like lactose and other milk-specific components can enter the blood. Milk proteins can be detected in the cow's blood during lactation and early involution.

Factors Affecting the Composition of Milk

Since the establishment of the quality purchase scheme for fresh milk on the basis of the fat and protein content interest in the factors influencing these two components has increased enormously. Variations in the composition of milk make it more difficult for milk plants to produce uniform products; variations in the composition of whole milk affect the properties of many other dairy products. The normal value of milk constituents are given in Table 5.2, 5.3, and 5.4. The ratio of fat to protein in a cheese is dependent upon the ratio in the milk. Variations in this fat: casein ratio may be responsible for the difference between a cheese of high quality and one of low quality. Lack of uniformity in the milk supply is a source of much trouble to the dairy industry. Because of variations in the composition of milk are of great practical importance. It should be remembered that most changes in composition are the result of many factors. There are various factors which affect the milk composition, include non-nutritional factors such as breed, age, stage of lactation, environmental factors, genetics, mastitis and nutritional factors. In cattle, fat is the most variable component while minerals and lactose are the least variable. Milk protein to milk fat ratio ranges from 0.78 to 0.85 depending on breed type. The composition of milk in dairy cows is generally ranges between 3.0-5.3% fat, 2.8-4.5% protein and 4.2-5.1% lactose.

Table 5.2 : Chemical composition of milk.

Constituent	Cow	Buffalo
Dry matter (%)	13.0	16.5
Fat (%)	4.0	6.7
Total protein (%)	3.4	4.5
Casein (%)	2.8	3.9
Whey protein (%)	0.6	0.6
Lactose (%)	4.8	4.5
Ash (%)	0.7	0.8

Adopted from Chakraborty (2005).

Table 5.3 : Approximate average values of different protein fractions of cows milk.

Type of protein	Concentration (g/L)
Casein fractions	
α_{s1}-casein	10
α_{s2}-casein	3.4
β-casein	10
κ-casein	3.9

Whey proteins	
α-lactalbumin	1.2
β-lactglobulin	3.0
Immunoglobulins	0.8
N-terminal β-casein fragments	0.8
Blood serum albumin	0.4
Lactoferrin	0.1-0.5
Lactoperoxidase	0.03
Lysozyme	0.0013

Table 5.4 : Average values of micronutrient content of cow whole milk (3.3% fat).

Minerals	Quantity per Liter	Vitamins	Quantity per Liter
Calcium (mg)	1277.3	Vitamin A (IU)	1299.5
Phosphorus (mg)	963.28	Vitamin B_1 (mg)	0.39
Chlorine (mg)	1031.36	Vitamin B_2 (mg)	1.67
Sodium (mg)	505.36	Vitamin B_3 (mg)	0.87
Potassium (mg)	1567.66	Vitamin B_6 (mg)	0.43
Magnesium (mg)	138.2	Vitamin B_{12} (mg)	3.68
Copper (mg)	0.1	Biotin (mcg)	19.6
Zinc (mg)	3.92	Vitamin C (mg)	9.69
Iron (mg)	0.52	Vitamin D (IU)	41.25
Manganese (mg)	0.04	Vitamin E (IU)	1.54
Molybdenum (mcg)	20.63	Folate (mcg)	61.57
Selenium (mcg)	15.47	Vitamin K (mcg)	41.25
Iodine (mcg)	237.21	Panthotenate (mg)	3.24

Adopted from Khanna (2005). Indian Dairyman., 57(7): 34.

Non-nutritional Factors

There are numerous factors which are non-nutriotional and can have an affect on the composition of milk such as genetics, breed, parity, stage of lactation, environmental factors, milk fraction and udder effect of mastitis.

1. Genetics

Fifty five percent of the variation in milk components is due to heredity and 45 % is due to nutrition. Heritability indicates the proportion of observed differences that are due to genetics, while the reciprocal is assumed to be due to environmental factors. *Heritability* is defined as the ratio of genetic variance to total phenotypic ratio. Protein and fat percentages are more highly heritable than milk yield. The fat content of milk from day to day exhibit greater fluctuation than other components, and has a repeatability of 0.60. Repeatabilities of protein and solid not fat (SNF) are higher - 0.85 and 0.90 respectively (Sharma and Singh, 2005). Milk yield is positively correlated to yield of fat and protein; however, milk yield is negatively correlated to fat and protein percentage. Heritabilities of fat, protein and lactose contents average 0.58, 0.49 and 0.55 respectively, while that of milk yield average 0.27. However, genetic selection has little effect on the lactose and mineral composition of milk (Legates, 1960).

Correlations between:

% Fat and % protein	r	=	.45 to .55
% Fat and % SNF	r	=	.40
% SNF and % protein	r	=	.81
Milk yield and % fat	r	=	- .15 to - .30
Milk yield and SNF	r	=	- .10
Milk yield and % protein	r	=	- .10 to - .30

2. Breed

There is a common tendency, within breeds, for high producing cows to produce milk with a low fat content. The composition of milk of individual cows of a particular breed can differ greatly e.g. milk from Holstein cows has a lower milk fat percent than milk from Jersey or Guernsey (Table 5.5). The effect of breed on milk constituents has been reported in various studies like Daley *et al.* (1986) found that milk fat percentage differed significantly among breed types. While Belcher *et al.* (1979) found no significant differences for milk fat percentage, but milk protein percentages had differences between breeds. Rahnefeld *et al.* (1990) reported breed effects on milk fat and protein percentages. Similarly Sharaby (1988) found breed differences for fat, protein and lactose content in milk in Jersey and Holstein cows. Milk of Jersey cows also has higher total solids than milk from other dairy cattle breeds. Milk color is also affected by breed. Milk from Jersey or Guernsey is more yellowish in color than other breeds. This is because these two breeds convert much less carotene (yellow pigment) to vitamin A than other breeds of dairy cattle. A difference in the breed of cows is the principal reason why the milk in some states averages as high as 4.5% of fat, in others as low as 3.65%.

3. Parity

Parity tends to cause both milk fat and protein to decline as the animal becomes older. The age of animal also influences the amino acid composition of casein as does the stage of lactation. Milk fat falls about 0.2% each year from the 1st to 5th lactation likely as a result of higher production and more udder infections. Protein decreases 0.02 to 0.05% each lactation as animals age. Quality of milk in terms of its composition influenced by the advancing age of lactating animals is evident from Table 5.6. The parity has a comparatively lower influence on the lactose, protein and dry fat free residual (Peeva, 2001).

Table 5.5: Variation in the composition of cows milk of different breeds.

Breed	Total solids	Fat	Protein	Lactose	Ash
Jersey	14.15	4.97	3.03	4.70	0.77
Holstein	11.91	3.56	3.02	4.61	0.3
Guernsey	13.69	4.58	3.49	4.78	0.75
Brown Swiss	12.69	3.80	3.18	4.80	0.72

Table 5.6 : Effect of age of lactating cows on the percent composition of milk.

Lactation no.	Fat	SNF	CP	Lactose
1	4.11	9.01	3.36	4.72
2	4.06	8.92	3.35	4.62
3	4.03	8.82	3.28	4.59
4	4.02	8.84	3.30	4.57
5	3.90	8.72	3.26	4.53
6	3.91	8.74	3.30	4.48
7	3.94	8.67	3.25	4.48
8	3.82	8.65	3.23	4.44
9	4.03	8.70	3.27	4.48
10	3.83	8.66	3.25	4.46
11	3.77	8.61	3.16	4.46

Adopted from Mudgal *et al.* (2003)

4. Stage of lactation

Stage of lactation also influences the composition and yield of milk. Stage of lactation affects milk protein and fat percentages very similarly. Milk production continues to increase after parturition and peak yield as obtained 4-8 weeks post partum. The peak yield may be held for a few weeks and starts declining afterwards. Fat percentage in milk decreases slightly during the early lactation and then increases as total production decreases with advancing lactation. Morgan (1991) reported the lowest values for milk fat percentage during the peak milk yield (middle of lactation) for Hereford cows.

This relationship of increased milk production and decreased fat percentage may be due "Dilution effect". Dilution effect is the inverse relationship between milk yield and percentage of milk constituents. This is supported by Pitcher *et al.* (1992) who reported that the dilution effect was responsible for the changes in milk composition in dairy cows and by Ibeawuchi and Dangut (1996) who found a significant inverse correlation between milk yield and milk fat in Zebu cattle. Milk protein content gradually increases with advancing lactation. Lactose and mineral concentrations increase slightly during advancing lactation. Milk is produced immediately after parturition to 5 days post partum is known as *colostrum*. The composition of colostrum is considerably different from the composition of normal milk. Cow's colostrum contains more minerals, protein and less lactose than milk. Fat percentage is usually higher in colostrum than in milk. Calcium, magnesium, phosphorus and chloride are high in colostrum, where as potassium is low. Iron is 10-17 times higher in colostrum than in milk. Colostrum contains 10 times as much vitamin A and 3 times as much vitamin D as that found in normal milk. The most remarkable difference between colostrum and milk is the extremely high levels of immunoglobulins (Ig) content of colostrum.

5. Environmental factors

The environmental temperature directly alters both milk yield and composition by affecting basal metabolism, feed intake, rate of passage of digesta, and nutrient requirements for maintenance. Moreover, reduced intake of forage during summer months may alter rumen fermentation and the acetate: propionate ratio and may be cause of reduce milk fat content. Similarly, milk protein and lactose percentages are lower during warm season. The hot and humid months depress fat and protein content. As temperature increase, through the spring, milk component levels are gradually decreased. In general, milk fat and SNF percentages are lower by 0.2 to 0.4% in summer than winter. Cows that are lactating appear to be more cold resistant but less heat tolerant than non lactating cows because of the metabolic heat produced by increased feed consumption.

6. Milk fraction

In dairy cattle an effect of milk fraction on some milk constituents has been found. Moore *et al.* (1981) reported that milk fat percentage was significantly higher at evening than at morning milking for foremilk, but significantly higher at morning than at evening milking for residual milk. Protein content was significantly higher at evening than at morning milking for machine milk and residual milk. Carlsson and Bergstrom (1994) reported that fat percentage was higher in residual milk than in foremilk.

7. Effect of mastitis

During the inflammatory process (mastitis), three mechanisms are involved in milk composition change: a decrease in synthesis, an increase in the permeability of the milk barrier and an increase in the proteolytic activities in milk (Roux *et al.*, 2003). The overall impact of mastitis on milk composition is presented in table 5.7.

Table 5.7 : The overall effect of mastitis on milk composition.

Decrease Milk constituent	Degree of change	Increase Milk constituent	Degree of change
Quarter milk yield	-(–)	Somatic cell count	+++
Dry matter	-	Whey proteins	+++
Lactose	-	Bovine serum albumin	+
Fat	-	Immunoglobulins	+++
Long-chained fatty acids	-	k-casein	+(+)
Total casein	--	Proteose peptones	++
α_{s1} casein	--	Free fatty acids	++
β- casein	---	Short-chained fatty acids	+
α-lactalbumin	-	Sodium	++
β-lactglobulin	---	Chloride	++
Calcium	--	Lactate	+++
Magnesium	---	Enzyme activity	
Phosphorus	---	Lipase	++
Zinc	-	Lysozyme	+++
Potssium	-	NAGase	+++
		β-glucuronidase	+++
		Plasmin	+++

Source: Pyorala, (2003).

a. Effect on Protein Content

It is generally accepted that during mastitis, there is an increase in milk proteins (Auldist and Hubble, 1998) particularly those originating from blood e.g. bovine serum albumin and immunoglobulins (Poutrell *et al.*, 1983; Baranova and Belov, 1993), while those milk proteins synthesized in the mammary gland e.g. α-casein, β-casein, κ-casein, α-lactalbumin and β-lactglobulin decreases (Lee *et al.*, 1991; Auldist *et al.*, 1995). As such, mastitis results in decrease of useable milk proteins i.e. caseins and increase in the undesirable whey protein fractions e.g. serum albumin, globulins (Sharma *et al.*, 2004) (Table 5.8). Serum albumin, immunoglobulins, transferrin, and other serum proteins pass into milk because vascular permeability changes. This increase in proteins of blood serum origin during mastitis is possibly due to a disruption to the integrity of the mammary epithelial by microbial toxins and opening of the tight junctions (Holdaway, 1990). The decrease in the casein concentrations during mastitis is largely due to post-secretory degradation of casein by proteinases originating from mastitis causing bacteria, leukocytes or the blood (Seaman *et al.*, 1988). The main caseinolytic enzyme in milk is *plasmin*, which normally found in milk in small quantities. Plasmin sensitive sites occur in α_{s1}-, α_{s2}-, and β-caseins, but k-casein is resistant to proteolytic hydrolysis (Fox, 1981). The plasmin is derived from plasminogen which originates in the blood and probably leaks into the milk in greater amounts due to disruption of the epithelium (Politis *et al.*, 1989). Schaar and Funke (1986) detected a close correlation between levels of sodium and plasmin in milk. Plasmin may contribute the leakage of sodium and presumably other blood constituents into milk by degrading membrane proteins of the epithelial lining. In part, it is the result of decreased synthesis and secretion of casein as a result of physical damage to the mammary epithelial cells by bacterial toxins during mastitis (Oliver and Calvinho, 1995). Singh *et al.* (1998) has been reported that protein content of milk increased by 5.05% and 17.05% in sub-clinical and clinical mastitis respectively. While in case of buffaloes milk protein content increased upto 10.51% than healthy buffaloes (Singh et al., 2006).

On the other hand, the whey proteins synthesized *de novo* are relatively resistant to proteolytic attack. However, in mastitis and high SCC milk, there is an evident decrease in a-lactalbumin and b-lactglobulin. This would be partly due to impaired cellular synthetic and secretory function, and partly due to leakage of these proteins out of the milk and into the extra cellular fluid via the paracellular pathway. *Lactoferrin*, the major antibacterial iron-binding protein in mammary secretions, increases in concentration during mastitis, likely because of increased output by the mammary tissue and a minor contribution from PMN. Mastitis is also associated with increases in the concentrations of many different enzymes in milk (Pyorala, 2003), which can play significant roles in the diagnosis of sub-clinical mastitis. Compared with normal milk, mastitis milk has higher levels of several enzymes, especially proteases (Heegaard *et al.*, 1994; Long *et al.*, 2001; Raulo *et al.*, 2002) that could potentially damage mammary tissue. The mechanisms responsible for mammary epithelium and tissue damage during mastitis are not well known (Mehrzad *et al.*, 2005).

b. Effects on Fat Content

Mastitis results in decreased in the concentration of fat in milk (Kitchen, 1981; Murno *et al.*, 1984) but some scientists recorded an increase in total fat content of mastitic milk (Pyorala, 2003; Bruckmaier *et al.*, 2004). According to

Bruckmaier *et al.* (2004) the increase in fat concentration indicates that there is a reduced lactose synthesis and therefore reduced milk volume while the fat synthesis is only slightly depressed. A decrease in fat concentration during mammary infection may be attributed to the reduced synthetic and secretory capacity of the mammary gland. Further, conditions within the infected mammary gland enhance the activity of milk lipoprotein lipase (mLPL) (Bansal and Randhawa, 2003), which attack the milk fat globule membranes. The leucocytes that invade the mammary gland in response to infection produce lipolytic enzymes, which breakdown the triglycerides, oxidation of fatty acids and lead to the development of rancid flavour in milk.

c. Effects on Lactose Content

It is well known that mastitis causes a decrease in the concentration of milk lactose (Auldist *et al.*, 1998; Nguyen and Neville, 1998). The decrease of lactose in milk is caused by leakage of lactose into the extracellular fluid and blood after the destruction of the normal lactose barrier (Mielke, 1975). The key role of lactose as the osmotic regulator of milk volume, the reduced lactose concentrations are unlikely to be due to reduced synthesis and secretion at the cellular level and can only be depressed; there is an increased influx of electrolytes during mastitis. This is because water would be drawn into the cells only in sufficient quantities to maintain osmotic equilibrium. The lower concentration of lactose in mastitic milk may be partly due to the lactose fermenting activities of the common mastitis causing bacteria.

d. Effects on Mineral Content

The concentrations of many minerals are altered during mastitis, and these changes can play significant roles in determining the produced quality of the milk and diagnosis of sub-clinical mastitis. *Potassium*, the most abundant mineral in milk, leaks out of milk through the paracellular pathway. Consequently, its concentration decreases (Auldist *et al.*, 1998). Conversely, *sodium*, found in the blood in high quantities, leaks into the milk increasing concentrations above normal. The concentrations of *chloride* in milk from cows with sub-clinical mastitis are elevated probably due to the influx of blood constituents into the milk during infection.

B. Nutritional Factors

Of all milk components, milk fat is the most influenced by dietary manipulations. Most of changes in milk composition due to dietary manipulation are related to changes in ruminal acetate: propionate ratio. Milk fat depression can be alleviated within 7 to 21 day by changing the diet. Milk protein changes may take 3 to 6 weeks or longer if the problem has been going on for a prolonged period. Nutrition or ration formulation changes are more strongly correlated to milk fat content than milk protein. Milk fat can be changed by 0.1 to 1.0%, while protein is seldom altered more than 0.1 to 0.4 percent by nutritional changes. But lactose content is not influenced by diet manipulation, except through over or under feeding. However Rodriguez *et al.* (1997) found that the lactose content of milk increased 1.4% with added fat and increased 1.6% with diets having high ruminally undegredable protein (RUP) content. Any diet or management factors that affect rumen fermentation can change milk composition. Consistently providing adequate energy and protein and balanced amounts of rapidly fermentable carbohydrate and effective fiber are keys to maintain optimum level of components. The challenge in feeding for milk components is that high energy; low fiber diets that increase milk protein are likely to reduce fat levels. Several nutritional factors can influence milk composition. These include plane of nutrition, roughage: concentrate ratio, forage quality, level and type of dietary fat.

Table 5.8 : Changes in the composition of mastitic milk from a normal cow milk.

Component	Level	
	Normal milk	Mastitic milk
Fat (%)	3.45	3.2
Lactose (%)	4.85	4.4
Total casein (mg/ml)	27.90	22.5
Total whey protein (mg/ml)	8.2	13.1
Whey protein components (mg/ml)		
β-lactglobulin	4-4.25	2.67-2.96
α-lactalbumin	1.03-1.22	0.58-0.65
Blood serum albumin	0.24	0.65
Total immunoglobulins	1.33	8.8
Sodium (mg/dl)	57	104.6
Potassium (mg/dl)	172.5	157.3
Chloride (mg/dl)	80-130	>250
Total calcium (mg/dl)	136	49
pH	6.65	6.9-7.1

Adopted from Kitchen, B.J. (1981). J. Dairy Res., 48: 167-188.

Both thin and fat cows tend to have low milk fat in later lactation. Protein can be depressed at calving if animals are overly obese or underweight. Underfeeding dairy cows reduce lactose percent and increase fat percentage.

Feeding imbalance rations (e.g. low energy: protein ratio). It has been proposed that the percentage of milk fat is affected by plasma insulin concentrations. The glucogenic-insulin theory proposes that increased insulin release which occurs when high starchy concentrate diets are fed, preferentially channels nutrients to adipose tissue, resulting in a shortage of nutrients at the mammary gland and thus milk fat depression (Griinari *et al.*, 1997). This theory has been questioned because injections of insulin in some cases did not result in a lower milk fat content (Mcguire *et al.*, 1995). A readily fermentable non-fiber carbohydrate like starch and sugar in the concentrate mixture affects the fat and protein level in milk. Increase in non-fiber carbohydrate results in increase in protein yield but fat percentage reduces. In contrast, as ration fiber levels increase and/or energy is reduced, milk protein is depressed and milk fat is increased. Lack of energy intake or lower ration digestibility may reduce milk protein by 0.1 to 0.4%. The excessive feeding of dietary protein does not increase milk protein, as most of the excess is excreted. However Pirlo *et al.* (1997) reported higher milk protein percentages in high protein diets. The use of non protein nitrogen (NPN) compounds like urea, as protein substitutes will reduce protein in milk by 0.1 to 0.3% if the NPN is a main provider of crude protein equivalent. The energy content of dairy ration affects the milk protein fraction. A 0.4% reduction in SNF can occur if energy is reduced by 40 percent. Amino acids required for milk protein synthesis are derived from microbes in the rumen. Thus, the protein content of milk is influenced by factors that regulate microbial growth and the process of the fermentation. Production of propionate in rumen increases milk protein synthesis by increasing the availability of certain amino acids like glutamate (Sharma and Singh, 2005).

The fermentation of feed stuffs in the rumen results into the production of volatile fatty acids like acetic acid (65-70%), propionic acid (18-20%), butyric acid (8-10%) and other fatty acids. Diets that alter fermentation affect fat content e.g. a low intake ratio of roughage to carbohydrate results in decreased acetate and butyrate, which are the major fat precursors and increases propionate which decreases milk fat. Types of concentrate used in the ration also affect the fat percentage. Processed grains used in concentrate, increases the digestion of starch in the rumen and the production of propionate which subsequently reduces milk fat. Feeding finely chopped forages has a negative impact on milk fat % and may cause milk fat depression syndrome (drop of milk fat % below 3%). Cows fed finely chopped forages spend less time chewing and therefore will produce less saliva. Ruminal pH will drops as less saliva is produced to buffer the acid production in the rumen. As the ruminal pH drops below 6, the activity of the cellulolytic bacteria is reduced and so is the production of acetic acid and butyric acid, which are the precursors of short chain fatty acid synthesis in the mammary gland. Incorporation of fat or oil in dairy cow ration can substantially alter the profile of milk fatty acids. Fats can be added in the diets of dairy animals at 5 to 6% of dietary dry matter to increase milk fat content. The effect of supplemented fat on milk fat percent depends on the type of supplemental fat. Feeding saturated fats can only increase fat percentage whereas, unsaturated fats decrease fat percentage.

Mammary Gland Involution

A dry period or stage of mammary involution is necessary during the lactation cycle for optimal milk production in the subsequent lactation. During dry period, adequate milk secretory cell proliferation and differentiation are essential to the success of the next lactation. The cessation of suckling or milking rapidly brings about mammary involution, which is characterized by a decrease in number of mammary epithelial cells and also in secretory activity per cell. Lysosomal enzymes are released, and many epithelial cells are lysed. Myoepithelial cells remain in the gland during involution and maintain the structure of the remaining epithelial cells. The space previously occupied by the degenerating alveoli is replaced with adipose cells (Swenson and Reece, 1996). It is generally accepted that lactation should be terminated 45 to 60 days prior to parturition. In cows given a 60 days dry period, mammary gland involution occurs during the early dry period and is characterized by 1) increased programmed cell death (apoptosis), 2) increased intramammary pressure and udder distention, 3) regression of secretory function of mammary epithelial cells (MEC), and 4) low levels of MEC proliferation (Holst *et al.*, 1987; Capuco and Akers, 1999). Concurrent pregnancy and advanced lactation at the time of milk stasis (dry-off) in dairy cows results in a rapid, but small increases in MEC apoptosis during involution and maintenance of alveolar structure and integrity occur throughout the dry period. By 25 d after dry-off, mammary DNA content (cell number) and luminal area of the alveoli are at a minimum and stromal components of the mammary gland are at a maximum, suggesting mammary involution is complete (Capuco *et al.*, 1997). Bush and Oliver (1987) used three methods of drying off the milking cows- I) abrupt cessation of milking by injecting the dry-off mammary antibiotic infusion, II) milking once daily for the last week of lactation, and III) milking once daily but feeding only hay for the last week. Out of these, the favored method of drying off is by abrupt cessation of milking, which forces the mammary gland to involute. The physiology of the mammary gland during the dry period differs markedly from that during lactation. For the sake of convenience, the dry period can be divided into three phases: first phase is active involution or early dry period, second steady state involution or mid-dry period, and third one is the period of colostrogenesis or late dry period.

After drying off, the udder continues to synthesize and secrete milk; maximum accumulation of fluid occurs in 2 to 3 days and then declines rapidly over the next week. Fluid accumulation triggers a period of active involution, which continues for 21 to 28 days (Sordillo and Nickerson, 1988). It is a transition phase of the mammary gland from the lactating to the non-lactating state. Changes in the mammary secretion composition and volume occur during active involution. During this phase the concentrations of antimicrobial components i.e. lactoferrin, NAGase, leukocytes, immunoglobulins and serum albumin in lacteal secretions increased while fluid volume decreases. The concentration of casein, α-lactalbumin, β-lactglobulin and milk fat decline slowly during the first 2 to 3 weeks of the dry period, but never completely disappear, while lactose concentrations decrease rapidly. The incidence of new intramammary infection is highest during the first 2 weeks of the dry period and during the first 2 weeks after parturition. The mid dry period is the time of lowest incidence of intramammary infection.

During the steady state involution, fluid volume is reduced to a few milliliters and milk constituents are at minimum concentrations. Antimicrobial defense components continue to be maintained at high concentrations compared with concentrations found during lactation. The length of the steady state period depends on the total length of the dry period. The cows with a 45 to 60 days dry period probably have a very short steady state phase or no steady phase of involution at all. When the dry period is <40 days, the gland tissue is undergoing active involution and beginning the colostrogenensis phase concurrently.

The last phase of the dry period is the period of colostrogenesis, which begins 2 weeks prepartum and continues several days into lactation. This phase of the dry period marks the transition from the non-lactating to lactating state. During this phase fluid volume increases along with concentrations of colostral immunoglobulins while lactoferrin and leukocyte concentrations decreases. Selective transport of IgG1 is a major activity of the epithelial cells in the last 2 weeks prior to parturition. Capuco *et al.* (1997) states that period of colostrogenensis begin 5 weeks prepartum. As involution progresses, the udder becomes more resistant to infection. Mammary gland resistance during the middle and late dry period is attributed to the keratin plug, which prevents multiplication and physical movement of bacteria. Continued movement of cornification of the teat canal epithelium as involution progressed led to the formation of a keratin plug.

Milk Removal from the Gland

The physiology of milk removal or ejection has been thoroughly studied. In 1910, Ott and Scott (1910) discovered that extracts from the posterior pituitary could cause an increase in milk flow from a cannulated teat. Some years later it was observed that the extracts from the posterior pituitary could cause an increase in intra mammary pressure (Gaines, 1915). In 1941, it was observed that milk ejection was a neuroendocrine reflex (Ely and Peterson, 1941), and a year later it was observed that a factor called oxytocin, detected in the blood, caused contraction of the myoepithelial cells surrounding the alveoli (Peterson and Ludwick, 1942). The role of oxytocin was then further demonstrated by Andersson, (1951), who discovered that the reflex included a terminal hormonal component.

Milk removal from the lactating mammary gland is the major factor in maintaining milk secretion. During the inter-milking period, milk accumulates in the storage spaces of the mammary gland i.e. the alveoli, ducts, gland and teat cisterns. A small amount of milk may be removed from the teat cistern, the gland cistern, and the large ducts of a cow by *passive milk removal* in the absence of milk ejection reflex, but milk stored within the alveoli and small ducts can not be harvested until letdown or the forceful expulsion of milk occurs, which can be achieved by the stimulation of milk ejection reflex.

There is a passive pressure inside the cow's udder of about 0.4 pounds per square inch (psi) before the cow is stimulated, after stimulation the pressure increases to about 0.8 psi. The sphincter muscles at the end of the teat is tight enough to keep the milk inside, but if the muscle is not strong enough, milk will leak out even before the cow is stimulated. For removal of the milk, the opening of the streak canal is must. The streak canal opening depends on the pressure produced inside or outside the udder. The outside pressure on the teat is 14.6 psi. The act of hand pressure and internal pressure forces open the teat sphincter and the milk is removed. This can open by- negative pressure (with milking machine), positive pressure (with hand milking), and both positive and negative pressure (during calf suckling). Milking machine usually applies 12.5 to 15 inches Hg of vacuum to the outside of the teat. This produces a pressure differential of 12.5 to 15 inches Hg negative vacuum pressure on the outside of the teat compared with the 0.8 psi positive pressure inside the teat. This pressure differential is great enough to open the teat sphincter and the milk is removed, even at the end of milking when the internal pressure diminishes.

Milk Ejection Reflex

Inside the udder filled with milk, usually less than 20% of the milk is stored in the cisternal compartment (udder and teat cisterns and the bigger milk ducts) (Bruckmaier *et al.*, 1994b), while the rest of the milk is stored in the smaller ducts and the alveolus. From a milking point of view this has to be considered, since removal of alveolar milk is only possible through activation of the milk ejection reflex, while the cisternal milk can be removed by overcoming the teat sphincter barrier. The importance of activation of the milk ejection reflex for optimal milk removal from alveolar compartments was demonstrated by Pfeilsticker *et al.* (1996), who observed that cisternal milk yield and fraction were significantly higher in teat-stimulated cows than in unstimulated controls. The milk ejection reflex actually is a *neuroendocrine reflex*. The milk ejection reflex has two pathways-1) an afferent (neural) pathway, 2) an efferent (hormonal) pathway.

1) Afferent pathway

The greatest amount of innervation (sympathetic) in the mammary glands is in the teats, where there are pressure sensitive receptors in the dermis. The milking stimuli, such as physical touch by milker hands or suckling, cleaning towels, activate nerve receptors in the dermis of the teats. Impulses are then carried from these receptors to the spinal cord, to the paraventricular nuclei (PVN) and supraoptic nuclei (SON) of the hypothalamus. When the cell bodies of the oxytocin containing neurons are stimulated by these impulses originating in the teat, an action potential moves down the oxytocin-containing neurons from the cell body in the hypothalamus down the axon to the neuron ending in the posterior pituitary. It is also apparent that oxytocin release can be induced by higher brain centers via conditioned responses (e.g. cry of her calf) or external stimuli (e.g. audiovisual and olfactory cues). When an impulse reaches the hypothalamus from the nerve endings of the teat or from visual and auditory sources, a secondary message is carried to the posterior pituitary where oxytocin is stored and released into the blood.

2) Efferent pathway

An efferent pathway begins with the release of oxytocin into the blood. The blood is then carry the oxytocin to the mammary gland in approximately 19 to 22 seconds (Nickerson, 1994). The oxytocin binds to receptors on the myoepithelial cells, causing the myoepithelial cells to contract (in 6 seconds), and resulting in increased intra-luminal (intramammary) pressure and ejection of milk from the alveolar lumen. Oxytocin receptors are associated with the myoepithelial cells, not the smooth muscle of the mammary gland. The time that passes from the movement of the stimulation to the letting down of milk varies with individual cows between 60 seconds to 90 seconds. Oxytocin has a half life of approximately 3-5 minutes and disappears rapidly from the blood serum via clearance through the kidney and liver (Wacks *et al.*, 1984).

To harvest all the milk from the udder, you must have the cow's cooperation. To achieve this cooperation, it is very important to treat the cows in a routine and gentle manner, both before and during milking. In certain situations (e.g. pain, excitement or fear), the milk ejection reflex can be inhibited. If a cow is stressed in any way prior to milking, adrenaline released into the blood by the adrenal gland. The hormone adrenaline inhibit the milk ejection or let down of milk by different mechanisms-

a) It constrict the blood vessels and capillaries in the udder, resulting decreased blood flow to udder, ultimately decreases the amount of oxytocin reaching the myoepithelial cells and no let down occur.

b) Adrenalin also acts directly on the myoepithelial cells by blocking oxytocin binding, thereby preventing contraction of myoepithelial cells, resulting no let down occur.

c) The adrenalin also partial or complete blocks the release of oxytocin from the posterior pituitary. There is no contraction of myoepithelial cells and no let down of milk.

For a complete milk removal, firstly the circulating oxytocin needs to reach a threshold level. Secondly, continuously elevated oxytocin concentrations are necessary (Svennersten-Sjaunja, 2004). Therefore appropriate teat stimulation throughout the milking is important for the milking process (Bruckmaier *et al.*, 1994a). In addition to the importance of the circulating levels of oxytocin it has been observed that anatomical changes occur in the structure of the PVN during lactation, giving increased possibilities for contact between the oxytocinergic neurons (Theodosis *et al.*, 1986).

References

Andersson, B. (1951). Acta. Physiol. Scand., 23: 8-23.

Auldist, M.J. and Hubble, I.B. (1998). The Aust. J. of Dairy Tech., 53: 28-36.

Auldist, M.J., Coats, S., Rogers, G.L. and McDowell, G.H. (1995). Aust. J. Exp. Agri., 35: 427-436.

Bansal, B.K. and Randhawa, S.S. (2003). In: compendium of 4th Round Table Conf. on Mastitis, 14-15 April, 2003, Palampur (H.P.), India., pp. 137-146.

Baranova, V.S. and Belov, A.D. (1993). Voprosy Veterinarnoi Biologii., 33-35.

Bauman, T.E. (1992). J. Dairy Sci., 75(12): 3432-3451.

Belcher, C.G. and Frahm, R.R. (1979). J. Anim. Sci., 49: 1195-1206.

Blackwood, J.H. and Stirling, J.D. (1932). Biochem. J., 26: 353, 772, 1127.

Bleck, G.T., Choi, B.K, Wheeler, M.B. and Flores, R.J. (1998). Illini Dairynet Press, 8 may, 1998.

Bruckmaier, R.M., O., C. E. and Blum, J.W. (2004). Veterinary Medicine-Czech., 8: 283-290.

Bruckmaier, R.M., Rothenanger, E. and Blum, J. W. (1994b). Milchwissenschaft. 49: 543 – 546.

Bruckmaier, R.M., Schams, D. and Blum, J.W. (1994a). J. Dairy Res., 61: 323-334.

Bushe, T. and Oliver, S.P. (1987). J. Dairy Sci., 70:696.

Capuco, A.V. and Akers, R.M. (1999). J. Mam. Gland Bio. Neoplasia., 4:137-144.

Capuco, A.V., Akers, R.M. and Smith, J.J. (1997). J. Dairy Sci., 80:477-487.

Carlsson, J. and Bergström, J. (1994). Acta Vet. Scand., 35: 67-77.

Chakraborty, G.C. (2005). Indian Dairy Industry. Annual dairy resource book vol. 1. Edn. 1st, Dr. Chawla dairy information centre Pvt. Ltd, Delhi, India.

Daley, D.R., McCuskey, A. and Bailey, C.M. (1986). In: Proc. 3rd Wld. Cong. Genet. Appl. Livest. Prod: 308-313.

Ely, F. and Petersen W.E. (1941). J. Dairy Sci., 24: 211- 223.

Fleishaker, J. and Mcnamara, P. (1988). J. of Pharmacol and Expe. Therapeutics., 244: 919-924.

Fox, P.F. (1981). Neth. Milk Dairy J., 35: 233.

Gaines, W.L. (1915). Am. J. Physiol., 38: 285-312.

Graham Jr., W.R. (1937). J. Biol. Chem., 122:1.

Griinari, J.M., McGuire, M.A., Dwyer, D.A., Bauman, D.E. and Palmquist, D.L. (1997). J. Dairy Sci., 80: 1076-1084.

Harvatine, K.J., Boisclair, Y.R. and Bauman, D.E. (2009). Animal, 3(1): 40–54.

Heegaard, C.W., Rasmussen, L.K. and Andreasen, P.A. (1994). Biochim. Biophys. Acta., 1222:45–55.

Herman, H.A., Graham Jr., W.R. and Turner, C.W. (1938). Mo. Agri. Expt. Sta. Research Bull., 275.

Herrington, B.L. (2000). In: milk and milk processing. 1st edn. Green world publisher, Lucknow (U.P.), India. Pp.16.

Holdaway, R.J. (1990). A comparison of methods for the diagnosis of bovine sub-clinical mastitis within Newzealand dairy herds. Ph.D. Thesis. Massey University.

Holst, B.D., Hurley, W.L. and Nelson, D.R. (1987). J. Dairy Sci., 70:935-944

Hurst, V. and Turner, C.W. (1942). Endocrinology., 31: 334.

Ibeawuchi, J.A. and Dangut, A.J. (1996). Disc. Inn., 8: 249-256.

Jensen, R.G. (2002). J. Dairy Sci., 85: 295–350.

Karg, H. and Schams, D. (1974). J. Reprod Fert., 39:463-472.

Khanna (2005). Indian Dairyman., 57(7): 34.

Kitchen, B.J. (1981). J. Dairy Res., 48: 167-188.

Lee, S.C., Yu, J.H., Jeeng, C.L., Back, Y.J. and Yoon, Y.C. (1991). Korean J. Dairy Sci., 13: 217-223.

Ligates, J.E. (1960). J. Dairy Sci., 43: 1527.

Linzell, J. and Peaker, M. (1971). Physiological Reviews., 51(3): 564-597.

Linzell, J. L. and Peaker, M. (1975). Journal of Physiology., 244: 771-782.

Long, E., Capuco, A. V., Wood, D. L., Sonstegard, T., Tomita, G., Paape, M. J. and Zhao, X.. (2001). Cell Death Differ., 8:808–816.

McGuire, J.G. and Bauman, D.E. (2002). In Encyclopedia of dairy science (ed. H Roginski, JW Fuquay and PF Fox), pp. 1828–1834. Elsevier Science Ltd., London, England.

Mcguire, M.A., Griinari, J.M., Dwyer, D.A. and Bauman, D.E. (1995). J. Dairy Sci., 78: 816-824.

McManaman, J.L. and Neville, M.C. (2003). Advances Drug Delivery Reviews. 55(5): 629.

Mehrzad, J., Desrosiers, C., Lauzon, K., Robitaille, G., Zhao, X. and Lacasse, P. (2005). J. Dairy Sci., 88:211-222.

Mielke, H. (1975). Veterinaermed., 30:334.

Moore, R.K., Ng-Kwai-Hang, K.F., Sabler, J. and Moxley, J.E. (1981). Res. Rep. Dep. Anim. Sci. McGill Univ.: 35-38.

Morgan, J.H.L. (1991). Wld. Rev. Anim. Prod., 26: 59-64.

Mudgal, V.D., Singhal, K.K. and Sharma, D.D. (2003). In: Advances in dairy animal production. Edn. 2nd , International Book Distributing Co., Lucknow (U.P.), India. Pp. 362-364.

Murno, E.L., Grieve, P.A. and Kitchen, B.J. (1984). Aust. J. Dairy Tech., 39: 7-16.

Neville, M.C. and Peaker, M. (1981). J. Physiol., 313: 561-570.

Nguyen, D.-A.D. and Neville, M.C. (1998). J. Mammary Gland Biol. And Neoplacia., 3(3): 233-246.

Nickerson, S.C. (1994). Dairy Research Report., Hill Farm Research Station, Lousiana State University :278.

Nickerson, S.C. (1994). Dairy Research Report., Hill Farm Research Station, Lousiana State University :286.

Oliver, S.P. and Calvinho, L.F. (1995). J. Anim. Sci., 73 (supp.2): 18-33.

Ott, I. and Scott, J.C. (1910). Proc. Soc. Exp. Biol. Med., 8: 48-49.

Peeva, Tz. (2001). Bulg. J. Agric. Sci., 7: 329-335.

Petersen, W.E. and Ludwick, T.M. (1942). Fed. Proc., 1: 66-67.

Pfeilsticker, H.U., Bruckmaier, R.M. and Blum, J.W. (1996). J. Dairy Res., 63: 509-515.

Pirlo, G., Capelletti, M. and Marchetto, G. (1997). J. Dairy Sci., 80: 730-739.

Pitcher, P.M., Ferguson, J.D., Galligan, D.T. and Chalupa, W. (1992). J. Dairy Sci., 75 (Suppl. 1): 291 (Abstrc.).

Plaut, K., Bauman, D.E., Agergaard, N. and Akers, R.M. (1987). Dom. Anim. Endocrinol., 4:279-290.

Politis, I., Lachance, E., Block, E. and Turner, J.D. (1989). J. Dairy Sci., 72: 900-906.

Poutrel, B., Caffin, J.P. and Rainard, P. (1983). J. Dairy Sci., 66: 535-541.

Pyorala, S. (2003). Vet. Res., 34(5): 565-578.

Rahnefeld, G.W., Weiss, G.M. and Fredeen, H.T. (1990). Can. J. Anim. Sci., 70: 409-423.

Ralston, N.P., Cowsert, W.C., Ragsdale, A.C., Herman, H.A. and Turner, C.W. (1940). Mo. Agr. Expt. Sta. Res. Bull., 317.

Raulo, S. M., Sorsa, T., Tervahartiala, T., Latvanen, T., Pirila, E., Hirvonen, J. and Maisi, P. (2002). Vet. Immunol. Immunopathol., 85:137–145.

Reece, R.P. and Turner, C.W. (1937).Mo. Agri. Expt. Sta. Research Bull., 266.

Rodriguez, L.A., Stallings, C.C., Herbein, J.H. and McGilliard, M.L (1997). J. Dairy Sci., 80: 353-363.

Roux, Y.L., Laurent, F. and Moussaoui, F. (2003). Vet. Res., 34: 629-645.

Sakamoto, K., Komatsu, T., Kobayashi, T., T. Rose, M., Aso, H., Hagino, A. and Obara, Y. (2005). Growth hormone acts on the synthesis and secretion of a-casein in bovine mammary epithelial cells. J. Dairy Res., 72: 264-270.

Schaar, J. and Funke, H. (1986). J. Dairy Res., 53: 515-528.

Schalm, O.W. and Mead, S.W. (1943). J. Dairy Sci., 26: 823.

Seaman, A.I., Verdi, R.J., Galton, D.M. and Barbano, D.M. (1988). J. Dairy Sci., 71: 505-512.

Sharaby, M.A. (1988). J. Dairy Res., 55: 171-177.

Sharma, Neelesh and Singh, Rajiv (2005). Indian Dairyman., 57(7): 43-47.

Sharma, Neelesh, Maiti, S.K. and Singh, R. (2004). Dairy Planner., 1(1): 40-41.

Shennan, D.B. and Peaker, M. (2000). Physiol. Rev., 80(3): 925-951.

Singh, A.K., Singh, Y., Chaudhary, R.N. and Shrivastava, A.K. (2007). J. Res., SKUAST-J., 6(1): 1-8.

Singh, R., Bansal, B.K., Randhawa, S.S. and Sudhan, N.A. (2006). Indian J. Anim. Res., 40(1): 30-33.

Singh, R., Bansal, Singh, K.B., Khera, S.S. and Sudhan, N.A. (1998). Indian Vet. J., 75(5): 462-465.

Sordillo, L.M. and Nickerson, S.C. (1988). Am. J. Vet. Res., 49:1112.

Svennersten-Sjaunja, K. (2004). In: Proceedings of NMC Annual Meeting. Pp. 215-228.

Swenson, M.J. and Reece, W.O. (1996). In: Dukes' physiology of domestic animals. 11th edn., Panima Publishing Corporation, New Delhi, India. Pp. 711-727.

Theodosis, D.T., Chapman D.B., Montagneses, C., Poulain, D.A. and Morris, J.F. (1986). Neurosci., 17: 661-678.

Tucker, H.A. (1985). Endocrine and neural control of the mammary gland. In B.L.Larson, ed., Lactation. Iowa State University Press, Ames. Pp. 39-79.

Tucker, H.A. (1994). Lactation and its hormonal control. In: The Physiology of Reproduction, Eds Knobil E, Neill JD, 2nd ed, Raven Press, NY, pp 1065-1098.

Tucker, H.A. (2000). J. Dairy Sci., 83(4): 874-884.

Wacks, E.A., Gorewit, R.C. and Currie, W.B. (1984). Domestic Animal Endocrinology., vol. 1(2): 121.

Wilde, C.J. and Knight, C.H. (1989). J. Dairy Sci., 72: 1679-1692.

Wilde, C.J. and Peaker, M. (1990). J. Agric. Sci., 114: 235-238.

Wilde, C.J., Addey, C.V.P., Boddy, L.M. and Peaker, M. (1995). Biochem. J. 305:51-58.

Wilde, C.J., Henderson, A.J., Knight, C.H., Blatchford, D.R., Faulkner, A. and Vernon, R.G. (1987). J. Anim. Sci., 64: 533-539.

□□□

CHAPTER

6

Udder Immunity

Mastitis is an inflammation of the mammary epithelium, that mainly develops in response to intramammary infection (IMI) by mastitis causing organisms (Bannerman *et al.*, 2004). Through genetic selection and technological advances in milk removal, the bovine mammary gland yields far more milk than is needed to nourish the newborn calf. Factors associated with the intense management of dairy cattle can profoundly affect mammary gland defense mechanisms and the ability of the host to resist mastitis. *Mammary gland immunity*, defined as the protection and resistance to infectious disease, is facilitated through a variety of immune and non-immunological factors. To understanding the immune defenses of the mammary gland is instrumental in devising and developing measures to control mastitis (Pascal and Riollet, 2006).

The interaction between mastitis causing bacteria and epithelium, endothelium, and mammary gland immune system cells is complex. For this reason, the study and complete characterization of the mammary gland, innate and acquired immune response to different etiological agents are necessary to understand in detail the pathophysiology of mastitis, and also to design efficient approaches to the diagnosis, treatment and control of mastitis (Boyso *et al.*, 2007). Knowledge of the mammary gland immune response during infection by pathogenic bacteria at the molecular level, is fundamental to design of effective therapy to control and eradicate bovine mastitis.

Technological advances in immunology have provided new research tools that have facilitated the study of mammary gland immunity and pathogenesis. As consequence, the last two decades have been major progress in understanding the bovine mammary gland defense system and its function in preventing disease (Sordillo and Streicher, 2002). Mammary gland immunity is a rapidly evolving field of research in veterinary medicine. According to dairy researchers (Kumar, 1988; Maiti *et al.*, 2003), incidence of mastitis is higher in cows compared with buffaloes. This difference between two species (cow and buffalo) might be due to the difference in anatomical and cellular defense mechanisms of these species. Understanding natural udder defense has led to further advances and may provide practical implication towards preventing IMI in bovine.

In general, the immune system is characterized by its capacity to recognize and discriminate foreign invading agents (Janeway and Medzhitov, 2002). Defense of the mammary gland against mastitis causing pathogens is mediated by several anatomical, cellular and soluble protective factors.

Mammary Defense Mechanisms

Bovine udder remains in constant touch with mud, manure and urine, and is therefore continuously exposed to environmental contaminants including microbial pathogens. These factors make the udder highly susceptible to pathogenic invasions. The mammary gland is protected by a variety of defense mechanisms. Craven and Williams (1985) divides udder defense into two broad categories viz. *non-phagocytic* and *phagocytic defenses*. The non-phagocytic defense comprises teat duct defense, non-specific humoral defense, phagocyte activity in mammary gland and immunoglobulins. The phagocytic defense consists mainly of phagocytic cells in the mammary gland and those recruited in response to inflammatory reactions. These mechanisms may operate individually or interact with each other to protect udder against infections. Sordillo *et al.* (1997) classified udder defenses as *innate immunity* (non-specific responsivness) and *acquired immunity* (specific responsiveness) (Figure 6.1). Innate immunity of the mammary gland is mediated by physical barriers of the teat end, phagocytic macrophages and neutrophils, natural killer (NK-) like cells and other soluble defense components e.g. lactoferrin, lactoperoxidase, cytokines, b-defensins and complement system etc. Acquired immunity comprising antibodies, macrophages and lymphocytes. Specific immune system recognizes, specific determinants of a pathogen that facilitate selective elimination. Because of the *"memory"* of certain lymphocytes, specific immune response can be augmented by repeated exposure to a pathogen. In the mammary glands, both innate and acquired protective factors are coordinated to provide optimal protection from mastitis.

According to Adams and Templeton (1998), there are atleast three phases of mammary defense to overcome mastitis causing organisms. The *first defense* mechanism is the skin and epithelial barrier. The skin and epithelium provide a physical barrier blocking entry of pathogenic organisms, but the epithelium also provides cell surface receptors for attachment of some organisms, which are the first step in the establishment of mastitis. The *second phase* of mammary defense is innate or non-specific, immune mechanism. The *third phase* of mammary defense is acquired or specific immunity. Antibacterial defense of the mammary gland depends upon a combination of non-specific and specific systems including anatomical features of the mammary gland and, humoral and cellular defense mechanisms. The innate and acquired immune systems interact closely in an attempt to provide protection against mastitis microorganisms (Rivas *et al.*, 2002; Burvenich *et al.*, 2003). *First,* the innate immune responses stimulate the acquired immune response and influence its activity. *Second,* the acquired immune response uses many innate immune effector mechanisms to eliminate microorgansms, and its action frequently increases innate immune response antimicrobial activity. The efficiency of these responses determines mammary gland susceptibility or resistance to infection (Boyso *et al.*, 2007).

Innate udder immunity is the predominant defense mechanism during the early stages of infection. Non-specific factors do not require prior exposure to infective organisms and represent the natural disease resistance factors (Rupp and Boichard, 2003). On the most global scale, resistance could be defined as the ability to avoid any infection or the quick recovery from an infection. If innate defense mechanisms function adequately, most pathogens are readily eliminated within a short period of time, before the specific immune system is activated. The field of innate immunity can be conceived as having two arms, the *sensing arm* and the *effector arm* (Beutler, 2004). The sensing arm deals with how the host perceives infection and the effector arm deals with how the organism combats infection. Each arm of the innate immunity can be sub divided into humoral and cellular components. The innate defenses or non-specific immune factors of the mammary gland are mediated by four reactive barriers (Deitemeyer, 2003) viz. anatomical or physical barriers, phagocytic barriers, soluble barriers and inflammatory barriers of the mammary gland (Figure 6.1). If a pathogen is able to evade or is not completely eliminated by the innate defense system, the acquired immune system is triggered. Acquired immune responses recognize specific antigenic determinants of a pathogen. In comparison to the first exposure to a bacterial antigen, a memory response would be much faster, considerably stronger, longer lasting, and often more effective against the mastitis causing organisms. Vaccination protocols are based on these unique features of the specific immune response (Sordillo and Streicher, 2002).

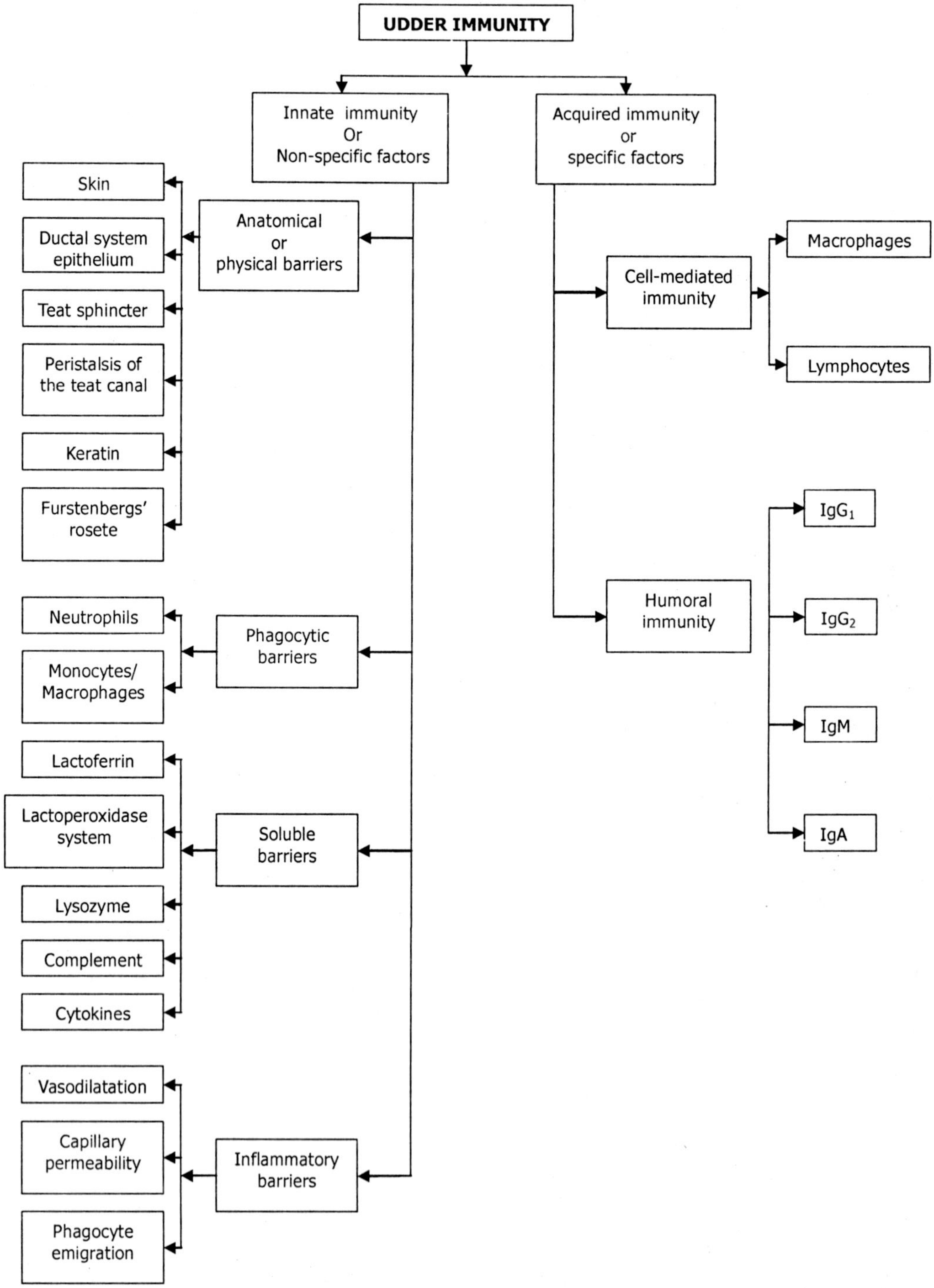

Figure 6.1 : Illustration of different types of mammary gland defense mechanisms.

A. Anatomical or Physical Defenses

The anatomical barrier comprised of the skin, duct system of the mammary gland and closing mechanisms of the teat sphincter and physical barrier include milking frequency. To maintain the integrity of the physical barriers, a cow need to be protected from trauma because teat lesions and injuries provides a site for pathogenic organism's entrance, growth and causing mastitis.

Skin

The teat skin is covered with a normal squamous cell epithelium and is hairless. It covers the underlying tissues, protects them from injury and extreme temperature. The sweat glands or sebaceous glands are absent on the teat skin of the cow (Kiro, 2005). Due to this, teat skin is very sensitive to drying off, and subsequently increase the risk of teat injury (sun burned, frost bite, chapped teats). It is well proven that teat ends with severe erosions or broken skin will have an increased risk of mastitis (Francesca, 2005).

Teat Canal or Streak Canal

The bovine teat canal is highly specialized in its unique function of preventing both leakage of milk and entry of bacteria and thereby plays a major role in the udder first defence line against mastitis. The teat canal is a longitudinally folded cylinder-shaped body opening, covered with approximately the same type of epithelium as the normal skin and surrounded with a net-like integrated musculoelastic system facilitates its opening and closure (Paulrud, 2005). The structures of the end of the teat and the papillary duct (teat canal) are marked as the *"Nipple barrier"* which represents the first line of defense of the mammary gland against the penetration of the pathogenic microorganism. Morphologically, the nipple barrier consists of: a papillary duct with its epithelium, *Fürstenberg's rosette*, an elastic connecting tissue and smooth muscle elements which surround the papillary duct, and structural and biochemical elements of the keratinous layer. The papillary duct (ductus papillaris) has a form of vertical straight lines coated by keratin. The main route of mastitis organisms to enter in the mammary gland is streak canal, through organisms enter to cause mastitis and therefore streak canal acts as the first line of defense. The streak canal acts as both a physical barrier and a source of antimicrobial sources (presence of keratin). The physical barrier is provided by the smooth muscle sphincter surround the teat end which inhibits bacterial penetration by maintaining tight closure and limiting bacterial entry through the teat orifice between milking. The teat canal is dilated during milking and after milking, on an average two hours are required for the teat sphincter to contract and close the streak canal (Schultze and Bright, 1983). The teat sphincter muscle tone varies considerably between individuals.

Increased susceptibility to mastitis in early involution or in the prepartum period, partially may, be due to changes in potency of the streak canal, including a reduction in length and an increase in diameter of the teat canal (Oldham *et al.*, 1991). The length and diameter of teat canal varies with age. The diameter of teat canal affects susceptibility to intramammary infection. Wider diameters being associated with increased bacterial penetration and increased incidence of mastitis (Motomura *et al.*, 1994). However Kartashova *et al.* (1992) reported no significant correlation between teat diameter and incidence of mastitis. The diameter of the teat canal itself has been shown to be associated with teat shape, with flat or inverted teats having a large diameter and pointed or round teats having a smaller diameter (Jorstad *et al.*, 1989). Motomura *et al.*, (1994) stated that large teat gradient (the base diameter minus the apex diameter of teat) is also associated with mastitis. Streak canal length also is an important factor in mastitis susceptibility with intramammary infections increasing in probability with decreasing streak canal length (Lacy-Hulbert and Hillerton, 1995). An inverse relationship between teat duct length and mastitis has been recognized by Grindal *et al.* (1991), but these authors considered that it was of secondary importance to peak flow rate. Quarters with a high peak flow rate showed a 12-folds increase in mastitis incidence compared to quarters with a low peak milk rate (Grindal and Hillerton, 1991). Machine milking is also change morphology of the teats, ultimately affect the udder immunity. Teats with >5% change in thickness have significantly increased teat duct colonization rates and IMI rates. Positive pressure milking increases PMNs content and decreases macrophages content of teat secretion. Some enzymes such as N-acetyl-β-D-glucosaminidase (NAGase) and lysozyme were decreased by positive pressure milking, the concentration of same enzymes are higher after no pulsation milking (Zecconi *et al.*, 2002). A better knowledge on the interaction between the teat apex immune defense mechanisms and the machine milking process is necessary to reduce the new infection rate of the mammary gland.

When the pathogenic organisms pass the teat orifice and colonize the teat canal then the next defense factor is the presence of *keratin,* antimicrobial substances within the teat canal. The teat canal is lined with keratin, which is crucial to the maintenance of the barrier function of the teat end. Teat keratin is a waxy material that is derived from stratified squamous epithelium of the teat canal. The epithelium is thicker in buffaloes than in cattle (Kumar, 1990) which provides an extra resistance against penetration of pathogens through epithelium. The importance of teat canal keratin in preventing intramammary infection was first suggested by Murphy in 1959. Teat keratin is a waxy material and it forms mesh like structure which enables trapping of invading bacteria, thus hindering their migration into the gland cistern (Hibbitt *et al.*, 1969). In fact, the keratin structure can completely occludes the teat duct during the dry period (Nickerson, 1987). The keratin is able to bind and immobilize most strains of non-encapsulated mastitis causing bacteria (Craven, 1985). The keratin layers in the teat canal are thicker in buffaloes in comparison with cows. Some fissures in the keratin layers have been reported through which organisms can enter into teat cistern. These fissures may be one of the factors responsible for intramammary infections in cows (Nickerson and Pankey, 1983). These fissures in buffaloes are narrower and smaller than cows, which could be one of the reasons for lower incidence of mastitis in buffaloes. The esterified and non-esterified fatty acids present in teat keratin, such as myristic , palmitoleic and linoleic acid are bacteriostatic (Treece, 1966). Keratin from mastitis resistant quarters contained high concentrations of lauric, myristic and palmitoleic acid, whereas stearic, linoleic and oleic acids are higher in concentration in mastitic susceptible quarters (Lojda *et al.*, 1980). The presence of sub clinical mastitis did not affect the lipid content of teat duct keratin (Miller *et al.*, 1992).

McDonald (1970) found that in mastitic quarters keratin layers are thinner, less dense and detached from the epithelium, compared with mastitis resistant quarters. Miller *et al.* (1991) demonstrated the importance of teat duct keratin in protection against mastitis, when removal of 70% of teat canal keratin significantly reduce the ability of cows to resist infection for two days following keratin removal. Inadvertent loss of teat duct keratin may result from incorrect administration of intramammary antibiotics when the syringe tip is inserted fully rather than partially into the teat canal (Boddie and Nickerson, 1986; Nickerson, 1987). Full insertion of antibiotic syringe tip may push portions of keratin colonized by bacteria into the teat cistern and induce intramammary infection. Full insertion of syringe tip can result in temporary dilatation of the teat duct lumen beyond the normal diameter (upto 8 times the normal diameter). Therefore, intramammary syringe should not be used with more than 3.1 mm diameter canula. A single use intramammary (IM) antibiotic tube with short tip (3-5mm) is recommended. The teat duct diameters range from 0.40 to 1.63mm for distal through proximal portions of the duct. Loss of teat duct keratin occurs during machine milking. Controversy about machine milking was fewer intramammary infections recorded with the group milked with pulsation despite of greater keratin loss (Capuco *et al.*, 1994). Approximately 40% of the keratin lining in teat canals of the Holstein dairy cattle is removed during the milking process, thus requiring continuous regeneration. A major factor allowing the invasion of pathogenic organisms into the mammary gland during the dry period may be that there is often a significant delay in the formation of a complete keratin plug in the teat canal (Godden *et al.*, 2003). Teat duct keratin also contain bactericidal cationic protein (e.g ubiquitin), which can bind electrostatically to mastitis pathogens (e.g. *Streptococcus agalactiae* and *Staphylococcus aureus*), alters the bacterial cell wall, thus rendering them more susceptible to osmotic pressure. The inability to maintain osmolarity causes lysis and death of the invading pathogens (Murphy and Stuart, 1953).

Furstenberg's Rosette

Fürstenberg's rosette is a fold of the mucous membrane at the boundary between the teat canal and the teat cistern. The mucosal epithelium of Furstenberg's rosette is stratified cuboidal or columnar and sub-epithelial connective tissue is thrown into folds which are rich in blood vessels. It has the shape of a fold of the mucous membrane, 0.7 to 1.2 mm in thickness, mechanically closing the teat canal proximally preventing spontaneous milk flow. Kumar (1990) reported 10 to 14 folds in rosette of buffaloes and 10 to 13 in cows. It has protective leukocytes population which are thought to leave the teat wall and enter the teat cistern via Furstenberg's rosette. It also contains bactericidal cationic proteins (e.g. ubiquitin).

Milking frequency

Milk is perfect medium for the growth of microorganisms. Accumulation of milk in the udder is also diminished the phagocytic activity of phagocytic cells. About 15 to 25% of the total amount of milk in the udder is not removed during milking; this milk is referred to as residual milk or complementary milk. Therefore, dairy farmer's advised to try the complete milking. Regular and complete flushing or milking support the accretion of large number of phagocytic cells in the udder and its phagocytic activity. Moreover, frequent milking helps to prevent mastitis because flushing helps to wash out mastitis causing bacteria colonizing the ductal lining and teat orifice. Milking frequency and complete milking is also affects the total milk yield e.g. milking twice daily yields atleast 40% more milk than milking once daily; milking 3 times a day may yield a 5 to 20% increase over twice-a-day milking; and milking 4 times a day may yield an additional 5 to 10%. Incomplete milking has been demonstrated to increase the risk of new IMI and severity of the disease in affected quarters. The large number of bacteria and toxins left in the gland after milking impair local mammary gland defense mechanisms leading to an exacerbation of mammary inflammation. On the other side completely different situation such as over-milking can definitely have an adverse effect on the teats condition, which in turn, may lead to an increased risk of new IMI (Edmondson, 2001). It is generally accepted that teats over-milked for 5 minutes show a higher level of damage to the mammary epithelial lining and more extravasations of red blood cells (McDonald, 1971). Over-milking for a long period removes more keratin and causes teat sinus injury (Edmondson, 2001). Extreme periods of over-milking are known to increase teat damage, either at the orifice or to the mucous membrane lining the teat sinus.

Cellular factors

Mastitis causing organisms that are able to overwhelm the anatomical defense must escape the antibacterial activities of the mammary gland microenvironment in order to establish the IMI. Neutrophils, macrophages, lymphocytes, erythrocytes and epithelial cells are found in normal bovine milk (Table 6.1). Leukocytes are more abundant in the tissue at the distal end of the teat cistern and at the junction with the teat canal Furstenberg's rosette (Nickerson *et al.*, 1983). Cellular defense mechanism is act as *"second line of defense"* of the mammary gland. Percentages of each cell type vary depending on the stage of lactation, health of the udder and milk secretion. In milk from normal uninfected lactating gland the macrophage is the predominant cell type (35%), followed by neutrophils (26%), lymphocytes (24%) and epithelial cells (15%) (Miller *et al.*, 1991; Paape and Tucker, 1966). Lee *et al.* (1980) reported much lower values for neutrophils (3%) and epithelial cells (2%), and higher values for macrophages (79%). Because of the presence of epithelial cells in milk, Paape *et al.* (1963) coined the phrase *"milk somatic cells"*, which is now internationally accepted terminology when referring to cells in milk. The term milk somatic cells include neutrophils, macrophages, lymphocytes, erythrocytes and epithelial cells. Erythrocytes can be found at concentrations ranging from 0 to 1.51 X 10^6/ml (Paape and Weinland, 1988). During early and late lactation the percentage of neutrophils tends to increase while the percentage of lymphocytes decreases (McDonald and Anderson, 1981). The proportion among various cell types in milk changes drastically during inflammation. The PMN increases with severity of mastitis and occasionally can approach 100% of the total somatic cells (Schalm *et al.*, 1971). In chronic mastitis, the number of mononuclear cells may increase (Schalm *et al.*, 1971). The somatic cell count (SCC) is a measure of the number of these cells per milliliter of milk. Total milk SCC from non-infected glands of cattle ranging from 1 to 3 X 10^5 cells per ml and the predominant cell is the macrophage, while during clinical mastitis this can rise to many millions per milliliter of milk (Nickerson, 1985). Sub clinically infected quarters contain 750,000 cells per ml. SCC tend to be slightly increased during early and late lactation (Sheldrake *et al.*, 1983). Total milk cell count in uninfected glands at the beginning of the dry period are usually <1 X 10^5 cells/ml (Concha *et al.*, 1978), but by day 7 of the dry period cell numbers can be as high as 2 X 10^5 cells/ml (Lascelles and Lee, 1978). In most uninfected uninflammed quarters, SCC is appreciably <1 X 10^5 cells/ml, with a low proportion of neutrophils. During involution of the gland neutrophils are the predominant cell type (60%) during the first 4 weeks after cesation of milking, followed by macrophages (25%), and lymphocytes (15%) (Miller *et al.*, 1990). During the first two weeks before parturition lymphocytes predominate (60%), followed by macrophages (30%) and neutrophils (10%) (McDonald and Anderson, 1981). At parturition SCC are usually higher than one million per ml, and decrease to 100,000 cells/ml in the 7 to 10 days postpartum (Jensen and Eberhart, 1981). The normal composition of milk somatic cells varies with the type of secretion or lactation cycle (Table 6.1).

Table 6.1 : Composition of somatic cells in different mammary secretions.

Type of mammary secretion	Milk somatic cells (%)			
	PMN	Macrophage	Lymphocytes	Epithelial cells
Milk	3	80	16	2
Colostrum	61	35	4	0
Dry gland secretion	3	89	7	1

Inspite of the presence of considerable numbers of immune cells in the local mammary gland environment, it has been suggested that the mammary gland is generally immunologically compromised when compared to the rest of the body (Hurley *et al.*, 1990). Upto such extent it may be due to the reduced phagocytic and viability of polymorphonuclear (PMN) cells in the milk compared to the blood and other body tissue. The milk somatic cells regulate both innate and acquired immune responses (Sordillo *et al.*, 1997; Sordillo and Streicher, 2002; Soltys and Quinn, 1999).

Neutrophils

Polymorphonuclear neutrophils (PMNs) forms the *first line of cellular defense* against that penetrates the physical barrier of the teat canal. The PMN and macrophages constitute professional phagocytes of bovine mammary gland. The PMN is characterized by a polymorphic segmented (multilobulated) nucleus, numerous cytoplasmic granules that provide constituents for killing bacteria, large stores of glycogen for energy and a highly convoluted surface that is used for phagocytosis of bacteria and formation of intracellular phagocytic vacuoles (Paape *et al.*, 2003). The multilobulated nucleus is important because it allows PMN to line up its nuclear lobes in a straight line, allowing rapid migration (diapedesis) between endothelial cells. Neutrophils usually comprise <8% of the cells in milk and secretion from fully involuted glands, but in colostrum and early involution secretion, they may comprise 40 to 80% of milk cells (Lee and Outteridge, 1976). Jensen and Eberhart (1981) reported that the proportion and concentration of neutrophils was high initially at drying off and was shown to reduce from the 2 to 4 week of the dry period. During mastitis or involution, the PMN are the first cells to enter the mammary gland alveoli (Kelly, 2000). The PMN acts rapidly but only for short periods in the early stages of IMI. These nonspecific cells migrate from the blood to the mammary gland in response to a variety of inflammatory mediators such as cytokines, complement and the prostaglandins (Baumann and Graudie, 1994; Persson *et al.*, 1993; Lin *et al.*, 1995). Neutrophils reach to the mammary gland by the diapedesis, where they survive for 1 to 2 days. The PMN diapedesis can occur within one hour of infection and within 4 hours large number can be presented in the milk. However, the diapedesis of PMNs into infected gland is delayed in recently fresh cows, potentially explaining greater susceptibility of cows in early lactation to peracute coliform mastitis. Neutrophils exert their bactericidal effect through a respiratory burst (phagocytosis). In addition to their phagocytic capabilities, neutrophils are a source of small antibacterial peptides, called the *"defensins"*, which are able to kill the mastitis causing organisms (Selsted *et al.*, 1993). It has reported that four important physiological functions of neutrophils in the mammary defense viz. chemotaxis, diapedesis, phagocytosis and finally intracellular killing (Burvenich *et al.*, 1994).

When the mastitis causing bacteria enter into the teat canal, there is production of chemoattractants, which increase the diapedesis of leukocytes at the site of infection to eliminate the pathogenic bacteria. If somatic cells move rapidly from the blood stream and are able to eliminate the inflammatory stimuli (bacteria), then recruitment of leukocytes ceases, and SCC returns to healthful levels (Sordillo *et al.*, 1997). If bacteria are able to survive this immediate host response, then the inflammation continues, resulting in SCC diapedesis between adjacent mammary secretory cells toward the alveolar lumen (Capuco *et al.*, 1986). Prolonged diapedesis of leukocytes causes damage to mammary parenchyma tissue, which leads to fibrosis and decreased production of milk (Sordillo and Nickerson, 1988). Neutrophils promote tissue injury and disturbed mammary function via reactive oxygen metabolite generation (the respiratory burst) and granular enzyme release (degranulation) (Miller *et al.*, 1993; Kehrli and Shuster, 1994). Peroxynitrite, produced during inflammation, has recently been implicated as a major cytotoxic agent. Peroxynitrite ($ONOO^-$) is the reaction product of superoxide (O^{2-}) and nitric oxide (NO). PMN cytoplasm contains numerous bactericidal granules that are used by PMN in killing of bacteria (Figure 6.2). The azurophilic or primary granules have antibacterial activity due to presence of peroxidase (Klebanoff, 1970). Peroxidase in the presence of hydrogen peroxide and halide ions kill engulfed bacteria. Bovine azurophilic granules also contain less amount of lysozyme (Rausch and Moore, 1975). Specific or secondary granules are peroxidase negative and appear during the myelocyte stage (Jain, 1986). Third "novel" peroxidase negative granules are larger than primary and secondary granules, first appear in myelocytes and are the predominant granules in mature bovine PMN (Baggiolini *et al.*, 1985). These granules contain lactoferrin and potent microbicidal arginine-rich peptides which are structurally distinct from defensins termed as *"bactenecins"* which efficiently kills several Gram-positive and Gram-negative bacteria in-vitro. "Novel" granules are also the exclusive store of powerful oxygen independent bactericidal compounds called "*β-defensins*". Recently, the isolation and characterization of a novel tridecapeptide amide from bovine neutrophils was reported. Termed "*indolicidin*", this cationic peptide was shown to be unusually rich in tryptophan, and to have potent bactericidal activity against *E. coli* and *S. aureus*.

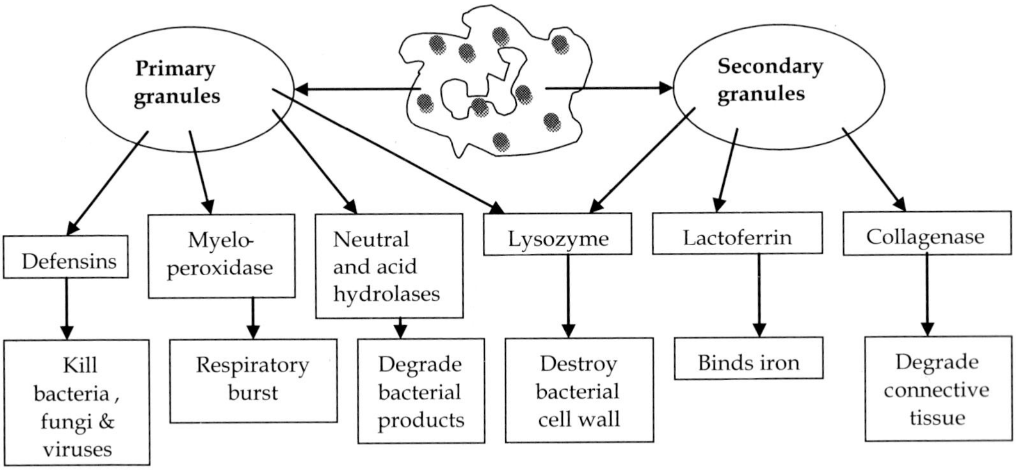

Figure 6.2 : The contents of cytoplasmic granules and their function in neutrophils. (Adopted from Tizard, 1977).

Mastitic milk is characteristically rich in PMNs but milk PMNs are less effective phagocytes than blood PMNs (Paape *et al.*, 2003). A negative correlation has been reported between the presence of clinical mastitis and the ability of milk to support phagocytosis. This reduced phagocytic activity of milk PMN is due to the many factors like- I) lower energy reserves in the form of stored glycogen (Rainard and Riollet, 2003), II) ingestion of milk fat and coating of the neutrophili with casein (Hoeben *et al.*, 1997), III) a decrease in the supply of hydrolytic enzymes within the PMNs following ingestion of fat and casein, IV) low levels of opsonins and complements in milk (Kenny *et al.*, 1995). Milk PMNs contain 38% less glycogen than blood PMN (Newbould, 1973). Diapedesis utilizes the energy reserves of a PMN which are needed for efficient phagocytosis and killing of invading mastitis causing organisms. Talos *et al.* (1975) have also been observed that blood glucose level was low in the blood of cattle 10 days after parturition, which is limiting factor associated with the phagocytosis of *S. aureus* by PMN leukocytes of milk. Diapedesis of PMN across mammary epithelium *in-vitro* reduces reactive oxygen species (ROS) production of PMN, and also contributes to reduced bactericidal activity of milk PMN (Smits *et al.*, 1999). A striking change in morphology occurs when PMN leave blood and enter milk. These milk PMNs after reaching the mammary gland ingest milk fat globules, casein and other milk components indiscriminately that result in large intracellular membrane bound vacuoles. Internalization of cell membrane leads to loss of pseudopodia and cell rounding. Cytoplasmic granules migrate and fuse to vacuoles forming phagolysosomes. Milk PMNs also have reduced numbers of secondary and "novel" granules compared to blood PMN. This loss of membrane and cytoplasmic granules results in diminishment of PMN phagocytic and bactericidal activities. Casein exerts an inhibitory effect on both phagocytosis and antimicrobial activity of PMN due to interfering with the oxygen radical generating pathway and depressing the oxidative burst (Rainard and Riollet, 2003).

It has also been reported that indiscriminate use of antibiotics alters neutrophil function for generating sufficient amount of reactive oxygen species (ROS) (Hoeben *et al.*, 1997). Oxidative burst activity of PMN is influenced by therapeutic agents at concentrations observed after intramammary treatment. Enrofloxacin increases chemuliminescence activity whereas neomycin, lincomycin, dihydrostreptomycin, oxytetracycline, danofloxacin, penicillin, ceftiofur, spiramycin, erythromycin and chloramphenicol reduce oxidative burst activity of bovine PMN (Hoeben *et al.*, 1997; Hoeben *et al.*, 1998; Paape *et al.*, 1990). Glucocorticoids shows no adverse effect on oxidative burst activity of PMN at therapeutic concentrations (Hoeben *et al.*, 1998). Because functional activity of milk PMN is already impaired as a result of ingestion of milk components, use of antibiotics that will not cause further impairment of PMN function becomes more critical in the ability to clear invading bacteria from the mammary gland (Paape *et al.*, 2003). Therefore, choice of antibiotic should depend not only on the sensitivity of the organism to the drug, but also to the effect of the drug on host defense mechanisms. During periparturient period the number and function of PMNs altered or impaired (Heyneman *et al.*, 1990; Cai *et al.*, 1994; Zecconi *et al.*, 1994). During the periparturient period, the decrease in neutrophil activity is associated with a higher incidence of mastitis (Yamaguchi *et al.*, 1999). At this time the number of immature neutrophils in the bovine blood decreases, while the number of mature neutrophils in the blood and mammary secretions is lowest. The PMNs also exhibit impaired function of major defense related activities, such as phagocytosis, respiratory burst activity, superoxide anion production, random cellular migration, and chemotaxis, around parturition (Kehrli *et al.*, 1989). Chemotactic neutrophil migration from blood could be impaired further due to the decreased production of cells expressing the adhesion receptor CD62L (L-selectin) that is necessary for penetration through the endothelium to sites of infection (Lee and Kehrli, 1998).

Macrophages

Once monocytes leave blood and enter tissue they mature and become macrophages. Macrophages are major cell type in milk, secretion of the involuted udder and mammary tissue. During bacterial pathogenesis, macrophages may serve to facilitate either innate or acquired immune responses. A considerable population of macrophages exists beneath the alveolar and ductal epithelium. During lactation, the proportion of macrophages is highest (68%) in the early postpartum period and lowest (21%) in late lactation (Park *et al.,* 1992). Similar to neutrophils, the non specific functions of macrophages are phagocytosis of invading bacteria and destroy them with proteases and ROS. Macrophages are less active than milk neutrophils at phagocytosis, and both milk cell types are less efficient than their blood counterparts (Mullan *et al.,* 1985). Although a direct defensive role of the milk macrophage is doubted, they are potential antigen presenting cells, and they are implicated in the detection of the inflammatory response. The mammary gland macrophage in milk functions as an "early detection device" in the initiation of the inflammatory process. The phagocytic rate of these cells can be increased dramatically in the presence of opsonic antibodies against particular pathogens (Magnusson, 1999). However, mammary macrophage numbers tend to be lower during inflammation and they posses fewer Fc receptors. Therefore, the ability of macrophages to secrete substances that facilitate the migration and bactericidal activities of neutrophils is believed to be of great importance to the non specific defense of the mammary gland than acting as professional phagocytes. These cells are long lived, and play several roles, from clearing the infection to repairing tissue (Kenny *et al.,* 1995). When macrophages recognize bacteria, they secrete proinflammatory cytokines e.g. TNF-α and IL-1β. Stimulating the bactericidal activity of neutrophils and also producing prostaglandins and leukotriens, which increase the local inflammatory response (Boulanger *et al.,* 2003; Stein *et al.,* 2003; Banner *et al.,* 2004; Kampen and Mallard, 1997). Besides neutrophils, macrophages are important factors of the inflammatory response. The PMN population subsides after the elimination of invading bacteria and followed by a predominantly macrophages influx. Macrophages do not only replace neutrophils but also actively participate in their removal. The rapid elimination of neutrophils by macrophages is essential to minimize inflammatory derived injury to the mammary secretory epithelium, which can result in scaring and can lead to a permanent loss of quarter and subsequently decrease in milk production (Paape *et al.,* 2003; Burvenich *et al.,* 2003). Bovine mammary macrophages bear the receptors for IgG_1 and IgG_2 (Rossi and Kiesel, 1977). Bovine macrophages express mCD14 on their surface and are potential source of sCD14 (Sohn *et al.,* 2004). Macrophages also play a role in the development of specific immune responses through antigen processing and presentation in association with major histocompatibility complex (MHC) class II antigens (Politis *et al.*, 1992). The phagocytic and bactericidal activities of these cells are especially reduced during the periparturient period (Paape *et al.*, 1981). This decrease could be mediated by a decrease in IgM, which facilitates phagocytosis by both macrophages and neutrophils, and MHC-II expression by macrophage is decreased during the periparturient period, which causes poor antigen presentation and results in weaker specific immune response from mammary gland lymphocytes (Fitzpatrick, 1992). The quality and quantity of phagocytic cells are important in the normal defense system of the cow (Daley *et al.*, 1991). The antibacterial functions of phagocytic cells have attracted a lot of attention, because they play important role in the control of mastitis.

Lymphocytes

Lymphocytes comprise the non-phagocytic cells of the mammary gland. They are the only cells of the immune system that recognize a variety of antigenic structures through membrane receptors, which define the specificity, diversity, and the immune system memory characteristics (Boyso *et al.*, 2007). Lymphocytes can be divided into two distinct subsets viz. T-lymphocytes and B-lymphocytes, that differ in function and protein products. Depending on their T-cell receptors, T-lymphocytes can be subdivided into ab T-lymphocytes and gd T-lymphocytes, where both T-helper cells ($CD4^+$) and T-cytotoxic/suppressor cells ($CD8^+$) express the ab T-cell receptors. Depending on stage of lactation and tissue lactation, the percentages of these cells can vary significantly. The concentration of lymphocytes in dry secretions is about 3000 to 6000 times that in normal milk (Lee *et al.*, 1980). The proportion of B-lymphocytes and T-lymphocytes in dry secretions is 28% and 47% respectively and, in milk 29% and 45% respectively (Concha *et al.*, 1980). The proportion of lymphocytes increased during involution and then decrease around parturition (Jensen and Eberhart, 1981).

The T-lymphocytes are responsible for cell mediated immune response by producing lymphokines that act as chemoatractants for PMN and macrophages and for stimulating leukocyte microbicidal activity. Targowski and Berman (1975) suggest that bovine mammary gland tissue lymphocytes are responsible for priming the udder against subsequent antigenic stimulation. The main function of T-helper cells is the production of cytokines. After recognition of specific antigens bound to MHC class-II molecules on antigen presenting cells, $CD4^+$ cells become activated and start to produce and release cytokines (Roitt, Brostoff and Male, 1998). The relative proportion of $CD4^+$ cells from the total T-lymphocyte population of the mammary gland contrasts with that in peripheral blood (Shafer-Weaver and Sordillo, 1996; Park *et al.*,

1992). T-cytotoxic cells recognize specific antigens in conjunction with MHC class-I molecules on the cell surface of the infected cells. Therefore, cytotoxic cells may act as scavengers, removing old or damaged secretory cells, the presence of which could increase the susceptibility of mammary gland to infections (Taylor *et al.*, 1994). The $CD4^+$ lymphocytes are the predominant phenotype in both tissue and secretions of healthy mammary glands; resulting in a $CD4^+ : CD8^+$ ratio is <1. Cells obtained from blood have a higher ratio of $CD4^+$ to $CD8^+$, which is consistently >1 (Sordillo *et al.*, 1997). The $CD4^+ : CD8^+$ ratio in mammary secretions shifts to >1 at drying off, stages >1 during the dry period and shifts back to <1 just before calving (Asai *et al.*, 1998). However, the functional significance of the CD8+ dominance is not fully understood. One hypothesis is that mammary $CD8^+$ T-cells is an activated cell type, different from blood $CD8^+$ T-cells, with a potential role in maintaining the integrity of epithelial linings by removal of damaged or infected cells (Taylor *et al.*, 1994). During acute and chronic *Staphylococcus aureus* mastitis, $CD4^+$ T cells become the dominating sub-population of T-lymphocytes (Rivas *et al.*, 2000; Riollet *et al.*, 2001). The functional significance of the elevated frequency of $CD8^+$ over $CD4^+$ lymphocytes in milk and mammary tissues has not been defined thoroughly. However, it is well established that $CD8^+$ cells can exert either cytotoxic or suppressor function. It is very difficult to distinguish T-suppressor cells from T-cytotoxic cells (Tizard, 2000). The $CD8^+$ lymphocytes immediately following parturition are of the suppressor type but from mid to late lactation are more of the type that have a cytotoxic nature (Sordillo *et al.*, 1997).

The function of γδ T-lymphocytes are primarily associated with the protection of epithelial surfaces. The cytotoxic ability of γδ T-lymphocytes suggests that they may be able to destroy altered epithelial cells (Mackay and Hein, 1991). Pollock and Welsh (2002) suggest that γδ T-lymphocytes can act as antigen presenting cells and produce an array of cytokines, and that they are cytotoxic to infected cells, but not necessarily MHC-restricted. These cells may also play a role in infectious diseases and therefore provide an important line of defense against bacterial infections. The number of γδ T-cells decreases significantly in the mammary gland during times of increased susceptibility to mastitis (Shafer-Weaver *et al.*, 1996) suggests that these lymphocytes may constitute an essential line of defense against the bacteria causing mastitis. β-lymphocytes have two important functions as they can both respond to specific antigens and act as a antigen presenting cells. β-lymphocytes recognize specific antigens through their surface receptors, which are antibodies, and become activated when the antigen has bound to the receptor. Upon presentation of the processed antigen to T-helper lymphocytes, IL-2 is secreted by the T-lymphocytes, which in turn induce proliferation and differentiation of the β-lymphocytes into either plasma cells or memory cells. The primary role of plasma cells is to produce large amounts of antigen specific antibodies which are a soluble form of the receptor molecule.

NK-cells

The lymphocytes consist of T- and B-cells together with a population of lymphoid cells, which do not consistently carry markers of either T- or B-cells, the so called *NK or Null cells*. These cells are large, granular lymphocytes that have cytotoxic activity independent of MHC and possess Fc receptors that enable these cells to participate in antibody-dependent, cell mediated cytotoxicity. Once the destruction of target cells is mediated by degranulation of granules containing perforin. These cells also can secrete inflammatory mediators, such as tumor necrosis factor (TNF)-α. NK-cells can destroy both Gram-positive and Gram-negative bacteria. NK-cells are critical to the removal of intracellular pathogens (Rainard and Riollet, 2006). For this reason, they could be important in the prevention of mastitis (Shafer-Weaver and Sordillo, 1996). Lymphoid cells that are isolated from mammary gland with NK-like activity also exhibit a novel antibacterial property (Sordillo *et al.*, 1991). Bovine NK-like cells ($CD2^+$, $CD3^-$, T Lc) express bactericidal activity against *S. aureus* upon stimulation with IL-2 (Sordillo *et al.*, 2002). The mechanism by which these cells mediated bactericidal activity is not fully elicited. Neutrophils and macrophages are the functional phagocytes of the body (Paape *et al.*, 2002), whereas NK-cells recognise cells that fail to express major histocompatibility complex (MHC) class molecules, and lyse these cells through various killing mechanisms (Paape *et al.*, 2000). There is no more study on the changes in NK-cell population during the periparturient period, but the potent bactericidal activity of these cells makes them worthy of future study.

Epithelial cells

For many years, it was considered that the main cell type found in the milk of healthy quarters was epithelial in origin (Schalm *et al.*, 1971). However, in 1980, it was reported that no secretory epithelial cells from teat and lactiferous sinuses of dairy cows were capable of ingesting milk fat globules and casein, and the ingested milk constituents are partly digested. The mammary epithelial cells are able to produce a variety of inflammatory mediators such as cytokine, chemokines, host defense peptides and arachdonic acid metabolites. The mammary epithelial cells may play a protective role in prevention of infection via ingestion and possible digestion of phagocytosed microbes, the opposite could also occur. The epithelial cells play a important role in neutrophil recruitment to the infection site. Adhesion of bacteria to epithelial cells as well as the interaction of bacterial toxins with them induces the synthesis of TNF-α, IL-6 and the chemokine IL-8 (Rainard and Riollet, 2003). Epithelial cells may also have phagocytic capabilities as an added defense against bacteria during the dry period (Nickerson, 1989).

B. Soluble Factors

The soluble factors of the mammary defense mechanism are associated with cellular factors. Each factor modifies the functions of the other factors involved in the mammary gland defense mechanism. These soluble factors can be divided into non-specific and specific factors. Milk itself contains several non-specific antibacterial components called *"lactenins"*. These factors include lactoferrin, lactoperoxidase system, lysozyme, b-defensins, complement system and cytokines etc. While immunoglobulins function as the soluble effector of the specific immune response.

Lactoferrin

Bovine lactoferrin is a monomeric metal (iron) binding glycoprotein synthesized as a 708-amino acid protein with a 19-amino acid signal peptide (Pierce *et al.*, 1991), which exerts several functions related to non-specific immune responses. It was first isolated from cow,s milk and subsequently from human milk, which is produced by epithelial cells, macrophages and neutrophils. Neutrophils which contain lactoferrin in their secondary and large granules, can account for about 5% of lactoferrin in milk during acute mastitis. The concentration of lactoferrin in bovine milk from normal quarter in very less amount (0.02 to 0.35 mg/ml of milk) compared with human milk (1 to 2 mg/ml) or sow's milk (0.5mg/ml) (Rainard and Riollet, 2006). Bovine colostrum contains very high concentration of lactoferrin (2 to 5mg/ml). The lactoferrin concentration increases with process of mammary involution with maximum concentration (<10 to 100mg/ml) attain after 1 to 2 weeks of involution (Welty *et al.*, 1976, Schanbacher *et al.*, 1993) (Table 6.2). The concentration of lactoferrin in mammary glands derived from *Staphylococcal* clinical mastitis is significantly higher than in normal mammary glands (Lomine *et al.*, 2005). Kawai *et al.* (1999) found that mean lactoferrin concentration was significantly higher in *M. bovis* or *S. aureus* infected quarter milk samples than that of quarters infected with coagulase negative staphylococci (CNS). In *E. coli* mastitis, lactoferrin concentration was significantly lower in milk from peracute mastitis than that from cows with acute mastitis. This decreased level of lactoferrin in peracute *E. coli* mastitis may be associated with the progress of inflammation in the early phase of mastitis.

Lactoferrin has an important function in the mammalian host defence mechanism (Figure 6.3). Lactoferrin has many proposed biological functions but it was first known for iron chelating properties, the basis of two of its activities, bacteriostasis and protection against oxygen radicals catalyzed by free iron (Legrand *et al.*, 2004). Lactoferrin is bacteriostatic *in vitro* for *S. aureus, Psedomonas aeruginosa, S. albus* (Masson and Heremans, 1966), *Bacillus stearotbermophilus,* and *Bacillus subtills* (Reiter and Brock, 1975). Bacteria which have high iron requirements are susceptible to the bacteriostatic activity of lactoferrin. One molecule of lactoferrin binds to two molecules of iron and when not fully saturated with iron, it inhibits a range of microorganisms in the presence of bicarbonate that require iron for their growth. In addition to binding iron, lactoferrin can directly kill certain bacterial strains and weaken adherence to the cellular membrane (Arnold *et al.,* 1977). Among mastitis causing pathogens, *E. coli* are the most susceptible followed by *S. aureus* which have the iron requirement for growth. Withholding iron from bacteria may enhance killing by phagocytes by preventing the production of dimutase, a bacterial enzyme that inactivates superoxide radicals. While *S. agalactiae* is resistant because it use lactoferrin as an iron source. The main function of lactoferrin is to protect the mammary gland against infection by coliforms, especially in the involution stage, due to the activation of phagocytosis and the complement system (Lee *et al.,* 2004). In addition, the bacteriostatic activities of lactoferrin can be abolished in the presence of citrate, a buffer produced by mammary epithelial cells which chelates iron and making available to the organisms (Hibbit *et al.,* 2002). In the mammary gland, efficacy of lactoferrin is negatively correlated with citrate content of milk (Bishop *et al.* 1976); citrate concentration varies greatly depending on the time of lactation. It is at its highest after parturition and during mid-lactation (2.38 mg/ml), and at its lowest in the dry period (about 0.50 mg/ml) i.e. during the dry period concentrate of citrate in the mammary secretion is low and lactoferrin is high (Green *et al.,* 2002). Bicarbonate, which is required for the binding of iron by lactoferrin, mole per mole, can overcome the effect of citrate especially during the dry-cow period, when citrate is absorbed from the udder secretion to blood, while bicarbonate diffuses from blood to the udder secretion. The molar ratio of citrate to apo-lactoferrin decreases with udder involution and increases with lactogenesis. The molar ratio has been found to be more important in the inhibition of the growth of Gram-negative bacteria *in vitro* than the absolute concentration of either component. Thus it is considered that the role of lactoferrin in the defense of mammary gland is more important during the dry period than lactation, especially against coliforms (Sordillo *et al.,* 1997). Evidence from a number of studies indicates that the antimicrobial activity of lactoferrin is more complex than simple Fe chelation. Lactoferrin has direct bactericidal activity and can kill susceptible bacteria by a mechanism distinct from sequestering of Fe, which is mediated through peptides known as *lactoferricins.* The smallest size of lactoferricins renders access to target sites on microbial surfaces easier than it is for native lactoferrin, which may explain the superior bactericidal effectiveness of lactoferricin as compared to native lactoferrin. Bacteriostatic and bacteriocidal activities of lactoferrin and its fragments are less efficient during lactation, but are likely to be significant in fully involuted mammary gland. Besides antibacterial activities, lactoferrin is endowed with immunomodulating and anti-inflammatory properties. Bovine lactoferrin also is able to reduce the endotoxin induced response of inflammatory cells. Iron deficient or iron free lactoferrin is called as *'apolactoferrin'* which also is iron binding glycoprotein. It has been reported that the antibacterial activity of apolactoferrin is greater than that of lactoferrin (Batish *et al.*, 1988). Apolactoferrin alter bacterial cell membrane function, or integrity and permeability, directly damaging the outer membrane of Gram-negative bacteria by binding to lipopolysaccharide endotoxin (LPS) and blocking its detrimental effects. The bacterial killing happened through osmotic damage, and the destabilization of the bacterial cell wall is thought to occur through a non-specific binding of calcium and magnesium to lactoferrin (Ellison *et al.*, 1988). LPS release was blocked by iron saturation of lactoferrin, and exogenous calcium and magnesium blocked the activity of lactoferrin as well (Ellison *et al.*, 1988). The bacteriostatic form of lactoferrin is either apo-lactoferrin or partly saturated lactoferrin, while the fully Fe^{3+} -saturated form has no antimicrobial activity (Arnold *et al.*, 1982). Approximately 6-8% of lactoferrin in milk is iron-saturated, which means that most of the lactoferrin in milk is present in the apo-form.

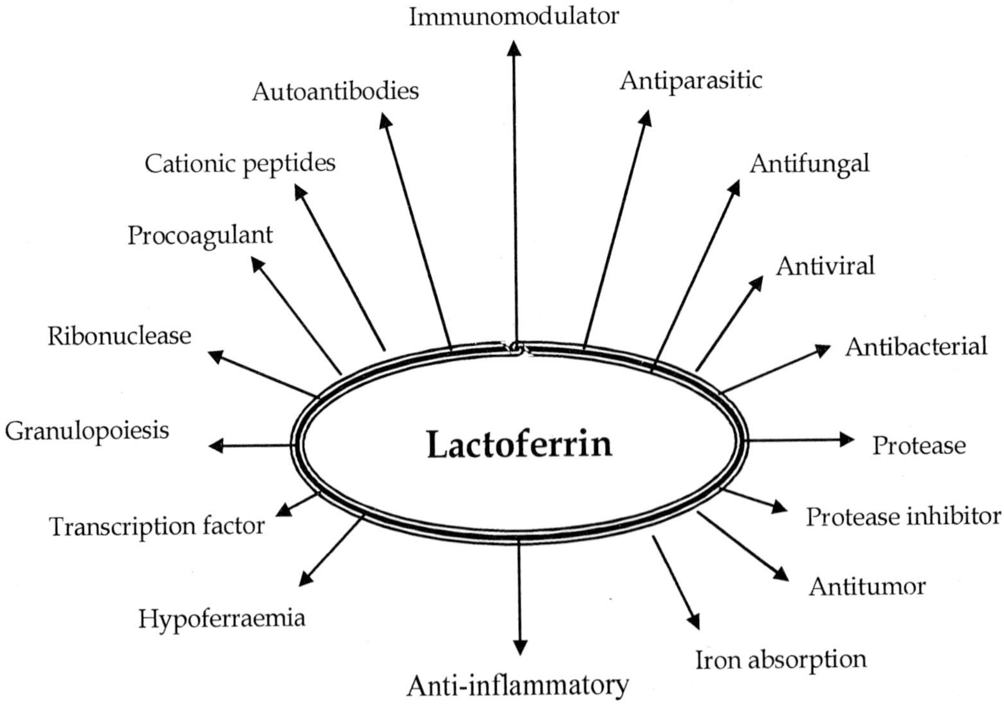

Figure 6.3: Functions of lactoferrin.

Table 6.2 : Concentration of lactoferrin in healthy and mastitic cows milk.

Lactation stage	Lactoferrin concentration (mg/ml)	Reference
Immediately after parturition	about 2.4	Nonnecke & Smith 1984
Lactating cow	0.02 to 0.35	Welty *et al.*, 1976
After 2 to 4 days of involution	0.52 to 3.0	Welty *et al.*, 1976
After 5 to 7 days of involution	2.6 to 17.8	Welty *et al.*, 1976
After 10 days of involution	<10 to 100	Welty *et al.*, 1976, Schanbacher *et al.*, 1993
Cows with sub-clinical mastitis	0.2 to 1.2	Kawai *et al.*, 1999, Hagiwara *et al.*, 2003
Cows with clinical mastitis	0.3 to 2.3	Harmon *et al.*, 1976, Kawai *et al.*,1999

Transferrin

Transferrin is another iron binding protein which is found in milk. Bovine milk contains low concentration of transferrin, from 1mg/ml in colostrum to 0.02-0.04mg/ml in milk compared to 4-5mg/ml in serum (Sanchez *et al.*, 1988). Transferrin is not synthesized in the bovine mammary gland, it comes from blood serum, by transcytosis in the normal gland and through exudation of plasma during mastitis. It is evidence by the study of Sanchez (1988), transferrin:albumin ratio is 4 times greater in colostrum than in mature or mastitic milk, suggesting a specific transport of transferrin from blood to milk. Transferrin may provide a first iron chelating bacteriostatic agent to milk, before lactoferrin concentrations augment. But lactoferrin bind iron 300 folds better than tranferrin.

Lactoperoxidase

Lactoperoxidase is a basic glycoprotein that has a molecular weight of 78,000 and contains a heme group. The enzyme has an iron content between 0.068 to 0.071% in combination with certain co-factor, forms a potent antimicrobial system. Lactoperoxidase in the presence of thiocyanate and hydrogen peroxide form the "lactoperoxidase system" (lacroperoxidase-thiocyanate-hydrogen peroxide system). Lactoperoxidase system is bacteriostatic for Gram-positive bacteria such as *S. aureus* and *streptococci*, and bactericidal for Gram-negative bacteria such as coliform. Lactoperoxidase is produced in small concentration by mammary epithelial cells. Bovine milk contains about 30mg peroxidase/ml (Reiter, 1985). It constitutes about 1% of the total serum proteins. In colostrum, the lactoperoxidase content is very low, but increases rapidly after 4 to 5 days postpartum. Thiocyanate concentrations vary with the feeding plane of the animal, feed containing the thiocyanate precursors (1 to 10ppm). Hydrogen peroxide produced by invading bacteria such as streptococci (2 to 4 ppm) or by oxidation of ascorbic acid. The low oxygen tension of the mammary gland can inhibit the production of peroxides, thus probably limiting the effectiveness of the peroxidase system against mastitis causing pathogens. The antimicrobial property of the lactoperoxidase system is based upon inhibition of vital bacterial metabolic enzymes due to oxidation by hypothiocyanate.

Lysozyme (N-acetylmuramyl hydrolase)

Lysozyme is bactericidal protein and that functions by destroying peptidoglycans from the cell wall of the Gram-positive bacteria as well as the outer membrane of Gram-negative bacteria. Lysozyme, famously discovered by Alexander Fleming as a component of his own nasal secretions, is found in other secreted fluids (milk, saliva, egg white and blood) as well and destroys the cell wall of Gram-negative and Gram-positive bacteria through an enzymatic mechanism. Bovine milk normally contains very low level (0.13 mg/ml) of lysozyme, compared with 0.1mg/ml in woman milk. During mastitis lysozyme concentration is higher (1-2 mg/ml) compared to normal milk. Lysozyme may be derived from blood or locally synthesized in the mammary gland (Nickerson, 1985). During inflammation, leukocytes appear to be the source of lysozyme (Persson *et al.*, 1992). There are two types of lysozyme. One type is found in the hen egg white and is known as *chicken type* or *c-lysozyme*. The other type is found in the goose egg white and is known as *goose type* or *g-lysozyme*. Cow,s milk may contain both c- and g-lysozymes. Lysozyme possesses antimicrobial activity against a number of mastitis causing organisms. It cleaves the glycosidic bond between N-acetylemuramic acid and N-acetylglucosamine in bacterial peptidoglycans, which constitute the major part of the bacterial cell wall of Gram-positive bacteria. Gram-positive bacteria are generally more susceptible because they have a much simple cell wall containing a more amount (90%) of peptidoglycan. Staphylococci, on the other hand, are more resistant. This is probably due to the presence of teichoic acid in their cell wall. In Gram-negative bacteria the peptidoglycan concentration in the cell wall is much lower (5-10%) and it is protected by an outer layer of lipopolysaccharide, which prevents lysozyme from reaching its substrate. Lysozyme, in combination with complement and secretory IgA, shows significant bactericidal activity to *E. coli* (*in-vitro*) in porcine and human milk, in comparison with bovine milk (Reiter, 1985). Because bovine milk contains only a small concentration of IgA and considerable less lysozyme than human milk. Lysozyme may enhance the binding of lactoferrin to bacterial cell wall. Lysozyme is not considered a significant defense of the bovine mammary gland.

Cytokines

Soluble factors released by lymphocytes are termed *"lymphokines"* and those from monocytes and macrophages are termed *"monokines"*, although they are now more commonly given the collective term *"cytokines"*. Cytokines are often referred to as hormones because they are usually produced transiently and locally with potent biological activity at extremely low doses. Because of their extreme potency, elevated levels of certain cytokines can be detrimental to the host as well. More than 30 cytokines have been identified, purified and characterized. Sometimes the term cytokine has been used to refer to biological mediators that are produced from non lymphoid cells; however, cytokine is generally used as an umbrella term to denote protein biological mediators that participate in immune regulation (Blecha, 1991). Cytokines play an important role of the host defense by regulating the activity of cells that participate in all aspects of specific and non-specific immunity (Hibbit *et al.*, 1995). Pathogen specific recognition is accomplished by a series of receptors known a *"Toll-like receptors"* (Yang *et al.*, 2008). These receptors recognise bacterial signals and their activation regulates cytokine expression in the host immune cells. Cytokines may exert their effects in the mammary gland by recruitment of effector cells, enhanced bacterial clearance by phagocytic cell populations and regulation of acute inflammation. Cytokines also accelerate the normal physiology of involution of the mammary gland and thus reduce the time when the gland is particularly susceptible to infection (Nickerson *et al.*, 1993). Cytokines influence different aspects in the maturation and differentiation of cells of the immune system (e.g. B-lymphocytes, NK-cells) and in the host's response to disease. Colostrum contains low concentration of cytokines and diminished immune cell function, therefore increasing the susceptibility to new IMI. The major cytokines those play important role in udder defense mechanism are- interleukins (IL-1β, IL-2, IL-6, IL-8, IL-12), colony stimulating factors (CSF), interferon (IFNγ) and tumor necrosis factor (TNFα) (Table 6.3). It is known that altered endogenous IL-2 production contributes to diminished immune capabilities. In fact, studies have shown that during last week of gestation there is reduced IL-2 activity, which correlates with the diminished immune cell function and increased susceptibility to mastitis during this period.

Interleukins

The term "interleukin" was originally introduced to describe cell free soluble factors that function as communicator molecules between leukocytes. Interleukin (IL-1β) is a term defining a group of low molecular weight (~17kDa) glycoprotein cytokines produced during inflammatory responses by macrophages and epithelial cells. During the inflammatory response, IL-1β regulates the expression of adhesions by endothelial cells and neutrophil chemotaxis in infections caused by *S. aureus* is important only in the early stages (Zlang and Issekutz, 2002). Upon inflammatory stimuli, monocytes produced IL-1, which not only affects temperature regulating center of the hypothalamus, leading to fever, but also stimulates the bone marrow to increase hematopoiesis, stimulates B-cells to produce antibodies, T-lymphocytes to produce IL-2 and IFNγ leads to a release of acute phase proteins from the liver and activates other macrophages. IL-1β also appeared to be an important mediator for the release of IL-8 from mammary epithelial cells (Boudjellab *et al.*, 2000). IL-2 is the most extensively characterized of all the bovine cytokines. This is produced by $CD4^+$ lymphocytes and was initially described as T-cell growth factor. IL-2 regulates the acquired immune response, because it stimulates growth and differentiation of B-lymphocytes, enhances thymocyte proliferation, activates NK-cells and induces cytotoxic T-cell activation. It has been reported that decreased endogenous IL-2 production cause a decrease in the udder immune response capacity, which can leads to the development of mastitis.

Interleukin-6 (IL-6) is proinflammatory cytokine produced by macrophages. IL-6 is involved in acute septic shock during coliforms or *S. aureus* mastitis. Hagiwara *et al.* (2001) suggests that serum IL-6 concentrations may be of prognostic value in the early diagnosis of severe mastitis in dairy cows. This cytokine also facilitates the exchange of neutrophils for macrophages in the udder, which is necessary for reduction of the deleterious effects of neutrophils on the secretory tissue of mammary gland. Interleukin-8 (IL-8) is a chemikine, which produced by monocytes, T-lymphocytes and macrophages, as well as epithelial and endothelial cells. The term "chemokine" is similar to lymphokines or monokines, represents those cytokines which have chemotactic activities, known as *"chemokines"*. Chemokines attract leukocytes to infection sites. IL-8 has several biological activities, including recruiting and activating neutrophils (Harda *et al.*, 1994), inducing neutrophil degranulation (Schroder *et al.*, 1987), stimulating phagocytosis of opsonised particles (Detmers *et al.*, 1991) and recruiting T-lymphocytes (Jinquan *et al.*, 1995). IL-8 stimulates the transmigration of PMN through the endoepithelial barrier in a dose dependent manner suggesting that the production of IL-8 by mammary endothelial cells at the site of inflammation plays an important role in the recruitment of PMN into the infected gland (Lee and Zhao, 2000). IL-8 is actively produced in mastitis caused by *E. coli*, whereas in mastitis caused by *S. aureus* it is present in low concentration (Persson *et al.*, 2003; Alluwaini, 2004). It indicates that, concentration of IL-8, can give the idea of type of mastitis whether *E. coli* or *S. aureus* mastitis. Interleukin-12 (IL-12) act as a mediator between innate and acquired immunity. The difference of T-cells is the main function of IL-12.

Table 6.3 : Role of cytokines in the mammary gland.

Cytokine	Source	Target cell	Function
IL-1	Macrophages and Epithelial cells	Neutrophils	- Increase neutrophil recruitment to the mammary gland. - Enhance neutrophil phagocytosis and bactericidal activity
IL-2	$CD4^+$ lymphocytes	Activated T- and B-lymphocytes	- Enhance growth and differentiation of B-lymphocytes. - Increases plasma cell numbers. - Enhances cytotoxic and bactericidal activities of lymphocytes. - Activates NK-cells. - Effective mastitis vaccine adjuvant.
IL-6	Macrophages	Activated B-cells, plasma cells and monocytes	- Enhance differentiation of B-cells into plasma cells. - Increase antibody secretion. - Favours the influx of monocytes to mammary gland.
IL-8	Macrophages, Endothelial, Epithelial and T-lymphocytes.	Neutrophils	- Increases neutrophil recruitment to the mammary gland. - Induces inflammation.
IL-12	Dendritic cells and T-lymphocytes	Activated T-cells	- Regulates the differentiation of T-lymphocytes.
TNFα	Macrophages, Neutrophils and Epithelial cells	B-lymphocytes, Neutrophils and Tumor cells	- Enhances B-cell maturation. - Enhances neutrophil phagocytosis and bactericidal activity - Enhances acute phase inflammatory response.
INFγ	$CD4^+$, $CD8^+$ and Nk-cells.	Macrophages and activated B-cells.	- Activates the T-lymphocytes. - Induce production of IL-12. - Reverses suppressive effect of mammary gland secretions. - Activation of neutrophils. - Effective mastitis vaccine adjuvant.
CSF	Macrophages, T-cells, Fibroblasts and Endothelial cells	Progenitor cells and Neutrophils.	- Promote the growth and differentiation of progenitor cells. - Increases milk SCC. - Enhances cytotoxic activity. - Potent macrophage chemoattractant.

Tumor necrosis factor (TNF)

When macrophages comes in contact with endotoxin, they produce a substance called *"tumor necrosis factor"*, that is able to kill certain tumor cells. TNFα is produced by macrophages, neutrophils and epithelial cells. It is main cytokine produced during the early stage of infection and is responsible for endotoxic shock in acute *E. coli* mastitis. Apart from its antiviral effects, TNF stimulates B-cell maturation, induction of natural killer cells and maturation of thymocytes (Lawman *et al.*, 1989). TNFα also upregulates PMN phagocytosis, adherence, chemotaxis and release of ROS. TNFα and IL-1β affect tight junctions between the epithelial cells, lowering the transepithelial resistance (Royal *et al.*, 1989) and allowing exchange of inflammation metabolites and cells between the two blood-milk barrier compartments. Another function of TNFα and IL-1 is to activate fibroblasts of the mammary gland.

Interferon (INF)

Interferon-gamma (INFγ) is another T-cell derived cytokine often produced in response to antigen stimulation. It is produced by $CD4^+/CD8^+$ lymphocytes and NK-cells. INFγ activates the acquired immune response, T-lymphocytes and IL-12 production. Interferons play a major role in the defense against virus infection. This cytokine also increases the phagocytic capacity of neutrophils recruited to the mammary gland. The pronounced influences of INFg on phagocytic cell populations suggests possible clinical application in the prevention of mastitis.

Colony stimulating factors (CSF)

The colony stimulating factors are a group of glycoproteins (cytokines) that regulate differentiation, proliferation and maturation of variety of hemopoietic stem cells and functional activity of mature cells. The CSFs are distinct glycoproteins that bind to cells by a common receptor and are produced by a variety of cells, including fibroblasts, endothelial cells, macrophages and T-cells. Granulocyte-maccrophage colony stimulating factor (GM-CSF) promotes the growth, differentiation of myeloid progenitor cells to granulocytes (neutrophils) and macrophages. The Granulocyte-colony stimulating factor (G-CSF), which targets the neutrophils, causes dramatic increases of neutrophil numbers in blood and milk, stimulates the phagocytic and bactericidal activities of neutrophils (Rainard and Riollet, 2006). The pronounced effect of G-CSF on phagocytic cell populations suggest possible clinical application in the prevention of mastitis. The G-CSF enhance the natural resistance to *S. aureus* infections of the mammary gland (Kehrli *et al.*, 1990).

Complement system

Complement is a group of different proteins found in both serum and milk that can influence the immune response and constitute a bridge between innate and acquired immunity. The biological properties of the activated complement, notably cytolysis, attraction of polymorphonuclear leucocytes by chemotactic factors derived from C3 and C5 and its participation in the ingestion and intracellular killing of bacteria indicate that it could play an important role in the prevention of mammary infections (Poutrel, 1982). The lowest concentrations of complement are observed in the milk of healthy mammary glands during lactation, while highest concentrations of complement are observed in colostrum, mastitic milk and during involution, presumably due to the mobilization of complement components by transudation from blood (Riollet *et al.*, 2000) (Table 6.4).

Table 6.4 : The concentration of complement components in the serum and milk of dairy cows.

Component	Serum concentration	Mature normal milk	Mastitic milk		Reference
			Sub-clinical	Clinical	
BSA (mg/ml)	40-50	0.2-0.3	0.3-0.6	1-20	Harmon *et al.* (1976) Mueller *et al.* (1982)
C1q (µg/ml)	200	0.2	ND	ND	Rainard and Poutrel (1995)
C3 (% of serum)	100	ND	5	5-18	O'Gairbhidhe *et al.* (1970) Mueller *et al.* (1982)
C5a (ng/ml)	15.4	0-0.12	0.18	5.5-50	Rainard and Poutrel (2000) Shuster *et al.* (1997)
Potential C5a (ng/ml)	4280	0.76-12.30	2.5	>50	Rainard *et al.* (1998)
fB (µg/ml)	350	2.1	ND	ND	Rainard, (2002) Tabeletal, (1984)

ND- Not determined

The complement system is composed of at least 29 distinct plasma and membrane proteins. The proteins that comprise the complement system are synthesized mainly by hepatocytes, but other sources include monocytes and macrophages. Effector functions of complement system include opsonization, attraction of phagocytes to the site of complement activation and lysis or intracellular killing of engulfed bacteria. The bactericidal activity of the complement was first investigated in milk of dairy cows (Rainard, 2003).

Sordillo *et al.* (1997) stated that complement is not generally considered as a significant antimicrobial system in bovine milk. The complement components assemble in a cascade process called *complement activation*, and adhere to the bacterial surface. The activation of the complement system results in a sequence of biochemical reactions in which one component activates another component in a cascade manner. Rainard (2003) describes the three activation pathways of complement system are- the classical pathway, alternative pathway and lectin pathway. The classical pathway in milk is not functional due to the lack of the classical pathway in milk is not functional due to the lack of C1q, but the alternative pathway can operate with two consequences- 1) deposition of opsonic C3b and C3bi on bacteria, and generation of the pro-inflammatory fragment C5a (Rainard *et al.*, 1998). Milk concentrations C5 vary widely between cows (0.2 to 1.9% of blood values), resulting in very different capacities to generate C5a (Rainard and Poutrel, 2000). C5a play the role in initiation of inflammatory response of the mammary gland by increasing neutrophil migration. C5a is a potent stimulator of the phagocytic function of neutrophils. While the overall significance of the complement system in mammary gland defense has yet to be fully defined, available information does suggest a predominant role as a proinflammatory mediator during coliform mastitis. Gram-negative bacteria (e.g. *E. coli*) are sensitive to complement lytic action, while Gram-positive bacteria (e.g. *S. aureus*) are resistant; however, all bacteria are susceptible to the opsonizing action of C3b and C3bi (Boyso *et al.*, 2007). The hemolytic activity and C3 concentration is higher in mastitic milk than healthy mammary gland milk (Korhonen *et al.*, 2000).

Immunoglobulins

Immunoglobulins (Ig) are the most important specific humoral factors in mammary gland immune defense. Immunoglobulins or antibodies in the mammary gland can be produced locally or are selectively transported from the serum (Hibitt *et al.*, 1995). There are four main types of antibodies founds in milk including IgG1, IgG2, IgA and IgM (Hurley *et al.*, 2002). IgG1 is transported preformed from the blood. IgA and IgM are produced in the mammary gland by activated plasma cells. Immunoglobulin concentrations in the mammary gland vary with the lactation stage, the highest concentration occurring near parturition (Concha *et al.*, 1980), and at the end of lactation (Guidry *et al.*, 1980). The immunoglobulin content of milk and colostrum also increases during mastitis (Nickerson, 1985). IgG1 concentration increases in clinical mastitis (Caffin *et al.*, 1983; Guidry *et al.*, 1980), which is thought to be the result of three mechanisms: I) disruption of the blood-milk barrier with leakage of serum proteins, including IgG1, into milk (Guidry *et al.*, 1980); II) an increase in selective transport of IgG1 into milk (Darton and McDowell,

1980); and III) a marked decrease in milk volume in infected glands, leading to an increase in the concentration of IgG1 (Maunsell *et al.*, 1998). Total imuunoglobulin concentration in normal milk is <1mg/ml, but during mastitis it increases to 80mg/ml in colostrum and milk (Nickerson, 1998). Bovine colostrum contains IgG1, IgA and IgM in concentrations exceeding those in blood. For IgG1 the colostrums : blood ratio is approximately 4:1, for IgA, 13:1, and for IgM, 2:1. IgG1 is major immunoglobulin in milk (0.5 mg/ml) due to selective transport. Colditz and Watson (1985) and Wiston *et al.* (1972) reports the immunoglobulin levels in lacteal secretion (Table 6.5).

Table 6.5: Concentration of immunoglobulins in lacteal secretions (mg/ml).

	IgA	IgM	IgG1	IgG2
Serum	0.37	3.0	11.2	9.2
Colostral whey	4.7	7.1	48.2	4.0
Milk whey	0.08	0.08	0.5	0.06

There are several mechanisms possible to protection by immunoglobulins against mammary infections, these mechanisms intervening at different stages of the infection process. The main function of immunoglobulin in milk is opsonization, phagocytosis, toxin neutralization, prevention of bacterial adhesion to mammary tissue and direct bacteriolysis (norcross *et al.*, 1991). IgG1, IgG2 and IgM are probably main opsonins for bovine milk. IgA does not aid in bacterial opsonization, but IgA contribute to prevention of adherence to the epithelial lining and colonization of organisms, agglutination and toxin neutralization.

Other soluble factors

In addition to above described antibacterial milk proteins, there are also some other milk proteins or factors which contribute the antibacterial function in the milk. The total antibacterial effect in milk is greater than the sum of the individual contributions of immunoglobulins and non-immunoglobulin defense proteins. The basic glycopeptides have bactericidal activity against various strains of *S. aureus* and *Streptococcus* (Lahov *et al.*, 1971). The bioactive peptides viz. casecidin, casocidin-I and isracidin inhibit the growth of *Staphylococcus, Streptococcus, Sarcina, Diplococcus* and *E. coli* (Zucht *et al.*, 1995; Lahov and Regelson, 1996). A potent bactericidal peptide specifically generated by pepsin degradation of lactoferrin, namely "lactoferrin-B" also have antimicrobial activity against both Gram-positive and Gram-negative bacteria (Tomita *et al.*, 1991; Jones *et al.*, 1994). Indolcidin, a cationic peptide isolated from bovine neutrophils, which is rich in tryptophan and to have potent bactericidal activity against *E. coli* and *S. aureus* (Selsted *et al.*, 1992).

Xanthine oxidase, an enzyme present in milk, much of the amount is found associated with the membrane surrounded the milk fat globule (Zittle *et al.,* 1956). It represents >8% of the intrinsic protein of the bovine milk fat globule membrane. Xanthine oxidase catalyses the formation of nitric oxide from inorganic nitrite, which under aerobic conditions leads to the generation of peroxinitrite, a powerful bactericidal agent (Rainard and Riollet, 2006).

β-defensins constitute a structural group of the broad variety of bactericidal peptides (Schroder, 1999). b-defensin was first isolated from bovine respiratory tract (Diamond *et al.,* 1991). They are present in PMN and epithelial cells. -defensin-like bactericidal activity was isolated from bovine teats >30 years ago (Hibbitt *et al.,* 1971) but no recent account has been given on the significance of b-defensin activity to counteract mastitis inside the udder. Bovine b-defensins are usually active against both Gram-negative and Gram-positive bacteria (Schonwetter *et al.,* 1995). The mechanism of antimicrobial activity of many of these peptides is via selective membrane disruption, leading to a characteristic broad spectrum of antibiotic activity which includes Gram-negative and Gram-positive bacteria, fungi and certain membrane enveloped viruses (Boman, 1995).

Phagocytosis

Phagocytosis is an evolutionarily conserved mechanism to remove apoptotic bodies and invading pathogens. It is a complex process by which phagocytes (neutrophils, macrophages, dendritic cells) move from the blood to the site of infection (chemotaxis) recognize invading pathogen or foreign material, ingest them and kill or destroy the ingested material. Phagocytosis can be divided into four discrete stages: 1) chemotaxis, 2) recognition, 3) ingestion, and 4) digestion (Figure 6.4).

Chemotaxis

Neutrophils normally circulate in the blood. Following bacteria entry into the gland, neutrophils are the first cells recruited into the milk and then represent the predominant cell type. Activation of complement at the site of injury results in the production of the pro-inflammatory mediators that is chemoattractants, the most important being complement components C5a and C3a, lipopolysaccharides (LPS), IL-1, IL-2 and IL-8 (Lee and Zhao, 2000; Deley *et al.,* 1991). The directed cellular migration of neutrophil along a concentration gradient of chemoattractants is called chemotaxis. Leukocyte chemotaxis is initiated by binding of chemoattractants to plasma membrane receptors. The binding alters transmembrane potential and activates ionic influxes. Consequently, the altered metabolic processes lead to rearrangement of cytoskeletal elements that is manifested by orientation and migration of

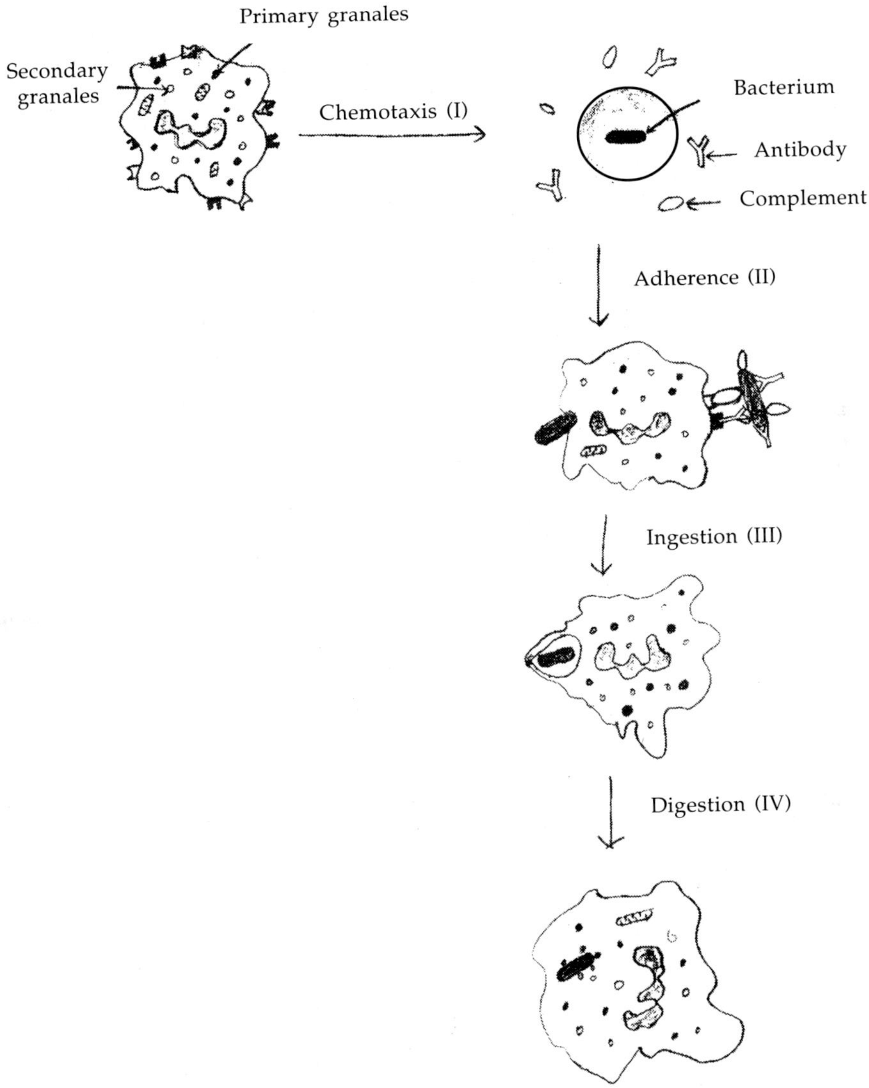

Figure 6.4 : Different stages of phagocytosis.

the cells toward the chemotactic source (Targowski, 1983). Several receptors on neutrophils participate in the migration from blood to milk. L-selectin (CD 62L) plays a role in the first step of egress from the blood flow (Rainard and Riollet, 2003). Chemoattractants bind to receptors on the PMN membrane, induce changes in the PMN cytoskeleton, and direct movement of PMNs along concentration gradient of the chemoattractants into mammary gland. C5a is the most biologically significant peptide and increase vascular permeability. It is a potent chemoattractants for neutrophils, eosinophils, basophils, macrophages and sub population of lymphocytes and it also induces the increased oxidative metabolism, release of ecosanoids and degradative enzymes, and stimulation of cytokine synthesis (IL-1 and IL-6) (Frank and Fries, 1991; Damereau, 1987). The C5a concentration in the milk of healthy quarters is ranged from 0.6ng/ml to 20ng/ml (Rainard and Poutrel, 2000) while in the milk of quarters suffering from clinical mastitis can exceed 50ng/ml (Shuster *et al.*, 1997). Neutrophil recruitment from the blood to the site of infection is essential in the defense of the mammary gland against invading bacteria and the promptness of the recruitment and the amount of recruited neutrophils are determining for the outcome of the infection (Rainard and Riollet, 2006). For instance, a 1 hour delay in neutrophil recruitment into an infected gland could result in an 8 fold larger number of E. coli to kill and much more endotoxin to detoxify (Burvenich *et al.*, 2003). Chemotaxis is largely responsible for bringing PMNs and monocytes into contact with particle and is, thus crucial in initiating the recognition phase of the phagocytic process.

Recognition

The recognition and attachment is the most important step of the phagocytosis. In order for phagocytosis to precede recognition must be conferred between the bacterium and the phagocyte. The main opsonising antibodies for bovine PMNs are IgG_2 and IgM (Anderson *et al.*, 1986) which recognize the bacterium through Fab region and bind to the neutrophils via their Fc receptors on the plasma membrane. In general, Fc receptors on phagocytic cells are responsible for binding and subsequent ingestion of opsonized particles with IgG, whereas C3b receptors are primarily responsible for binding but do not trigger ingestion of particles opsonized with C3b. In contrast, complement receptors on PMNs participate in both binding and ingestion of opsonized *Staphylococci* (Verhoef *et al.*, 1977). Molecules that coat foreign particles in this way and so promote phagocytosis are called *"opsonins"*. An important phagocytic mechanism for control of intramammary infection by Gram-negative bacteria is non-opsonic phagocytosis (Dosogne *et al.*, 1998). Non-immunological recognition consists of lectins and hydrophobic properties of cell surfaces. Carbohydrate receptors on the cell surface of bovine PMN mediate interaction with carbohydrate rich pili of Gram-negative bacteria. This lectin-carbohydrate interaction results in recognition and phagocytosis of Gram-negative bacteria in the absence of specific opsonins (Paape *et al.*, 2003). Toll-like receptors (TLR) have been identified as a major class of receptors recognizing conserved bacterial structures called *"pathogen-associated molecular patterns (PAMPs)"*. The term *"pattern recognition receptors" (PRRs)* has been applied to denote those host molecules that recognize microbial infection, and PAMPs has been applied to denote the structural features of microbes that are recognized (Janeway, 1989). They are crucial for recognition of microbes by the innate immune system and for bridging the innate and acquired immune responses (Netea *et al.*, 2004). The TLR2 receptors recognize peptidoglycan and lipoteichoic acid of Gram-positive bacteria, and TLR4 recognizes lipopolysaccharides (LPS) of Gram-negative bacteria. After recognition of antigen by specific receptors, they adhere to the surface of neutrophils. Some pathogens possess an antiphagocytic substances on their surfaces that prevents recognition and consequently, phagocytosis.

S. aureus resist recognition because protein A on its surface binds the Fc portion of IgG, prevents opsonization, and coating the bacterium with host antibody which is not recognized as foreign particle.

Ingestion

Ingestion begins with the firm attachment of particle or immunological complex (antigen-antibody complex) to surfaces of phagocytic cells. Once contact is made, a cohesive force prevents their separation despite the flow of extracellular fluid (Targowski, 1983). As phagocyte crawl to ward a chemotactic source, a pseudopod contain a filamentous network of proteins, actin and myosin, whose state determines the fluidity of the cytoplasm (Tizard, 1998). The pseudopods join together resulting in formation of an intracellular vacuole is called *"phagosome"*, containing the foreign body. Immediately after formation of the phagosome, cytoplasmic lysosome vesicles fuse with the phagosome and release their contents into the phagosome vacuole to form a phagolysosomes. The process of fusion of lysosomes to the phagosome and release of their contents is called *degranulation*. Within the phagolysosomes the viable organism may be killed and digested.

Killing and Digestion

There are two fundamental mechanisms for killing and digesting phagocytized foreign material, an oxygen dependent and an oxygen independent mechanism. Oxygen dependent killing mechanism is also known as *"respiratory burst"* (McCall and Vallance, 1992).

Oxygen Dependent Mechanism

Once complement components and immunoglobulins bind to receptors on the PMN surface, the cells become activated and increase their oxygen consumption nearly 100 folds, which results in the activation of NADPH-oxidase system on the cell surface. This activated NADPH-oxidase converts NADPH (the reduce form of NADP) to $NADP^+$ with the electron. One molecule of oxygen accepts a single donated electron, resulting in the one molecule of superoxide anion ($.O_2^-$).

$$NADPH + 2O_2 \xrightarrow{\text{NADPH oxidase}} NADP^+ + H^+ + 2.O_2^-$$

The superoxide anion is not itself a reactive oxidant, but is a substrate for the production of other reactive oxygen species, by way of the production of H_2O_2. In turn, H_2O_2 is an abundant substrate for the generation of more violent oxidants. Two molecules of $.O_2^-$ interact simultaneously to generate one molecule of hydrogen peroxide (H_2O_2) with the presence of an enzyme superoxide dismutase (SOD). This is the key reaction that permits the subsequent generation of reactive oxygen species.

$$2\ .O_2^- + 2\ H^+ \xrightarrow{\text{Superoxide dimutase}} H_2O_2 + O_2$$

Because this reaction occurs so rapidly or due to very short life span of superoxide anion, it does not accumulate but H_2O_2 does. This H_2O_2 is converted to bactericidal compounds through the action of myeloperoxidase. Myeloperoxidase is found in large amount in the primary or zymogen granules of the neutrophils, which is the most important respiratory burst enzyme. This enzyme catalyzes the reaction between hydrogen peroxide and intracellular halide ions (Cl^-, I^- Br^-, HCN^-) to generate hypohalides.

$$H_2O_2 + Cl- \xrightarrow{\text{Myeloperoxidase}} H_2O + OCl-$$

These hypohalides rapidly attack many biological molecules by oxidizing bacterial proteins and enhance the bactericidal activities of lysosomal enzymes. On the other hand the ROS are also very important in inhibiting reabsorption of toxins from inflamed udder (De and Mukherjee, 2006). Myeloperoxidase mediated system also forms singlet oxygen, which may kill bacteria by disrupting double bonds in the structure of the microbial cell wall. Hypochlorite (OCl-) can generate singlet oxygen ($^1O_2$).

$$OCl^- + H_2O_2 = {}^1O_2 + Cl- + H_2O$$

Hypochlorous acid (HOCl) can react with superoxide to yield the extremely reactive hydroxyl radical:

$$O_2^{\bullet -} + HOCl = O_2^{\bullet -} + OH^{\bullet} + Cl^-$$

The hydroxyl radical ($OH^{\bullet}$) can be produced independently from H2O2 and superoxide, via the Fenton reaction, which is catalyzed by iron.

$$O_2^{\bullet -} + H_2O_2 = OH^{\bullet} + OH^- + O^2$$

Reactive nitrogen species are also produced though a spontaneous reaction, using superoxide as a substrate (Beutler, 2004).

$$NO^{\bullet} + O_2^{\bullet -} = ONOO^-$$

During the respiratory burst, there is production of several microbicidal oxidizing agents in the phagolysosomes, including superoxide anions, hydrogen peroxide, singlet oxygen and hydrogen peroxide etc. These radicals oxidize the lipids such as in the bacterial membranes causing the lysis of the bacteria, and will oxidize or crosslink protein destroying their function. Bovine PMN release amounts of superoxide and hydrogen peroxide when their plasma membrane is perturbed (Leino and Paape, 1993; Lohuis and Burvenich, 1997).

Oxygen Independent Mechanism

The oxygen independent mechanism itself indicates that in this mechanism oxygen is not required for the destruction or killing of the engulfed foreign particle. In this mechanism, the engulfed organism killed and digested by several oxygen independent reactants such as lactoperoxidase, lysozyme, hydrolytic enzyme, lactoferrin etc. These enzymes present in primary granule of PMNs are able to kill the engulfed pathogens by digesting their bacterial cell wall. The acids are formed in the phagosomes, this directly kill acid sensitive bacteria, but also provides an acidic environment for the lysosomal hydrolases (their optimum pH is ~4.5). The functions of all aforesaid digesting or killing enzymes already have been discussed under the soluble factors of udder immunity of this chapter.

The majority of bacteria are destroyed promptly by phagocytic cells using these mechanisms. However, some organisms such as *S. aureus*, *L. monocytogenes* and *M. tuberculosis* can survive and even multiply within the phagocytic cells (Targowski, 1983). These microorganisms can be destroyed by activated "angry" macrophages (North, 1978; Adams, 1982).

Udder Immunosuppressive Agents

The udder immunosuppressive agents are those agents or factors which suppress the innate udder immunity results increase the susceptibility to mastitis. There is little knowledge about the role of immunosuppressive agents in susceptibility to mastitis, but it is well recognized that cattle suffering from chronic disease often have bone marrow suppression resulting in abnormalities of circulating leukocytes.

Some mastitis pathogens themselves may produce toxins that have an adverse effect on host immunity. One of the most contagious pathogenic bacteria causing bovine mastitis is *S. aureus*. This bacterium produces toxins that damage host cell membranes, and molecules that act as superantigens (Foster, 2004; Zecconi *et al.*, 2005). The ability of the *S. aureus* to escape from the immune response and survive inside different cells is fundamental for this bacterium to persist for longer periods, mastitis caused by *S. aureus* tends to become sub clinical and chronic, and has a low response to conventional antibiotic therapy due to its intracellular localization in mammary gland epithelial cells (Dego *et al.*, 2002). *S. aureus* secretes a number of proteins or toxins that inhibit or delay the effects of the innate immune system. For instance, staphylokinase (SAK) binds to α-defensins and inhibits their bactericidal activity (Jin *et al.*, 2004). Also, SAK transforms plasminogen to plasmin, which binds to IgG and C3b leading to an antiopsonic function. *S. aureus* produces other proteins, such as leucocidin, α-toxin, aureolysin, V8 proteinase (acts as an anti-defensin) and enterotoxins that function as superantigens (stimulate T-lymphocytes and macrophages) (Rooijakkers *et al.*, 2005). Enterotoxin is the most commonly secreted toxin of *S. aureus* strains causing bovine mastitis.

Bacteria possess a wide array of defense mechanisms in order to avoid phagocytosis and digestion by phagocytes. Protein A, a component of the Fc region of immunoglobulins, thus inhibiting phagocytosis (Ohman *et al.*, 1988). The capsule of *S. aureus* will cover immunoglobulin and complement ligands bound to its surface, thus preventing their binding to receptors on phagocytes. Decreased hydrophobicity of the bacterialsurface of encapsulated bacteria is another mechanism for resisting phagocytosis. Once internalized, *S. aureus* will resist oxidative killing by neutrophils through generation of catalase. In contrast to the chemotaxis of neutrophils in response to LPS, there is evidence that staphylococcal α-toxin and leucocidin will impede migration of neutrophils towards chemoattractants (Wilkinson, 1980). Phagocytic recognition is impaired by capsular antigens and LPS of *E. coli*. Some organisms like the mycoplasmas have the facility to attach proliferate on the leukocyte surface.

Bovine Virus Diarrhoea Virus (BVDV), Bovine Leukaemia Virus (BLV), Bovine Immunodeficiency Virus (BIV) may affect the ability of cows to resist mastitis. Immunosuppression is a feature of both transient primary BVDV infections in immunocompetent animals and occasionally of permanent immune disfunction in some animals persistently infected with BVDV (Johnson and Muscoplat, 1973). Immunosuppression in primary BVDV infections is probably of more relevance to susceptibility to mastitis than immuno-suppression in persistently infected cattle (Baker, 1995). In primary BVDV infections, transient reductions in absolute numbers of T and B lymphocytes and in the percentage of B cells have been recorded (Bolin *et al.*, 1985), whereas in persistently infected cattle absolute lymphocyte numbers remain similar to normal values (Johnson and Muscoplat, 1973). Fetrow and Ferrer, (1982) reported that cows that were BLV antibody positive did not have an increased prevelance of mastitis compared to uninfected cows. Infection of cows with BLV has been associated with lymphoid tissue depletion and multiple secondary infections including mastitis, and its possible influence on the chronicity of mastitis has also been suggested (Snider *et al.*, 1996). Some of the immune functions that may be adversely affected by BLV include temporary decreases in neutrophil function but not in lymphocyte blastogenesis or mononuclear cell numbers (Flaming *et al.*, 1997).

References

Adams, D. (1982). Today., 3:285.

Adams, L.G. and Templeton, J.W. (1998). In: Rev. Sci. Tech. Off. Int. Epiz., 17 (1): 200-219.

Alluwaimi A.M. (2004). Res Vet. Sci., 77: 211-22.

Anderson, K.L., Smith, A.R., Shanks, R.D., Whitmore, H.L., Davis, L.E. and Gustafsson, B.K. (1986). Am. J. Vet. Res. 47: 2405–2410.

Arnold, R.R., Cole, M.F. and McGhee, J.R. (1977). Scince. 197: 263-265.

Arnold, R.R., Russell, J.E., Champion, W.J., Brewer, M. and Gauthier, J.J. (1982). Infect. Immun. 35: 792-799.

Asai, K., Kai, K., Rikiishi, H., Sugawara, S., Maruyama, Y., Yamaguchi, T., Ohta, M. and Kumagai, K. (1998). Veterinary Immunology and Immunopathology., 65: 51-61.

Baggiolini, M., Horisberger, U., Gennaro, R. and Dewald, B. (1985). Ultrastructure of circulating and maturing cells, Lab. Invest. 52: 151–158.

Baker, J. C. (1995). Vet. Clinics of North Am. Food Anim. Practice., 11(3): 425-45.

Bannerman, D.D., Paape, M.J., Lee, J.W., Zhao, X., Hope, J.C. and Rainard, P. (2004). Clin Diagn Lab Immunol., 11: 463-472.

Batish, V.K., Chander, H., Zumdegni, K.C., Bhatia, K.L. and Singh, R.S. (1988). Aust. J. Dairy Technol., 5: 16.

Baumann, H. and Graudie, J. (1994). Immunol. Today., 15: 74.

Beutler, B. (2004). Mol. Immunol., 40: 845–859.

Blecha, F. (1991). J. Dairy Sci., 74(1): 328-339.

Boddie, R. L. and Nickerson, S. C. (1986). J. Dairy Sci., 69(1): 253-7.

Bolin, S. R., McClurkin, A. W. and Coria, M. F. (1985). Am. J. Vet. Res., 46(4): 884-6.

Boman, H. G. (1995). Annu. Rev. Immunol., 13: 61–92.

Boudjellab, N., Chan-Tang, H.S. and Zhao, X. (2000). Comp Biochem Physiol A Mol Integr Physiol., 27:191-199.

Boulanger, D., Bureau, F., Me´lotte, D., Mainil, J. and Lekeux, P. (2003). J. Dairy Sci., 86: 1259-67.

Boyso, J.O., Alrcôn, Juan J.V., Juârez, M.C., Zarzosa, A.O., Meza, Joel E.L., Patino, A.B. and Aguirre, Victor M.B. (2007). J. Infection., 54: 399-409.

Burvenich, C., Paape, M.J., Hill, A.W., Guidry, A.J., Miller, R.H., Heyneman, R., Kremer, W.D.J. and Brand, A. (1994). Vet. Q., 16(1): 45-50.

Burvenich, C., Van Merris, V., Mehrzad, J., Diez-Fraile, A. and Duchateau, L. (2003). Vet Res., 34: 521-64.

Caffin, J.P., Poutrel, B. and Rainard, P. (1983). J. Dairy Sci., 66: 2161–2166.

Cai, T.Q., Weston, P.G., Lund, L.A., Brodie, B., McKenna, D. J. and Wagner, W.C. (1994). Am. J. Vet. Res., 55: 934–943.

Capuco, A. V., Mein, G. A., Nickerson, S. C., Jack, L. J., Wood, D. L., Bright, S. A., Aschenbrenner, R. A., Miller, R. H. and Bitman, J. (1994). J. Dairy Sci., 77(1): 64-74.

Capuco, A. V., Paape, M. J. and Nickerson, S. C. (1986). Am. J. Vet. Res., 47: 663.

Concha, C., Holmberg, O. and Morein, B. (1978). J. Dairy Res., 45(2): 287-90.

Concha, C., Holmberg, O. and Morein, B. (1980). J. Dairy Res., 47(3): 305-11.

Craven, N. (1985). Forschung., 37: 554–558.

Craven, N. and Williams, M.K. (1985). Vet. Immunol. Immunopathol. 10: 71-127.

Daley, M. J., Oldham, E. R., Williams, T. J. and Coyle, P. A. (1991). Am. J. Vet. Res., 52(3): 474-9.

Daley, M.J., Coyle, P.A., Williams, T.J., Furda, G., Dougherty, R. and Hayes, P.W. (1991). J. Dairy Sci., 74: 4413–4424.

Damereau, B. (1987). Rev. Physiol. Biochem. Pharmacol. 108: 151–206.

Darton, P.J. and McDowell, G.H. (1980). Aust. J. Exp. Biol. Med. Sci., 58: 149–157.

De, U.K. and Mukherjee, R. (2006). Intas Polivet., 7(I): 29-33.

Dego, O.K., van Dijk, J.E. and Nederbragt, H. (2002). Vet. Quart. 24: 181-98.

Deitemeyer, K. (2003). In: Intuitive Immunology, Part 5. VetScript. New Zealand Veterinary Association. NZ. Pp 16-18.

Detmers, P.A., Powell, D.E., Walz, A., Clark-Lewis, I., Baggionlini, M. and Cohn, Z.A. (1991). J. Immunol., 147: 4211–4217.

Diamond, G., Zasloff, M., Eck, H., Brasseur, M., Maloy, W.L. and Bevins, C.L. (1991). Proc. Natl. Acad. Sci. U.S.A., 88: 3952–3956.

Dosogne, H., Burvenich, C. and Paape, M.J. (1998). Comp. Haematol. Int., 8: 82–86.

Edmondson, P. (2001). In Practice., 23(3): 150-159.

Ellison, R.T. III, Giehl, T.J. and Laforse, F.M. (1988). Infect. Immun. 56: 2774-2781.

Fetrow, J. and Ferrer, J. F. (1982). J. Dairy Sci., 65(5): 881-2.

Fitzpatrick, J. L., Cripps, P. J. Hill, A. W. Bland, P. W. and Stokes, C. R. (1992). Vet. Immunol. Immunopathol. 32: 13–23.

Flaming, K.P., Frank, D.E., Carpenter, S. and Roth, J.A. (1997). Vet. Immunol. and Immunopathol., 56: 27-38.

Foster, T.J. (2004). J. Clin. Invest., 12: 1693-6.

Francesca, N. (2005). Teat condition in dairy cows. Mastitis Newsletter (IDF)., 26: 34-35.

Frank, M.M. and Fries, L.F. (1991). Today., 12: 322–326.

Godden, S., Rapnicki, P., Stewart S., Fetrow, J., Johnson, A., Bey, R. and Farnsworth, R. (2003). J. Dairy Sci., 86: 3899-3911.

Green, M., Huxley, J. and Bradley, A. (2002). In Practice. Journal of Veterinary Postgraduate Clinical Study. British Veterinary Association. UK. Pp 582-587.

Grindal, R. J. and Hillerton, J. E. (1991). J. Dairy Res., 58(3): 263-8.

Grindal, R. J., Walton, A. W. and Hillerton, J. E. (1991). J. Dairy Res., 58(4): 383-8.

Guidry, A. J., Paape, M. J. and Pearson, R. E. (1980). Am. J. Vet. Res., 41(5): 751–753.

Hagiwara, K., Yamanaka, H., Hisaeda, K., Taharaguchi, S., Kirisawa, R. and Iwai, H. (2001). Vet. Res. Communi., 25(2): 99-108.

Harda, A., Sekido, N., Akahoshi, T., Wada, T., Mukaida, N. and Matsushima, K. (1994). J. Leukocyte Biol., 56: 559–564.

Harmon, R.J., Schanbacher, F.L., Ferguson, L.C. and Smith K.L. (1976). Infect. Immun., 13: 533–542.

Heyneman, R., Burvenich, C. and Vercauteren, R. (1990). J. Dairy Sci., 73: 985–994.

Hibbitt, K.G. (1985). In: Proceedings of Immunology in Clinical Practice. Continuing Education. NZVA. Pp 206-219.

Hibbitt, K.G., Brownlie, J. and Cole. C.B. (1971). J. Hyg. (London), 69: 61-68.

Hibbitt, K.G., Cole, C.B. and Reiter, B. (1969). J. Gen. Microbiol., 56: 365.

Hoeben, D., Burvenich, C. and Heyneman, R. (1997). J. Dairy Sci., 80: 403-410.

Hoeben, D., Burvenich, C. and Heyneman, R. (1998). J. Dairy Sci., 81: 403–410.

Hoeben, D., Burvenich, C. and Massart-Leen, A.M. (1998). Eur. J. Pharmacol., 354: 197–203.

Hoeben, D., Dosogne, H., Heyneman, R. and Burvenich, C. (1997). Eur. J. Pharmacol., 332: 289–297.

Hurley, D. J., Kensinger, M. H., Mastro, A. M. and Wilson, R. A. (1990). Vet. Immunol. and Immunopathol., 25(2): 177-93.

Jain, N.C. (1986). Schalm's Veterinary Hematology, 4th ed., Lee and Febiger, Philadelphia, PA, pp. 676–730.

Janeway, Jr. C.A. and Medzhitor, R. (2002). Annu. Rev. Immunol., 20:197-216.

Jensen, D. L. and Eberhart, R. J. (1981). Am. J. Vet. Res., 42(5): 743-747.

Jin, T., Bokarewa, M., Foster, T., Mitchel, J., Higgins, J. and Tarkowski, A. (2004). J. Immunol., 172: 1169-76.

Jinquan, T., Deleyran, B., Gesser, B., Maare, H., Delevran, M., Larsen, C. G. and Thestrup-Pederson, K. (1995). J. Immunol., 154: 3742–3752.

Johnson, D. W. and Muscoplat, C. C. (1973). Am. J. Vet. Res., 34(9): 1139-41.

Jones, E. M., Smart, A., Bloomberg, G., Burgess, L. and Millar, M. R. (1994). J. Appl. Bacteriol., 77: 208–214.

Jorstad, A., Farver, T. B. and Riemann, H. (1989). Acta Vet. Scand., 30(3): 239-45.

Kampen, C.V. and Mallard, B. A. (1997). Vet. Immunol. Immunopathol., 59: 79–91.

Kartashova, V., Kasyanchuk, V. and Skorokhodov, Y. (1992). Molochnoe i Myasnoe Skotovodstvo., No.1: 34-35.

Kawai, K., Hagiwara, S., Angri, A. and Nagahata, H.C. (1999). Vet. Res. Communication. 23(7): 391-398.

Kehrli Jr., M.E., Nonnecke, B.J. and Roth, J.A. (1989). Am. J. Vet. Res., 50: 207–214.

Kehrli, M. E., Jr., and Shuster, D. E. (1994). J. Dairy Sci., 77: 619.

Kehrli, M.E., Cullor, Jr. J.S. and Nickerson, S.C. (1990). J. Dairy Sci., 73: 235

Kenny, K., Bastida-Corcvera, F. and Norcross, N.L. (1995). In: Andrews AH, Blowey RW, Boyd H, Eddy RG (eds) Bovine Medicine. Blackwell Scientific Publications, Oxford, UK. Pp 335-350.

Kiro, P. (2005). The defense mechanisms of the udder- Part one. Published: 02 May 2005. http//www.milkproduction.com/library.

Klebanoff, S.J. (1970). Biochemistry of the phagocytic process, North-Holland Publishing Company, London, , pp. 89–114.

Komine, K., Komine, Y., Kuroishi, T., Kobayashi, J., Obara, Y. and Kumagai, K. (2005). J. Vet. Med. Sci., 67(7): 667-677.

Korhonen, H., Marnila, P. and Gill, H.S. (2000). Br. J. Nutr. Supply, 84: S75-80.

Kumar, B. (1988). Studies on incidence, chemotherapy and control of mastitis in cattle and buffalo. M.V.Sc. Thesis, Punjab Agric. Univ., Luthiana, India.

Kumar, S. (1990). Studies on mastitis in buffaloes with emphasis on resistance, chemotherapy and control. M.V.Sc. Thesis, P.A.U., Ludhiana, India.

Lacy-Hulbert, S. J. and Hillerton, J. E. (1995). J. Dairy Sci., 62(3): 395-404.

Lahov, E. and Regelson, W. (1996). Food Chem. Toxicol., 34: 131–145.

Lahov, E., Edelsten, D., Sode-Mogensen, M. T. and Sofer, E. (1971). Milchwissenschaft., 26: 489–495.

Larsen, C.G., Anderson, A.O., Oppenheim, J.J. and Matsushima, K. (1989). Immunology., 68: 31-36.

Lascelles, J. and Lee, C.S. (1978). Lactation: a comprehensive treatise. Academic Press, New York, IV, 115-117.

Lawman, M.J.P., Campos, M., Bielefeldt, O.H., Griebel, P. and Babiuk, L.A. (1989). Recombinant cytokines and their potential therapeutic value in Veterinary medicine. Animal Biotechnology, London. Pergamon press., 64-106.

Lee, C. S. and Outteridge, P. M. (1976). Aust. J. Expe. Biol. and Medical Sci., 54(1): 43-55.

Lee, C. S., Wooding, F. B. and Kemp, P. (1980). J. Dairy Sci., 47(1): 39-50.

Lee, E.K. and Kehrli Jr., M.E. (1998). Am. J. Vet. Res., 59: 37–43.

Lee, J.W. and Zhao, X. (2000). Cell Biol Int. 24: 889-895.

Lee, N.Y., Kawai, K., Nakamura, I., Tanaka, T., Kumura, H. and Shimazaki, K. (2004). J. Vet. Med. Sci., 66: 1267-9.

Legrand, D., Elass, E., Pierce, A. and Mazurier, J. (2004). Biometals., 17: 225–229.

Leino, L. and Paape, M.J. (1993). Am. J. Vet. Res., 54: 1055–1059.

Lin, Y., Xia, L., Turner, J. D. and Zhao, X. (1995). Am. J. Vet. Res., 56(2): 203-7.

Lohuis, J.A.C.M. and Burvenich, C. (1997). Flem. Vet. J., 66: 205–215.

Lojda, L., Stavikova, M. and Zakova, M. (1980). In: Proc. Conf. Resistance Factors and Genetic Aspects of Mastitis Control., 242-248.

Mackay, C. R., and Hein. W.R. (1991). Curr. Top. Microbiol. Immunol. 173: 107.

Magnusson, U. (1999). Am. J. Vet. Res. 60: 546–548.

Masson, P. L. and Heremans, J. F. (1966). Prot. Biol. Fluids, 14:115.

Maunsell, F.P., Morin, D.E., Constable, P.D., Hurley, W.L., McCoy, G.C., Kakoma, I. and Isaacson, R.E. (1998). J. Dairy Sci., 81(5):1291-1299.

McCall, T. and Vallence, P. (1992). Trend Physiol. Sci., 13:1-6.

McDonald, J.S. (1971). J. Am. Vet. Med. Assoc., 158(2):184-190.

McDonald, J.S. and Anderson, A.J. (1981). Am. J. Vet. Res., 42: 1366-1368.

McDonald, T. J., McDonald, J. S. and Rose, D. L. (1970). Am. Vet. Medical Assoc. 31(11): 1937-41.

Miller, J.K., Brzezinska-Slebodzinska, E. and Madsen, F.C. (1993). J. Dairy Sci., 76: 2812.

Miller, R. H., Bitman, J., Bright, S. A., Wood, D. L. and Capuco, A. V. (1992). J. Dairy Sci., 75(6): 1436-42.

Miller, R. H., Pankey, J. W., Bright, S. A., Bitman, J., Wood, D. L. and Capuco, A. V. (1991). In: Proc. of the USDA, Agricultural Research Service.

Miller, R.H., Paape, M.J. and Fulton, L.A. (1991). J. Dairy Sci., 74(11): 3782-3790.

Miller, R.H., Paape, M.J., Peters, R.R. and Young, M.D. (1990). J. Dairy Sci., 73(7): 1751-1755.

Motomura, Y., Yugi, H., Kamimura, S. and Hamana, K (1994). J. Japan Vet. Medical Assoc., 47(6): 387-389.

Mueller, R., Carroll, E.J. and Panico, L. (1982). Veterinarmed. B., 29: 99–106.

Mullan, N.A., Carter, E.A. and Nguyen, K.A. (1985). Res. Vet. Sci., 38: 160–166.

Murphy, J.M. (1959). Cornell Vet., 49: 411.

Murphy, J.M., and Stuart, O.M. (1953). Cornell Vet., 43: 290.

Netea, M.G., Van Der Graaf C., Van Der Meer, J.W. and Kullberg, B.J. (2004). J. Leukoc. Biol., 75: 749–755.

Newbould, F.H. (1973). Can. J. Comp. Med., 37 189–194.

Nickerson, S. C. (1985). J Am. Vet. Medical Assoc., 187(1): 41-5.

Nickerson, S. C. (1987). J Am. Vet. Medical Assoc., 191(11): 1484-1488.

Nickerson, S.C. (1988). Agri. Pract., 9: 32.

Nickerson, S.C. (1989). J. Dairy Sci., 72:1665-1678.

Nickerson, S.C. and Pankey, J.W. (1983). Am. J. Vet. Res., 44: 1433–1441.

Nickerson, S.C., Owens, W.E. and Boddie, R.L. (1993). J. Dairy Sci., 76: 1290-1297.

Norcross, N.L., Burvenisch, C., Vandeputte-Van-Messom, G. and Hill, A.W. (1991). Rijkuniver-Siteit Gent., 129-139.

North, R.J. (1978). J. Immunol., 121: 806.

O'Gairbhidhe, C.P., Jain, N.C., Carroll, E.J. and Schalm, O.W. (1970). J. Dairy Sci., 53: 602–604.

Ohman, L., Maluszynska, G., Magnusson, K.E. and Stendahl, O. (1988). Prog. Drug. Res., 32: 132-147.

Oldham, E. R., Eberhart, R. J. and Muller, L. D. (1991). J. Dairy Sci., 74(11): 3775-81.

Paape, M.J. and Tucker, H.A. (1966). J. Dairy Sci., 49: 265-267.

Paape, M.J. and Weinland, B.T. (1988). J. Dairy Sci., 71: 250-256.

Paape, M.J., Bannerman, D.D., Zhao, X. and Lee, J.W. (2003). Vet. Res., 34: 597–627.

Paape, M.J., Hafs, H.D. and Synder, W.W. (1963). J. Dairy Sci., 46: 1211-1216.

Paape, M.J., Miller, R.H. and Ziv, G. (1990). J. Dairy Sci., 73: 1734–1744.

Paape, M.J., Wergin, W.P. and Guidry, A.J. (1981). Adv. Exp. Med. Biol., 137: 555.

Park, Y. H., Fox, L. K., Hamilton, M. J. and Davis, W. C. (1992). J. Dairy Sci., 75(4): 998-1006

Pascal, R. and Riollet, C. (2006). Vet. Res., 37: 369-400.

Paulrud, O.C. (2005). Vet. Res. Communication., 29(3): 215-245.

Persson Waller, K., Colditz, I.G., Lun, S. and O¨stensson, K. (2003). Res Vet Sci., 74: 31-6.

Persson, K., Carlsson, A., Hambleton, C. and Guidry, A.J. (1992). Journal of Veterinary Medicine Series B-Zentralblatt fur Veterinarmedizin Reihe B-Infectious Diseases and Veterinary Public Health., 39: 165-174.

Persson, K., Larsson, I. and Hallen Sandgren, C. (1993). Vet. Immunol. Immunopathol., 37: 99.

Pierce, A., Colavizza, D., Benaissa, M., Maes, P., Tartar, A., Montreuil, J. and Spik, G. (1991). Eur. J. Biochem., 196: 177-184.

Politis, I., Zhao, X., McBride, B.W. and Burton, J.H. (1992). Vet. Immunol. Immunopathol., 30: 399–410.

Poutrel, B. (1982). Ann. Rech. Vet., 13(1): 85-99.

Rainard, P. (2002). J. Dairy Res., 69: 1–12.

Rainard, P. and Poutrel, B. (1995). Infect. Immun., 63: 3422–3427.

Rainard, P. and Poutrel, B. (2000). Generation of complement fragment C5a in milk is variable among cows. J. Dairy Sci., 83: 945–951.

Rainard, P. and Riollet, C. (2003). Reprod Nutr. Dev., 43: 436-57.

Rainard, P., Sarradin, P., Paape, M.J. and Poutrel, B. (1998). Vet. Res., 29: 73–88.

Rausch, P.G. and Moore, T.G. (1975). Blood., 46: 913–919.

Reiter, B. (1985). Bull. Int. Dairy Fed., 191: 1–35.

Reiter, B., and Brock, J. H. (1975). Immunology, 28:171.

Riollet, C., Rainard, P. and Poutrel, B. (2000). Clin. Diagn. Lab. Immunol., 7: 161–167.

Riollet, C., Rainard, P. and Poutrel, B. (2001). J. Dairy Sci., 84: 1077-1084.

Rivas, A.L., Tadevosyan, R., Quimby, F.W., Coksaygan, T. and Lein, D.H. (2002). Can J Vet Res., 66:165-72.

Rooijakkers, S.H.M., van Kessel, K.P.M. and van Strijp, J.A.G. (2005). Trends Microbiol., 13: 596-601.

Rossi, C. R. and Kiesel, G. K. (1977). Am. J. Vet. Res., 38(7): 1023-5.

Royall, J.A., Berkow, R.L., Beckman, J.S., Cunningham, M.K., Matalon, S. and Freeman, B.A. (1989). Am J Physiol., 257: L399-410.

Rupp, R. and Boichard, D. (2003). Veterinary Research., 34: 671–688.

Sanchez, L., Aranda, P., Perez, M.D. and Calvo, M. (1988). Biol. Chem. Hoppe Seyler., 369: 1005–1008.

Schalm, O.W., Carroll, E.J. and Jain N.C. (1971). In: Jain N.C. (Ed.), Bovine Mastitis, Lea and Febiger, Philadelphia., pp. 94–127.

Schanbacher, F.L., Goodman, R.E. and Talhouk, R.S. (1993). J. Dairy Sci. 76: 3812-3831.

Schonwetter, B.S., Stolzenberg, E.D. and Zasloff, M.A. (1995). Science., 267: 1645–1648.

Schroder, J. M. (1999). Cell. Mol. Life Sci., 56: 32-46.

Schroder, J. M., Morwietz, U., Morita, E. and Christophers, E. (1987). J. Immunol., 139: 3474–3483.

Schultze, W.D. and Bright, S.C. (1983). Am. J. Vet. Res., 44: 2373–2375.

Selsted, M.E., Nonotny, M.J., Morris, W.L., Tang, Y.Q., Smith, W. and Cullor, J. S. (1993). J. Biol. Chem., 267: 4292-4295.

Selsted, M.E., Tang, Y.Q., Morris, W.L., McGuire, P.A., Nonotny, M.J., Smith, W., Henschen, A.H. and Cullor, H. S. (1993). J. Biol. Chem., 268: 6641.

Shafer-Weaver, K. A. and Sordillo, L.M. (1996). J. Dairy Sci., 79: 1347.

Shafer-Weaver, K. and Sordillo, L.M. (1996). J. Dairy Sci., 79:1347–1352.

Shafer-Weaver, K.A., Pighetti, G.M. and Sordillo, L.M. (1996). In: Proc. Soc. Exp. Biol. Med., 212: 271.

Sheldrake, R.F., Hoarse, R.J.T. and McGregor, G.D. (1983). J. Dairy Sci., 66(3):542.

Shuster, D.E., Kehrli, M.E., Jr Rainard, P. and Paape, M. (1997). Infect. Immun., 65: 3286–3292.

Singh, P.J. (1991). Studies on mastitis in cattle at machine milked farms in Punjab. M.V.Sc. Thesis, Punjab Agric. Univ., Ludhiana, India.

Smits, E., Burvenich, C., Guidry, A.J., Heyneman, R. and Massart-Leen, A. (1999). Vet. Immunol. Immunopathol., 68: 169–176.

Snider, T. G., Luther, D. G., Jenny, B.F., Hoyt, P.G., Battlesm J.K., Ennis, W.H., Blas-Machado, U., Lemarchand, T.X. and Gonda, M.A. (1996). Comparative Immunolog, Microbiology and Infectious Diseases., 19: 117-31.

Sohn, E.J., Paape, M.J., Peters, R.R., Fetterer, R.H., Talbo,t N.C. and Bannerman, D.D. (2004). Vet. Res., 35: 597–608.

Soltys, J. and Quinn, M.T. (1999). Infect Immun., 67: 6293-302.

Sordillo, L.M. and Nickerson, S.C. (1988). Am. J. Vet. Res., 49: 1112.

Sordillo, L.M. and Streicher, K.L. (2002). J. Mammary Gland Biol Neoplasia., 7:135-46.

Sordillo, L.M., Campos, M. and Babiuk, L.A. (1991). J. Dairy Sci., 74:3370.

Sordillo, L.M., Kendall, J.T., Corl, C.M. and Cross, T.H. (2005). J. Dairy Sci., 88: 1378–1390.

Sordillo, L.M., Shafer-Weaver, K. and DeRosa, D. (1997). J. Dairy Sci., 80:1851-65.

Stein, B.N., Gamble, J.R., Pitson, S.M., Vadas, M.A. and Khew-Goodall, Y. (2003). J Immunol., 171: 6097-104.

Talos, V.G., Roth, P.P. and Trif, A. (1975). Deutsche Tierarztliche Wochenchrift, 82: 286.

Targowski, S.P. (1983). J. Dairy Sci., 66:1781-1789.

Targowski, S.P. and Berman, D.T. (1975). Am. J. Vet. Res., 36:1561.

Taylor, B.C., Dellinger, J.D., Cullor, J.S. and Scott, J.L. (1994). Cell. Immunol., 156: 245.

Tizard, I.R. (1998). Veterinary immunology:An introduction, 5th edn. Harcourt brace & Company Asia Pte Ltd., New Delhi, India.

Tomita, M., Bellamy, W.R., Takase, M., Yamauchi, K., Wakabayashi, H. and Kawase, K. (1991). J. Dairy Sci., 74: 4137–4142.

Treece, J. M., Morese, G. E. and Llevy, C. (1966). J. Dairy Sci., 49: 1240.

Verhoef, J., Peterson, P.K. and Quie, P.G. (1977). Immunolog., 33:231.

Welty, F.K., Smith, K.L. and Schanbacher, F.L. (1976). J. Dairy Sci. 59: 224–231.

Wilkinson, P.C. (1980). Rev. Infect. Dis., 2: 293-318.

Yamaguchi, T., Hiratsuka, M., Asai, K., Kai, K. and Kumagai, K. (1999). J Dairy Sci., 82:1459-64.

Yang, W., Zerbe, H., Petzl, W., Brunner, R.M., Gunther, J., Draing, C., Von Aulock, S., Schuberth, H.J. and Seyfert, H.M. (2008). Mol. Immunol., 45: 1385-1397.

Zecconi, A., Binda, E., Borromeo, V. and Piccinini, R. (2005). J. Dairy Res., 72: 203-8.

Zecconi, A., Bronzo, V., Piccinini, R., Spreafico, G. and Ruffo, G. (1994). J. Dairy Res., 61: 271–279.

Zecconi, A., Hamanno, J.A., Bronzo, V., Maroni, P., Giovannini, G. and Piccinini, R. (2002). Biol. Mamm. Gland., 480: 287-293.

Zhang, H. and Issekutz, A.C. (2002). Am. J. Pathol., 160: 2219-30.

Zittle, C.A., Dellamonica, E.S., Custer, J.H. and Rudd, R.K. (1956). J. Dairy Sci., 39(5): 528-535.

Zucht, H.D., Raida, M., Adermann, K., Magert, H.J. and Forssman, W.G. (1995). FEBS Lett., 372: 185–188.

❑❑❑

CHAPTER

7

Etiology

Mastitis is defined as an inflammatory reaction of the parenchyma of the mammary gland that can be of an infectious, traumatic or toxic nature (International Diary Federation, 1987). Previously, the mastitis researchers associated the mastitis with physical factors like cold and mechanical injuries. Frank in the year 1876, transmitted the disease by inoculating inflammatory secretions from diseased quarters into the canals of healthy quarters. He thus proved the infectious nature of this disease and put forward an entirely new concept in the investigation of mastitis etiology. An association between mastitis and pathogenic micro-organisms was established in 1887. Most major pathogens were identified by the 1940s. When antimicrobial therapy became available for production animals in 1945, it proved effective in the control of some, but not all, mastitis pathogens. In the 1960s, the multifactorial etiology of bovine mastitis was commonly recognized. Today's, mastitis is considered to be a multifactorial disease. The most common cause of mastitis is infection with mastitis causing organisms. Whilst over 200 microbial species, sub species and serotypes have been isolated from bovine mammary gland (Mallikarjunaswamy and Krishnamurthy, 1997) and identified as causative agents of mastitis. Apart of different species of bacteria, several other groups of micro-organisms such as virus, fungi, yeast, algae and Chlamydia can cause mastitis in cattle and buffeloes (Table 7.1). Mastitis bacteriology provides relevant information for the farmer and veterinarian to inform mastitis treatment and prevention strategies and should be carried out as a routine irrespective of mastitis incidence and bulk milk quality. Selecting the correct cows and quarters to sample, the correct number of samples, sampling technique and result interpretation are important to ensure an accurate assessment of the causes of mastitis in a herd.

Despite intensive aetiological research, still around 20-35% of clinical cases of bovine mastitis have an unknown etiology. Etiology of mastitis may be two types *"nonspecific type"* and *"specific or infectious type"*. The importance of various mastitis pathogens has also markedly changed throughout the past 50 years as a result of different control and husbandry methods used. Mastitis in India is usually caused by bacteria; non-bacterial organism's occurrence is rare.

Nonspecific mastitis was described as a deterioration of the mammary gland in the absence of a demonstrable etiologic agent. As first used, the name referred to mammary glands producing milk of above normal chlorine content and pH. Nonspecific mastitis has been expanded to include instances of mastitis from which commonly recognized bacterial pathogens are not isolated. During the recovery period of acute coliform mastitis, as well as in chronic coliform mastitis, the organisms frequently can not be demonstrated unless the milk is incubated before being cultured. When leukocyte count or screening test for mastitis are used, some mammary quarters will be found to be producing milk of above normal somatic cell count from which pathogenic bacteria are not isolated. Mammary quarters that have recovered from acute mastitis often require many weeks and months to return to normal. In veracity, nonspecific mastitis is misnomer.

With the proliferation of international trade, globalization, and global warming, the importance of the control of contagious and infectious diseases has increased dramatically (Barkema *et al.*, 2009). Mastitis causing organisms can be categorized as: *contagious or environmental pathogens*. The mastitis, which is caused by contagious organisms, called as *contagious mastitis*, and caused by environmental organisms known as *environmental mastitis*. Contagious mastitis is the "cow associated" form where infected cows are the reservoirs for bacteria and spread occurs cow to cow at milking time. As the name suggests, environmental mastitis comes from the cow's world or environment. One difference between contagious and environmental pathogens is that the primary reservoir for contagious pathogens is the infected udder and exposure is during milking. In contrast, the environmental pathogens survive and multiply readily in extra-mammary sites, especially bedding, and exposure to these organisms usually occur between milkings.

1. Contagious Pathogens

There are certain pathogenic bacteria which are contagious in nature. They transmit the infection from animal to animal through milking machine, milker's hand, clothes etc. Several contagious mastitis pathogens are endemic in most countries with a dairy industry, but not necessarily within every farm. The organisms which are mainly responsible for contagious mastitis are *Staphylococcus aureus, Strptococcus agalactiae* and *Mycoplasma spp. Corynebacterium pyogenes* is an opportunistic, contagious mastitis pathogen, usually spread by flies. *Staphylococcus aureus* and Mycoplasma have reservoirs outside the mammary gland and therefore cow's can develop *Staphylococcus aureus* and Mycoplasma mastitis themselves. Mycoplasma exists as a commensal organism in many cows, which are the bacteria lives in the lungs or reproductive tract without causing clinical disease. It can recrudesce, or flair up, and go to the mammary gland and cause mastitis at any time. *Staphylococcus aureus* is mostly an udder pathogen, but some cows with the mastitis strain of *Staphylococcus aureus* on their skin. These out of mammary gland reservoirs can provide bacteria for new infections.

2. Environmental Pathogens

The environment (e.g. soiled bedding material, dung, other waste material, dairy water etc.) of the cows and buffaloes is rich in mastitis pathogens and poses a constant threat to udder health. Environmental mastitis bacteria include a large number of both Gram positive and Gram negative species. *Streptococcus dysgalactiae, Streptococcus uberis, S. faecalis, S. bovis, Coagulase negative staphylococcus (CNS), Enterococcus fae*calis and *Enterococcus faecium* of the Gram positive species and *Escherichia coli, Klebsiella spp. Enterobacter spp.* and *Serratia spp.* of the Gram negative are the most common environemental pathogens of the bovine udder. However, *Escherichia coli* and *S. dysgalactiae* represents large proportion of the identified intramammary infections caused by the environmental pathogens in India.

3. Opportunistic Pathogens

These organisms get upper hand when there is poor hygienic condition, lower nutritional status and injury to the udder. The opportunistic organisms are- *Corynebacterium bovis, Pseudomonas* spp., *Nocardia* spp., *Yeast* etc.

There is description of some important mastitis causing microorganisms:-

Staphylococci

The genus Staphylococcus includes *Staphylococcus aureus*, the pathogenic form, and the *Staphylococcus epidermidis*, which is commonly regarded as being nonpathogenic or only mildly so. The *Staphylococcus epidermidis* together with other nonpathogenic organisms of the family Micrococaceae are commonly referred to as "*micrococci*" to distinguish them from the pathogenic *Staphylococcus aureus*.

Table 7.1: Common mastitis causing microorganisms.

Bacteria	Fungi / Yeast	Algae	Viruses
Staphylococcus aureus, Streptococcus agalactiae, Escherichia coli, Streptococcus dysgalaciae, Streptococcus uberis, Streptococcus zooepidermidis, Streptococcus faecalis, Streptococcus pyogenes, Corynebacterium pyogenes, Pseudomonas aeruginosa, Mycoplasma bovis, M. Canadensis, M. californicum, M. bovihirnis, M. dispar, M. bovigenitalium, M. alkalescens, Campylobacter jejuni, Haemophilus somnus, Streptococcus pneumoniae, Corynebacterium ulcerans, Klebsiella pneumoniae, K. oxytocia, Enterobacter aerogenes, Mycobacterium bovis, M. tuberculosis, M. lacticola, M. fortuitum, Bacillus cereus, Pasteurella multocida, P. Haemolytica, Bacteroides funduliformis, Serratia marceseens, Acholeplasma laidlawii, Yersenia pseudotuberculosis, Mannheimia haemolytica.	*Aspergillus fumigatus, A. nidulans, Trichosporon cutaneum, Trichosporon beigelii, Pichia spp., Geotrichum candidum, Nocardia asteroids, N. brasiliensis, N. farcinica. N. neocaledoniensis, Candida krusei, C. tropicalis, C. paratropicalis, C. quillermondii, C. rugosa, Crptococcus neoformans, Saccharomyces spp., Torulopsis etc.*	*Protothecal zopfii, P. trispora, P. wickerhamii, P. blaschkeae etc.*	*Adeno virus, Herpes virus, Rota virus, Reo virus, Mammilitis virus, Pseudocowpox virus, Parainfluenza virus, Apthovirus, R.P. virus, Bovine immunodeficiency virus etc.*

Facultative bacteria:
Peptococcus indolicus, Bacteroides melaninogenius, Eubacterium combesii, Clostridium sporogene, C. perfringens type A and Fusobacterium necrophorum, Citrobacter, Proteus.

Staphylococcus aureus

Staphylococci are Gram positive, aerobic, catalase positive, oxidase negative, non-motile, non spore forming and fermentative organisms. *Staphylococcus aureus* is part of the coagulase positive group that includes *Staphylococcus intermedius* and some strains of *Staphylococcus hyicus*. *Staphylococcus aureus* is one of the most important worldwide including India common causes of mastitis in bovines. It is responsible for major financial losses in dairy farming and for the culling of many cows. The pathogenicity of *Staphylococcus aureus* depends on the combined action of more than 40 different extracellular toxins, enzymes and cell surface proteins. *Staphylococcus aureus* virulence factors comprise structural components, secretory products and mechanisms that contribute to the ability of the bacteria to survive in the host cause mastitis. Structural components are peptidoglycan, teichoic acid and protein A, present in the cell wall and various cell surface associated molecules e.g. exopolysaccharides and proteins. Protein A is distributed as discrete patches throughout the cell wall in most strains of virulent *Staphylococcus aureus.* It has been detected on 50-60% of *Staphylococcus aureus* strains isolated from bovine mammary gland infection. The protein is believed to have antiphagocytic activity especially during the later stage of intramammary infection (Forsgren *et al.*, 1983). *Staphylococcus aureus* secreted or produces different exotoxins and enzymes that destroy tissue and protect bacteria from host immune response. *Staphylococcus aureus* isolated from bovine mastitis express a, b, g and d hemolytic toxins (Bramley *et al.*, 1989) and all are antigenically distinct. *Staphylococcus aureus* produces a-toxins during growth or multiplication in the mammary gland and it is produced by about 20-50% of strains from bovine intramammary infections. Bovine teat cells are the most resistant to damage by a-toxin and secretory cells are the least resistant (Cifrian *et al.*, 1995). b-toxin is a sphingomyelinase-C and is produced by 75-100% of *Staphylococcus aureus* strains from bovine intramammary infection. It hydrolyses the sphingomyelin present in the exoplasmic leaflet of the plasma membrane resulting in increased permeability with progressive loss of cell surface charge. β-toxin damages bovine mammary secretory epithelial cells, increases the damaging effects of α-toxin, which in turn increases the adherence of *Staphylococcus aureus* to mammary epithelial cells and increases the proliferation of *Staphylococcus aureus*. The role of γ, δ and exfoilative (A and B) toxins in intramammary infection are not known. Other toxins include enterotoxins (serotypes A, B, C1, C2, C3, D,E, and H), leukocidin and toxic shock syndrome toxin-1. Leukocidin toxin has cytolytic effects on bovine polymorphonuclear neutrophils and macrophages. *Staphylococcus aureus* also produces numerous extracellular enzymes including coagulase, collagenase, acid and alkaline phosphatase, catalse, proteases, nuclease, elastase, lipasehyaluronate lyase, thermonuclease, lipase, betalactamase, glycerol-ester-hydrolase, fatty acid modifying enzymes and staphylokinase that have been implicated in the pathogenesis of bovine mastitis. Enzymes could allow *Staphylococcus aureus* to use milk substrates for their metabolism.

Staphylococcus aureus is the cause of contagious mastitis that is mainly sub-clinical and chronic but may be peracute and lead to gangrene of affected quarter. The chronic and sub-clinical forms predominate and on a herd basis are most important. Clinically infected quarters often show moderate to severe swelling and visible signs of garget or chunks of milk, especially in fore stripping. Acute *Staphylococcus aureus* infections generally develop late in the lactation or just prior to calving. Chronic and sub-clinical mastitis are often associated with fibrosis, abscessation and blocked ducts within the gland. As few as 10 CFU (colony forming units) of *Staphylococcus aureus* can infect the udder (Newbould and Neave, 1965). Major reservoirs of these organisms are infected udder, teat canals and teat lesions, but these bacteria also have been found on teat skin, muzzles, nostrils and vagina. The bacteria are spread to uninfected quarters by teat cup liners, milker's hand, wash cloths and flies. There is some evidence that aerosols play some role in the spread of this organism.

The most notable features of the *Staphylococcus aureus* surround its ability to evade and influence the host immune system. *Staphylococcus aureus* produce various toxins that destroy all membrane and can directly damage milk producing tissue. Coagulase is one such product, which is useful in the coagulase test to distinguish pathogenic from nonpathogenic strains of Staphylococci. Leucocytes are attached to the area of inflammation where they attempt to fight off the infection. Initially, the bacteria damage the tissue lining, the teat and gland cisterns within the quarter. Then they move up into the duct system and establish deep seated pockets of infection in the milk secreting cells (alveoli). This is followed by walling-off of bacteria by scar tissue and the formation of abscesses, which is responsible for the poor response to antibiotic treatment. A small part of the antibiotic failure may be due to the production of penicillinase by some strains of Staphylococci. Only

20-70% of the antibiotic treatments during the dry period therapy are effective and only 10-30% of cases of *Staphylococcus aureus* mastitis are cured by antibiotic treatment during lactation. Alveolar and duct cells may be destroyed and milk yield is reduced. Grohn *et at.* (2004) evaluated the effect of pathogen specific (Staphylococcus) clinical mastitis on milk yield and reported that about 8.4 kg/day and 5.5 kg/day reduction in milk yield in primiparous and pluriparous cows, respectively after clinical mastitis outcome. Piccinni *et al.* (2003) reported total loss of 5.778 tons of milk/year in Lombardia (Italy). The degenerated cells may combine with leucocytes and clog the milk ducts that drain the alveolar areas, contributing to further scar tissue formation. The ducts may reopen and release *Staphylococcus aureus* organisms to other areas of the mammary gland and subsequently abscess formation may occurs.

The *Staphylococcus aureus* strains are more dangerous to dairy farmers world wide because it have so many properties (Green and Bradley, 2004) like-

1. Production of various enzymes and toxins, some of which cause damage to mammary tissue and allow tissue invasion. The alpha-toxin is potentially the most damaging, because it causes vasoconstriction leading to ischemic necrosis of affected tissues and gangrene. Combination of β- and δ-toxins are more irritating than either toxin alone (Slanetz and Barley, 1953)
2. An ability to survive in the keratin of the teat canal of healthy cows, a substance normally inhibitory to bacterial growth.
3. A capability to resist phagocytosis, e.g. protein 'A' in the cell wall of some *Staphylococcus aureus* strains binds to the Fc portion of antibody molecules making the bacteria unrecognizable to neutrophils. Even if phagocytosed, *Staphylococcus aureus* may survive and even multiply inside phagocytes.
4. Low level of complement and opsonizing antibodies specific to *Staphylococcus aureus* in milk.
5. An ability to resist antibiotic therapy due to-

- Production of beta-lactamase, an enzyme that inactivates penicillin and closely related antibiotics. Probably around 50% of mastitis *Staphylococcus aureus* strains produce beta-lactamase and there is evidence that these strains are more difficult to cure with all antibiotics.
- The ability of the bacteria to survive inside polymorphonucleocytes (PMN), macrophages and mammary epithelial cells, protected from antibiotic action, may significantly contribute to their antibiotic therapy

resistance. Additionally, the pathological changes, notably granulomata and fibrosis, induced in chronic *Staphylococcus aureus* infections renders chronically infected cows essentially incurable.

- An existence of L-forms that are resistant to antibiotics.

Glands harboring non-phathogenic *Staphylococci* commonly exhibit mild leucocytosis in milk without clinical mastitis. This leucocytosis is protective against coliform organisms (Schalm and Lasmanis, 1968). Indiscriminate treatment of cows for *Staphylococcal* infections will lead to removal of the non-pathogenic *Staphylococci* and may predispose the herd to infection by coliform organisms or other mammary pathogens.

Coagulase negative Staphylococci (CNS)

Coagulase negative Staphylococcus (CNS) refers to staphylococcus bacteria that are not *Staphylococcus aureus*. The name *"coagulase-negative"* refers to a laboratory test that differentiates this species of bacteria from the "coagulase-positive" *Staph aureus*. These bacteria are also some times referred to an *"environmental staphs"*. Coagulase-negative *Staphylococcal* spp. including *Staphylococcus epidermidis, Staphylococcus xylosus* and other staphylococci have low virulence and are considered opportunistic causes of mastitis, but they can cause microscopic lesions in the mammary gland (Morresey 1999), and can induce moderate increases in somatic cell count (SCC). *Staphylococcus hyicus* and *Staphylococcus chromogenes* are commonly isolated from milk samples and the teat canal; *Staphylococcus xylosus* and *Staphylococcus sciuri* are found free-living in the enviroment; *Staphylococcus warneri, Staphylococcus simulans* and *Staphylococcus epidermidis* are part of the normal flora of the teat skin (Radostits *et al.*, 2000). Boddie *et al.* (1987) found that *Staphylococcus xylosus* and *Staphylococcus hyicus* subspecies *chromogenes* were the predominant flora isolated from the teat skin. The prevalence of these pathogens is higher in first lactation animals than older cows, and higher immediately after calving than in the remainder of the lactation. They have also been found in the teat canal and in intramammary infections in nulliparous heifers. A study by Matthews *et al.* (1991) suggested that quarters harbouring coagulase negative Staphylococcal infection suppressed bacterial invasion by mastitis-causing pathogens. Indeed the presence of *Staphylococcus epidermidis* may be beneficial as it tends to occupy attachment sites in the teat duct required by coagulase positive pathogenic staphylococci (Quinn *et al.*, 1994).

In many countries with intensive dairy production CNS have been identified as *"emerging mastitis pathogens"*. The CNS has often been referred to as minor pathogens because infections tend to be mild with minimal economic loss (Smith and Hogan, 1995a). These infections only modestly elevated SCC and infrequently cause clinical mastitis. It is generally held that in clinical CNS mastitis, only mild local signs are usually seen, such as slight swelling and changes in the milk appearance, but thorough investigations of clinical characteristics of mastitis caused by CNS are rare (Taponen *et al.*, 2006). The predominant species of CNS associated with intramammary infection are a part of the normal skin flora of cows and as such the exposure of teat ends is very high. The CNS are generally the leading cause of intramammary infection in herd's practicing post-milking teat infection and total dry cow therapy (Smith and Hogan, 1995b). Infections with CNS are usually highest immediately after calving, decline in mid lactation and decrease again in late lactation until the cow receives dry cow therapy. It is generally assumed that spontaneous cure rate of CNS mastitis is high, and in many countries, mastitis caused by CNS is commonly left untreated. The observed spontaneous cure probability varies from 60–70% to 16–49% (Taponen *et al.*, 2006). However, several studies have shown that CNS mastitis may persist during lactation, with 76% to 85% persisting until cessation of milking (Taponen and Payorala, 2009).

Streptococci

An identification of Streptococci as a cause of bovine mastitis was first recorded towards the end of the 19th century. Streptococci are Gram positive, most are facultatively anaerobic and some are strictly anaerobic, catalase-negative, oxidase-negative, non-motile, non-spore forming, and fermentative. Streptococci were the first bacteria to be incriminated as the cause of an infectious and contagious form of chronic mastitis of worlwide distribution. Refinements in bacteriological techniques for identification of different streptococci were developed between 1920 to 1935. Three species, *Strpetococcus agalactiae, Streptococcus dysgalactiae* and *Streptococcus uberis*, were identified as the main streptococci involved in the mastitis, with *Streptococcus agalactiae* being the most prevalent. Under special circumstances, other species of streptococci may produce herd problems of mastitis but are not of worldwide significance. Recently an outbreak of *Streptococcus canis* mastitis in dairy cows from Israel had been reported (Chaffer *et al.*, 2005). The occurence of *Streptococcus canis* was 38% of cows and 20% of all quarters. They can be classified into six principal categories based on growth characteristics, type of haemolysis, and biochemical activities or classified by virtue of Lancefield groups (Carter *et al.*, 1995).

Streptococcus agalactiae

Streptococcus is a general name for a class of bacteria capable of causing mastitis in dairy animals. *Streptococcus agalactiae* is a common cause of sub-clinical and mild to moderate clinical mastitis in dairy cows. It was a major cause of chronic mastitis in pre-antibiotic era. *Streptococcus agalactiae* is a highly infectious obligate parasite of the udder and, unlike coliform organisms, it does not survive in the environment of the cow i.e. totally dependent upon the mammary gland for survival in nature, because of this host-parasite relationship, it is relatively easy to eradicate. It is contagious organism and transmits from infected cows (udder) to healthy cows (udder) during milking. Cows with *Streptococcus agalactiae* mastitis usually have elevated somatic cell counts but normal milk. Occasionally the cow may progress from sub-clinical to clinical mastitis. During episodes of clinical mastitis the signs are usually limited to abnormal milk and udder swelling. Incomplete milking aggrevates *Streptococcus agalactiae* mastitis and may intensify the injury to secretory tissue and hasten secretory destruction of the gland (Schalm and Mead, 1943). *Streptococcus agalactiae* multiplies in the milk and on the mammary epithelial surfaces, generally causing a subacute or chronic inflammatory reaction with periodic acute flareups. The affected tissue eventually is destroyed resulting in reduced milk production or agalactia. The presence of *Streptococcus agalactiae* in a herd suggests that there are defects in milking hygiene, postmilking teat disinfection and/or dry-cow therapy. Since *Streptococcus agalactiae* is easily eliminated by intramammary antibiotic therapy it is eliminated from herds employing teat disinfection and dry-cow therapy effectively and routinely. It is possible to include the elimination of infection by blitz therapy during lactation. *Blitz therapy* is where all quarters of infected cows are treated with intramammary antibiotics. It is important to confirm that *Streptococcus agalactiae* is the cause of the high cell count before embarking on blitz therapy. The incidence of *Streptococcus agalactiae* mastitis seems to increase with the lactation age of cows in an infected herd, fourth or more lactations showing a 75% or more infection rate (Schalm *et al.*, 1971). In many countries, IMI with *Streptococcus agalactiae* is still common (Zadoks and Fitzpatrick, 2009). In individual cows, the loss of production caused by *Streptococcus agalactiae* mastitis is about 25% during the infected lactation, and in affected herds the loss may be of the order of 10-15% of the potential production. The duration of infection is shorter than staphylococci, primarily because of the better response to therapy.

Environmental Streptococci

The term *"environmental streps."* often is used to replace the terms *"non-ag. Streptococci"* and refers to all forms of streptococcal bacteria other than *Streptococcus agalactiae* that are capable of causing mastitis in dairy cows and buffaloes. The most common mastitis causing environmental streps are two- *Streptococcus dysgalactiae* and *Streptococcus uberis*. Other environmental streps. are *Streptococcus faecalis* and *Streptococcus bovis*, *Streptococcus pyogenes*, *Streptococcus pneumoniae* etc.

Streptococcus dysgalactiae is not as infectious as *Streptococcus agalactiae* and is not an obligate pathogen. This organism has both contagious and environmental characteristics often associated with poor teat skin condition. It can cause acute infection with systemic illness with outbreaks often associated with an increase in teat lesions. Mammary infection with *Streptococcus dysgalactiae* often follows teat injury. *Streptococcus dysgalactiae* is commonly isolated from dry cows and heifers and is one of the most prevalent pathogens in summer mastitis cases.

The esculin hydrolysing streptococci are an important cause of bovine mastitis and, in some herds, are the major cause of clinical mastitis. Several species can be involved but the predominant one (>70 per cent) is *Streptococcus uberis*. Others include *Streptococcus bovis, Streptococcus faecalis* and *Streptococcus faecium*. Infection with these organisms is not controlled by postmilking teat disinfection although dry-cow antibiotic therapy reduces infection rates by about 50%. However, *Streptococcus uberis* remains the commonest cause of infection in the dry period and susceptibility to infection has been shown to increase following dryingoff (Marshall *et al.*, 1986). The high infection rates in the dry period and the failure of post milking teat disinfection to control disease emphasize the independence of milking and transmission. *Streptococcus uberis* is considered to be an opportunistic pathogen that can survive and multiply in extramammary sites, including lips, haircoat, tonsils and the rectum of cows. It is known that *Streptococcus uberis* can invade bovine mammary epithelial cells *in vitro* (Matthews *et al.*, 1994), and that it has anti-phagocytic properties (Oliver *et al.*, 1998). *Streptococcus uberis* proliferates in most bedding material, but especially in straw (Ward *et al.*, 2002). Faecal contamination of the teats is an important factor in the development of *Streptococcus uberis* mastitis. Excessive use of water to wash udders without proper drying of the udder before milking has been associated with increased *Streptococcus uberis* infection during lactation. *Streptococcus uberis* is the pathogen that is most frequently isolated from clinical cases that occur in the dry period (Jayarao *et al.*, 1999), and the incidence increases with advancing age (Jayarao *et al.*, 1999; Sharma, 2003). Smith *et al.* (1985b) and Todhunter *et al.* (1995) reported that the rate of streptococcal infection was higher during the summer in lactating and dry cows and the prevalence of *Streptococcus uberis* is also high near calving or during early and late lactation (Jayarao *et al.*, 1999). Infection characteristics of environemental streptococci include- 1) 40% infection will persist for less than 8 days; 2) 60 to 70% will persist for less than 30 days; 3) 18% will persist for more than 100 days; 4) 40-50% will become clinical; and 5) 50% will develop during the dry period, especially during the 2 weeks before parturition. *Streptococcus uberis* is considered by some to be the major weakness in mastitis control recommendations, due to its' ubiquitous nature and a lack of knowledge of the pathogenesis of *Streptococcus uberis* infections.

The difficulty in control of this pathogen was recognised by Dodd and Neave (1970), who concluded that complete elimination of *Streptococcus uberis* was unlikely but the infection can be maintained at a low level and control improved by virtue of better dry period therapy and by better management of existing milking machines.

The primary sources of environmental strep. bacteria that cause mastitis are environmental sites on the farm such as bedded housing, calving areas, standing water and soil in open corrals and pens. The most frequent and significant sites for teat end exposure are dry cow lots or pens and fresh cow pens, lots or stalls. In addition, outside dirt lots or yards, ponds and low wet areas increases the risk of environmental strep. infections. An other important source of environmental streps. are deposited on to the bedding from belly skin and uterine discharges. Most mammary gland infections caused by environmental streps. occur during the intervals between milkings when the teat ends comes in contact with highly contaminated bedding or other surfaces. Because of their many environmental sources, environmental strep. bacteria can not be totally eliminated from a dairy herd. Environmental strep. infections can range from mild, clinical cases to severe, life threatening infections. About 50% of infections by environmental streptococci cause clinical mastitis.

Coliform pathogens

"Coliform" is a general term for fermentative Gram-negative bacilli that inhabit the intestinal tract of man and other animals normally without causing disease and that are contained within the family Entcrobacteriaceae. The term has not been defined strictly; some workers include in it all the enteric bacteria; others limit it to the lactose-fermenting members. In reference to bovine mastitis, the term usually has the latter meaning because the gram-negative bacteria commonly causing udder disease are lactose fermenters and includes *Escherichia coli, Klebsiella* and *Enterobacter* species (*aerogenes* and *cloacae*). Enterobacteria are Gram negative, aerobic and facultative anaerobic medium sized rods, catalase positive, oxidase negative, non-spore forming, fermentative and usually motile organisms. The term coliform mastitis frequently is used incorrectly to identify mastitis caused by all Gram negative bacteria. Genera classified as coliforms are *Escherichia, Klebsiella* and *Enterobacter.* Other Gram negative bacteria frequently isolated from intramammary infections include species of *Serratia, Pseudomonas* and *Proteus.* Specifically *Escherichia coli* and *K. pneumoniae* are most commonly isolated coliforms from intramammary infections. Coliform bacteria occupy many habitats in the cows environment. They are ubiquitous in the environment of dairy cows, manure and infected quarters are the primary source of *Escherichia coli*. Infection is more common among housed cows and occurs particularly around calving. The bacteria

survive poorly on skin and are rapidly eliminated from the mammary gland. They are viable at 15-45°C and grow optimally at 37°C. They thrive in acidic conditions but can tolerate alkalinity up to pH 9.5. Sub-clinical infection is less common and peracute mastitis occurs frequently around calving. About 50 per cent of these peracute infections die. *Escherichia coli* was first recorded in bovine mastitis milk in 1896 (Kitt, 1896). *Escherichia coli* are normal inhabitants of the gastrointestinal tract of warm blooded animals. Both *Klebsiella spp.* and *Enterobacter spp.* populate soils, grains, water and intestinal tracts of animals (Hogan and Smith, 2003). *K. pneumoniae* is cause of mastitis when dairy farmer's use saw dust bedding, especially rough cut saw dust that contain bark or soil. Newman and Kowalski, (1973); and Bramman *et al.* (1973) reported that saw dust bedding is a source of *Klebsiella spp.* in several herds with mastitis due to this organism. *K. pneumoniae* is responsible for causing acute chronic mastitis in dairy animals (Tijare *et al.*, 2002). A serious outbreak of mastitis *K. pneumoniae* had been reported by Sampimon *et al.* (2006). *Serratia marcesens* share many environmental sources with *Klebsiella spp.* and *Enterobacter spp. Pseudomonas spp.* and *Proteus spp.* commonly contaminate drop hoses used to wash udders before milking. Although the mammary gland is not considered a natural habitat for coliform bacteria, many strains are capable of surviving and multiplying in the mammary gland. Coliform mastitis is typically acute or per acute, but chronic and sub-clinical infections accompanied with periodic acute flare-ups also occurs. Coliform mastitis is generally self limiting and does not cause extensive damage to the mammary parenchyma; hence, milk production does not decrease significantly following recovery (Jain, 1979). Per-acute cases of coliform mastitis may result in a loss of function of the affected gland, agalactiae affecting all quarters and, occasionally, death of the cow within a few days due to endotoxaemia, with clinical signs including pyrexia, marked depression, dehydration, rumen dysfunction, anorexia and recumbency. Peracute cases only comprise around 10% of all coliform infections (Bushnell, 1974); the more common presentation being acute cases characterized by hard, swollen quarters with brief period of pyrexia, anorexia and rumen atony. A major difference between intramammary infections caused by coliform bacteria and those caused by other Gram negative bacteria, is the duration that bacteria persist in the mammary gland. The majority of infections with Gram negative organisms are of short duration (<28 days), but *Klebsiella* spp., *Pseudomonas* spp. and *Serratia* spp. may result in infections of significantly longer duration (chronic infection) than infections with *Escherichia coli*. The average duration of *Escherichia coli* intramammary infections during lactation is <10 days (Todhunter *et al.*, 1991). Infection characteristics of coliforms include- 1) 57% infection will persist for <10 days; 2) 70% will persist for <30 days; 3) 2% will persist for more than 100 days, with most being Klebsiella spp.; 4) 90% will become clinical; and 5) 10% will cause peracute clinical mastitis. Since coliform bacteria are widespread in the environment of the dairy cow, the question arises as to why this form of mastitis is relatively uncommon and why it is so severe when it does occur. The coliforms are not pathogens in the true sense. They will multiply rapidly in normal milk but are inhibited by milk containing leukocytes and other products of inflammation. As long as the more common mastitis pathogens are available to invade mammary glands and stimulate a leukocytosis in the milk, coliform organism seems unable to establish themselves within such glands. The rates of new intramammary infections caused by coliforms are greater during the dry period than during lactation. The rate of new intramammary infection is about four times higher in the dry period than during lactation (Figure 7.1), the two weeks after drying off and the two weeks prior to calving (Smith *et al.*, 1985a). While during lactation is highest at calving and decreases as days in milk advances. Severity of the disease depends on the virulence of invading organism. Gram negative bacteria isolated from bovine mammary infections posses a myriad of virulence factors. Endotoxin is the primary virulence factor of Gram negative bacteria responsible for damage to the cow. Endotoxin refers to the lipopolysaccharide portion of the Gram negative bacterial wall. Locally, endotoxin does not directly affect secretory cell but disrupts the blood flow. The ability of strains to evade neutrophils is a key virulence factor for coliform bacteria. Difference in susceptibility to phagocytosis among coliform strains is related to variability of surface exposed antigens. Capsules produced by *K. pneumoniae* isolated from bovine intramammary infections block deposition of complement and camouflage against antibody mediated opsonization. Capsule producing strains of *Escherichia coli* (Hill *et al.*, 1983). *Pseudomonas* spp. and *Proteus* spp. produce capsular material associated with reduced phagocytosis and chronicity of disease.

Coliform bacteria do not appear to colonize inside the mammary gland, but multiply in the secretion without attachment to epithelial surfaces. Once coliforms enter the mammary gland, they often multiply rapidly or may remain dormant for several days. As they multiply, coliforms produce endotoxins, which are subsequently released when the bacteria are destroyed by leucocytes. Once released from the bacteria, the toxins are absorbed into the blood stream. A cow affected by the toxins will show signs of high fever, depressed appetite, rapid weight loss, abnormal milk and decreased production within a few hours.

Proteus species

Proteus species are Gram negative bacteria that are found in the cows environment in bedding, manure, feed and water. Generally, *Proteus* spp. is not a common mastitis pathogen, it is generally contamitant. However, rare infections can occur between milkings when teat ends are indirect contact with contaminated surfaces. Mastitis due to *Proteus* spp. is often chronic, difficult to cure, and unresponsive to antibiotics.

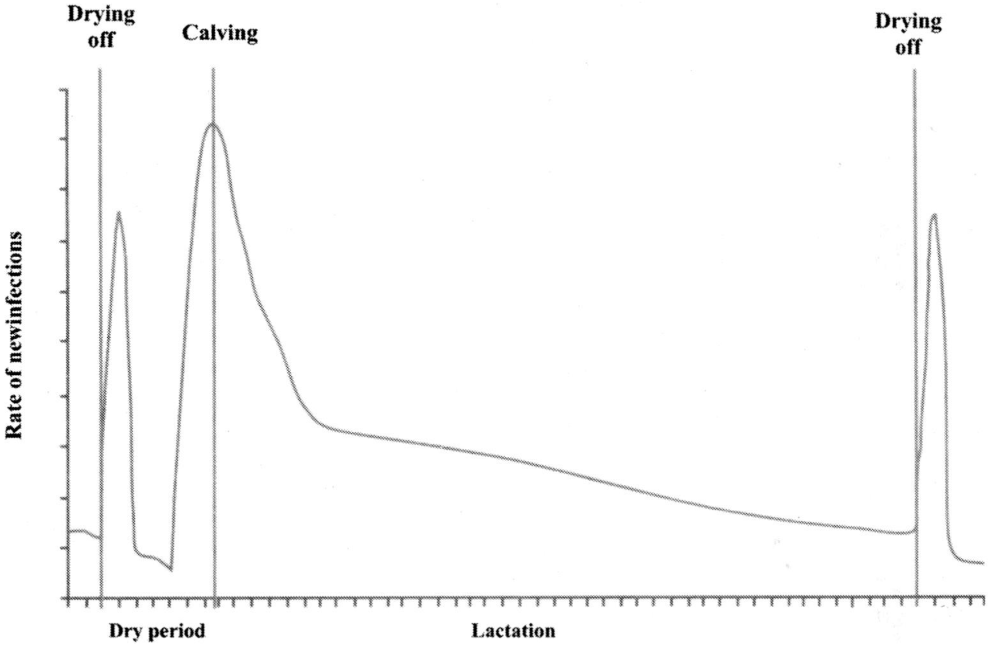

Figure 7.1: Schematic representation of the frequency of new coliform intramammary infections during the lactation cycle.

Serratia species

Serratia species are Gram negative bacteria that are commonly found in soil and water. *S. marcescens* causes mild chronic mastitis in which swelling of the quarters with clots in the milk appear periodically. *S. liquefaciens* can also cause similar mastitis. However, *Serratia* spp. may cause clinical mastitis that does not respond well to lactating cow antibiotic treatment.

Corynebacteria species

Diphtheroid organisms are commonly encountered in milk and, with the exception of *Corynebacterium pyogenes*, are pathogenic. *Corynebacterium pseudotuberculosis* infection is also prevalent in many Israeli dairy herds (Aroch *et al.*, 2003). The corynebacteria are small pleomorphic Gram positive rods.

Corynebacterium bovis

Corynebacterium bovis are Gram positive, aerobic, non-spore forming, non-motile, catalse positive, fermentative, small pleomorphic rods with club shaped swelling at one or both ends. Pallisade or *"picketfence"* alignment of cells is common. It belongs to a genus sub grouping (composed of 10 species) whose principal characteristic is that their growth in vitro is enhanced by the addition of lipid to growth media. These species are referred to as "lipophilic". *C. bovis* is one of the most prevalent organisms isolated from bovine milk. It is a commensal organism of the reproductive tract of some cows and bulls, and on the squamous cell epithelium of the teat duct of as many as 20% of the quarters of the cows. The primary site of *C. bovis* infection within the bovine mammary gland is thought to be the teat canal. Numbers of organisms appear to fall rapidly above ad around Furstenberg's rosette, although infection can exist in the teat cistern and udder tissues. *C. bovis* is considered to be mildly pathogenic (sub-clinical disease) often inducing moderate increases in SCC and can spread rapidly from cow to cow in the absence of adequate teat dipping (Quinn *et al.*, 1994). Despite its limited pathogenicity it is highly infectious, even more so than *Staphylococcus aureus* and *Streptococcus agalactiae* (Pankey *et al.*, 1985). A study in U.K. by Huxley *et al.* (2002) has suggested that the presence of *C. bovis* may have a protective role against sub sequent infection with a major mastitis pathogen. The role of *C. bovis* in intramammary infection dynamics is contentious. Since 1972, literature has produced much conflicting data on the protective effect of *C. bovis*. Some researchers suggest that *C. bovis* protect the quarters against subsequent infection with *Staphylococcus aureus* (Berry and Hillerton, 2002), *Streptococcus agalactiae* (Viseslava and Vera, 1989), *Streptococcus uberis* (Zadoks *et al.*, 2001), *Escherichia coli* (Hogan *et al.*, 1988) and major pathogens (Honkanen-Buzalski *et al.*, 1984). Conversely other workers suggested that quarters infected with *C. bovis* were at significantly at greatest risk of suffering concurrent infection with environemental *Streptococci* (Berry and Hillerton, 2002), and *Staphylococcus aureus, Streptococcus agalactiae,* other *Streptococci* and all major pathogens (Brooks *et al.*, 1983).

Black *et al.* (1972) postulated various possible reason in the protective role of *C. bovis*, including competitive growth/antagonism induced leucocytosis or an increase in host immunity. *C. bovis* infections may protect quarters by interfering with the ability of other pathogens to invade or multiply within the quarter. Bacteria can produce a wide range of molecules and substances that can inhibit the growth of and in some circumstances kill other bacteria.

Corynebacterium pseudotuberculosis

The mastitic form of the disease varies from being chronic, mild and sub-clinical to a subacute, severe clinical mastitis. In mild cases milk production is not affected, but the consistency of the milk is abnormal, and it contains flakes and clots. In severe cases the course of the disease is subacute to chronic, and it is associated with a progressive decline in production.The affected quarters become extremely swollen, hard and tender, with large amounts of purulent secretion and the complete cessation of milk production from all quarters, although no other systemic signs are observed and the cows appetite remains normal. Both the mild and the more severe clinical forms of the disease do not respond to antimicrobial treatment. The pathogenesis of *C. pseudotuberculosis* mastitis is uncertain, although it has been suggested that flies (House fly) play a role in its transmission (Braverman *et al.*, 1999). It is not known whether the udder is infected by haematogenous or lymphogenous spread, or whether it is inoculated via the teat canal. An experimental study was conducted by Aroch *et al.* (2003), the inoculation of 2000 colony-forming units of Corynebacterium pseudotuberculosis into one teat canal of each of three cows resulted in severe, chronic, pyogranulomatous mastitis. Within three days the cows had a reduced haematocrit, haemoglobin concentration and red cell count. The anaemia was initially normocytic, normochromic and non-regenerative, and was associated with a brief peak of neutrophilia; a regenerative response became evident two to three weeks later.

Mycoplasma species

Mycoplasma is a term for a group of organisms (bacteria like) that are classified as neither bacteria nor viruses. The *Mycoplasmas* are the smallest and simplest prokaryotic cells capable of self replication, they stain poorly Gram negative and can be seen in smears as coccobacilli, coccal forms, ring forms, spirals and filaments. It is a very fastidious organism; their infections are persistent, difficult to cure, and frequently challenging to detect and diagnose. Distinguishing characteristics of mycoplasma organisms are that they have no cell walls, permitting total assistance to any bacterial substance that interferes with cell walls such as penicillin, and upon visual inspection of cultured agar plates they appear to have a fried egg appearance. *Mycoplasma* mastitis was first reported in England in 1960 (Dairy Digest, 2004), while in United States, this disease was first reported in 1961 (Hale *et al.*, 1962). First it got the name *Mycoplasma bovimastitidis* then *Mycoplasma agalactiae subsp. bovis*, because of the similar clinical picture to the contagious agalactia of sheep caused by *M. agalactiae*. Several species of *Mycoplasma* (*M. bovis, M. Californicum, M. canadense, M. bovigenitalium, M. alkalescens, M. arginini, M. bovihirnis, M. dispar*, unnamed species (bovine group 7 and F-38) can cause mastitis in dairy cows (Alexander *et al.*, 1985; Jasper, 1981; Kumar and Garg, 1991) but *M. bovis* is the most frequent cause of *Mycoplasma* mastitis. Garg (2001) has been reported various species of Mollicutes from different parts of the India. Mollicutes are classified in three groups: *Mycoplasma, Acholeplasma* and *Ureaplasma*. Under *Mycoplasma* are *Mycoplasma bovis, M. canadense,*

M. bovigenitalium, M. californicum, M. alkalecens, M. bivirhinis, M. arginini, M. dispar, M. mycoides var. Capri, M. capricolum ss. capricolum, M. capricolum ss. Capripneumoniae. Acholeplasma are *Acholeplasma laidlawi axanthum, A. oculi* and *A. modicum*, and Ureaplasma is *U. diversum*. Ghazaei (2006) has been reported 48.75% prevalence of *M. bovis* in Ardabil state of Iran.

Entry of the disease to a herd is usually by the purchase of animals, and their introduction without quarantine. Mastitis causing *Mycoplasma* organisms are commonly found in the mucus membranes of the respiratory tract and urogenital tracts of healthy cows. Stresses such as calving, transportation, other diseases and external trauma may weaken the animal's immune system and allow the organisms to enter other body tissues such as the mammary gland, causing clinical mastitis. The most common cow-to-cow transmission of mastitis causing mycoplasma organisms occurs during the milking process through teat cups, milkers hands and mastitis therapy products and devices. Current data suggest that a significant number of new outbreaks may occur via internal or animal-to-animal transmission of *Mycoplasma* by asymptomatic carriers within the herd (Fox *et al.*, 2005). Failure to clean and sanitize the teat ends properly before administering mastitis treatments may actually spread mycoplasma from infected animals to uninfected animals (Hay, 2002). *Mycoplasma* bovine mastitis is a highly contagious and economically important disease of dairy animals. Mycoplasma mastitis may occur in two forms- clinical and sub-clinical form. Clinical form is characterized by a sudden onset of swelling in the udder of lactating cows with abnormal milk (tannish or brownish discolouration) usually observed from 1 to 3 days later. Milk often becomes watery in appearance and may contain small flakes of "sand like" material, when milk samples are left to stand; sandy particles usually sink to the bottom and leave whey like supernatant. Between days 4 to 6, discharge often appears yellowish brown which later (between 4 to 14 days) becomes very purulent (cottage cheese like appearance) (Larry, 1997). Even though milk production often decreases rapidly during infection, affected animals usually continue to eat and drink normally. *M. bovis* may also cause arthritis in affected cows, recently a report of arthritis in *M. bovis* mastitic cows has been reported by Houlihan *et al.* (2007) and they also reported that affected cows were aborted during hight of mastitis. *M. bovis* was even also isolated from aborted fetus. Sub-clinical form, is confirmed on the basis of somatic cell count (SCC). Normally SCC is elevated in mycoplasma infection but Janus (2009) reported that sub-clinical infections do occur with or without elevated SCC. Unremarkable SCC results may allow sub-clinically infected carrier animals to remain in the herd undetected for long period of time. These carrier animals act as reservoirs of infection and are a source of mycoplasma organisms for other cows. *Mycoplasma* mastitis due to *M. bovigenitalium* may be very mild and disappear from the herd spontaneously and without causing loss of milk production (Jackson and Boughton, 1991). Prevalence of *Mycoplasma* mastitis has increased in several countries (Fox *et al.*, 2005). Fortunately, mastitis due to *Mycoplasma* species is not a major problem in India, there major mastitis organisms are *Staphylococcus*, *Streptococcus* and Enterobacteriaceae.

Summer mastitis complex

Summer mastitis is complex infection caused by aerobic-anaerobic organisms, that is defined as *"acute suppurative mastitis"* occurs in heifers and non lactating cows predominantly during the summer (June, July, August and September) months in Britain. In India and U.S., the disease has been reported to occur irrespective of season, climate or weather. Microaerophilic *Actinomyces pyogenes* (formerly *Corynebacterium pyogenes*) predominates and produces toxic factors to allow synergestic growth of anaerobic bacteria such as *Peptococcus(Micrococcus) indolicus, Fusobacterium necrophorum, Streptococcus dysgalactiae, Bacillus* (Bacteroides) *melanonogenicus*. Other microaerophilic like Stuart-Schwan cocci, other Bacteroidaceae and *Micrococcus spp.* are also involved. *Corynebacterium pyogenes* is a potent toxin and pus producing organism. The serum of healthy cattle, sheep, goats and pigs contains *A. pyogenes* antitoxin (Lovell, 1939). In cattle the amount of antitoxin increases as the animal becomes older. Mastitis caused by *A. pyogenes* is always peracute with a severe systemic reaction including fever (105-106°F), rapid heart rate, complete anorexia, and severe depression and weakness. Abortion may occur during this stage. The clinical signs are characteristic and initially include lethargy and a swollen quarter(s) rapidly progressing to a hard, swollen and painful quarters. The characteristic of summer mastitis is watery secretion with clots early and later thick and creamy purulent exudate, with characteristic extremely foul odor and is frequently accompanied with a severe systemic reaction. The foul odor is not due to only *A. pyogenes* but rather to an accompanying organism, *Peptococcus indolicus.* Lameness in the hind limb on the affected sides is a common presenting sign. The affected quarters of the cows always destroyed; often indurated with subsequent abscesses that rupture through the floor of the udder, frequently at the base of the teat. The main method of transmission is by the sheep head fly *Hydrotea irritans.* These flies have been shown to carry mastitis pathogens and their control has reduced the incidence of summer mastitis. It is a sucking fly that feeds on discharges and the blood of the cattle and will be attracted to any wounds on the skin and teats of the cows already infected and carry the infection from infected site to the teats of healthy cows. The *Hydrotea irritans* tends to concentrate on front teats more than back, perhaps because the swishing tail discourages them from back teats. Infections are often associated with teat end damage, which suggest a direct mode of infection. Summer mastitis is a serious disease in that the mortality rate without adequate treatment is probably about 50% (Radostits *et al.*, 2000) and causes heavy economic losses. In a year of 1992, estimate of the cost of summer mastitis was about £270 per case in Europe (Berry, 1998). Milk production in subsequent lactations can be reduced by 5-60%. Adult flies are more commonly present during July, August and September, the months that summer mastitis is most common. Dry cow therapy and good fly control are still two of the most important and effective control measures available.

Mycobacterium

Mycobacteria are acid fast, non-motile, non-spore forming, aerobic, oxidative and thin rods of varying lengths and sometimes branching filamentous forms occur but these easily fragment into rods. *Tuberculous mastitis* mastitis in cows is usually due to *Mycobacterium bovis*, but *M. tuberculosis and M. avium* are also involved. Tuberculous mastitis is of major importance due to public health concern, risk of spread to calves, and difficulty in differentiating it from other causes of mastitis. *Mycobacterium lacticola*, have been isolated from cases of mastitis in cattle which occur after the intramammary infusion of therapeutic agents in oils (Richards *et al.*, 1980) and *M. chelonei* (Menard *et al.*, 1983) are encoured rarely as a cause of a severe outbreak of bovine mastitis. Five cases of mastitis, three due to M. lacticola and two due to unidentified acid fast bacilli, were described for the first time in England (Stuart and Harvey, 1951). An excellent treatise on the pathogenesis, morbid anatomy and histology of tuberculous mastitis in the cow was published in 1917 by M'Fadyean. Tuberculosis of the udder is generally described as a slowly progressive, painless induration. Clinical characteristic of tuberculous mastitis is marked induration followed by hypertrophy of the upper part of the udder and there is enlargement of the supramammary lymph nodes. The induration is characteristic, it has a stony hard, roughish feel. In the early stages the milk is often normal in appearance, but very fine floccules are apparent later which precipitate out to leave a clear, amber fluid when the milk is left to settle.

Pseudomonas species

Pseudomonas species are Gram-negative rods, oxidase positive, strict aerobic, oxidase, catalase-positive, oxidase positive and most are motile with exception *Ps. mallei*. The numbers of *Ps. aeruginosa* in mastitis milk are commonly minimal, and therefore milk must be incubated overnight before culturing on blood agar in order to detect the organism. These bacteria are not typically a major cause of mastitis, but in certain herds under certain conditions they may create a troubling mastitis problem. *Pseudomonas aeruginosa* is one of the species that has been associated with significant mastitis problem in certain herds. *Ps. aeruginosa* is widespread in the environment of dairy cows because it requires few nutrients to grow and multiply. Water supplies of all types (wells, troughs, ponds, parlor, wash hoses and sprinkler pens), contaminated teat dips and contaminated drugs and infusion equipment are the major sources of *Pseudomonas aeruginosa* on dairy farms. It has also been isolated from waste feed, soil, manure and animal skin.

The *Pseudomonas aeruginosa* infection rate in dairy herds is usually <1% of cows and rarely >3%. The infections range from sudden, very acute, life threatening clinical cases to non-clinical infections. Chronic mastitis is more characteristic of the infection with periodic acute flare-ups. The organism has persisted in a gland for as long as five lactations, but spontaneous recovery may occur. *Pseudomonas aeruginosa* has a tendency to cause sudden outbreaks of clinical mastitis in several cows and buffaloes within a few days despite to i) apparent changes in management practices. Necrosis of the involved quarter may occur leading to erosion of the vascular system with serious intrglandular hemorrhage, the secretion in such cases contains blood, or ii) occlusion of the teat cistern by scar tissue with conversion of the parenchyma into sac-like structures filled with purulent exudates. The role of various products of *Pseudomonas aeruginosa* in its pathogenesis has been studied (Liu *et al.*, 1961). The slime layer appears to be the most important factor in pathogenesis. Hemolysin and the extracellular enzymes played some role, whereas the bacterial cells, endotoxin, and the pyocyanin appeared to have negligible or significant effects. The virulence of the organism depends both on the toxigenicity and the ability to grow in the serum of animals.

Pasteurella species

The pasteurellae are small Gram negative rods or coccobacilli, non-motile, non-spore forming, facultatively anaerobic, oxidase positive and catalase positive bacteria. Mastitis due to *Pasteurella* spp. is rare in cattle, but can occur with severe toxemia and gangrenous changes (Morresey, 1999). In cattle *Pasteurella haemolytica* and *Pasteurella multocida* are causative organisms of mastitis. In cattle the mastitis is severe with fever, profound toxaemic shock, weak pulse, tachycardia and recumbency. The affected quarter is very swollen, the milk is watery, red tinged and contain flakes (Radostits *et al.*, 2000). The outbreaks have been reported caused by *Pasteurella haemolytica* as the sole pathogen or in addition to other significant pathogens such as *Actinopyogenes* and *Streptococcus dysgalactiae* in dry cows (Roberts, 1990; Teale *et al.*, 1990).

Brucella species

Brucella abortus caused bovine mastitis is more common than *B. melitensis* and *B. suis* (Horning, 1935). The occurrence of *B. abortus* in the milk of naturally infected cows was first reported by Schroeder and Cotton in 1911.

B. abortus causes causes a nonpurulent interstitial mastitis, not apparent apparent on clinical examination. The quality of the milk is not altered significantly because the damage to the secretory tissue is comparatively small.

Listeria species

Listeria species are Gram positive rods, catalase positive, oxidase negative, non-spore forming and non-acid fast bacteria. *Listeria monocytogenes* is being recorded more commonly as a cause of bovine mastitis because of the zoonotic importance. *L. monocytogenes* causes a mild mastitis with a decrease in milk production. Bourry and Poutrel (1996) found that intramammary infections with *L. monocytogenes* are mostly sub-clinical, with abnormalities in the milk being rare. However, Kalorey *et al.* (2008) had been isolated various species of *Listeria* (6.75% of milk samples) including *L. monocytogenes* (5.1%), *L. seeligeri* (0.1%), *L. innocua* (0.9%) and *L. welshimeri* (0.1%).

Leptospira species

Leptospirosis is now identified as one of the emerging infectious disease, caused by infection with Spirochaete of the genus Leptospira which consists of 60 or more species classified as serogroups and serotypes, affecting domestic and wild animals worldwide (Hatem *et al.*, 2008). It has been associated with serious financial losses for dairy farmers due to infertility, abortions, higher culling rates, clinical mastitis and decrease in milk yield (Quinlan and McNicholl, 1993; Guitian *et al.*, 1999). It may also be responsible for high mortality among young calves, decreased milk production, and blood-contaminated milk. Leptospires, are shed in urine and survive in surface water, streams, or moist, alkaline soil. The source of infection is most often urine containing leptospires that splashes into the eyes of susceptible animals or contaminates pasture, drinking water, or feed. Swine may act as carriers, often infecting cattle. Leptospirosis may be transmitted to cattle by many infected species- rats and other rodents, raccoons, skunks, foxes, opossums, and dogs. Leptospiral mastitis is popularly known as *"flabby udder"* in cattle. It is caused by a number of serovars of Leptospirae especially serovar *hardjo* (Balakrishanan *et al.*, 2009). Lactating animals may fail to produce milk, or they coud hve a leptospiral infection in the mammary gland affecting all four quarters that may result in the formation of yellow, clotted, colostrums like or bloody milk. The udder is flaccid with no signs of inflammatory swelling. This manifestation is due to endotoxins. Hatem *et al.* (2008) have been reprted *Leptospira interrogans* serovars: Pomona, Canicola, Icterohaemorrhagiae, Grippotyphosa and Wolffi at rates 51, 37, 16.2, 16.2 and 13.5% respectively from cattle suffering from mastitic. Oliveira *et al.* (2001) recorded agglutinins against *L.* Canicola, *L.* Grippotyphosa, *L.* Icterohaemorrhagiae and *L.* Pomona in 0.21%, 0.86%, 1.08% and 0.80% respectively in dairy cattle suffering from mastitis. Recently *L. hardjo* have also been reported in a cow suffering from haemorrhagic mastitis in Chennai, India (Balakrishanan *et al.*, 2009).

Yersenia pseudotuberculosis

Yersinia pseudotuberculosis is a Gram-negative, coccoid to pleomorphic rod which is frequently found in the gastrointestinal tract of wild small mammals and birds, which are considered to be its natural reservoirs. Bleul *et al.* (2002) reported a case of *Y. pseudotuberculosis* in a four year old Jersey cow in Switerland with subcutaneous growth on the caudal aspect of the left rear quarter of the udder. However, the milk from all four quarters was macroscopically normal and the yield was only 1 litre/day.

Bacillus species

Bacillus species are large, Gram positive or Gram variable, endospore forming rods, aerobic or facultative anaerobic, catalase positive and motile with exception of *B. anthracis* and *B. mycoides*. *B. cereus* and *B. subtilis* are saprophytic organisms and when they get the chance cause an acute haemorrhagic mastitis in cattle. Mastitis due to *B. anthracis* has also been reported in 6 years old cow in mid lactation with acute swelling in the udder and copious exudation of serosanguinous like fluid from the teat (Ngeleka *et al.*, 2008). *B. cereus* cases are often associated with teat injury. *B. anthracis* endospores can survive in soil for upto 50 years.

Clinically there is acute to peracute mastitis affecting one or more quarters. *B. anthracis* has a plasmid encoded 'triparite' protein toxin with protective, lethal and edema factors. There is severe swelling and pain with high fever (104-106°F) and severe toxaemia. Secretions are red tinged and serous in consistency. Gangrene may occur and in cows which survive, portions of affected gland will slough out and a chronic relapsing mastitis will persist (Radostits *et al.*, 2000).

Haemophilus somnus

H. somnus may cause mild, chronic, an acute form with high fever and blood stained milk, and a ganrenous mastitis (Hazlett *et al.*, 1983). It also has zoonotic importance. Amrstrong *et al.* (1986) confirmed the report of Hazlett *et al.* in the field by reporting a clinical case of peracute mastitis in a two year old cow by *H. somnus*.

Clostridium species

Clostridium species are large Gram-positive, anaerobic, fermentative, oxidase negative, catalase negative and endospore producing rods. *Clostridium perfringens* type-A may rarely cause mastitis but may cause a peracute gangrenous mastitis, characterized by high fever, swelling and superficial hyperemia of the affected quarter, followed later by gangrene, enlargement of the supramammary lymph nodes and subcutaneous emphysema involving the vulva (Johnston, 1986). The secretion from the udder is thin, brown, blood tinged and frequently contains numerous gas bubbles. The cow may die within 1 or 2 days due to septicemia or toxemia, but if prompt therapy is given she may survive. Goncalves *et al.* (2006) isolated *Clostridium perfringens* type-A for first time in Brazil from the milk of clinically affected quarter, which showed necrosis of papilla mammary and ventral portion of the affected quarter.

Fungi and Yeast

Generally, the mastitis due to fungi and yeast is uncommon or rare. Kirk and Bartlett (1986) have been mentioned a prevalence of fungal mastitis of 2 to 7%. The prevalence of mycotic mastitis is usually very low (1-12% of all mastitis causes), but some times it can occur in enzootic proportions (Krukowski and Saba, 2003). In tropical countries percentage can be more elevated (Costa *et al.*, 1993). The percentage of fungal isolation in surveys carried out in many countries varies considerably, with 6.1% rates reported in Egypt (Awad *et al.*, 1980), 1.3% in South Korea (Yeo and Choi, 1982),1.3% in Denmark (Aalbaek *et al.*, 1994), 9.6% in Poland (Krukowski *et al.*, 2000), and 12.07% (Costa *et al.*, 1993) to 25.4% (Santos and Marin, 2005) in Brazil. In India, bacteria are the major mastitis etiological agents, prevalence of Mycotic mastitis is less but upto 60% of cases of Mycotic mastitis has been reported (Vimalraj *et al.*, 2006). Isolation of yeast like fungi from bovine milk was reported as early as 1901 (Beck, 1957). Between 1934 and the early 1950's, several species of yeast were isolated from cows with mastitis (Santos and Marine, 2005; Beck, 1957; Pouden *et al.*, 1952; Murphy and Drake, 1947). During the 1950's and 1960's, reports of yeast induced mastitis and identification of the involved species became much more common (Clarke, 1960; Galli, 1954). Mycotic mastitis had been documented to be caused by various genera od moulds and yeasts, however, the most frequently encountered mycobiota are *Candida* spp., *C. albicans, C. krusei, C. parapsilosis, C. pelliculosa, C. pseudotropicalis, C. steatolytica, C. tropicalis, C. guilliermondii, C. zeulanoide, C. vini, C. famata* (Santos and Marin, 2005), *Cryptococcus* spp., *Cryptococcus neoformans, Pichia farinose, Rhodotorulla mwilaginosa* (Monga, 2000), *Nocardia asteroids, N. brasiliensis, N. farcinica, N. neocaledoniensis, Aspergillus* spp., *Trichosporon* spp., *Saccharomyces* spp., *Penicillium* spp. etc. (Carter, 1995), but the involvement of *Geotrichum candidum* in bovine mastitis is very rare (Chahota *et al.*, 2001). *G. candidum* is an opportunistic, keratinophilic yeast like fungus that is widely distributed in nature i.e. soil, fodder etc. In 1918, an organism identified presumptively as *Streptothrix hominis* III (Claypole) was isolated from a number of milk samples (Evans,

1918). This organism later became known as *Nocardia asteroids*. Nocardia are found naturally in the soil, water, air and herbage, and on the skin of the udders of healthy cows (Heidrich and Renk, 1967). Recently, a *Nocardia neocaledoniensis* mastitis outbreak has been reported in Italian dairy herd by Pisoni *et al.* (2008). However, *Nocardia* spp. are an uncommon cause of mastitis, and outbreaks have typically been reported in dairy farms with poor hygienic and managemental conditions.

A primary means by which yeast are spread is by contaminated intramammary tubes, syringes and teat canulae, where aseptic technique has not been followed. Spread can also be cow-to-cow but is rare. It may occur at milking time when improper procedure or faulty milking equipment is used. With the exception of *Cryptococcus* spp., yeast intramammary infections are usually self limiting with spontaneous recovery and the infections usually have no systemic consequences.

Severity of clinical mastitis appears to be related to genus of the yeast involved. *Cryptococcus* and *Nocardia* infections usually cause acute clinical mastitis. *C. neoformans*, caused acute mastitis in cattle and buffaloes, which is characterized by initial marked swelling of the affected quarter and supramammary lymph nodes, febrile spikes, milk (secretion) appears viscid, mucoid and gray-white coloration. The severe loss of milk production, which may continue indefinitely. There may be loss of appetite and a rise in temperature but the absence of toxaemia. The swelling may occur in severe form in all four quarters within 12 hours of the administration of antibiotics accompanied by cessation of milk production, subcutaneous edema of the udder, perineum and sternum, and swelling of the supramammary and internal iliac lymph nodes, but no rise in temperature. *Trichophyton* spp. and *Candida* spp. may cause severe local inflammation (swelling of the quarter) and clots in the milk. The infection rate is low and the fungi may disappear spontaneously. Many other types of yeast including *A. funigaus*, *Saccharomyces* spp., *Pichia* spp. and *Torulopsis* can also caused mastitis in cattle. Treatment of yeast induced mastitis has in general been unsuccessful. Most species are resistant to common antibiotics, an exception is *C. krusei*, which was reported to be sensitive to the neomycin (Beck, 1957).

Algae

The Prototheca genus of algae is an important which mainly cause the mastitis in bovines since 1952. The genus *Prototheca* includes unicellular yeast-like colorless (without chlorophyll) microalgae (phylogenetically related to *Chlorella*) and comprises 4 accepted species (*Prototheca zopfii*, *Prototheca stagnora*, *Prototheca whickeramii*, and *Prototheca ulmea*) and a fifth not generally accepted species (*Prototheca moriformis*) (Ueno *et al.*, 2003). These microorganisms reproduce only asexually; the cytoplasm splits, forming 2 to 16 daughter cells. *Prototheca* spp. was first described as a cause of mastitis by Lerch in 1952. Protothecal mastitis in cows is mostly caused by *P. zopfii* (Janosi *et al.*, 2001) and sometimes by *P. trispora* and *P. wickerhamii* (Gonzalez, 1996). The mastitis caused by *P. zopfii* algae is a disease of high-producing, machine-milked dairy cows. It occurs worldwide in tropical and temperate climatic areas, and mostly appears sporadically in a therapy-resistant form. However, in poorly managed dairy herds it may be endemic, causing serious economic losses as a result of decreased milk quality and quantity and culling of infected animals. Outbreaks of bovine mastitis attributable to *P. zopfii* have been described as a global problem, with reported occurrences in North America (Anderson and Walker, 1988; Higgins and Larouche, 1989), South America (Almeraya, 1994; Vargas *et al.*, 1998), Europe (Legneau, 1996; Aalbaek *et al.*, 1998; Buzzini *et al.*, 2004), Japan (Osumi *et al.*, 2008) and India (Katoch *et al.*, 1997).

Prototheca spp. are considered as opportunistic and environemental pathogen. *Prototheca* spp. are often associated with wet areas containing decaying manure and plant matter. They can also be found in flowing, standing, tank and well water, manure, teat dip containers, milking machine and feed troughs. Prototheca infections are thought to occur when the teats of cows are exposed to high populations of algae in environmental sites during the intervals between milking; however spread during milking time is not significant. The common belief is that the transmission of an infection caused by *P. zopfii* occurs by means of direct (and constant) contact of mammary glands with other contaminated sources on the dairy farm (Scaccabarozzi *et al.*, 2008). Only one study has been devoted so far to the exploration and characterization of environmental sources of *Prototheca* spp. in dairy herds (Costa *et al.*, 1997). Recent report of Osumi *et al.* (2008) has also been suggested that cow-barn surroundings (drinking water, sewage and feces) are the source of *P. zupfii*. They have been isolated *P. zupfii* genotype 2, from milk of mastitis cases and 90.62% *P. zupfii* genotype 1 and 9.38% *P. zupfii* genotype 2 from isolates of cow-barn surroundings.

Prototheca mastitis can occur in clinical and sub-clinical form. Most infections with prototheca are clinical with the milk being grossly abnormal (watery and clots) but without severe systemic signs such as off feeds, depression or a high fever. Cattle appear to be equally susceptible to new infections, regardless of the stage of lactation, including the dry period (Furuoka *et al.*, 1989). In cows, the infection may be restricted to the udder or disseminated to the lymph nodes (McDonald *et al.*, 1984). A key feature of Prototheca mastitis is the progressive drop in milk production in affected quarter because Prototheca damage the quarter (induration). Due the detrimental impact of prototheca infections on milk quality and lack of response to treatment (Shahan and Pore, 1991), culling is advised for known infected cows.

Viruses

Bovine herpesvirus (BHV)-1 (Gourlay *et al.*, 1974), BHV4 (Wellenberg *et al.*, 2000), foot-and-mouth disease virus (Burrows *et al.*, 1971), and parainfluenza 3 virus (Kawakami *et al.*, 1966) have been detected in milk from cows with clinical mastitis. A possible role of viruses in bovine sub-clinical mastitis has been suggested before (Fuchs, 1994). However, the detection of virus in milk from cows with mastitis obviously does not prove that these agents are the cause of mastitis, or that they are involved in an indirect way. Viruses when inoculated into the bovine mammary gland may not persist, or may multiply for a few days without causing udder irritation or may produce mastitis. The virus of poliomyelitis does not propogate in the mammary gland or give rise to antibody in the milk or blood (Mitcheli *et al.*, 1953).

BHV-1, a member of the *Alphaherpesvirinae* subfamily within the *Herpesviridae* Family. In 1974, BHV1 was isolated from a cow with mastitis in the USA. Although, bacterial culture was negative and only BHV1 was isolated from the milk, the evidence that the virus caused the mastitis. In France, BHV1 was isolated from milk samples from cows with mastitis in combination with *Mycoplasma agalactiae* (Espinasse *et al.*, 1974). BHV1 was also isolated from one of the milk samples obtained from one out of 96 cows with mastitis (Bilge, 1998). A possible role of BHV1 in the etiology of bovine mastitis, without or in combination with bovine viral diarrhoea virus (BVDV), was also suggested by Siegler *et al.* (1984). After experimental intramammary inoculation of BHV1 has been shown to replicate in the bovine mammary gland and to induce signs of clinical mastitis after an intramammary inoculation (Greig and Bannister, 1965; Corner *et al.*, 1967). An intramammary inoculation of one young heifer with a BHV1- IBR (Infectious bovine rhinotracheitis virus) or a BHV1-IPV (Infectious pustular vulvovaginitis virus) strain induced swollen quarters, hard and tender to the touch (Greig and Bannister, 1965). A strong reduction in milk yield was recorded, and milk samples showed abnormal morphology, with clots and blood, after the intramammary inoculation of cows with the BHV1-IBR strain.

BHV-4, a Rhadinovirus and member of the *Gammaherpesvirinae* subfamily within the *Herpesviridae* family, has been isolated from cows with various clinical signs, including mammary pustular dermatitis (Reed *et al.*, 1977). Although, BHV4 probably does not appear to play an important role as primary udder pathogen in the etiology of clinical mastitis, it may play a role in sub-clinical mastitis cases, or in an indirect way. A specific role for bovine herpes virus 4 (BHV-4) in mastitis has been suggested (Wellenberg *et al.*, 2002). Other authors state that BHV-4 does not play a role in causation of mastitis, but that reactivation of the virus by mastitis may contribute to more severe or prolonged mastitis episodes (Kalman *et al.*, 2004). More research is warranted to establish a possible indirect role of BHV4 infections in bovine mastitis, e.g. as a result of immunosuppression.

Foot-and-mouth disease (FMD) virus, a member of the *Aphthovirus* genus within the family of the *Picornaviridae*. Although, a primary infection of the mammary gland is unlikely to be a common occurrence in the pathogenesis of FMD, the virus can also replicate in the secretory epithelial cells of the mammary gland. Many researchers have isolated FMD virus from milk of FMD affected cows (Ray *et al.* 1989; Fuchs, 1994), and also teat and udder lesions have been reported in FMD-affected cattle during an outbreak with an Asia-1 serotype (Firoozi *et al.*, 1974). FMD virus is not the cause of a viral clinical mastitis as such, but secondary bacterial infections may result in clinical mastitis. After intramammary inoculation, affected quarters became swollen and tender to the touch. The milk showed abnormal morphology (with clots), and a drop in the milk yield of approximately 60% was recorded (Burrows *et al.*, 1971). After an infection of lactating cows with FMD virus, *Arcanobacter pyogenes* had been isolated from 15 quarters showing purulent mastitis (Saini *et al.*, 1992). Mastitis associated with FMD virus is assumed to be due to secondary bacterial infections. Field studies also support a secondary role of FMD in bovine mastitis. An increased incidence of bovine mastitis cases with secondary bacterial pathogens has been reported after an infection with FMD virus (Seinhorst *et al.*, 1991).

Parainfluenza 3 (PI3) virus, a member within the *Paramyxoviridae* family. The cows from which PI3 virus was recovered from the milk did not show signs of clinical mastitis, but an increased milk SCC was recorded in many milk samples. The affected udders developed swelling and induration. The milk showed a color change, an increased pH and increased numbers of glandular epithelial cells, neutrophils, lymphocytes and monocytes.

Bovine leukaemia virus (BLV), belonging to the *Deltaretrovirus* genus and member of the family of *Retroviridae*. A possible association of BLV infections and mastitis in dairy cows has been investigated on individual and on herd level, however with contradictory results. A positive association has been reported (Milojevic *et al.*, 1991; Rusov *et al.*, 1994), that the occurrence of mastitis and increased cell counts are more often recorded in cows with enzootic leukosis than in healthy cows. No experimental studies have been reported to investigate whether BLV is able to induce sub-clinical or clinical bovine mastitis. Such experiments are necessary to gain more insight into the role of BLV in the etiology of bovine mastitis.

Bovine herpes mammillitis virus (BHV2), vaccinia, cowpox, pseudocowpox, FMD viruses, and to a lesser extent vesicular stomatitis virus can cause a local dermatitis, often with ulcerations in the ductus papillaris, leading to secondary bacterial infections in the sinus lactiferus and the corresponding mammary gland (Francis, 1984).

Distribution of mastitis causing organisms in India and Worldwide

In any geographical location, knowledge of species level distribution of mastitis pathogens is important for disease control and epidemiological studies. In most countries, the major mastitis pathogens are *Staphylococcus aureus, Streptococcus agalactiae, Streptococcus dysgalactiae* and *Streptococcus uberis,* and *Escherichia coli.* The main organisms associated with clinical and sub-clinical mastitis in India are *Staphylococcus aureus, Streptococcus agalactiae, Streptococcus dysgalactiae* and *Streptococcus uberis* and *Escherichia coli.*

ASIA

India

The main organisms associated with clinical and sub-clinical mastitis in India are *Staphylococcus aureus, Streptococcus agalactiae, Streptococcus dysgalactiae* and *Streptococcus uberis* and *Escherichia coli.* By contrast, Klebsiella, *Listeria monocytogenes, Geotrichum candidum* and *Candida guilliermondi* mastitis outbreaks are only occasionally reported (Katoch *et al.*, 2003; Chahota *et al.*, 2001) from India. Mycoplasma mastitis is also occasionally reported from India and reason may be that all workers do not try to isolate Mycoplasma from mastitis cases.

Prevalence of major pathogens is decreasing, the relative importance of other organisms, particularly coagulase negative staphylococci (CNS), increasing. In India, the prevalence of CNS among bacterial isolates from milk samples increased from 9.91% in 2003 (Sharma and Prasad, 2003) to 72.13% in 2009 (Dutta, 2009). CNS are now among the most commonly isolated organisms from milk samples of cows with sub-clinical mastitis in many countries (Rajala-Schultz *et al.*, 2004; Østerås *et al.*, 2006). In 2007, the first international symposium on CNS in bovine mastitis was organised, reflecting the increasing recognition of the potential importance of this group of pathogens (De Vliegher *et al.*, 2009). Molecular methods for identification of CNS provide accurate tools for epidemiological studies at CNS species level and future development of species-specific recommendations for treatment and prevention of CNS mastitis (Zadoks and Fitzpatrick, 2009).

Jammu & Kashmir

A total of 43 milk samples from clinical mastitic cows were subjected to cultural examination, results revealed presence of *Staphylococcus aureus*

(30.76%), *Streptococcus* spp. (21.15%), *Staphylococcus albus* (7.69%), *Micrococcus* spp. (7.69%), *Bacillus cereus* (5.77%), *Escherichia coli* (5.77%), *Klebsiella* spp. (3.85%), *Pseudomonas* spp. (3.85%), *Nocardia* spp. (3.85%), Yeast (3.85%), *Corynebacterium* spp. (1.92%), *Proteus* spp. (1.92%) and *Bacillus subtilis* (1.92%) (Hussain *et al.*, 2006). Singh *et al.* (2000) have been isolated *Staphylococcus* spp. as chief mastitis causal agent followed by *Micrococcus* spp., *Bacillus* spp., *Klebsiella* spp., *Escherichia coli* from sub-clinical and clinical mastitis cows in Srinagar. A study in Jammu by Sudhan *et al.* (2005) suggests that *Staphylococcus aureus* (56.89%) is major pathogen followed by *Micrococcus* spp. (15.51%), *Bacillus cereus* (12.06%), *Staphylococcus epidermidis* (8.62%), *Klebsiella* spp. (3.44%), *Escherichia coli* (1.72%), and *Corynebacterium* spp. (1.72%). A total of 28 isolates were recovered from 32 cross bred cows positive to sub-clinical mastitis. Inthis study *Staphylococcus* spp. was observed to be major causative agent (71.43%), followed by *Streptococcus* spp. (14.28%), *Escherichia coli* (7.14%), *Pseudomonas* spp. (3.57%) and Gram negative rods (3.57%) (Singh *et al.*, 2005). Sharma *et al.* (2007) isolated *Staphylococcus aureus* and *Escherichia coli* from acute clinical mastitis in buffalo. Peer *et al.* (2007) have also been isolated *Staphylococcus, Streptococcus, Escherichia coli, Corynebacterium* spp., *Klebsiella* spp., *Pseudomonas* and *Nocardia* spp. from mastitis milk samples from Srinagar.

Himachal Pradesh

Nagal *et al.* (1999) studied over 9 years (1987-1995) and cultured 728 mastitis milk samples. They isolated *Staphylococcus aureus* (61.76%), *Streptococcus pyogenes* (12.03%), *Staphylococcus epidermidis* (2.40%), *Escherichia coli* (5.61%), *Corynebacterium* spp. (4.01%), *Bacillus* spp. (1.53%), *Pasteurella multocida* (0.80%), *Pseudomonas aeruginosa* (0.53%), *Nocardia asteroides* (0.26%), *Proteus* spp. (0.26%), *Candida* spp. (1.87%) and *Prototheca* spp. (0.14%). Prasad (2000) had also been isolated *Staphylococcus* spp. (68.83%), *Streptococcus* (16.88%), *Escherichia coli* (7.80%), *Klebsiella* (2.59%), *Diplococcus* spp. (1.30%), *Proteus* spp. (1.30%) and *Corynebacterium* (1.30%) from mastitic dairy cows. In a work carried out by Sharma and Prasad (2002) the samples of cows yielded the prime causative agents viz. *Staphylococcus spp.* (54.05%) and *Escherichia coli* (11.71%). The microbial profile obtained from milk samples of buffaloes was similar to that of cows where primarily *Staphylococcus spp.* (63.15%) was involved followed by *Escherichia coli* (15.79%) and *Enterobacter aerogena* (10.53%). A broad range of bovine mastitogens have been isolated from Himachal Pradesh- *Staphylococcus aureus* (Major mastitogen), *Streptococcus* spp., *Escherichia coli, Corynebacterium* spp., *Candida* spp., *Pseudomonas* spp., *Proteus* spp., *Klebsiella* spp., *Pasteurella* spp., *Nocardia* spp., *Bacillus* spp., *Diplococcus* spp., *Aspergillus* spp., *Prototheca* spp. Other important mastitogens had isolated from Himachal Pradesh are *Listeria monocytogenes*,

Geotrichum candidum and *Candida guilliermondi* (Katoch *et al.*, 2003). Chahota *et al.* (2001) have also been isolated the *Geotrichum candidum* from clinical bovine mastitis. Sharma and Prasad (2003) studied on 81 cows and 12 buffaloes suffering from clinical mastitis. The microorganisms isolated from cows were *Staphylococcus aureus* (44.14%), CNS (9.91%), *Escherichia coli* (11.71%), *Streptococcus* spp. (14.41%), *Bacillus* spp. (9.01%), *Corynebacterium* spp. (7.21%), *Proteus* spp. (1.80%), *Nocardia* spp. (0.90%) and *Klebsiella* spp. (0.90%) and from buffaloes *Staphylococcus aureus* (47.37%), CNS (15.97%), *Escherichia coli* (15.79%), *Enterobacter aerogenes* (10.53%), *Bacillus* spp. (5.26%) and *Corynebacterium* spp. (5.26%).

Punjab

Singh *et al.* (1994) have been isolated *Staphylococci* (73.08%), *Streptococci* (14.61%), *Escherichia coli* (5.38%), *Corynebacterium* spp., *Proteus* spp. and *Klebsiella* spp. The findings of Saini et al. (1994) are similar to previous reports. They found *Staphylococcus aureus* (48.57%) as major pathogen followed by CNS (17.14%), *Streptococcus* spp. (11.42%), *Escherichia coli* (11.42%), *Klebsiella* spp. (4.28%), *Corynebacterium* (2.85%), *Proteus* (1.42%) and *Bacillus* (2.85%). Study on 154 dairy cows and 117 buffaloes milk samples and isolated the *Staphylococci* (59.40%), *Streptococci* (27.27%), *Corynebacterium* spp (6.67%), *Escherichia coli* (3.64%), *Proteus* spp. (1.22%), *Bacillus* spp. (0.61%) and mixed infections of *Staphylococci* and *Streptococci* (1.22%) from cows and *Staphylococci* (41.51%), *Streptococci* (35.85%), *Corynebacterium* spp. (20.75%) and *Escherichia coli* (1.89%) from buffaloes (Bansal *et al.*, 1995). Prabhakar *et al.* (1995) isolated and identified the organisms responsible for clinical mastitis in Buffaloes. Distribution of organisms was *Staphylococcus aureus* (34.21%), CNS (13.16%), *Streptococcus agalactiae* (14.47%), *Escherichia coli* (10.53%), *Pseudomonas* spp. (7.89%), *Streptococcus pyogenes* (3.95%), *Klebsiella* spp. (3.95%), *Streptococcus dysgalactiae* (2.63%), *Proteus* spp. (2.63%), *Streptococcus uberis* (1.31%), *Diptheroids* (1.31%) and mixed infections (1.31%).

Haryana

Study was conducted on 868 clinical mastitis quarters of buffaloes and microorganisms isolated were *Staphylococcus aureus* (26.30%), *Staphylococcus epidermidis* (19.10%), *Micrococci* (1.89%), *Streptococcus agalactiae* (8.13%), *Streptococcus dysgalactiae* (17.0%), *Streptococcus uberis* (0.54%), *Streptococcus bovis* (1.62%), *Streptococcus* spp. (2.84%), *Enterococci* (0.81%), *Corynebacterium pyogenes* (5.96%), *Corynebacterium* spp. (12.87%), *Escherichia coli* (6.5%), *Klebsiella* spp. (2.16%), *Pseudomonas aeruginosa* (0.67%), *Proteus* spp. (0.27%), *Bacillus* spp. (1.21%), *Diplococcus pneumoniae* (0.54%), *Candida* spp. (1.53%) and *Aspergillus* spp.(0.13%). *Streptococcus agalactiae* was of serotypes 11 and 11/R, and included some non-typable strains. *Escherichia coli 0.* serotypes were 017, 020, 028, 029, 030, 036, 039, 031, 068, 073, 074, 075 and 0116 (Kapur *et al.*, 1992). Tuteja *et al.* (1993) reported that amongst 307 isolates from 697 apparently healthy quarters, *Staphylococci* were the most dominant (44.3%) followed by *Micrococci* (30.0%), *Streptococci* (18.9%), *Corynebacterium sp.* (5.5%), *Bacillus sp.* (1.0%) and *Enterococci sp.* (0.3%). Serotyping of 37 Streptococcus agalactiae strains showed that types R (9), Ib (8), X (5), IIR (4), IbR (4), NT (3), IIIR (1), IVR (1), I I (1) and IIIX (1) were prevalent in the cows. Sharma and Kapur (2000) isolated *Staphylococci* (70.37%, Streptococci (20.99%) and *Diphtheroids* (8.64%) from buffaloes mastitic milk. Kumar and Sharma (2002) studied a total of 613 isolates obtained from infected udder of cows and buffaloes. Of these, non-hemolytic *Staphylococcus* spp. (48.94%) was the most prevalent organism followed by hemolytic *Staphylococcus* spp. (12.89%), *Corynebacterium* spp. (9.14%), *Coliforms* and other gram negative bacilli (10.93%), *Bacillus sp.* (2.12%), *Pseudomonas auruginosa* (1.46%) and mixed infection (3.90%). Twenty one milk samples from clinical mastitic buffaloes were evaluated for bacterial isolates. Major bacterial isolates detected in culture were *Staphylococcus* spp. (57%), followed by *Escherichia coli* (9.5%) and *Streptococcus* spp. (9.5%), and mixed infection (*Staphylococcus spp.* and *Escherichia coli*) in 23.8% isolates (Phogat and Dahiya, 2003). According to Tuteja *et al.* (2003) amongst 161 isolates from 420 apparently healthy cow quarters examined, *Staphylococcus epidermidis* was the most predominant (55.88%) followed by *Corynebacterium* spp. (12.42%), *Micrococci* (11.80%), unclassified *Streptococci* (7.45%), *Staphylococcus aureus* (6.83%), *Streptococcus dysgalactiae* (4.97%) and *Streptococcus agalactiae* (1.24%). The report of Sharma *et al.* (2006) is also in the support of this study, they found *Staphylococcus epidermidis* as major (46.67%) organism followed by *Staphylococcus aureus* (36.67%), *Streptococcus agalactiae* (10%), *Streptococcus dysgalactiae* (5%) and *Streptococcus uberis* (1%) from sub-clinical mastitis affected cross bred cows (Sahiwal and Jersey). Sharma and Sindhu (2007) isolated 3447 isolates from infected buffaloes quarters. Out of these, 38.81% were *Staphylococcus* spp., 32.4% *Streptococcus* spp., 11.80% *Escherichia coli*, 5.2% *Corynebacterium* spp., 1.36% *Bacillus* spp., 2.03% *Klebsiella* spp., 0.78% *Pseudomonas aeruginosa*, 0.14% *Proteus* , 0.14% yeast. As per all previous reports *Staphylococcus* spp. was the chief mastitis etiological agent in Haryana state but in the recent report of Kumar *et al.* (2009) *Streptococcus dysgalactiae* was major (50.00%) organism isolated from the cases of sub-clinical mastitis in cows followed by *Staphylococcus aureus* (27.27%), *Staphylococcus epidermidis* (15.91%), *Streptococcus agalactiae* (4.55%) and *Corynebacterium payogenes* (2.27%).

Rajasthan

Chahar *et al.* (2008) reported that *Staphylococcus* spp. was the most frequent isolate (47.06%) followed by *Streptococcus* spp. (19.12%), *Bacillus* spp.

(11.76%), *Escherichia coli* (2.94%) and *Corynebacterium* spp. (2.94%) from Rajasthan. Sharma *et al.* (2010) also reported that Staphylococcal mastitis incidence is high, they found *Staphylococcus aureus* in 55% samples followed by *Escherichia coli* (27.5%), *Streptococcus* spp. (12.5%) and *Klebsiella* spp. in 5% samples.

Uttar Pradesh

Singh *et al.* (1982) reported that *Staphylococci* was major (74.71%) bacterial isolate followed by *Streptococci* (21.13%) and other (4.15%) from cows and buffaloes. The report of Maiti *et al.* (1996) is also in the favour of previous study, they isolated *Staphylococcus* as a chief etiological agent in bovine mastitis and other organisms were *Streptococcus dysgalactiae, Streptococcus uberis, Escherichia coli* and *Corynebacterium payogenes.* Ranjan *et al.* (2003) isolated 57.14% Gram positive bacteria and 42.86% Gram negatives. *Staphylococcus* spp. accounted for 75% of Gram positive and *Escherichia coli* accounted for 66.66% of Gram negative isolates from clinical mastitic cross bred cows. The organisms isolated from 111 milk samples collected from sub-clinical mastitis and clinical mastitic cows were *Staphylococcus aureus* (17.0%), other *Staphylococcus* (*Micrococci*) (40%), *Streptococcus* spp. (29.0%) and *Coliform* organism (11%) (De and Mukharjee, 2009).

Uttarakhand

Shukla *et al.* (1998) screened the cows and buffaloes for mastitis in Tarai region and founf that *Staphylococcus aureus* was the major (60.32%) pathogen followed by *Streptococci* (31.98%). Nauriyal *et al.* (2003) on bacteriological examination of buffaloes and cows milk samples from cases of sub-clinical mastitis recovered 223 monomicrobic isolates. Thirty-eight isolates were of mixed infection involving two or more pathogens. Major mastoid contributed (89.23%) to the total monomicrobic isolates in case of cows, which included *Staphylococcus aureus* (66 isolates), *Bacillus* spp. (27), *Streptococcus agalactiae* (20), *Streptococcus uberis* (17), *Escherichia coli* (9), *Streptococcus dysgalactiae* (8) and *Corynebacterium pyogenes* (3). Contagious pathogens (*Staphylococcus aureus* and *Streptococcus agalactiae*) had 38.56% share while environmental pathogens (*Escherichia coli, Streptococcus uberis, Streptococcus dysgalactiae*) accounted for 15.24% of total isolates. A minor pathogen *Micrococcus sp.* had a share of 24 isolates.

Madhya Pradesh

Tijare *et al.* (1999) reported that out of a total 159 isolates, 62 (38.99%) belonged to *Staphylococcus spp.* causing sub-clinical mastitis. Amongst these 4 (2.52%) were of *Staphylococcus aureus* and 58 (36.48%) were coagulase negative *Staphylococcus spp.* Other isolates in descending order in frequency of isolation were *Bacillus sp.* (18.24%), *Escherichia coli* (18.24%), *Klebsiella pneumoniae* (11.32%), *Serratia marcescens* (6.92%), *Corynebacterium bovis* (6.29%), *Micrococcus sp.* (1.89%), *Streptococcus uberis* (1.89%), *Streptococcus agalactiae* (1.26%) and *Streptococcus bovis* (0.63%). Ghose *et al.* (2003) cultured bacteriologically 162 milk samples of cows and isolated 209 bacterial strains including *Staphylococci* (58.85%), *Streptococci* (32.53%), *Micrococci* (5.74%), *Corynebacteria* (1.91%) and *E.coli* (0.95%). Ghose and Sharda (2003) studies on 1060 milk samples from 272 cows and isolates identified as *Staphylococcus epidermidis* (52.48%), *Staphylococcus aureus* (39.01%) and *Micrococcus* spp. (8.51%). A work was conducted by Das and Joseph (2005) at 15 dairy farms in Jabalpur and isolated *Staphylococcus* spp. (coagulase positive) (27.9%), *Staphylococcus* spp. (coagulase negative) (16.28%), *Streptococcus agalactiae* (6.98%), *Corynebacterium bovis* (4.65%), *Corynebacterium pyogenes* (5.81%), *Bacillus cereus* (4.56%), *Escherichia coli* (17.44%), *Klebsiella pneumonie* (5.81%), *Pseudomonas aeruginosa* (3.49%), *Trichisporon spp.* (3.49%) and *Cryptococcus neoformans* (3.49%) from clinical mastitis buffaloes.

Chhattisgarh

A total of 110 isolates were obtained from 75 quarters of buffaloes positive to sub-clinical mastitis. Among the various microorganisms isolated, the *Staphylococcus spp.* occupied prime position with 63 (57.27%) isolates out of 110. Other Gram-positive microbes in descending order of their frequency were *Streptococcus spp.* (15.45%), *Corynebacterium spp.* (10.00%) and *Diplococcus* (4.54%). *Escherichia coli* (12.73%) was the only Gram-negative organism isolated from milk (Sharma *et al.*, 2007). Sharma (2008) isolated *Staphylococuus spp.*, *Streptococcus spp.* and *Escherichia coli* from 6 cross bred cows suffering from acute clinical mastitis preceded by Foot and Mouth disease in all study animals. Vishwakarma (2008) also found that the *Staphylococcus spp.* occupied the prime position (39.53%) closely followed by *Streptococcus sp.* (20.93%). Other pathogens isolated were *Micrococccus sp.* (16.27%), *E.coli* (9.30%), *Klebsiella sp.* (6.97%) and *Pseudomonas sp.* (6.97%).

Gujarat

Patel *et al.* (2000) reported that out of 1175 quarters, 683 quarters (58.13%) were culturally positive. The organisms isolated were *Staphylococci* (74.04%), *Bacillus sp.* (7.32%), *Streptococci* (6.00%), *Corynebacterium sp.* (2.93%) and Gram-negative (5.71%). Kalyani *et al.* (2003) reported that out of 53 milk samples, 36 samples yielded bacterial growth. The organisms identified were *Staphylococcus spp.* (20), Gram negative bacilli (15) and one milk sample revealed mixed infection of Gram positive and Gram negative bacteria. Goswamy *et al.* (2003) reported that out of 217 culturally positive samples from 86 milking cows in different lactation status from organized farms in and around Anand and isolated a total of 232 bacteria. The organisms isolated were coagulase positive and negative *Staphylococcus spp., Streptococcus agalactiae, Streptococcus bovis, Streptococcus uberis, Streptococcus lactis, Streptococcus dysgalactiae, Streptococcus duran, Micrococcus spp., Bacillus spp., Corynebacterium spp., Listeria spp., Nocardia spp., Escherichia coli, Pasteurella multocida, Klebsiella spp., Enterobacter spp., Pseudomonas spp. and Proteus spp.* Nauriyal and Verma (2008) have been isolated *Staphylococcus aureus* 30%, *Streptococcus agalactiae* 25%, *Escherichia coli* 15%, *Proteus* spp. 10% and mixed infections were *Streptococcus agalactiae* with *Micrococcus* spp. 10%, *Staphylococcus aureus* with *Bacillus* spp. 5% and *Escherichia coli* with *Micrococcus* 5% from clinical mastitis cases of cows. Nauriyal and Verma (2009) were also carried out a study on 33 lactating pure bred Kenkrej cows and found that 94.12% samples showed monomicrobic isolates and remaining 5.88% samples had mixed growth. Contagious pathogens contributed 33.33% to total bacterial isolates. Among these, coagulase-positive *Staphylococci* and *Streptococcus agalactiae* had a share of 30.56 and 2.78% respectively. Out of 5.56% isolates of environemental pathigens, *E. colli* and *Pseudomonas* spp. contributed 2.78% each. Minor pathogens had maximum (61.12%) contribution to total bacterial isolates. Of these, CNS and *Micrococcus* spp. had a share of 38.89 and 16.67% respectively, and *Corynebacterium* spp. and *Bacillus* spp. were isolated 2.78% each.

Bihar

A total of 160 milk samples from 40 cross bred cows suffering from clinical mastitis were subjected to bacteriological isolation and found *Staphylococcus aureus* (49.23%), *Streptococcus agalactiae* (26.92%), *Streptococcus payogenes* (12.30%), *Escherichia coli* (7.69%), *Klebsiella pneumoniae* (2.31%) and *Corynebacterium pyogenes* (1.54%) (Akhtar *et al.*, 2003). Cultural examination of 104 milk samples revealed growth in 95 samples and *Staphylococcus* spp. (70.97%) was the predominant organism both in cow and buffaloes, including *Stapph. epidermidis* (63.6%) and coagulase negative staphylococci (36.36%) (Sahay *et al.*, 2007).

Jharkhand

Bacteria responsible for bovine mastitis were isolated from 209 clinical mastitis cases. However, in 3 samples no growth was seen. Out of 206 positive samples, *Staphylococcus* spp.(28.15%), *Streptococcus* spp. (8.74%), *Bacillus cereus* (1.45%), *Corynebacterium pyogenes* (0.97%%), aerobic Gram positive rods (1.94%), *Escherichia coli* (17.47%), *Pseudomonas pyogenes* (1.45%), *Pasteurella haemolytica* (0.48%), *Proteus* spp. (0.48%), *Prototheca* spp. (1.45%) and in 6.31% cases pure fungal growth were observed (Thakur *et al.*, 2001). Jha *et al.* (2004) screened 258 milk samples and isolated *Staphylococcus* spp. in 18.99%,

Streptococcus spp., in 15.50%, Gram positive *Bacilli* in 16.28%, Gram negative *Bacilli* in 17.05% of samples. Mixed isolates were found in 32.17% samples. Munda *et al.* (2007) has been reported *Staphylococci* (50%), *Streptococcus agalactiae* (12.50%), *Streptococcus dysgalactiae* (8.33%), *Streptococcus uberis* (4.16%), *Proteus* spp. (8.33%) and *Pseudomonas* spp. (4.16%). Recently Ranjan *et al.* (2010) have been isolated *Staphylococcus aureus*, coagulase negative *Staphylococcus spp., E. coli, Pseudomonas spp., Streptococci spp., Klebsiella spp, Bacillus spp.* and Yeast from bovine mastitis milk samples.

West Bengal

Chand *et al.* (1989) isolated the *Staphylococci* spp. (57.70%), *Streptococci* (35.40%), *Corynebacterium* spp. (5.31%) and *Escherichia coli* (1.77%) out of 113 isolates from sub-clinical mastitis cows and *Staphylococci* spp. (56%), *Streptococci* (32%), *Corynebacterium* spp. (8%) and *Escherichia coli* (4%) from clinical mastitis cows. Dutta *et al.* (2003) studied a total 124 samples, of which 121 (96.77%) were bacteriologically positive and 3 (3.23%) negative. Coagulase negative *Staphylococci* were the predominated isolates (50.65%) followed by *Streptococci* and least was *E.coli* (1.30%).

Orissa

Misra et al. (1993) reported *Staphylococcus aureus* (42.10%), *Escherichia coli* (18.95%), *Streptococcus* spp. (5.26%), *Klebsiella* spp. (3.16%), *Pseudomonas* spp. (4.74%), *Proteus* spp. (5.26%), *Klebsiella* spp. (3.16%) and *Candida albicans* (2.10%) out of 190 bovine mastitic milk samples. A study was carriedout on 542 pooled milk samples and found *Staphylococcus aureus* as predominant pathogen from 59.37% samples followed by *Streptococcus agalactiae* (16%), Staph. albus (10.63%), *Staphylococcus epidermidis* (4.9%), *Streptococcus dysgalactiae* (1.1%), *Escherichia coli* (2.9%), *Klebsiella spp.* (2.2%), *Bacillus cereus* (1.8%), *Corynebacterium bovis, Corynebacterium pyogenes* and *Pseaudomonas* spp. (1.1%) (Sahoo *et al.*, 2009).

Assam

Studies of Saxena *et al.* (1993) reprted the *Staphylococcus aureus* (27.58%), CNS (23.45%), *Bacillus* spp. (14.48%), *Streptococcus uberis* (9.65%), *Pneumococcus* spp. (8.27%), *Streptococcus* spp. (6.21%), *Corynebacterium* spp. (5.56%), *Micrococcus* spp. (4.14%) and *Streptococcus bovis* (0.69%) from 191 quarters milk samples of cows. Rahman and Baxi (1982) isolated a total of 252 strains of different bacterial organisms from milk samples of cows and buffaloes. The organisms isolated were *Staphylococcus spp., Streptococcus* spp., *Escherichia coli, Enterobacter sp., Citrobacter sp., Klebsiella aerogenes, Corynebacterium sp., Pseudomonas aeruginosa and Salmonella sp.* Bhattacharya and Rahman (1995) collected milk samples from Arunachal Pradesh and Assam and found that the *Staphylococcus spp.* (47.26%) was found to be the chief etiological agent of bovine mastitis. Other isolates were *Streptococcus* spp. (42.66%), *Corynebacteria* spp. (19.86%), *Escherichia coli* (3.42%), *Pseudomonas aeruginosa* (1.37%) and *Bacillus* spp. (3.42%). Nath and Dutta (2005) had been reported that *Staphylococcus aureus* is the major mastitogen followed by *Streptococcus dysgalactiae* and *Streptococcus bovis* in Khanapara region of Assam and Meghalaya. Dutta (2009) was found CNS 72.13% isolates comprising *Staphylococcus warneri, Staphylococcus hominis, Staphylococcus chromogens, Staphylococcus simulans,* and *Staphylococcus aureus* in 27.86% isolates.

Mizoram

Lalrintluanga *et al.* (2003) have been isolated coagulase negative staphylococci (55.10%), Streptococci (22.45%), *Staphylococcus aureus* (7.14%), *Corynebacterium* spp. (6.12%), *Escherichia coli* (3.06%), *Proteus* spp. (2.04%), *Klebsiella aerogenes* (2.04%) and *Citrobacter* spp. (2.04%) from the cow milk samples.

Maharashtra

Dhote et al. (1999) reported a higher incidence of Staphylococcal mastitis in cows belonging to various dairy farms located in districts adjacent to Nagpur. Milk samples were collected from 30 cross bred (Holstein or Jersey with Gir) cows and subjected to microbial isolation, *Staphylococci* were major (54.55%) pathogens followed by *Streptococci* (36.36%), *Escherichia coli* (4.55%) and *Klebsiella* (2.27%) (Bhalerao *et al.*, 2000). Sarode (2002) reported the percentage of different organisms among 104 isolates of mastitis milk samples as *Staphylococcus* spp. (74.04%) *Streptococcus* spp. (13.46%), Gram-negative rods (7.69%), *Bacillus* spp. (2.88%) and *Micrococcus* spp. (1.92%). Chavan *et al.* (2007) reports showed *Staphylococcus epidermidis* was chief (34%) pathogen while in most of reports either from India or other countries *Staphylococcus aureus* is main mastitis causing pathogen. Other pathogens were *Staphylococcus aureus* (24.58%), *Streptococcus agalactiae* (11.64%) and *Corynebacterium diphtheriae* (8.84%). From the studies on 24 buffaloes during dry period showed 100% bacterial growth of mammary secretions, CNS were dominant organisms (40.47%) followed by *Staphylococcus aureus* (16.66%), *Streptococcus spp.* (33.33%) and *Micrococcus* spp. (9.52%) (Ahire *et al.*, 2008). On microbial investigation of milk from clinical mastitis buffaloes revealed *Staph.* spp., *Strep.* spp., *Escherichia coli, Candida* spp. and *Aspergillus* spp. (Patil *et al.*, 2009).

Goa

Barbuddhe *et al.* (2001) culture a total of 141 cows milk samples from bacteriological study and reported that *Psedomonas aeruginosa* (60.46%),

Staphylococcus aureus (32.25%), *Streptococcus* spp. (11.63%), *Escherichia coli* (10.47%), *Listeria* spp. (5.81%), *Bacillus* spp. (8.14%) and *Proteus* spp. (9.30%). Of the 48 milk samples of clinical mastitis, 27 yielded single causative agents (56.25%) and 21 had multiple etiological agents (43.75%).

Andhra Pradesh

Ramachandraiah *et al.* (1990) reported the occurrence of mastitis due to *Staphylococcus* spp. was highest (52.9%) followed by *Streptococcus* spp. (20.3%), *Yeast* (5.6%), *Bacillus* spp. (3.4%), *Corynebacterium* spp. (3.4%), *Pseudomonas* spp. (2.2%) and *Diplococcus* spp. (2.2%). Mastitis due to single isolate occurred in 90% while mixed infections recorded in 10% of the cases tested. Kumari and Gupta (2002) subjected a total of 81 milk samples collected from post-parturient cows to cultural isolation. The percentage distribution of different isolates were *Staphylococcus* spp. (35.21%) the most prevalent organism in the samples followed by *Escherichia* spp. (28.39%), *Streptococcus* spp. (18.51%), *Pseudomonas* spp. (4.91%), *Corynebacterium* spp. (2.46%), and *Klebsiella* spp. (2.46%). According to Choudhuri (2000) cultural examination of the milk samples of cows from SCM revealed 69 isolates, which were as follows- *Staphylococcus* spp. (55.07%), *Micrococcus* spp. (27.53%), *Escherichia coli* (8.69%), *Klebsiella* spp. (2.89%), *Proteus* spp. (1.49%) and *Streptococcus* spp. (1.49%). Ramani Pushpa (2010) isolates *Staphylococcus aureus* ((70.76%), *Escherichia coli* (15.38%), *C. jejuni* (10.75%) and *Streptococcus agalactiae* (3.07%) from 65 clinical mastitis milk samples of Buffaloes.

Karnataka

Milk samples from 26 clinical cases of bovine mastitis were subjected to cultural isolation and yielded 32 bacterial isolates. Of these 32 isolated *Staphylococcus aureus* (34.38%) was main pathogen responsible for clinical mastitis followed by CNS (25%), *Escherichia coli* (21.87%), *Streptococcus* spp. (9.38%), *Pseudomonas* spp. (6.25%) and *Proteus* spp. (3.12%) (Yathiraj *et al.*, 2007). Sumathi *et al.* (2008) a total of 75 bacterial isolate were recovered from 60 milk samples obtained from 60 clinical cases of mastitis cows from Bangalore. Out of 60 samples, 21 samples (35%) yielded pure cultures of which 6 were gram positive and 15 were Gram negative organisms and the remaining 39 (65%) yielded mixed cultures. The predominant bacterial isolates *Staphylococcus aureus* (24%) and *Escherichia coli* (20%) followed by *Staphylococcus epidermidis* (16%), *Streptococcus* spp. (16%), *Klebsiella* spp. (10.67%), *Bacillus* spp. (5.33%), *Corynebacterium* spp. (4%), *Proteus* spp. (2.66%) and *Pseudomonas* spp. (1.33%). Rajeev *et al.* (2009) obtained 100 milk samples from clinical mastitis cows and isolated 121 isolates. Out of these 121 isolates, 70 (57.85%) were Gram positive bacteria, 36 (29.75%) Gram negative bacteria and 15 (12.39%) were yeast. The majority of the bacterial isolates recovered belonged to the genus *Staphylococcus* (35.54%) consisting of 13 different species like *Staphylococcus aureus* (6), *Staphylococcus arlettae* (5), *Staphylococcus capitis subsp. ureolyticus* (5), *Staphylococcus haemolyticus* (4), *Staphylococcus felis* (4), *Staphylococcus equorum* (3), *Staphylococcus epidermidis* (2), *Staphylococcus sciuri* (2), *Staphylococcus intermedias* (1), *Staphylococcus chromogens* (1), *Staphylococcus schleiferi subsp. Coagulans* (1), *Staphylococcus caseolyticus* (1) and *Staphylococcus hyicus* (1). Seven *Staphylococcal species* could not be identified. Other organisms isolated were *Escherichia coli* (19), *Streptococcus* (17), *Yeast* (15), *Klebsiella* (8), *Pseudomonas* (7), *Bacillus* (6), *Corynebacterium* (4) and *Proteus species* (2).

Tamilnadu

Paul *et al.* (2000) studied a total of 83 milk samples from cows and 49 from buffaloes from different dairy farms in and around Chennai. Out of 132 samples collected, 45 (34.09%) and 7 (5.30%) samples revealed monobacterial and mixed bacterial infection respectively. The distribution of organisms showed the predominance of *Staphylococcus spp.* (38.46%) followed by *Streptococcus* spp. (13.46%) and *Escherichia coli* (19.23%). The less commonly detected bacteria were *Pseudomonas aeruginosa* (4.5%), *Bacillus subtilis* (4.5%) and *Corynebacterium* spp. (1.5%). Vijayalakshmi *et al.* (2001) studied 130 milk samples and reported that 40 (30.7%) were culturally positive for aerobic pathogens viz. *Staphylococcus aureus* (27.5%), *Streptococcus* spp. (22.5%), *Klebsiella* spp. (15%), *Escherichia coli* (7.5%), *Enterobacter* spp. (7.5%), *Proteus* spp. (5%) and *Pseudomonas* spp. (10%). Balakrishnan *et al.* (2004) isolated the organisms from clinically affected mastitis cows- *Staphylococcus aureus* (35%), *Escherichia coli* (27.5%), *Streptococcus agalactiae* (17.5%), *Pseudomonas aeruginosa* (12.5%), *Streptococcus dysgalactiae* (2.5%), *Pasteurella haemolytica* (2.5%) and *Actinobacillus capsulatus* (2.5%). A cultural isolation of 120 milk samples from clinical mastitic cows showed most frequent microorganism *Escherichia coli* (60.86%) followed by *Staphylococcus aureus* (41.73%), *Bacillus cereus* (15.65%), *Streptococcus agalactiae*(13.04%) and *Enterobacter cloacae* (0.86%) (Varma and Dorairajan, 2006). Here *Escherichia coli* is chief etiological agent of clinical mastitis, while in most of areas of India *Staphylococci* are more prevalent. Reetha *et al.* (2006) cultured milk samples of clinical mastitis cases and found that *Staphylococcus* spp. (53.3%) was the predominant causative organism and *Escherichia coli* (46.7%) the next and no bacteria could be isolated from 3 samples (10%).

Mycotic mastitis recorded in 60% of cases which was caused by yeasts and molds including *Candida* spp. (66.67%), *Aspergillus* spp. (66.67%), *Rhizopus* spp. (33.33%), *Cryptococcus* spp. (33.33%) and *Trichosporon* spp. (22.2%) (Vimalraj *et al.*, 2006). Senthilvelan *et al.* (2006) has been reported the occurrence of *Candida albicans* in the milk of mastitic cows from Chennai. Vijayalakshmi and Prathaban (2007) collected milk samples from clinically suspected cases of mastitis, 40 were found culturally positive. *Staphylococcus aureus* (27.5%) was the main causal agent followed by *Streptococcus* spp. (22.5%), *Klebsiella* spp. (15%), *Pseudomonas* spp. (10%), *Escherichia coli* (7.5%), *Enterobacter* spp. (7.5%), *Staphylococcus* spp. (5%) and *Proteus* spp. (5%). A survey was conducted by Palanivel *et al.* (2008) on 300 graded Murrah buffaloes in Chennai during the period April, 2002 to March, 2003, results revealed that the *Staphylococcus spp.* and *Coliform* spp. were main causative pathogens followed by Streptococcus, *Acranobacterium* and *Bacillus* spp. 'Rose Milk' (Haemorrhagic mastitis) is very frequent complaint by the dairy farmers and remains a therapeutic challenge for our practicing veterinarians. Etiological, epidemiological and clinicopathological study was conducted in Chennai by Selvaraj *et al.* (2008) and found Leptospirosis to be the most common cause of "Rose Milk" followed by *Streptococcus agalactiae* and *Staphylococcus aureus*.

Kerala

Ross *et al.* (2001) isolated *Staphylococcus aureus* (28.03%), *Escherichia coli* (20.56%), *Streptococcus agalactiae* (14.95%) *Bacillus subtilis* (13.08%), *Pseudomonas aeruginosa* (12.15%) and *Streptococcus dysgalactiae* (11.21%) from mastitic cow's milk. Mallikarjunaswamy and Krishnamurthy (1997) reported that the major pathogen of bovine mastitis was *Staphylococcus epidermidis* (37.38%) followed by *Staphylococcus aureus* (30.84%), *Streptococcus agalactiae* (15.88%), *Streptococcus dysgalactiae* (0.9%), *Streptococcus uberis* (0.46%), *Bacillus subtilis* (3.27%) and *Escherichia coli* (1.86%). Sebastian and Vijayakumar (2002) reported that the bacterial isolates (percentage distribution) from bovine mastitis milk as *Staphylococcus aureus* (23.8%), *Coagulase negative Staphylococcus* (6.4%), *Streptococcus agalactiae* (2.3%), *Escherichia coli* (3.0%), *Klebsiella pneumoniae* (0.8%), *Bacillus sp.* (1.1%) and *Chromobacterium violaccum* (0.3%). Rajendran *et al.* (2006) isolates were identified as *Staphylococcus* spp. (39.6%), followed by *Streptococcus* spp. (27.1%), *Escherichia coli* (10, 20.8%), *Corynebacterium* spp. (4, 8.3%) and *Bacillus* spp. (4.2%) from milk of mastitis cows. In a study on sub-clinical mastitis in cows, *Staphylococcus aureus* was chief pathogen (43.59%) followed by CNS (33.33%), *Streptococcus agalactiae* (12.82%) and *Escherichia coli* (10.26%) (Siji and Vijayakumar, 2007).

Other Asian Countries

Bangladesh

Kader *et al.* (2002) studied 55 bacterial isolates and observed that 43 (78.18%) had monobacterial and 12 (21.82%) had mixed bacterial infection. Monobacterial infection with *Staphylococcus spp.* were isolated in 29 samples (39.64%), *E. coli* in 9 (11.11%), *Bacillus sp.* in 3 (3.70%) and *Streptococcus* spp.

in 2 (2.47%), where as concurrent bacterial infection with *Staphylococcus spp.* plus *Streptococcus spp.* was noted in 4 (4.93%), *E.coli* plus *Staphylococcus spp.* in 2 (2.47%), *Staphylococcus spp.* plus *Bacillus* spp. in 5 (13.51%) and *Staphylococcus* spp. and *Corynebacterium* spp. in 1 (1.23%) cow.

Iran

Atyabi *et al.* (2002) have been reported *Streptococcus agalactiae* (22.11%), *Streptococcus disgalactiae* (11.43%), *Stap. aureus* (2.89%), *Staphylococcus beta haemolytic Dot aureus* (5.54%), *Staphylococcus* non haemolytic (24.72%), *Actinomyces pyogenes* (1.07%), *Bacillus cereus* (1.76%), *Escherichia coli* (10.16%), *Kelebsiella peneumoniae* (0.14%), *Pseudomonas aeroginosa* (0.21%), *Pasturella multocida* (0.03%), *Mycoplasma* spp. (0.03%) from 2904 milk samples, Tehran, Iran. However, no growth in 19.98% samples. Ebrahimi and Nikookhan (2005) Collected milk samples from acute and chronically mastitis affected cows reared under conventional and confined housing and subjected for fungal isolation. Out of positive samples *Fusarium* (28.26%) were most frequent one in chronic cases and followed by *Trichosporon* (26.08%), *Candida* spp. (17.39%), *Aspergillus fumigatus* (13.04%), *Rhodotorulla* (10.87%) and *Geotrichum* (4.35%) while in cases of acute mastitis the most frequent ones were *Trichosporon* (66.04%) and followed by *Candida* spp. ((11.20%), *Geotrichum* (5.66%), *Aspergillus fumigatus* (3.77%), *Fusarium* (1.89%) and *Rhodotorulla* (1.89%). From a total of 300 milk samples collected from Mashhad, Iran, 67 (22.33%) were positive for coagulase-negative *staphylococci*. CNS strains were identified as 18 (26.86%) strains of *Staphylococcus hyicus,* 14 (20.89%), strains of *Staphylococcus chromogenes,* 15 (22.39%) strains of *Staphylococcus epidermidis,* 10 (14.92%) strains of *Staphylococcus haemolyticus,* 3 (4.48%) strains of *Staphylococcus sciuri,* 4 (5.97%) strains of *Staphylococcus simulans* and 3 (4.48%) strains of *Staphylococcus xylosus* (Mohsenzadeh and Fallah Rad, 2007). Kheirabadi *et al.* (2008) from our studies concluded that sub-clinical mastitis is mainly caused by *Staphylococcus aureus,* in west central region of Iran. They isolated the *Staphylococcus aureus* (63.3%), *Streptococcus agalactiae* (0.4%), *Coliforms* (7.9%), *Staphylococcus* spp. (12%), *Micrococcus* spp. (5.8%), *Streptococcus* spp. (9.8%) and others (0.8%).

Israel

Jemeljanovs *et al.* (2002) had been isolated *Staphylococcus aureus* (62.50%) *Streptococcus agalactiae* (21.88%), *Escherichia coli* (12.50%) and *Diplococcus* (3.12%) from clinical mastitis milk samples, while from sub-clinical mastitis cases *Staphylococcus aureus* (54.90%), *Streptococcus agalactiae* (25.49%), Coccus and other microorganisms (19.61%) from Lativa. *Yersinia pseudotuberculosis* was isolated from mastitis cases in nine dairy cows in Israel by Shwimmer *et al.* (2007). Jemeljanovs *et al.* (2008) a total of 577 sub-clinical and clinical mastitis secretion samples from the different dairy farms in Lativa were analysed and found that *Staphylococcus aureus* and CNS prevail in sub-clinically (72.7%) and clinically (46.7%) diseased cow's udder secretion samples. *Staphylococcus aureus* were isolated from 41.1% of sub-clinically and 24.1% clinically diseased cow's secretion samples, but CNS from 27.0% and 20.4% respectively. *Streptococcus* spp. were isolated from 5.9% of sub-clinically and 33.6% of clinically mastitic cows, while in the 1980s *Streptococcus* spp. were isolated from 65.5% of sub-clinical and 64.8% of clinical mastitis cases. Therefore, present findings revealed that replacement of predominating agents of mastitis from the genus *Streptococcus* to the genus *Staphylococcus* has been occurred in Lativa.

Japan

Bacteria isolated from clinical mastitic cows milk included *Escherichia coli* (75%), *Klebsiella oxytoca* (13%), *Pseudomonas aeruginosa* (8%) and *Enterobacter* species (4%) by Nakajima *et al.* (1997). Miyano *et al.* (2004) have been confirmed that mammary lesions in clinical bovine mastitis was associated with bovine herpes virus type 4 in Japan, and found intranuclear eosinophilic inclusion bodies in lactiferous duct and epithelium of mammary tissue of a clinical mastitic cow.

China

A bacteriological analysis was carried out based on the quarter milk samples from 102 clinical and 187 sub-clinical mastitis cases. From clinical cases, 85.3% of the samples were detected to have bacteria, which were significantly more than those from the sub-clinical cases (72.2%). Contagious pathogens including *Streptococcus agalactiae, Staphylococcus aureus* and *Corynebacterium bovis,* accounted for the major part of the detected pathogens in the clinical (41.2%) as well as in the sub-clinical cases (39.5%). Environmental pathogens were the secondary important bacteria for the clinical cases in this study, in which *Streptococcus uberis, Streptococcus faecalis, Streptococcus bovis, Proteus* spp. and *Escherichia coli* were isolated. Significantly more quarters (20.6%) were found to have environmental bacteria infection in the clinical cases compared to the sub-clinical cases (2.2%). The detective rates of coagulase-negative staphylococci in the clinical and sub-clinical groups were 14.7% and 13.4%, respectively (Hu et al., 1998). Zhang et al. (2002) had been isolated Staphylococcus (23.81%), Streptococci (39.69%), Bacilli (25.39%) and others (11.11%) from mastitic dairy cows. Ma et al. (2005) investigated on 14 dairy cattle farms in Shandong, China. A total of 234 clinical mastitis milk samples and a total of 241 sub-clinical mastitis milk samples were collected for bacterial inspection. The results indicated that: The majority of bacteria which caused clinical mastitis in lactation cows were coagulase-negative

Staphylococcus, *Staphylococcus aureus*, Streptococcus, yeast and Corynebacterium. *Escherichia coli*, Streptococcus, coagulase-negative Staphylococci, *S. aureus* and yeast took major part in clinical mastitis milk samples of dry period cows. The bacteria which took high inspection rates in sub-clinical mastitis milk samples were coagulase- negative Staphylococci, *Staphylococcus aureus*, Streptococcus, yeast, Pseudomonas and Corynebacterium. The anaerobe infection rates in lactating clinical mastitis, sub-clinical mastitis and dry milk cows clinical mastitis milk samples were 5.82%, 4.17% and 10.16% respectively. While in the study of Liu et al. (2005) *Staphylococcus aureus* (78.98%) was chief etiological agent of mastitis instead of Streptococcus as in previous study. Besides, common environmental pathogrns such as salmonell and *Escherichia coli* decreased obviously with detecting rates of 21.1% and 9.24% respectively, contrarily, *P. aeruginosa* and *B. cereus* increased evidently, their detecting rated were 5.41% and 11.15% respectively. *P. aeruginosa* and Cryptococcus had caused outbreaks of clinical mastitis, and Cryptococcus, to some degree, had become another new pathogen causing pertinacious mastitis. Liu et al. (2006) isolate 91 strains of bacteria from the milk of dairy cows with sub-clinical mastitis in huhhot area of China. Of which 72 (79.12%) strains of *Staphylococcus aureus*, 8 (8.8%) *Staphylococcus hemolyticus*, 6 (6.59%) *Streptococcus epidermidis*, 1 (1.1%) *Streptococcus dysgalactiae*, 2 (2.2%) *Bacillus coli*, 1 (1.1%) Serratia and 1 (1.1%) Klebsiella. Wang and Niu (2009) isolated 110 strains of bacterium from 115 milk samples collected from 29 cows in 3 different scale dairy farms, including 29 of Streptococcus (25.22%), 26 of Staphylococcus (22.61%), 19 of Enterobacter (15.65%), 18 of Yeast (16.52%), 8 of Corynebacterium (6.96%). Positive rate of pathogen of milk samples was 79.13% and mixed infection rate was 20%. Zhang et al. (2009) had also been reported that more prevalent pathogens of bovine clinical mastitis are *Staphylococcus aureus*, Strpetococcus, *Escherichia coli* and *Pasteurella multocida*. Li *et al.* (2009) had also been reported that *Staphylococcus aureus* was major cause of clinical mastitis and other organisms were *Staphylococcus epidermidis*, *Staphylococcus saprophyte*, *Streptococcus agalactiae*, *Streptococcus udder*, *Streptococcus lactis*, *Streptococcus faecium*, *Corynevbacterium bovis*. Microzyme, *Escherichia coli*, *Klebsiella* spp., *Proteus* spp., *Shigella* spp., *Enterobacter aerogenes* and *Serratia* spp. The data of recent study revealed that *Escherichia coli* is the commonest organism in mastitis cases, being implicated in 82% cases, and *Streptococcus uberis* (53%) continues to be a prevalent pathogen closely followed by *Staphylococcus aureus* (41%), *Streptococcus dysgalactiae* (29%) and *Streptococcus agalactiae* (27%). In addition, *Streptococcus uberis* and *Staphylococcus aureus* were more frequently associated with clinical mastitis than sub-clinical case, while the infection rates of other bacteria were similar. Further more, *Staphylococcus epidermids* (15%) and *Staphylococcus saprophyticus* (10%), previously considered as naught pathogenic bacteria, were also detected in the diseased mammary gland of the problem cows (Cheng *et al.*, 2010).

Jordan

National cross-sectional study of mastitis in dairy cattle in Jordan (Lafi *et al.*, 1994), it was reported that the most estimates of prevalence of bacterial pathogens intramammary infections were: coagulase negative *Staphylococci* 16.04%, *Staphylococcus aureus* 9.41%, *Klebsiella* spp. 6.17%, *Corynebacterium* bovis 5.35% and *Brucella melitensis* 4.52%. Lafi and Hailat (1998) examined 30 milk samples of clinical mastitic cows and the microorganisms isolated by them were *Staphylococcus aureus* (36.7%), *Streptococcus agalactiae* (30%), *Escherichia coli* (16.7%), *Corynebacterium bovis* (10%) and *Klebsiella sp.* (6.6%). Milk samples were collected from 220 Holstein Friesian cows in 10 farms in Thuleil area, Jordan and isolated. In clinical mastitis the incidence of *Coliform* 26.1%, *Streptococcus* spp 8.7%, *Staphylococcus aureus* 40.6%, *Proteus* spp. 1.4%, *Corynebacterium* spp. 5.8%, *Pseudomonas* **spp.** 4.3% , mixed (*Coryne, Strept, Staph* and *Coliforms*) 7.3% and others 5.8%. While in sub-clinical mastitis *Coliforms* were 31.9%, *Streptococcus* spp. 7.2%, *Staphylococcus aureus* 42.7%, *Proteus* spp. 2.2%, *Corynebacterium* spp. 2.9%, mixed and others 13.1% (Hawari and Dabbas, 2008).

Nepal

Among the bacteriologically positive samples of mastitis milk from Nepal, single bacterial species was found in 79.6% of samples, while mixed bacterial growth was recorded in 20.3% samples. Among the isolated bacteria, *Staphylococcus aureus* was found in highest proportion followed by mixed infection of *Streptococcus* spp. with other organisms (Joshi and Joshi, 1997). A study conducted in western mid hills of Nepal on clinical bovine mastitis showed that single organism was involved in 68% of cases while mixed infection was recorded in 32% of the cases. Coliform infection (25%) followed by *Streptococcus* spp. (20%) and *Staphylococcus* spp. (10%) were the most commonly isolated organisms (Joshi *et al.*, 1997). Joshi *et al.* (1998) conducted epidemiological investigation on clinical mastitis (CM) in cows and buffaloes during 1994-1995 in the western hills of Nepal to identify microorganisms involved. Milk samples from infected teats were subjected to bacteriological examination. Bacteriological examination revealed that 112 (88.2%) teat milk sample had microbial growth, of which 76 (68.0%) had single microbial infections and 32.0 % had mix infections. Coliforms (particularly *Klebsiella pneumoniae* and *Escherichia coli*) were recorded in 25% followed by *Streptococcus* spp (19.6%) and *Staphylococcus* spp. (9.8%). Dhakal *et al.* (2006) a total of 200 buffaloes milk samples subjected to cultural isolation and found bacterial growth in 26% samples while 74% samples did not showed any cultural growth. Of these *Staphylococcus epidermidis* (57.69%), *Streptococcus bovis* (17.31%), *Staphylococcus aureus* (15.38%), *Streptococcus dysgalactiae* (7.69%), and *Escherichia coli* (1.92%). Dhakal *et al.* (2007) also studied on a total of 355 Murrah cross buffaloes, consisting of 23 sub-clinical and 332 clinical mastitis cases from 2002 to 2005. They isolated *Staphylococcus aureus* (11.1%), *Staphylococcus albus* (33.3%), *Staphylococcus epidermidis* (11.1%), *Micrococcus* (19.3%), *Streptococcus mitis* (2.8%), *Clostridium* spp. (5.6%), *Corynebacterium diphtheriae* (2.8%), *Escherichia coli* (2.8%), *Bacillus subtilis* (5.6%), *Micrococcus* plus *Bacillus subtitis* (5.6%) from sub-clinical cases and *Staphylococcus aureus* (26.8%), *Staphylococcus epidermidis* (8.9%), *Micrococcus* (23.2%), *Clostridium* spp. (10.7%), *Escherichia coli* (7.1%), *Klebsiella pneumoniae* (3.6%), *Providencia* spp. (3.6%), *Pseudomonas* spp. (3.6%), *Bacillus subtilis* (8.9%), *Micrococcus* plus *Bacillus subtilis* (3.6%) from clinical cases of mastitis. From the above studies in Nepal, it is concluded that pattern of bacterial distribution responsible for mastitis has been changed i.e. previously (1994-1998) *Escherichia coli* was predominating organism while recent reports showed that *Staphylococcus* spp. are more prevalent than *Escherichia coli* in mastitis case.

Pakistan

Javed and Siddique (1999) reported that major mastitis organism was *Staphylococcus aureus* (32.09%) followed by coagulase negative *Staphylococci* (12.06%), *Streptococcus uberis* (7%), *Streptococcus agalactiae* (3%), *Corynebacterium pyogenes* (3.5%), *Bacillus sp.* (3%) and *Escherichia coli* (10%) from Pakistan. Ahmad (2001) performed microbiological examination of 157 SCM milk samples and 46 clinical mastitis milk samples. There was a high occurrence of *Streptococcus pyogenes* (35.46%) followed by *Staphylococcus aureus* (33.99%), *E.coli* (27.09%), *Pseudomonas spp.* (1.97%) and *Corynebcterium pyogenes* (1.48%). Iqbal *et al.* (2004) reported *Escherichia coli* (30.12%), *Staphylococci* (16.87%), *Streptococci* (3.60%), *Pseudomonas* (14.51%), *Proteus* spp. (4.82%), *Pasteurella* (1.20%), *Salmonella* (2.41%), *Bacillus* spp. (2.41%) and mixed growth (24.09%) from buffaloes and *Escherichia coli* (46.98%), *Staphylococci* (13.42%), *Streptococci* (9.39%), *Pseudomonas* (14.77%), *Proteus* spp. (4.02%), *Pasteurella* (2.01%), *Salmonella* (1.34%) and mixed growth (8.02%) from cows milk samples from Peshawar, Pakistan. Milk samples collected from 50 dairy buffaloes and 50 crossbred cows from Pakistan. Among the isolates, *Staphylococcus aureus* showed the highest (45%) frequency, followed by *Streptococcus agalactiae* (23%), *Escherichia coli* (18%) and *Bacillus spp.* (14%) in buffaloes, while in case of crossbred cows, *Staphylococcus aureus* (48%), *Streptococcus agalactiae* (30%), *Escherichia coli* (13%) and *Bacillus spp.* (8%) (Khan and Mohammad, 2005). A total of 200 fore milk samples collected from 200 mastitis quarters of buffaloes from Pakistan were subjected to microbiological examination. Microbiological results showed *Staphylococcus aureus* was most prevalent (49.53%) bacteria, followed by *Streptococcus agalactiae* (23.83%), *Staphylococcus hyicus* (8.88%), *Staphylococcus epidermidis* (6.54%), *Bacillus* spp. (3.74%), *Staphylococcus huminis* (1.40%), *Escherichia coli* (1.4%), *Staphylococcus xylosus* (0.93%), *Streptococcus dysgalactiae* (0.93%), *Corynebacterium* spp. (0.93%), Yeast (0.47%), *Prototheca* (0.47%) and CNS (0.93%) (Ali *et al.*, 2008).

South Korea

Microorganisms from 296 mastitic quarters from Jeju, Korea Republic were isolated and identified as *Staphylococcus aureus* (51.4%), Coliforms (16.5%), *Streptococcus dysgalactiae* (15.8%), *Bacillus* spp. (5.1%), *Staphylococcus epidermidis* (2.7%), *Streptococcus agalactiae* (2.1%), *Enterococcus feacalis* (1.7%), *Corynebacterium* spp. (1.7%), *Streptococcus uberis* (1.0%), *Pseudomonas aeruginosa* (0.3%) and *Pasteurella multocida* (0.3%) (Kang *et al.*, 2001). Nam *et al.* (2009) carried out a 6 years (from 2003 to 2008) study on the trend in the distribution of Gram negative bacteria of bovine mastitis and unearth that *Escherichia coli, Pseudomonas fluorescens, Klebsiella pneumoniae, Enterobacter cloacae, Acinetobacter lwoffi/junii, Pseudomonas aeruginosa* and *Serratia marcescens* were the most commonly observed pathogens during this period. Nam et al. (2010) found that the most frequently isolated pathogen was coagulase-negative staphylococci (40.7%), followed by Gram-negative bacteria (19.5%) other than *Escherichia coli, Staphylococcus aureus* (12.2%), *Streptococcus uberis* (5.3%), *Enterococcus* spp. (4.8%), *E. coli* (4.5%), and environmental streptococci (3.1%) other than *S. uberis*. This study demonstrates that environmental pathogens were the vast majority of bacteria isolated from mastitic bovine milk samples in Korea.

Portugal

Information about the prevalence of mastitis pathogens in Portugal is scarce, and the previous epidemiological survey showed that 50% of the total infected quarters were caused by sub-clinical infections due to *Staphylococcus aureus* and *Streptococcus uberis* (Louza *et al.*, 1986). A study by Pinho *et al.* (2008) on 15,046 milk samples of 373 farms from January 2005 to January 2008 and found that environmental agents were the most prevalent (69.4%) compare to contagious agents (30.3%). *Streptococcus* spp. non-*agalactiae* (20.7%) were most frequently isolated followed by CNS (14.7%), coliforms (14.3%), yeast (9.4%), *Enterococcus* spp. (4.3%), *Bacillus* spp. (3.5%), fungi (0.2%) and 22.2% samples showed no growth or contaminated.

Kingdom of Saudi Arabia

Shathele *et al.* (2009) reported that *Escherichia coli* was major (21.1%) causal agent of clinical mastitis in cows, followed by *Streptococcus haemolyticus* (12.2%), *Corynebacterium bovis* (11.1%), *Streptococcus agalactiae* (10%) and other isolates were 45.5%. Fadlelmula et al. (2009) carried out an etiological study in a Saudi Arabian dairy farm with a capacity of 11,200 dairy cows and found most predominant bacterial isolates were *Streptococcus uberis* (28.8%), *Escherichia coli* (18.5%), *Streptococcus dysgalactiae* (10.8%) and *Staphylococcus aureus* (9.8%). Other bacteria and fungi were isolated in a range of 0.3 to 3.8%. This is the first report of bovine mycotic mastitis from the Kingdom of Saudi Arabia.

North America (U.S.A.)

A large scale study was conducted by the United State Department of Agriculture (Veterinary services) in 17 dairy states of U.S. including California, Idaho, New Mexico, Texas, and Washington (West) and Indiana, Iowa, Kentucky, Michigan, Minnesota, Missouri, New York, Ohio, Pennsylvania, Vermont, Virginia, and Wisconsin (East) to know the status of three major contagious mastitis pathogens and found that out of these three pathogens *Staphylococcus aureus* was more prevalent (43%), while *Streptococcus agalactiae* and *Mycoplasma* spp. were found in 2.6 and 3.2% samples, respectively (USDA-APHIS Info Sheet, 2008). However, *Mycoplasma* (Gonzalez and Wilson 2003; Fox *et al.*, 2005) and *Klebsiella* (Hoe and Ruegg, 2005; Munoz *et al.*, 2007; Paulin-Curlee *et al.*, 2007) mastitis are major concerns in the USA. Fox *et al.* (1995) collected the milk samples from California, Louisiana, Vermont and Washington dairy cattle and isolated the CNS (78.73%), *Staphylococcus aureus* (8.36%), Environmental bacteria (4.44%) and others (8.48%).

Ohio

Bartlett *et al.* (1992) found that the most common isolates from clinical mastitis cases of cows were coagulase-negative staphylococci and *Escherichia coli,* each present in 14.6% of samples taken. Estimates of population prevalence of intramammary infection for Ohio dairy farms were: coagulasepositive staphylococci (2%), coagulase-negative staphylococci (2%), *Escherichia coli* (1%), other coliforms (1%), *Streptococcus agalactiae* (2%) esculin-positive streptococci (5%) and other esculin-negative streptococci (3%).

Wisconsin

Bacterial pathogens isolated from 133 cows with mild or moderate mastitis *Streptococcus* spp., 35.3%; *Escherichia coli*, 26.3%; Coagulase-negative staphylococci, 19.5%; *Klebsiella* spp., 9.8; *Enterobacter* spp., 3.0%; *Pasteurella* spp., 1.5%; *Proteus* spp., 1.5%; *Corynebacterium* spp., 0.8%; *Staphylococcus aureus*, 0.8%; *Serratia* spp., 0.8% and Other gram-negative rods, 0.8% (Hoe and Ruegg, 2005).

Louisiana

Trinidad *et al.* (1990) reported the distribution of *Staphylococcus chromogenes* (43.1%), *Staphylococcus aureus* (19.9%), *Staphylococcus hyicus* (24.3%), *Staphylococcus hominis* (0.7%), *Staphylococcus simulans* (0.7%), *Staphylococcus xylosus* (1.1%), *Staphylococcus warneri* (0.4%), *Staphylococcus epidermidis* (0.4%), *Staphylococcus* spp. (0.4%), *Streptococcus dysgalactiae* (0.4%), *Streptococcus* spp. (3.3%), *Nocardia* spp. (0.4%), Unidentified (0.7%) and mixed infection (5.5%) from lacteal secretion of unbred and primigravid heifers from Louisiana.

California

A study was conducted in 1996 by Kirk *et al.* at California, milk samples were collected from 339 heifers for isolation of mastitis etiological agents. Isolated organisms were Coliforms 16%, *Streptococcus* spp. 11%, CNS 39%, *Strep.* spp. and CNS mixed 4% and others 1%. Roberson *et al.* (2004) isolated *Streptococcus uberis* (29.1%), *Escherichia coli* (19.4%), *Klebsiella pneumoniae* (14.6%), CNS (4.9%), *Klebsiella oxytoca* (3.9%), *Serratia marcescens* (3.9%), *Streptococcus dysgalactiae* (2.9%), *Staphylococcus aureus* (2.9%), Yeast (2.9%), *Citrobacter* spp. (1.0%), *Enterobacter* spp. (1.0%), *Enterococcus* spp. (1.0%) and *Streptococcus mutans* (1.0%) and no growth in 11.5% samples from Holistein and Jersey cows of Kansas State Unversity, dairy farm. Resende et al. (2009) Conducted a study on a total of 370,748 milk samples between January of 1999 and December of 2008. Multiple mastitis pathogens were isolated from 64.2% of the samples (n=237,968), and among these positive samples Environmental *Staphylococcus* spp were the most prevalent (44.8%) followed by Coliforms (33.5%), Environmental *Streptococcus* spp(14.8%), *Bacillus* spp (10.4%), Coagulase-negative *Staphylococcus* (5.6%), *Staphylococcus aureus* (5.6%) and *Streptococcus agalactiae* (0.1%).

Mexico

The findings of bacteriological milk sample examination during September to November 2007 showed that CNS was most (24.49%) prevalent organism, followed by *Staphylococcus aureus* (18.44%), *Streptococcus* spp. (6.91%), *Escherichia coli* (0.57%) and 35.46% samples were negative to bacterial growth (Bedolla *et al.*, 2008). Castaneda *et al.* (2008) study in 33 dairy herds of cattle in Jalisco, Mexico and reported that 53.8% of the examined milk samples were negative to bacterial growth and in rest samples CNS was prevalent organism (15.4%) followed by *Corynebacterium* spp. (13.9%), *Streptococcus agalactiae* (6.6%), *Staphylococcus aureus* (5.8%), Coliforms (3.6%) and other (*Bacillus* spp., *Nocardia* spp., *Candida* spp.) in 1.7% quarters.

Canada

Intramammary infection status was studied in 520 quarters of 131 cows in early lactation from July 1998 to April 1999 in different places of Canada. Distribution of microorganisms were divided into two groups as Major pathogens include Environmental streptococci (5.0%), *Klebsiella* spp. (1.0%), *Escherichia coli* (1.7%), mixed (0.2%), *Staphylococcus aureus* (1.9%), *Bacillus* spp. (2.9%), *Enterobacter* spp. (1.0%), *Pseudomonas* spp. (0.77%), *Citrobacter* spp. (0.38%) and *Proteus* spp. (0.2%), and minor pathogens contains CNS (17.9%), Corynebacterium bovis (1.2%) and mixed (1.9%) (Sargeant *et al.*, 2001). Bouchard *et al.* (2006) conducted a study on freshly calved and mastitic cows in Quebec province of Canada and found 27% and 59% culturally positive animals respectively. Bacterial distribution in freshly calved cows was *Staphylococcus aureus* (10%), *Staphylococcus* spp. (9%), *Streptococcus* spp. (3%), *Corynebacterium* spp. (2%), Coliform (1%), Yeast (1%), *Streptococcus agalactiae* (0.4%) and other (1%), and in mastitic cows *Staphylococcus aureus* (17%), Coliform (17%), *Streptococcus* spp. (12%), *Staphylococcus* spp. (6%), Yeast (3%) and other (4%). Recently *Bacillus anthracis* mastitis has also been reported in a beef cow from Saskatoon, Canada (Ngeleka *et al.*, 2008). A study of Olde Riekerink *et al.* (2008) at 106 dairy farms from 10 province of Canada and isolated *Staphylococcus aureus* (21.7%), *Escherichia coli* (17.6%), *Streptococcus uberis* (13.3%), CNS (10.7%), *Klebsiella* spp. (9.1%), *Streptococcus dysgalactiae* (8.4%), *Enterococcus* spp. (4.7%), *Streptococcus* spp. (4.4%), Yeast (4.0%), *Arcanobacterium pyogenes* (2.6%), *Bacillus* spp. (2.2%), *Pseudomonas* spp. (1.6%), *Serratia* (0.8%), *Corynebacterium bovis* (0.4%), *Staphyloccus* spp. (0.3%), *Streptococcus agalactiae* (0.3%), *Pasteurella* spp. (0.1%) and Other 3.5% of isolates.

South America

Brazil

Costa *et al.* (1996) were isolated *Prototheca spp.* from 14.55% of the milk samples and *Nocardia spp.* from 4.55%. *Prototheca spp.* was isolated from 8.06% of the secretion samples from dry cows and *Nocardia spp.* was isolated from 2.15% samples from Brazil. A total of 7902 cows milk samples from sub-clinical mastitis and 850 of clinical mastitis from Sao Paulo State of Brazil. *Staphylococcus* was isolated from 32% of sub-clinical samples and 19% of clinical samples, *Staphylococcus aureus* from 22% and 11% of sub-clinical and clinical mastitis respectively. Enterobacteriaceae were found in 12% of sub-clinical cases and 26% of clinical cases; *Escherichia coli* was the most frequent of the Enterobacteriaceae isolated (5% of sub-clinical cases and 7% of clinical cases). *Streptococcus* was isolated from 18% of sub-clinical cases and 16% of clinical cases; *Streptococcus agalactiae* from 14 and 11% respectively.

Corynebcaterium bovis was isolated from 16% of sub-clinical and 12% of clinical cases. Other bacteria isolated included *Rhodococcus equi, Actinomyces pyogenes, Nocardia asteroids* and *Bacillus cereus* (Langoni *et al.*, 1998). Corbellini *et al.* (2001) has been described the clinical, epidemiological and pathological aspects of protothecal mastitis in a Brazilian dairy herd, and *Prototheca zopfii* infection was diagnosed in 11 of 121 milking cows. Langoni *et al.* (2001) reported mastitis bacterial distribution in buffaloes in Brazil, as *Corynebacterium bovis* (31.3%), *Staphylococcus epidermidis* (30.1%), *Streptococcus agalactiae* (26.5%), *Staphylococcus aureus* (4.8%), *Acinetobacter calcoaceticus* (2.4%), *Pasteurella multocida* (2.4%) and *Bacillus spp.* (2.4%). A study was conducted on 37 dairy farms of Brazil by Santos and Marin (2005), and isolated *Escherichia coli* (26.5%), Coagulase-positive Staphylococcus (25.0%), *Candida* spp. (17.3%), *Streptococcus* spp. (8.1%), *Enterobacter* spp. (8.1%), other fungi (8.1%), *Proteus* spp. (1.9%), *Pseudomonas* spp. (1.1%), Gram negative *Bacillus* (1.1%), *Shigella* spp. (0.8%), *Serratia* spp. (0.4%), *Bacillus* spp. (0.4%), *Edwardsiela* spp. (0.4%), *Sarcina* spp. (0.4%), *Providencia* spp. (0.4%) from the milk of clinical and sub-clinical mastitic cows. Various species of Candida was also isolated in this study *C. krusei* (44.5%), *C. rugosa* (24.5%), *C. albicans* (8.9%), *C. guilliermondii* (8.9%), *C. parapsilosis* (4.4%), *C. zeulanoide* (2.2%), *C. vini* (2.2%), *C. famata* (2.2%) and *C. tropicalis* (2.2%). Oliviera *et al.* (2010) reported *Staphylococcus aureus* (42.85%), *Corynebaterium* sp. (42.85%), coagulase negative *Staphylococcus* (36.19%), *Pseudomonas* sp. (16.19%), *Escherichia coli* (15.23%), *Bacillus* sp. (15.23%), *Streptococcus* sp (13.33%), *Klebsiella* sp. (1.9%) and *Proteus* sp. (0.95%) occurrence from mastitis samples.

Uruguay

Gianneechini *et al.* (2002) study in Uruguay dairy farms and isolated *Staphylococcus aureus* (37.5%), *Escherichia coli* (12.5%), *Staphylococcus hyicus* (5.0%), *Staphylococcus chromogenes* (2.5%), *Streptococcus agalactiae* (5.0%), *Streptococcus uberis* (2.5%) and *Enterococcus spp* (2.5%) from clinical mastitis cases and *Staphylococcus aureus* (62.8%), *Streptococcus agalactiae* (11.3%), *Enterococcus spp.* (8.2%), *Staphylococcus hyicus* (2.54%), *Staphylococcus chromogenes* (2.15%), *Staphylococcus epidermidis* (0.59%), *Staphylococcus simulans* (0.39%), *Staphylococcus warneri* (0.19%), *Staphylococcus haemolyticus* (0.19%), CNS novobiocin resistant strains (1.17%), *Streptococcus uberis* (6.4%), *Streptococcus dysgalactiae* (1.8%), *Escherichia coli* (1.5%), *Staphylococcus hyicus* (coagulase-positive) (0.6%) and in 32.5% samples no growth, from sub-clinical mastitis samples.

Europe

It is the most common infectious disease in farmed animals. Around one million cases occur each year in the UK. It is painful, occasionally life threatening, and costs the dairy industry £200m every year in lost production and treatments. Within the UK alone it has been estimated that around 12m doses of antibiotic are used annually to control and treat mastitis in cattle. In some European countries, e.g. Belgium, Denmark, Norway and the UK, occurrence of *Streptococcus agalactiae* is now sporadic (Andersen *et al.*, 2003; Østeras *et al.*, 2006; Bradley *et al.*, 2007; Piepers *et al.*, 2007). In other areas, *Streptococcus agalactiae* is still quite common, e.g. in parts of Europe [Germany: 29% of herds positive (Tenhagen *et al.* 2006)] and the Americas [Brazil: 60% of herds positive (Duarte *et al.* 2004); Uruguay: 11% of herds positive (Gianneechini *et al.*, 2002); New York, USA: 10% of cows positive (Wilson *et al.*, 1997)] (Cited in Zadocks and Fitzpatrick, 2009).

Sweden

Study was carried out in 684 milk samples from organized dairy farm of Sweden and isolated Coagulase-negative Staphylococci 37 (13.65%), *Corynebacterium boris* (9.22%), *Staphylococcus aureus* (6.64%), *Streptococcus uberis* (3.32%), Other organsim (1.84%), *Streptococcus dysgalactiae* (0.74%), and unspecified mixed cultures (64.57%) among culturally positive samples (Emanuelson *et al.*, 1987).

Italy

Moretti *et al.* (1998) reported that the major mastitis pathogen was *Staphylococcus aureus* (34.3%) followed by *Streptococcus albo* (19.8%) and followed by yeasts *Trichosporon capitatum* (31.2%), *Trichosporon beigelii* (18.72%) and *Candida albicans* (12.48%), *Candia guillermondii* (12.48%), *Candida tropicalis* (12.48%) in Central Italy. A study was conducted by Ferguson *et al.* (2007) from 2000 to 2006 on 18,711 cow milk samples in Ragusa, Italy. They found that no growth was on 47.4% samples, CNS, 14.6%; *Staphylococcus aureus*, 12.5%; Environmental *Streptococcus* spp., 6.6%; *Streptococcuss agalactiae*, 1.4%; Coliform spp., 1.7%; Other bacteria, 3.3% and multiple bacterial isolates, 0.5%. Scaccabarozzi *et al.* (2008) isolated *Prototheca* spp. (11.9%), *Staphylococcus aureus* (2.2%), *Streptococcus uberis* (1.6%), *E. coil* (1.5%), CNS (1.5%), *Streptococcus dysgalactiae* (1.1%), mixed infections (10%) and 70.2% samples were negative to any growth from Northern Italy. Cremonesi *et al.* (2008) have also been isolated *Staphylococcus aureus* (7.6%), *Streptococcus* spp. (1.4%), other *Staphylococcus* spp. (30.4%) and *Mycoplasma bovis* (1.1%), *Escherichia coli* (0.8%) from milk samples.

France

Bourry *et al.* (1997) isolated *Listeria monocytogenes* 31.43%, CNS 14.28%, *Streptococcus uberis* 8.57%, *Staphylococcus aureus* 8.57% samples and no growth was observed in 37.14% samples.

Germany

Edinger *et al.* (1999) collected milk samples from heifer (Berlin, Germany) just prior to first milking and found that the most prevalent causal agent of bovine mastitis was *Staphylococcus spp.* (69%) followed by *Streptococcus spp.* (12%) and *Escherichia coli* (5%). Keller *et al.* (2000) has been identified five genera and 29 species of yeast from Hannover, Germany dairy cattles. Species of the genus Candida dominated with 77% of all samples. More than 25% of yeasts from milk were identified as *C. rugosa* and more than 20% as *C. catenulata*. The six species found most often represented 74% of all yeasts in this group. A report of Tenhagen *et al.* (2006) from Brandenburg, Germany showed that mastitis pathogens were isolated from 26.4% of the cow milk samples. Coagulase-negative staphylococci (9.1%) and *Corynebacterium bovis* (7.3%) were the pathogens most frequently isolated. Among the major pathogens, *Staphylococcus aureus* (5.7%) and *Streptococcus uberis* (1.0%) had the highest prevalence. *Streptococcus agalactiae* was isolated in samples from 29% of the herds. Mastitis bacteriological study from Thuringia, Germany has also been reported that *Staphylococcus aureus* was chief (35.5%) mastitiogen followed by CNS (32.7%), *Streptococcus dysgalactiae* (10.6%), other environmental streps. (9.0%), *E. coli* (3.6%), *Streptococcus agalactiae* (2.4%), *Corynebacterium* spp. (1.1%) and others (5.1%) (Fadlelmoula *et al.*, 2007). Tenhagen *et al.* (2008) found that CNS were the predominant group of bacteria isolated (46.8% of samples) from clinically healthy quarters of primiparous cows around parturition, followed by *Streptococci* (12.6%), *Escherichia coli* (4.7%) and *Staphylococcus aureus* (4.0%). In cases of clinical mastitis in primiparous and older cows, *Streptococci* were the predominant finding (32.1% and 39.2%), followed by CNS (27.4 and 16.4%), *coliforms* (10.3 and 13.1%) and *Staphylococcus aureus* (10.0 and 11.7%). While in the previous studies in Germany *Staphylococcus aureus* was major mastitis causing agent in dairy cattle.

Norway

Waage *et al.* (1999) in study included 1040 heifers with clinical mastitis in Norway, and the total number of quarters that were clinically affected was 1361 The organisms that were most frequently isolated from samples from these quarters were *Staphylococcuss aureus* (44.3%), *Streptococcus dysgalactiae* (18.2%), *Staphylococcus aureus* together with *Streptococcus dysgalactiae* (1.2%), coagulase-negative staphylococci (12.8%), *Arcanobacterium pyogenes* (3.5%), A. *pyogenes* together with *Streptococcus dysgalactiae* (0.5%) or *Staphylococcus aureus* (0.4%), and *Escherichia coli* (6.4%). Of the coagulase-negative Staphylococci, *Staphylococcus simulans* (53.7%), *Staphylococcus hyicus* (14.8%), and *Staphylococcus chromogenes* (14.8%) were the most prevalent species.

Except for a higher relative percentage of *A. pyogenes* in cases that occurred before parturition (8.2%) than in cases that occurred after parturition (2.7%). A study of Reksen *et al.* (2006) from 2492 sampled cows in Norway, reported no growth on 64.6% samples, *Staphylococcus aureus* (22.7%) followed by CNS (7.9%), *Streptococcus dysgalactia, Streptococcus uberis* and other *Streptococcus* spp. (4%) and other pathogens were 0.8%.

Turkey

Beytut *et al.* (2002) isolated from 105 cows, *Staphylococcus aureus* (43.75%), *Corynebacterium pyogenes* (19.79%), *Streptococcus agalactiae* (9.37%), *Staphylococcus epidermidis* (8.33%), *Escherichia coli* (7.29%), *Streptococcus dysgalactiae* (4.16%), *Bacillus subtilis* (3.15%), *Bacillus cereus* (2.08%) and *Candida* spp. (2.08%) from Turkey.

Greece

Zdragas *et al.* (2004) studied a total of 952 milk samples from cows with clinical bovine mastitis cases, from 269 farms in Noethern Greece. Among the microorganisms *Escherichia coli* was isolated in 49.30% of the samples followed by *Staphylococcus* spp., *Corynebacterium* spp., *Streptococcus* spp., *Pseudomonas* spp., *Proteus* spp. and *Klebsiella* spp. The bacteriological results from 4.3% of the samples were negative. Filioussis *et al.* (2007) isolated *Mycoplasma bovis* from 8.2% quarter milk samples collected from cases of bovine clinical mastitis. Major mastitis pathogens (*Staphylococcus aureus, Streptococcus agalactiae, Streptococcus dysgalactiae* and *Streptococcus uberis*) were isolated from 37% quarter milk samples, while non-major mastitis pathogens (coagulase negative Staphylococci, *Actinomyces pyogenes, Bacillus* spp., *Candida* spp., *Enterobacter* spp., *Klebsiella* spp., *Micrococcus* spp., *Pseudomonas* spp., *Citrobacter* spp., *Escherichia coli, Enterococcus faecalis* and *Mannheimia haemolytica*) were isolated from 46.6% samples.

Slovenia

Mijovic *et al.* (2006) isolated *Prototheca zopfii* from a case of sub-clinical bovine mastitis from Slovenia.

Poland

A study in Poland on 11224 quarters of 4850 cows was conducted by Malinowski *et al.* (2002) and isolated *Prototheca spp.* (28 strains) from 200 (0.4%) milk samples. Malinowski *et al.* (2006) also isolated *Staphlococcus aureus, Streptocouus spp.*, CNS, *Acranobacterium pyogenes, Corynebacterium spp.*, Gram positive bacilli and yeast like fungi from milk of mastitic dairy cattle from Poland. Kleczkowski *et al.* (2007) have been isolated *Staphylococcus aureus,*

Streptococcus agalactiae and *Escherichia coli*, from bovine mastitis in Poland. A study conducted by Szczubial *et al.* (2008) reported 100% growth of microorganisms from mastitic milk samples of cows from Lublin, Poland. The bacteria isolated from milk of cows with acute mastitis included *Streptococcus agalactiae* (1), *Staphylococcus aureus* (10), and *Escherichia coli* (3). In mild clinical cases, *Streptococcus dysgalactiae* (8), *Streptococcus uberis* (5), *Staphylococcus aureus* (2), CNS (1), and *Escherichia coli* (2) were identified. In cows with chronic clinical mastitis, *Streptococcus dysgalactiae* (6), *Streptococcus uberis* (2), and *Candida* spp. (8) were detected whereas in those with sub-clinical mastitis, *Streptococcus agalactiae* (9), *Streptococcus Dysgalactiae* (4), *Streptococcus uberis* (8), and CNS (5) were isolated. No microorganisms were demonstrated in milk from healthy cows. Baranski *et al.* (2008) studied on prevalence of bacteria and fungi during the drying off period in North-East Poland between October, 2003 to September, 2005. They found Coagulase-negative staphylococci (*Staphylococcus epidermidis, Staphylococcus chromogenes Staphylococcus haemoliticus, Staphylococcus hyicus Staphylococcus warneri Staphylococcus saprophiticus*) was major organism (5%), *Streptococcus agalactiae* (2.40%), *Streptococcus uberis* (1.80%), *Streptococcus dysgalactiae* (0.30%), *Staphylococcus aureus* (1.90), *Escherichia coli* (1%), *Arcanobacter pyogenes* (0.09) and *Fungi* (*Candida* spp., *Mucor* spp., *Penicilium* spp., *Aspergillus* spp.)- 4.20%.

Finland

Pitkala *et al.* (2004) isolated the organisms responsible for clinical and sub-clinical bovine mastitis during 1995 to 2001 in Finland, CNS (49.63%), *Staphylococcus aureus* (10.17%), *Streptococcus agalactiae*(0.07%), *Streptococcus dysgalactiae* (0.14%), *Streptococcus uberis* (1.94%), Other *Streptococci* (0.21%), *Enterococcus* spp. (1.20%), *Aerococcus viridans* (0.71%), *Lactococcus* spp. (0.73%), *Corynebacterium* bovis (34.41%), Coliforms (0.42%) and Other bacteria (0.37%). Bovine mastitis organisms isolate from 1017 cases of clinical mastitis during 2002-2003 from Finland. Coagulase negative *Staphylococci* (15.60%), *Streptococcus uberis* (13.70%), Coliforms (11.60%), *Staphylococcus aureus* (10.70%), *Streptococcus dysgalactiae* (9.50%), *Acranobaterium pyogenes* (3.80%) and other bacteria or mixed 7.90% samples (Nevala *et al.*, 2004). A study on milk samples of 3166 dairy cows from Finland revealed that Corynebacterium bovis was major mastitis pathogen followed by *Staphylococcus aureus* (21.0%), CNS (15.8%), other *Streptococci* and *Enterococci* (5.8%), *Streptococcus agalactiae* (3.1%), *Streptococcus uberis* (2.4%), *Streptococcus dysgalactiae* (1.9%), Coliforms (0.6%), *Actinomyces* spp. (0.2%) and other bacteria (1.9%) (Haltia *et al.*, 2006).

U.K.

The pathogen prevalence profile of clinical mastitis in the U.K. in late 1960's showed *Staphylococcus aureus* was responsible for 38%, *Streptococcus dysgalactiae* 20%, *Streptococcus uberis* 18%, coliforms (5%), *Streptococcus agalactiae* (3%) and other organisms 6% of intramammary infections while 15% of infections were not associated with a pathogen and were classified as "no growths" (Booth, 1997). The bacteriological results of the investigation of clinical mastitis prevalence in the early 1980's by Wilesmith *et al.* (1986) identified *Escherichia coli* in 18%, *Streptococcus uberis* in 17%, *Staphylococcus aureus* in 15%, *Streptococcus dysgalactiae* in 9%, *Streptococcus agalactiae* in 2%, other pathogens in 7%, minor pathogens in 4%, mixed pathogens in 5%, no growths in 15% and contamination in 8% of samples. In U.K. the distribution of the 1457 clinical cases according to the result of the culture was *Escherichia coli* 32%, *S. uberis* 23% *staph* 7%, *Corynpyogens* 1% mixed 10% and others 24% (Fauli *et al.*, 1983).

The main organisms associated with clinical mastitis in England and Wales are *Escherichia coli* and *Streptococcus uberis* (Milne *et al.*, 2002; Peeler *et al.* 2003; Bradley *et al.*, 2007). A steady increase in relative importance of *Streptococcus uberis* can be seen over the decades, with 15, 17, 21 and 24.5% of clinical mastitis cases attributed to this species in 1969, 1980, 1993 and 2005, respectively (Neave *et al.*, 1969; Bramley, 1984; Hillerton *et al.*, 1993; Bradley *et al.*, 2007). When accounting for the incidence of clinical mastitis per 100 cows per year, however, the absolute incidence of *Streptococcus uberis* mastitis decreased from 21 cases per 100 cows in 1969 (Neave *et al.*, 1969), to only seven or eight cases per 100 cows in 1980 (Bramley, 1984) and 1993 (Hillerton *et al.*, 1993).

A survey was conductd by Milne *et al.* (2002) from October, 1999 to February, 2001 to confirm the importance of environmental pathogens in dairy herds in mid-Devon, Great Britain. The bacteriological results of the study showed that the most prevalent isolates in descending order were *Staphylococcus uberis* (37%), Enterobacteriaceae (23%), coagulase negative Staph. spp. (10%), other bacterial species (9%), *Streptococcus dysgalactiae* (4%) and *Staphylococcus aureus* (3%). No growth was seen in 14% of the submitted samples.

Orpin (2000) isolated *Streptococcus uberis* (67%), *E. coil* (16%), CNS (12%), *Bacillus* spp. (3%) and *Streptococcus agalactiae* from 6% quarters from clinical cases and, *Staphylococcus aureus* (0.4%), CNS (43.6%), *Streptococcus uberis* (20.8%), *Streptococcus dysgalactiae* (8.8%), *Corynebacterium bovis* (15.5%), *Coliforms* (1.3%), *Streptococcus faecalis* (14.8%) and *Bacillus* spp. in 25.2% quarters of sub-clinical mastitic cattle from Leicester. Green *et al.* (2005) carried out a study during dry period and isolated *Corynebacterium* spp. 35·12%, CNS 6·25%, *Escherichia coli* 1·94%, Coagulase-positive staphylococci 1·52 %, *Streptococcus uberis* 1·09%, *Streptococcus dysgalactiae* subspecies *dysgalactiae*

0·57%, *Enterobacter* spp. 0·31%, *Citrobacter* spp. 0·10%, *Serratia* spp. 0·10% and *Arcanobacterium pyogenes* 0·05%.

Peeler *et al.* (2003) have also been reported *Coliform* spp. (30.33%), *Staphylococcus uberis* (20.33%), *Coliform* and *Staphylococcus uberis* mixed (1.67%), *Staphylococcus aureus* (2.67%), *Streptococcus dysgalactiae* (2.67%), CNS and *Corynebacterium bovis* (8.67%), yeasts (5.33%), other pathogens (16.33%) and no growth on 12% samples from Somerset, U.K. In recent years, reported *Streptococcus uberis* incidence has increased again, with 16 cases/100 cows/ year reported for 2005 (Bradley *et al.*, 2007). The second most common group of pathogens causing clinical mastitis in England and Wales consists of *Escherichia coli* and other Enterobacteriaceae (Milne *et al.*, 2002; Bradley *et al.*, 2007) (Cited in Zadoks and Fitzpatrick, 2009).

Newton *et al.* (2008) surveyed 10 dairy herds in South West of England and isolated the organism during the period of drying-off and found *Corynebacterium* spp. as chief mastitis pathogen (36.7%) followed by CNS (17.1%), *Streptococcus uberis* 36 (6.36%), *Bacillus* species (6.18%), Coagulase positive Staphylococci, (5.3%), *Escherichia coli* (1.77%), Other coliforms (1.59%), *Streptococcus dysgalactiae* (0.71%), *Pseudomonas* spp. (0.35%), Yeast species (0.35%) and others (7.07%).

The Netherlands

The prevalence of intramammary infection and distribution of mastitis pathogens were determined in The Netherlands in 1973, 1975, 1980 and in 1985 (Vecht *et al.*, 1989). In the 70's, *Streptococcus agalactiae* was the predominant mastitis pathogen (6.9% infected quarters), while in the 80's *Staph aureus* became the most frequently isolated pathogen (3.7% infected qurters). *Staphylococcus aureus* is the main pathogen associated with clinical mastitis in The Netherlands, followed by *Escherichia coli* and *Streptococcus dysgalactiae* (Barkema *et al.*, 1998).

Bacteriological examination of milk samples from clinical mastitis cases from randomly selected dairy herds in the Southern Netherlands showed that the most frequent isolates from clinical cases were *Escherichia coli* (16.9%), *Staphylococcus aureus* (14.4%), *Streptococcus uberis* (11.9%) and *Streptococcus dysgalactiae* (8.9%) (Miltenburg *et al.*, 1996). Sampimon *et al.* (2008) carried out a mastitis causing bacteriological study on 11,225 quarter milk samples of 2,873 cows, bacteriological growth occurred in 37% of these milk samples. Coagulase negative Staphylococci and *Staphylococcus aureus* were the most prevalent pathogens and were isolated in 11.9% and 8.6% milk samples respectively and followed by *Streptococcus uberis* (5.7%), *Streptococcus dysgalactiae* (5.0%), *Corynebacterium* spp. (3.6%), Other Streptococci (2.5%),

Coliform (1.1%), Yeast (0.4%), *Streptococcus agalactiae* (0.4%), *Arcanobacterium pyogenes* (0.2%) and 0.2% samples were contaminated.

Ireland

Toxic mastitis is caused by *E .coli, Klebsiella* spp., *Enterobacter* spp. and *Serratia* spp. various studies have been conducted on the toxic mastitis. A large scale study was carried out by Menzies *et al.* (2000) on 265 clinical cases of toxic mastitis from October, 1995 to May, 1997 in Northern Ireland. The milk samples were collected from from 6 countries (Antrim, Armagh, Down, Fermanagh, Londonderry and Tyrone) and organisms were isolated *Escherichia coli* (50.4%), *Citrobacter* spp. (0.8%), *Salmonella dublin* (0.4%), *Morganella morganii* (0.4%), *Proteus* spp. (0.4%), *Aeromonas* spp. (0.4%), *Pseudomonas* spp. (1.1%), *Mannheimia haemolytica* (0.8%), *Staphylococcus aureus* (2.7%), *Streptococcus dysgalactiae* (2.7%), *Actinomyces* spp. (2.7%), *Streptococcus uberis* (1.9%), *Enterococcus* spp. (0.8%), *Staphylococcus xylosus* (0.8%), *Candida* spp. (0.8%), *Aspergillus* sp. (0.4%), and mixed isolates *Escherichia coli* and *Streptococcus uberis* (3.8%), *E. coi* and *Enterococcus* spp. (2.7%), *Escherichia coli* and *Streptococcus dysgalactiae* (2.3%), miscellaneous isolates (6.9%) and no bacteria isolated in 11.5% samples. Six to five percent saples were contaminated. Byrne *et al.* (2001) has been isolated *Mycoplasma bovis* from 13.33% milk samples of cows from the Republic of Ireland.

Switzerland

Bluel *et al.* (2006) studied on 56 cows having toxic mastitis and isolated the *Escherichia coli* (46.42%), *Staphylococcus aureus* (19.64%), other *Streptococci* (14.28%), *Bacillus* species (7.14%), other *Staphylococci* (5.35%), *Klebsiella* spp. (1.78%), *Aspergillus fumigatus* (1.78%), *Yersinia pseudotuberculosis* (1.78%) and Yeast (1.78%) in all bacterial isolates.

Denmark

A total of 166 samples of secretions collected from Danish heifers suffering from clinically diagnosed summer mastitis were examined bacteriologically. One hundred and sixty three samples yielded positive findings whereas no growth was obtained from 3 specimens. The majority of samples revealed a mixed flora in which the predominant components were *Actinomyces pyogenes, Peptostreptococcus indolicus*, a *microaerophilic coccus* (Stuart-Schwan coccus), *Fusobacterium necrophorum, Bacteriodes melaninogenicus* and *Streptococcus dysgalactiae*. Pure cultures were recovered in only 7% of cases. *P. indolicus* was isolated from 875 of the cases, a *microaerophilic coccus* from 84%, *A. pyogenes* from 72%, *Fusobacterium necrophorum* from 52%, *Streptococcus dysgalactiae* from 37%, *B. melaninogenicus* from 33% and various unidentified obligate anaerobic Gram-negative rods from 31% (Madsen *et al.*, 1990). A one-year study of Aalbaek *et al.* (1994) on 2,896 mammary secretions from Danish (Denmark) cattle with clinical or sub-clinical mastitis revealed 45 strains of fungi and algae. The species of fungi were identified, *Candida krusei* (37.78%), *C. kefyr* (13.33%), *C. rugosa* (13.33%), *Geotrichum capitatum* (11.11%), *C. tropicalis* (6.67%), *C. catenulata* (4.44%) and *C. valida* (2.22%) and. The algal species *Prototheca zopfii* was demonstrated in 11.11%.

Belgium

Different species of Yeast have been isolated from bovine mastitis cases by Lagneau *et al.* (1996) from Belgium. A total of 436 milk samples from non-infected and 80 from infected quarters were investigated. Out of these 24.5% of the samples collected from non-infected and 55% of those collected from infected quarters were positive. Normal milk yielded not less than 16 different species and among them many potentially pathogenic yeast species such as *Candida parapsilosis, C. guilliermondii, C. tropicalis, C. glabrata* and *T. asahii*, all five able to grow at 40°C. In contrast, the yeasts isolated from infected quarters were from 3 species, *C. kefyr, C. catenulata* and *C. lambica*, which were also among the yeasts species recovered from normal milk. Among the three species, only one i.e. *C. kefyr* is able to grow above 40°C and from there can be considered as potentially pathogenic, even if bacterial association is necessary to cause mastitis.

Lithuania

In recent years *Streptococcus uberis* and other environmental pathogens, such as *Escherichia coli*, have been reported to be more prevalent in U.K., than the contagious pathogens, for example *Staphylococcus aureus* and *Streptococcus agalactiae*, as causes of clinical mastitis in dairy cows (Milne *et al.*, 2005). According to the data of National Veterinary Laboratory, Lithuania, the main agents of bacterial mastitis were *Staphylococcus aureus*, 59.74%, *Streptococcus agalactiae*, 15.1%, *Pseudomonas aeruginosa*, 0.62% and *Corynebacterium spp.*, 0.97% (Januskauskas and Riskeviciene, 2007).

Edward Island

Richard *et al.* (2006) were found *Staphylococcus aureus* as a major (74%) etiological agent for bovine mastitis and followed by *Streptococcus agalactiae* (1.6%), and *Mycoplasma* spp. (*M. bovis* and *M. alkalescens*) 1.9% from Edward, Island.

Oceania

New Zealand

Compton *et al.* (2007) conducted a study on 708 heifers of Waikato region of New Zealand and collected milk samples 3 weeks before and within 5 days after calving and trend of microorganisms distribution was studied. CNS were the predominant (13.5%) and other organisms were *Corynebacterium spp., Escherichia coli, Staphylococcus aureus, Streptococcus dysgalcatiae, Streptococcus agalactiae, Streptococcus uberis, Klebsiella spp., Pasteurella spp., Proteus spp.* and *Enterococcus spp. Streptococcus uberis* prevalence increased 4-fold on the day of calving compared with precalving period. Prevalence of all pathogens decreased rapidly following calving. Clinical mastitis cases were predominantly associated with *Streptococcus uberis* (64%). Parker *et al.* (2008) isolated *Streptococcus uberis* (68.22%), *Staphylococcus aureus* (5.04%), CNS (19.77%) and 3.6 (6.98%) other major pathogens (*Streptococcus dysgalactiae, Streptococcus agalactiae, Klebsiella* spp., *Pasturella* spp., *Enterococcus* spp., and *Escherichia coli*) of all isolated oraganisms from clinical cases of mastitis in cows. A recent study in Waikato, Taranaki, Canterbury and Sounthland regions of New Zealand, reported Srep. uberis was chief cause in clinical mastitis followed by Staph. aureus, *Strep. dysgalactiae, Escherichia coli*, CNS and other organisms (McDougall *et al.*, 2009).

Africa

Nigeria

Ameh *et al.* (1999) examined 154 milk samples from apparently normal cow udder and reported that bacteria were detected in 81 (53%) samples, while 73 (47%) samples had no bacterial growth. *Staphylococcus aureus* (34.6%) occurred more frequently in mastitis milk, (P<0.001) than in non-mastitis milk. This was followed by coagulase-negative *Staphylococci* (15.4%). Other bacteria isolated from mastitis milk were *Streptococcus spp.* (9.6%), *Escherichia coli* (6.7%), *Actinomyces pyogenes* (5.8%), *Bacillus spp.* (2.9%) and *Salmonella spp.* (1.9%).

Egypt

A total of 165 mastitic quarter milk samples collected from cows of Egypt. Of these 162 (98.1%) samples were bacteriologically positive. *Staphylococcus aureus* was isolated from 31.5% of the samples, *Streptococcus agalactiae* (16.4%), *Streptococcus dysgalactiae* (15.2%), *Escherichia coli* (12.7%), *Pseudomonas aeruginosa* (3.0%) and *Actinomyces pyogenes* (1.8%) were also isolated (Seleim *et al.*, 2002). El-Khodery and Osman (2008) carried out a study on 56 buffaloes suffering from acute clinical mastitis and isolated *Klebsiella pneumoniae* (28.57%), *Escherichia coli* (19.64%), mixed *Klebsiella pneumoniae* and *Escherichia coli* (32.14%), *Staphylococcus aureus* (12.50%), *Streptococcus uberis* (5.36%) and *Streptococcus agalactiae* from 1.78% cases. Ahmed *et al.* (2008) also found that *Escherichia coli* as chief etiological agent (75.76%) of sub-clinical mastitis in buffaloes followed by *Staphylococcus epidermidis* (59.10%), *C. bovis* (45.45%),

Klebsiella spp. (34.85%), *Staphylococcus aureus* (16.67%), *Streptococcus uberis* (13.64%), *Streptococcus dysgalactiae* (6.06%), *E. faecalis* (7.58%), *E. aerogenes* (6.06%) and *Streptococcus agalactiae* (3.03%).

Sudan

It would be of interest to note that in Sudan (Bagadi, 1970), the organisms isolated in clinical and sub-clinical mastitis in Zebu cattle were *Staph.* spp. 50 and 68.7%, *Streptococcus* spp. 15.3 and 12.6%, *Corynebacterium* spp. 11 and 00%, *Coliforms* 11 and 4.8% and mixed 10.2 and 13% respectively. Mohamed *et al.* (1993) reported *Staphylococcus aureus* (23.56%), *Staphylococcus epidermidis* (9.77%), *Escherichia coli* (6.32%), *Acinobacter anitratus* (7.47%), *Bacillus cereus* (6.86%), *Bacillus subtilis* (4.59%) and *Yeasts* (3.45%) during July 1990 to June 1992 from Sudan. Ibtisam *et al.* (2006) also reported that *Staphylococcus aureus* was major (23.56%) pathogen followed by *Staphylococcus epidermidis* (14.37%), *Actinomyces pyogenes* (9.77%), *Escherichia coli* (6.32%), *Acinetobacter antratus* (7.47%), *Bacillus cereus* (6.86%) and *Bacillus subtilis* (4.59%) in Sudan dairy farm. Madut *et al.* (2009), a total of 205 bacterial isolate were recovered from 2283 quarter milk samples examined. The isolated bacteria were *Staphylococcus spp.* 107 (52.5%), *Streptococcus* spp. 25 (12.3%), *Enterobacterium* spp. 4 (2%), *Lactobacillus* spp. 4 (2%), *Coryneform* bacteria 27 (13.2%), *Micrococcus* spp. 10 (4.9%), *Pseudomonas* spp., 11 (5.9%), *Bacillus* spp., 10 (4.9%) and *Aercoccus* spp., (Table 4). In this study isolated *Corynebacterium* were *Corynebacterium striatum* 9 (33.3%), *Arcanobacterium pyogene* 4 (14.8%), *Corynebacterium pseudotuberculosis* 2 (7.4%), *Corynebacterium ulcerans* 5 (18.5%), *Corynebacterium bovis* 7 (25.9%).

Ethiopia

Bovine mastitis bacteria were isolated from 243 lactating cows during Nov. 2002 to May 2003 from central Ethipia. The dominant bacterial isolates were *Staphylococcus* spp. (33.33%), *Micrococcus* spp. (26.67%), *Bacillus* spp. (15.00), *Streptococcus* spp. (8.33) and *Enterobacteriaceae* (6.67%) (Seyoum *et al.*, 2003). Sori *et al.* (2005) has been isolated the bacteria from bovine clinical and sub-clinical mastitis includes *Staphylococcus aureus* (44.03%), *Staphylococcus epidermidis* (14.93%), *Micrococcus* spp. (6.72%), *Streptococcus agalactiae* (3.73%), *Streptococcus dysagalactiae* (4.48%), *Streptococcus uberis* (2.99%), Other *Streptococcus* spp. (2.99%), *Actinomyces pyogenes* (5.97%), *Corynebacterium bovis* (5.97%), *Corynebacterium ulcerans* (2.24%), *Bacillus* spp. (4.48%), *Escherichia coli* (0.75%) and *Pseudomonas aeruginosa* (0.75%). Getahun *et al.* (2008) isolated most common isolates from the clinical mastitic quarters were *Streptococcus agalactiae* (30%), *S. dysgalactiae* (30%), *Staphylococcus aureus* (20%), *Staphylococcus epidermidis* (10%) and *Staphylococcus intermidius* (10%), while from sub-clinical cases were *Staphylococcus aureus* (42.6%), *Staphylococcus epidermidis* (22.1%), *Staphylococcus intermidius* (1.5%), *Strpt. agalactiae* (12.8%) and *Streptococcus uberis* (10.3%), *Streptococcus dysgalctiae* (1.5%), *Bacillus cerus* (2.1%), *Micrococcus* spp. (2.1%), *Actinomyces pyogenes* (2.1%), *Escherichia coli* (0.5%), *Corynebacterium bovis* (2.1%) and Mixed growths (0.5%) from Selalle area, Ethiopia. A study was carried out by Argaw and Tolosa (2008) in North Shoa Zone of the Oromia Regional state in central Ethiopia from March – April 2000. All positive quarters milk samples were cultured and 90 % yielded growth and in the remaining 10 %, there was no observation of growth. The microorganisms isolated in this study *Staphylococcus epidermedius* were 38.41%, *Staphylococcus intermedius* 23.19%, *Staphylococcus aureus* 9.42%, *Micrococcus* 5.80%, *Staphylococcus hyicus* sub spp *hyicus* 5.07%, *Staphylococcus saprophyticus* 2.17%, *Staphylococcus bovis* 2.17%, *Staphylococcus pygoneous* 1.45%, *Proteus mirables* 1.45%, *Provedercia alclificanis* 1.45%, *Corynebacterium bovis* 1.45%, *Corynebacterium hemolyticum* 1.45%, *Streptococcus pyogenes* 1.45%, *Aeromones hydrophileus* 0.72%, *Pasteurella multocida* 0.72%, *Alcaligens* spp. 0.72%, *Pasterella hemolyticum* 0.72%, *Candida krusei* 0.72%, *Corynebacterium pyogenes* 0.72% and *Pseudomonas aeroginosa* 0.72%. A short study was conducted by Lakew *et al.* (2009) and found *Staphylococcus* spp. (41.4 %), *Streptococcus* spp. (24.8 %), and other Gram positive rods and Gram negative enteric bacteria (33.8 %) from cattle.

Kenya

Shitandi *et al.* (2004) isolated mastitis causing bacteria from clinical mastitis milk samples of dairy cows from Rift Valley of Kenya and isolated *Staphylococcus aureus* (30.3%), CNS (17.8%), *Streptococcus* spp. (20.4%), *Escherichia coli* (10.5%), *Actinomyces* spp. (5.2%) and *Salmonella* spp. (0.5%). Bacteriological study of bovine mastitis in Kenya, showed *Staphylococcus aureus* (59.89%), CNS (17.03%), *Streptococcus* spp. (15.38%) and *Escherichia coli* (7.69%) of culturally positive samples (Shitandi and Kihumbu, 2004).

Uganda

Bacteriological analysis of mastitic milk in 304 milking cows in Uganda revealed, *Streptococcus* spp. (35.60%), *Staphylococcus aureus* (25.50%) and *Klebsiella* spp. (15.40%). *Escherichia coli, Corynebacterium pyogenes, Pseudomonas aeruginosa, Proteus* spp. and *Candida albicans* were the other isolated species (Tweyongyere and Kasirye, 1998).

Tanzania

A study was carried out to establish the prevalence and determinants of mastitis in smallholder dairy farms in Kibaha and Morogoro districts (Tanzania). Of the 919-quarter milk samples cultured, 8.2% were positive for aerobic bacteria with predominant isolates being *Staphylococcus epidermidis*

(2.8%), *Staphylococcus aureus* (1.7%), *Streptococcus agalactiae* (1.2%) and *Staphylococcus intermedius* (1.1%) and fungal growth was observed in 21.8% (n = 881) of the samples and the isolates were yeast (19.2%), Mucor (2.5%) and Aspergillus (0.1%) (Mdegela *et al.*, 2004). Bacteriological investigation was conducted on 96 randomly selected traditional herds in Dodoma rural and Mvomero districts of Tanzania showed that major isolates were *Staphylococcus aureus* (35.3%), other *Staphylococci* (20.8%), *Coliforms* (27.7%), *Microcci* (5.8%) and *Streptococci* (9.8%) (Karimuribo *et al.*, 2005).

A 31-year record-based retrospective study was carried out to determine the aetiology bovine clinical mastitis in smallholder dairy herds in the Dar es Salaam region of Tanzania, for the period November 1971-December 2002. The most prevalent bovine-mastitis pathogens were *Staphylococcus aureus* (25.7%); *Streptococcus agalactiae* (15.4%); *Klebsiella pneumoniae*(14.3%); *Escherichia coli* (14.1%). Other isolates included *Pseudomonas aeruginosa* (7.5%), *Streptococcus dysgalactiae* (5.2%), and *Streptococcus uberis* (4.2%). Mixed cultures were isolated from 9 (0.52%) of the culture positive. Contagious pathogens were isolated from 45.6% of the culture-positive samples, whereas environmental and miscellaneous pathogens were isolated from 48.2% and 5.7% of the culturepositive samples, respectively. Thirty per cent of the miscellaneous pathogens were *Candida* species and included *Candida albicans* (33%), *C. guillermondi* (29%), *C. tropicalis* (19%) and *C. pelliculosis* (19%). On the other hand, *Trichophyton verrucosum*, constituted 7% of the miscellaneous positive samples (Kivaria, 2006). Karimuribo *et al.* (2006) have also been reported *Stap. aureus* (23.4%), *Staphylococcus epidermidis* (23.0%), other *Staphylococcus* spp. (17.3%), *Micrococcus* spp. (12.7%) and *Streptococcus* spp. other than *Streptococcus agalactiae* (10.0%). Other isolates were coliforms (5.4% which included *Escherichia coli, Klebsiella* spp. and *Proteus* spp.), *Arcanobacter pyogenes* (3.5%), and *Streptococcus agalactiae* (3.3%). A cross sectional study was carried out in the Iringa and Tanga regions of Tanzania between January to March, 1999 and found bacteriological growth only on 27.9% samples, isolates were isolated *Stap. aureus* (5.9%), *Staphylococcus epidermidis* (5.7%), other *Staphylococci* (unidentified) (4.3%), *Streptococcus agalactiae* (0.8%), Other *Streptococci* (2.5%), *Escherichia coli* (0.7%), *Klebsiella* spp. (0.5%), *Proteus* spp. (0.3%), *Arcanobacterium pyogenes* (0.9%), Diplococci (0.8%) and 3.3% growth were contaminated (Karimuribo *et al.*, 2008).

Because distribution of pathogens changes over time, herd-level samples for bacteriological culturing must be taken regularly to monitor udder health. Additionally, national mastitis prevalence studies give important information through monitoring the national udder health status.

References

Aalbaek, B., Jensen, H.E. and Huda, A. (1998). Acta Pathol. Microbiol. Immunol. Scand., 106:483–488.

Aalbaek, B., Stenderup, J., Jensen, H.E., Valbak, J., Nylin, B. and Huda, A. (1994). APMIS., 102(6): 451-456.

Ahire, S.J., Nale, R.A., Dighe, D.G., Keskar, D.V. and Samad, A. (2008). Indian J. Vet. Medicine. 28(1): 61-62.

Ahmad, R. (2001). Pakistan Vet. J., 21(4): 220-221.

Ahmed, W.M., Sherein, I., Abd Ei-Moez and Nabil, M. (2008). Global Veterinaria, 2(1): 41-45.

Akhtar, M.H., Roy, G.P., Singh, A.P., Sinha, B.K., Kumar, A. and Kumar, R. (2003). In: Proceeding of 4th Round table conference on mastitis, Palampur, H.P. (India), 14-15 April, pp. 178-184.

Alexander, P.G, K.J. Slee, S. McOrist, L. Ireland, and P.J. Coloe. (1985). Aust. Vet. J., 62:135.

Ali, L, Mohammad, G., Arshad, M., Saqib, M. and Hassan, I.J. (2008). Pakistan. Pak. Vet. J., 28(1): 31-33.

Almeraya, A. P. (1994). Vet. Mexico, 25:65–67.

Ameh, J.A., Edgbe, N. and Zaria, L.T. (1999). Veterinarki Archiv., 69(2): 87-95.

Andersen, H.J., Pedersen, L.H., Aarestrup, F.M. and Chriel, M. (2003). J. Dairy Sci., 86(4): 1233-1239.

Anderson, K.L. and Walker, R.L. (1988). J. Am. Vet. Med. Assoc., 193:553–556.

Argaw, K. and Tolosa, T. (2008). The Internet Journal of Veterinary Medicine., Volume 5 Number 1. http://www.ispub.com/ostia/index.php?xmlFilePath=journals/ijvm/front.xml

Aroch, I., Harmelin, A., Saran, A., Levin, D. and Shpigel, N.Y. (2003). Vet. Rec, 153(12): 746-750.

Atyabi, N., Vojgani, M. and Gharagozloo, F. (2002). In: Book of abstracts of 27th World Veterinary. (Abstract No. 218), Tunis, Tunisia, 25-29 Sept., p. 107.

Awad, F.I., El Molla, A., Fayed, A., Abd el-Halim, M. and Refai, M. (1980). J. Egypt. Vet. Med. Ass., 40(3): 35–41.

Bagadi, H.O. (1970). Trop. Anim. Health Prod., 2: 28-34

Balakrishnan, G., Govindarajan, R., Roy, P., Gopu, P., Jayakumar, V. and Murali Manohar, B. (2009). Tamilnadu J. Vet. & Anim. Sci., 5 (2): 75-76.

Balakrishnan, G., Unny, M., Dorairajan, N. and Subramanian, M. (2004). Indian Vet. J., 81(10): 1166-1167.

Bansal, B.K., Singh, K.B., Rohan, R., Joshi, D.B. and Nauriyal, D.C. (1995). J. Res., PAU., 32(1): 79-81.

Baranski, W., Ras, M., Janowski, T., Zdunczyk, S., Dewulf, J., Kruif, A.D., Vliegher, S.D. and Opsomer, G. (2008). Medycyna Wet., 64(3): 301-305.

Barbuddhe, S.B., Chakurkar, E.B. and Sundaram, R.N.S. (2001). Indian J. Compa. Micro. Immunol. Inf. Diseases., 2292): 164-165.

Barkema, H.W., Green, M.J., Bradley , A.J. and Zadoks, R.N. (2009). J. Dairy Sci., 92(10): 4717–4729.

Barkema, H.W., Schukken, Y.H., Lam, T.J., Beiboer, M.L., Wilmink, H., Benedictus, G. and Brand, A. (1998). J Dairy Sci., 81(2): 411-419.

Bartlett, P.C., Miller, G.Y., Lance, S.E. and Heider, L.E. (1992). Prev. Vet. Med., 12: 59-71.

Beck, C.C. (1957). Mich. State Vet., 17: 82-88.

Bedolla, L.C., Mejia, R., Renteria, I., Bedolla, E., Garcia, E., Castaneda, H., Castaneda, M.A., Serratos, J.C. and Wolter, W. (2008). In: Lam, T.J.G.M. (2008). Mastitis control from science to practice. 1st edn., Wageningen Academic Publisher, The Netherlands. p. 86.

Berry, E. (1998). In: Proc. of the British Mastitis Conf., pp. 46-53.

Berry, E.A. and Hillerton, J.E. (2002). J. Dairy Sci., 85: 112-121.

Beytut, E., Aydn, F., Ozcan, K and Genc, O. (2002). Kafkas Universitesi Veteriner Fakultesi Dergisi., 8(2): 111-112.

Bhalerao, D.P., Jagdish, S., Keskar, D.V., Dangore, A.D. and Sharma, L.K. (2000). Indian Vet. J., 77(3): 244-246.

Bhattcharyya, D. and Rahman, H. (1995). Indian Vet. J., 72(4): 414-415.

Bilge, S. (1998). Vet. Fakultesi Dergisi, Ankara Turkey. 45: 313-321.

Black, R.T., Bourland, C.T. and Marshall, R.T. (1972). J. Dairy Sci., 55: 1016-1017.

Bleul, U., Bohler, K., Stephan,K., Pospischil, A. and Braun, U. (2002). Vet. Rec, 151(21/28): 767-769

Bluel, U., Sacher, K., Corti, S. and Braun, U. (2006). Vet. Rec, 159(11): 677-680.

Boddie, R.L., Nickerson, S.C., Owens, W.E. and Watts, J.L. (1987). Agri-Practice 8, 22-25.

Booth, J.M. (1997) In: Proceedings of the British Mastitis Conference, Stoneleigh, pp. 3-9.

Bouchard, E., Roy, J.P. and Tremlay, D.D. (2006). In: Comp. XXIV World buiatrics cong., Nice, France.

Bourry, A. and Poutrel, B. (1996). J. Dairy Sci., 79(12): 2189-95.

Bourry, A., Cochard, T. and Poutrel, B. (1997). J. Clin. Micro., 35(6): 1606-1608.

Bradley, A.J., Leach, K.A., Breen, J.E., Green, L.E. and Green, M.J. (2007). Vet. Rec., 160(8): 253-257.

Bramley, A.J. (1984). Br. Vet. J., 140(4): 328-335.

Bramley, A.J., Patel, A.H., O'Relly, M., Foster, R. and Foster, T.J. (1989). Infection and Immunity., 57: 481-512.

Bramman, S.K., Eberhart, R.J., Ashbury, M.A. and Herman, S.J. (1973). J. Am. Vet. Med. Ass., 162: 109.

Braverman, Y., Chizov-ginzburg, A., Saran, A. and Winkler, M. (1999). Scientific and Technical Review, 18: 681-690.

Brooks, B.W., Barnum, D.A. and Meek, A.H. (1983). Can. J. Comp. Med., 47: 73-78.

Burrows, R., Mann, J.A.,Greig, A.,Chapman, W.G. and Goodridge, D. (1971). J. Hyg. Camb., 69: 307-321.

Bushnell, R.B. (1974). In: Proc. of the National Mastitis Counc., pp. 62-69.

Buzzini, P., Turchetti, B., Facelli, R., Baudino, R., Cavarero, F., Mattalia, L., Mosso, P. and Martini, A. (2004). Mycopathologia, 158:427–430.

Byrne, W.J., Mccormack, R., Brice, N., Egan, J., Markey, B. and Ball, H. J. (2001). Veteriniary Record., 148(3): 331-333.

Carter, G.R. (1995). Diagnostic procedures in Veterinary Bacteriology and Mycology. 6th ed., (Carter, G.R. and Cole Jr., J.R. Eds) Academic Press inc., California. Pp. 457-467.

Carter, J. M., Hutcheson, A. M., and Quinlan, R. A. (1995). Exp Eye Res, 60(2): 181-92.

Castaneda, H., Wolter, W., Jager, S.P., Szchock, M., Castaneda, M.A., Prez, G. and Bedolla, C. (2008). In: Lam, T.J.G.M. (2008). Mastitis control from science to practice. 1st edn., Wageningen Academic Publisher, The Netherlands. p. 85.

Chaffer, M., Freidman, S., Saran, A. and Younis, A. (2005). J. Am. Vet. Med. Assoc., 15(6): 1994-1996.

Chahar, A., Gahlot, A.K., Tanwar, R.K. and Fakhruddin (2008). Indian J. Vet. Med., 28(2): 91-93.

Chahota, R., Katoch, R., Mahajan, A. and Verma, S. (2001). Veterinarski Arhiv. 71 (4) : 197-201.

Chand, A., Roy, C.R., Banerjee, P.K. and Guha, C. (1989). Indian vet. J., 66: 277-282.

Chavan, V.V., Digrakar, S.U., Dhonde, S.N. and Hase, P.B. (2007). In: Proc. of XXV Ann. Conv. Of ISVM, Pantnagar, Uttarakhand, India. P.28.

Cheng, D.R., Zhu, S.Y., Yin, Y., Ding, W.W., Mu, Z.X., Su, Z.R. and Sun, H.C. (2010). African J. Microbiol. Res., 4 (11): 1110-1116.

Choudhuri, P.C. (2000). In: Proceeding of 1st round table conference on Mastitis, Izatnagar, Bareilly, U.P. (India). Pp. 84-92.

Cifrian, E.A., Guiddry, A.J., O'Brein, C.N. and Marquardt, W.W. (1995). Res. Vet. Sci., 58: 20-25.

Clarke, R.T.J. (1960). Nz. Vet. J., 8: 79.

Compton, C. W. R., Heuer, C., Parker, K. and McDougall, S. (2007). J. Dairy Sci., 90(9):4157–4170.

Corbellini, L.G., Driemeier, D., Ruz, C., As, M.M. and Ferreiro L. (2001). Trop. Anim. Hlth. Prod., 33(6): 463-470.

Corner, A.H., Greig, A.S. and Hill, D.P. (1967). Can. J. Comp. Med. Vet. Sci., 31: 320-330.

Costa E.O., Melville P.A., Ribeiro A.R., Watanabe E.T., Parolari M.C.F.F. (1997). Mycopathologia, 137: 33-36.

Costa, E.O., Gandra, C.R., Pires, M.F., Coutinho, S.D. and Teixeira, C.M. (1993). Mycopathologia, 124: 13–17.

Costa, E.O., Ribeiro, A.R., Watanabe, E.T., Pardo, R.B., Silva, J.B. and Sanches, R.B. (1996). Vet. Res. Comm., 20(3): 237-241.

Cremonesi, P., Castiglioni, B., Moroni, P. and Pisoni, G. (2008). In: Lam, T.J.G.M. (2008). Mastitis control from science to practice. 1st edn., Wageningen Academic Publisher, The Netherlands. p. 84.

Dairy Digest (2004). Mycoplasma: An emerging problem in dairy herds. October issue, published by Pennisylia University.

Das, P.K. and Joseph, E. (2005). Buffalo Bulletin 24 (1): 3-9.

De Vliegher, S., Zadoks, R.N. and Barkema, H.W. (2009). Vet. Microbiol., 134(1-2): 1-2.

De, U.K. and Mukherjee, R. (2009). Indian Vet. J., 86(8): 858-859.

Dhakal, I.P. (2006). J. Vet. Med. B, 53: 81–86.

Dhakal, I.P., Dhakal, P., Koshihara, T. and Nagahata, H. (2007). J. Vet. Med. Sci., 69(12): 1241–1245.

Dhote, S.W., Kurkure, N.V., Kalorey, D.R. and Ganvir, P.T. (1999). Indian Vet. J., 76: 251-252.

Dodd, F.H. and Neave, F.K. (1970). Mastitis Control. National Institute of Research (NIRD) into Dairy Biennial Review Paper, 3359: 21-60.

Duarte, R.S., Miranda, O.P., Bellei B.C., Brito, M.A.V.P. and Teixeira, L.M (2004). J. Clin. Microbiol., 42(9): 4214-4222.

Dutta, J.B. (2009). In: Compendium of 27th ISVM International summit and convention at Chennai, Tamilnadu, India.. p. 19.

Dutta, R., Barua, A.J., Late Dutta, G.N. and Deka, D. (2003). Indian J. Vet. Med., 23(1): 46-47.

Ebrahimi, A. and Nokookhan, F. (2005). Indian Vet. J., 82(1): 52-54.

Edinger, D., Tenhagen, B.A., Hauwieser, W., Kalbe, P., Klunder, G. and Baumgartner, B. (1999). Deutsche Tierarztliche Wochenschrift., 106(11): 470-474.

El-Khodery, S.A. and Osman, S.A. (2008). Trop Anim Health Prod., 40: 93–99.

Emanuelson, U., Olsson, T., Holmberg, O., Hageltorn, M., Mattila, T., Nelson, L. and Astrom, G. (1987). J. Dairy Sci., 70(4):880-887.

Espinasse, J., Gilbert, Y. and Saurat, P. (1974). Revue de Medecine Veterinaire., 125: 1441-1452.

Evans, A.C. (1918). J. Inf. Dis., 23: 373.

Fadlelmoula, A.A., Fahr, R.D., Anacker, G. and Swalve, H.H. (2007). Res. J. Anim. Vet. Sci., 2: 24-27.

Fadlelmula, A., Al Dughaym, A.M., Mohamed, G.E., Al Deib, M.K. and Al Zubaidy, A.J. (2009). Bulg. J. Vet. Med., 12(3): 199-206.

Fauli, W.B., Walton, J.R., Bramly, A.J. and Huges, J.W. (1983). Vet. Rec., 29: 415-420.

Ferguson, J. D., Azzaro, G., Gambina, M. and Licitra, G. (2007). J. Dairy Sci., 90(12): 5798–5813.

Filioussis, G., Christodoulopoulos, G., Thatcher, A., Petridou, V. and Bourtzi-Chatzopoulou, E. (2007). The Vet. J., 173: 215–218.

Firoozi, M.R., Amighi, M., Mastan, M.B. and Maleknezad, P. (1974). In: Proceedings X Congress Reg.OIEFAO sur less Epiz. En Asie en Extr. Orient. Et Oceanie, Tehran (Iran), 20-27 Oct.

Forsgren, A., Ghetie, V., Lindmark, R. and Sjoquist, J. (1983). Protein A and its exploitation. In: Easmon CSF, Adlam, C. (Eds) Staphylococci and Staphylococcal infections, Vol. 2: The organisms in vivo and in vitro. 429-480, Academic Press, London.

Fox, L.K., Chester, S.T., Hallberg, J.W., Nickerson, S.C., Pankey, J.W. and Weaver, L.D. (1995). J. Dairy Sci., 78(7): 1619-1628.

Fox, L.K., Kirk, J.H. and Britten, A. (2005). J. Vet. Med. B Infect. Dis. Vet. Public Health, 52:153–160.

Fox, L.K., Kirk, J.H. and Britten, A. (2005). J. Vet. Med. B Infect. Dis. Vet. Public. Health., 52(4): 153-60.

Francis, P.G. (1984). Teat skin lesions and mastitis. Br. Vet. J. 140: 430-436.

Fuchs, H.-W. (1994).Mastitiden:Virusinfectionen. In: Wendt,K., Bostedt, H., Mielke, H., and Fuchs, H.-W. (Editors), Euter- und Gesáugekrankheiten. Gustav Fisher Verlag Jena (Stuttgart), pp. 422-425.

Furuoka, H., Anri, A., Arita, Y., Tuzuki, N., Satoh, H. and Itakura, C. (1989). Jpn. J. Vet. Sci., 51:197–199.

Galli, G. (1954). Vet. Ital., 5: 587-604.

Garg, D.N. (2001). In: Proceeding of 2nd Round table conference on mastitis. pp. 1-9.

Getahun, K., Kelay, B., Bekana, M. and Lobago, F. (2008). Trop. Anim. Hlth. Prod., 40(4): 261-268.

Ghazaei, C (2006). J. Anim. Vet. Adv., 5 (4): 280-283.

Ghose, B. and Sharda, R. (2003). In: Proceeding of 4th Round table conference on mastitis, Palampur, H.P. (India), 14-15 April, pp. 171-174.

Ghose, B., Sharda, R., Chhabra, D. and Sharma, V. (2003). Indian Vet. J., 80(6): 499-501.

Gianneechini, R., Concha, C., Rivero, R., Delucci, I. and López J. M. (2002). Acta Vet. Scand., 43: 221-230.

Gonclaves, L.A., Freitas, T.D., Assis, R.S., Filho, E.J.F. and Lobato, F.C.F. (2006). Ciência Rural, 36(4): 3131-1333.

Gonzalez, R.N. (1996). In: Proc. 35th Annual Meeting of National Mastitis Council. Nashville, Tennessee, 82-89.

González, R.N. and Wilson, D.J. (2003). Vet. Clin. North. Am. Food. Anim. Pract., 19(1): 199-221.

Goswami, S.N., Roy, A. and Kalyani, I.H. (2003). In: Compendium of XXI ISVM Convention and National Symposium at Anand, Gujarat, India.. p. 236-237.

Gourlay, R.N., Stott, E.J., Espinasse, J. and Barle, C. (1974). Vet. Rec., 95: 534-535.

Green, M. and Bradley, A. (2004). UK Vet. (Cattle Practic), 9(4): 1-9.

Green, M.J., Green, L.E., Bradley, A.J., Burton, P.R., Schukken, Y.H. and Medley, G.F. (2005). Vet. Rec., 156(1): 71-77.

Greig, A.S. and Bannister, G.L. (1965). Can. J. Comp. Med. Vet. Sci., 29: 57-62.

Grohn, Y.T., Wilson, D.J., Gonzalez, R.N., Hertl, J.A., Shulte, H., Bennet, G. and Schukken, Y.H. (2004). J. Dairy Sci., 87: 3358-3374.

Guitian, F.J., Thurmond, M.C. and Hietala, F.K. (1999). J. Am. Vet. Medical Assoc., 215: 515-518.

Hale, H.H., Helmboldt, C.F., Plastridge, W.N. and Stula, E.F. (1962). Cornell Vet., 52: 582.

Haltia, L., Honkanen-Buzalski, T., Spiridonova, I., Olkonen, A. and Myllys, V. (2006). Acta Vet. Scand., 48:22-27.

Hatem, M.E., Attia, E.R., Ata, N.S. and Ibrahim, E.S. (2008). Am-Euras. J. Agric. & Environ. Sci., 3(2): 205-210.

Hawari, A.D. and Dabbas, F. (2008). J. Anim. Vet. Sci., 3 (1): 36-39.

Hay, G.M. (2002). Mycoplasma mastitis. Luisiana: Dairy Digest, Nov.-Dec., pp.3-5.

Hazlett, M.J., Litte, P.B. and Barnum, D.A. (1983). Canadian Vet. J., 24: 135-136.

Heidrich, H.J. and Renk, W. (1967). Diseases of the mammary glands of domestic animals. W.B. Saunders Co., Philadelphia.

Higgins, R., and Larouche, Y. (1989). Med. Vet. Quebec, 19:140–141

Hill, A.W., Heneghan D.J.S., Williams M.R. (1983). Vet. Microbiol., 8: 293–300.

Hillerton, J.E., Shearn, M.F., Teverson, R.M., Langridge, S. and Booth, J.M. (1993). J. Dairy Res., 60(1): 31-41.

Hoe, F.G. and Ruegg, P.L. (2005). J. Am. Vet. Med. Assoc., 227(9): 1461-1468.

Hoe, Fernanda G.H., and Ruegg, Pamela L. (2005). J.Am.Vet. Med. Assoc., 227(9 suppl.1): 1461-1468.

Hogan, J. and Smith, K.L. (2003). Vet. Res., 34: 507-519.

Hogan, J.S., Smith, K.L., Todhunter, D.A. and Schoenberger, P.S. (1988). J. Dairy Sci., 71: 2520-5.

Honkanen-Buzalski, T., Griffin, T.K. and Dodd, F.H. (1984). J. Dairy Res., 51: 371-378.

Houlihan, M.G., Veenstra, B., Christian, M.K., Nicholas, R.and Ayling, R. (2007). Vet. Rec., 160(1): 126-127.

Hu, S.H., Du, A. and Cai, W. (1998). Chinese J. Prev. Vet. Med., 1998-04.

Hussain, S.A., Willayat, M.M., Peer, F.U. and Rashid, R. (2006). Indian J. Vet. Med., 26(20): 104-105.

Huxley, J. N., Green, M. J., Green, L. E., and Bradley, A. J. (2002). J. Dairy Sci., 85(3): 551-561.

Ibtisam, E.M., El Zubeir and El Owni, O.A.O. (2006). Res. J. Anim. Vet. Sci., 1(1): 25-29.

International Dairy Federation (1987).Bovinemastitis.Definitions and guidelines for diagnosis. Brussels, Belgium. 211: 3-8.

Iqbal, M., Ali Khan, M., Daraz, B. and Siddique, U. (2004). Pakistan Vet. J., 24(4): 161-164.

Jackson, G. and Boughton, E. (1991). Vet. Rec., 129: 444.

Jain, N.C. (1979). J. Dairy Sci., 52: 128-134.

Jánosi, S., Rátz, F., Szigeti, G., Kulcsár, M., Kerényi, J., Lomkó, T., Katona, F.and Huszenicza, G. (2001). Vet. Quart., 23: 58-61.

Janus, A. (2009). Vet. World., 2(1): 38-39.

Januskauskas, A. and Riskeviciene, V. (2007). In: Proc. Mastitis Symp. St Petersburg State Academy of Veterinary Medicine, Russia, January 10-12, p.25.

Jasper, D.E. (1981). Bovine mycoplasmal mastitis. In: Cornelius, C.E., and B.F. Simpson, eds. Advances in veterinary sciences and comparative medicine. Academic Press, New York. p. 121.

Javed, Iqbal and Siddique, M. (1999). Pakistan Vet. J., 19(3): 149-154.

Jayarao, B.M., Gillespie, B.E., Lewis, M.J., Dowlen, H.H. and Oliver, S.P. (1999). J. Vet. Med. Series B, 46(7): 433-442.

Jemeljanovs, A., Bluzmanis, J. and Konosonoka I.H. (2002). In: Book of abstracts of 27th World Veterinary. (Abstract No. 437), Tunis, Tunisia, 25-29 Sept., p. 208.

Jemeljanovs, A., Konosonoka, I.H., Bluzmanis, J. and Ikauniece, D. (2008). In: Lam, T.J.G.M. (2008). Mastitis control from science to practice. 1st edn., Wageningen Academic Publisher, The Netherlands. p. 83.

Jha, N.K., Sinha, O.P. and Thakur, D.K. (2004). In: Proc. of 5th Round table conference on mastitis, IVRI, Izatnagar (India), 27-28 Feb., pp. 49-55.

Johnston, A.M. (1986). Vet. Rec., 116: 111.

Joshi, H.D. and Joshi, B. R. (1997). Vet. Rev., 12(1): 1-6.

Joshi, H.D., Joshi, B.R. and Shrestha, H.K. (1998). Vet. Rev., 13: 12-15.

Joshi, H.D., Joshi, B.R. and Shrestha, H.K. (1997). In: Proc. of the IInd National workshop on Livestock and Fisheries Research in Nepal. NARC / NASRI Lalitpur : 85-92.

Kader, M.A., Samad, M.A., Saha, S. and Taleb, M.A. (2002). Indian J. Dairy Sci., 55(4): 218-223.

Kalman, D., Janosi, S. and Egyed, L. (2004). Microb. Pathog., 37:125–129.

Kalorey, D.R., Warke, S.R., Kurkure, N.V., Rawool, D.B. and Barbuddhe, S.B. (2008). Food Control, 19(2): 109-112.

Kalyani, I.H., Roy, A., Purohit, J.H. and Jhala, M.K. (2003). In: Comp. XXI ISVM Convention and National Symposium at Anand, Gujarat, India. p. 238.

Kang-Hee, J., Kim-Ik, Chun, Kim-Jin, H, Son-Won, G, Lee-Du, S., Kang, H.J., Kim, I.C., Son, W.G. and Lee, D.S. (2001). Korean J. Vet. Res., 41(4): 511-521.

Kapur, M.P., Sharma, A. and Bhardwaj, R.M. (1992). Buffalo Bulletin, 11(2): 32-35.

Karimuribo, E.D., Fitzpatrick, J.L., Bell, C.E., Swai, E.S., Kambarage, D.M., Ogden, N.H., Bryant, M.J. and French, N.P. (2006). Preventive Veterinary Medicine, 74: 84–98.

Karimuribo, E.D., Fitzpatrick, J.L., Swai, E.S., Bell, C., Bryant, M.J., Ogden, N.H., Kambarage, D.M. and French, N.P. (2008). Vet. Record, 163: 16-21.

Karimuribo, E.D., Kusiluka, L.J., Mdegela, R.H., Kapaga, A.M., Sindato, C. and Kambarage, D.M. (2005). J. Vet. Sci., 6(3):213-221.

Katoch, R.C., Nagal, K.B., Sharma, M. and Sharma, M. (1997). Indian J. Anim. Sci., 67:292–193.

Katoch, R.C., Sharma, M., Verma, S., Chahota, R. and Dhar, P. (2003). In: Proc. 4th Round table conference on mastitis, Palampur, H.P. (India), 14-15 April, pp. 195-203..

Kawakami, Y., Kaji, T., Kume, T., Omuro, M., Hiramune, T., Murase, N. and Matumoto, M. (1966). Japan J. Microbiol., 10: 159-169.

Keller, B., Scheibl, P., Bleckmann, E. and Hoedemaker, M. (2000). Mycoses., 43(1):17-19.

Khan, A.Z. and Mohammad, G. (2005). Pakistan Vet. J., 25(1): 9-12.

Kheirabadi, P., Ebrahimi, A. and Barati, F. (2008). Indian Vet. J., 85(4): 375-377.

Kirk, J. H., Wright, J. C., Berry, S. L., Reynolds, J. P., Maas, J. P.and Ahmadi, A. (1996). Preventive Veterinary Medicine, 28: 187-198.

Kirk, J.H. and Bartlett, P.C. (1986). Comp. Food. Anim., 8: 106–110.

Kitt, T. (1896). Deutsch Zeit. Fur Tiermed. Vergl. Path., 12: 1-36.

Kivaria, F.M. (2006). Epidemiological studies on bovine mastitis in smallholder dairy herds in the Dar es Salaam region, Tanzania. Dissertation Utrecht University, Faculty of Veterinary Medicine.

Kleczkowski, M., Klucinski, W., Shaktur, A. and Sikora, J. (2007). Bull. Vet. Inst. Pulawy, 49: 203-207.

Krukowski, H. and Saba, L. (2003). Folia Veterinaria, 47(1):3-7.

Krukowski, H., Tietze, M., Majewski and Ro´zanski, P. (2000). Mycopathologia, 150: 5–7.

Kumar, A. and Garg, D.N. (1991Vet. Rec., 128:429.

Kumar, M., Goel, P., Sharma, A. and Kumar, A. (2009). In: Compendium of 27th ISVM International summit and convention at Chennai, Tamilnadu, India.. p. 4.

Kumar, R. and Sharma, A. (2002). Indian J. Anim. Sci., 72(5): 361-363.

Kumari, P.M. and Gupta, B.J.R. (2002). Indian Vet. J., 79(1): 89.

Lafi, S., Al-Rawashdeh, O., Na'Was, T. and Hailat, N. (1994). Trop. Anim. Health Prod. 26: 168-174.

Lafi, S.Q. and Hailat, N.Q. (1998). Veterinarski Archiv, 68(2): 51-57.

Lagneau, P.E., Lebtahi, K. and Swinne, D. (1996). Mycopathologia., 135(2):99-102.

Lakew, M., Tolosa, T. and Tigre, W. (2009). Trop. Anim. Hlth. Prod., 41(7): 1525-1530.

Lalrintluanga, C., Ralte, E.L. and Hmarkunga (2003). Indian Vet. J., 80(9): 931-932.

Langoni, H., Domingues, P.F., Molero-Filho, J.R. and Baldini, S. (2001). Ars-Veterinaria, 17(3): 213-217.

Langoni, H., Silva, A.V., Cabral, K.G., Dominques, P.F. and Silva, A.V. (1998). Revista Brasileira Medicina Veterinaria, 20(5): 204-209.

Larry, J. (1997). Michigan Dairy Review, 2(2): 4.

Legneau, P. E. (1996). J. Mycol. Med. 6:145–148.

Lerch, M. (1952). Einen durch Algen (*Prototheca*) hervorgerufene Mastitis der Kuh. Berl. Münch. tierärztl. Wschr., 65: 64-69.

Li, T., Liu, X., Zhang, Y.Q. and Yang, M.Q. (2009). Progress in Vet. Med., 2009-07.

Liu, D.C.,Cheng, Y. and Zhang, Z.Y. (2006). China Anim. Husb. Vet. Med., 2006-07.

Liu, W.J., Chen, C.F., Teng, W.J., Wu, J. and Ren, X.Y. (2005). Ecology of Domestic Animal, 2005-04.

Louza, A.C., Viegas, F.J.T. and Branco, F.N.A.B. (1986). Rev. Port. Ciencias Vet., 81: 263-285.

Lovell, R. (1939). J. Path. Bact., 49: 329.

M'Fadyean, J. (1917). J. Comp. Path., 30: 139.

Ma, B.C., Niu, J.H., Gao, Y.J., Qin, Z.M., Chai, T.J., Li, J.J. and Wang, C.A. (2005). Ecology of Domestic Animal, 2005-06.

Madsen, M, Hoi Sorensen, G and Aalbaek, B. (1990). Vet Microbiol., 22(4):319-28.

Madut, N.A., Gadir, A.E.A. and El Jalii, I.M. (2009). J. Cell and Animal Biology, 3 (5): 71-77.

Maiti, S.K., Parai, T.P. and Pandey, H.S. (1996). Indian Vet. J., 73(11): 1172-1174.

Malinowski, E., Lassa, H., Klossowska and Klossowska, A. (2002). Bull. Vet. Inst. Pulawy, 46: 295-299.

Malinowski, E., Lassa, H., Klossowska, A., Markiewicz, H., Kaczmarowski, M. and Smulski, S. (2006). Bull. Vet. Inst. Pulawy, 50: 349-352.

Mallikarjunaswamy, M.C. and Krishnamurthy, G.V. (1997). Indian Vet. J., 74(10): 885-887.

Matthews, K.R., Almeida, R.A. and Oliver, S.P. (1994). Infection and Immunity, 62: 12, 5641-5646.

Matthews, K.R., Harmon, R.J., and Langlois, B.E. (1991). J. Dairy Sci., 74(6): 1855-1859.

McDonald, J. S., Richard, J. L. and Cheville, N. F. (1984). Am. J. Vet. Res., 45:592–595.

McDougall, S., Bryan, M.A. and Tiddy, R.M. (2009). J. Dairy Sci., 92(9): 4421-4431.

Mdegela, R.H., Kusiluka, J. M., Kapaga, A.M., Karimuribo, E.D., Turuka, F.M., Bundala, A., Kivaria, F., Kabula, B., Manjurano, A., Loken, T. and Kambarage, D.M. (2004). J. Vet. Med.. Series B, 51(3): 123-128.

Menard, L., Vanasse, C., Diaz, C. and Rivard, G. (1983). Can. Vet. J., 24(10): 305-307.

Menzies, F.D., Mcbride, S.H., Mcdowell, S.W.J., Mccoy, M.A., Mcconnell, W. and Bell, C. (2000). Vet. Rec., 147(7): 123-128.

Mijovic, A., Leban, M. and Staric, J. (2006). In: Comp. 7th Middle European Buiatric Congress and Convention Centre Radin, Rdenci, Slovenia, 29th -1st April, 2006, pp.71-75.

Milne, M.H., Barrett, D.C., Fitzpatrick, J.L. and Biggs, A.M. (2002). Vet. Rec, 151: 241-243

Milne, M.H., Biggs, A.M., Barrett, D.C., Young, F.J., Doherty, S., Innocent, G.T. and Fitzpatrick, J.L. (2005). Vet. Rec, 157(27/8): 245-250.

Milojevic, Z., Rusov, C., Zivkovic, R., Stojicevic, S., Jojic-Malicevic, L. and Bozovic, V. (1991). Vet.Glasnik 45: 691-696.

Miltenburg, J.D., Lange, D.De., Crauwels, A.P.P., Bongers, J.H.. Tielen, M.J.M., Schukken, Y.H. and Elbers, A.R.W. (1996). Vet. Rec, 139: 204-207.

Misra, P.R., Roy, P.K. and Das, K.L. (1993). Indian J. Dairy Sci., 46: 543.

Mitchell, C.A., Walker, R.V.L. and Bannister, G.L. (1953). Can. J. Comp. Med., 18: 426.

Miyano, H., Haritani, M., Sentsui, H., Tsuboi, T., Tanimura, N., Kimura, K.M., Kobayashi, M., Obara, N. and Akimoto, Y. (2004). J. Vet. Med. Sci., 66(4): 457-460.

Mohamed, I.E., Mohamed, G.E. and El-Owni, O.A.O. (1993). In: Proc. 2nd Scientific Cong. Egyptian Society for Cattle Diseases. 5-7 Dec, 1993. Assiut, Egypt. Volume 2: 326-336.

Mohsenzadeh, M. and Fallah Rad, A.H. (2007). J. Anim. Vet. Adv., 6 (8): 981-985.

Monga, D.P. (2000). In: Proc. of 1st round table conf. on mastitis, 18-19 Feb., 2000. Izatnagar, Bareilly, India. Pp. 93-97.

Moretti, A., Pasquali, P., Mencazoni, G., Boncio, L. and Fioretti, D.P. (1998). J. Vet. Medicine. Series-B, 45(3): 129-132.

Morresey, P.R. (1999) Bovine mastitis. In: Current Veterinary Therapy for Food Animal Practice, ed. Howard, J.L. and Smith, R.A., W.B. Sauders Company, Philadelphia, pp. 563-566.

Munda, V., Prasad, A., Tiwary, B.K. and Mahto, D. (2007). Vet. World., 5(12): 375-376.

Munoz, M.A., Welcome, F.L., Schukken, Y.H. and Zadoks, R.N. (2007). J. Clin. Microbiol., 45(12): 3964-3971.

Murphy, J.M. and Drake, C. (1947). Am. J. Vet. Res., 8(1): 43-51.

Nagal, K.B., Sharma, M. and Katoch, R.C. (1999). Indian J. Anim. Sci., 69(3): 150-152.

Nakajima, Y., Mikami, O., Yoshioka, M. and Motoi, Y. (1997). Res. Vet. Sci., 62: 297-298.

Nam, H.M., Kim, J.M., Lim, S.K., Jang, K.C. and Jung, S.C. (2010). Res. Vet. Sci., 88(3): 372-374.

Nam, H.M., Lim, S.K., Kang, H.M., Kim, J.M., Moon, J.S., Jang, K.C., Kim, J.M., Joo, Y.S. and Jung, S.C. (2009). J. Dairy Sci., 92: 2020-2026.

Nath, K. and Dutta, J.B. (2005). Intl. J. Cow Sci., 1(1): 63-65.

Nauriyal, D.S. and Verma, A.K. (2008). In: Comp. of XXVI annual convention of ISVM, Ranchi, Jharkhand, India. pp. 13-14.

Nauriyal, D.S. and Verma, A.K. (2009). In: Compendium of 27th ISVM International summit and convention at Chennai, Tamilnadu, India.. p. 9.

Nauriyal, D.S., Chaturvedi, V.K. and Pachauri, S.P. (2003). In: Compendium of XXI ISVM Convention and National Symposium at Anand, Gujarat, India. p. 236.

Neave, F.K., Dodd, F.H., Kingwill, R.G. and Westgarth, D.R. (1969). J. Dairy Sci., 52(5): 696-707.

Nevala, M., Taponen, S. and Pyorala, S. (2004). Suomen Elainlaakarilehti., 110 (7/8): 363-369.

Newbould, F.H.S. and Neave, F.K. (1965). J. Dairy Res., 32: 171.

Newman, L.E. and Kowlski, J.J. (1973). Am. J. vet. Res., 34: 979.

Newton, H.T., Green, M.J., Benchaoui, H., Cracknell, V., Rowan, T. and Bradley, A.J. (2008). Vet. Rec,162(5): 678-684.

Ngeleka, M., Hawkes, R. and Pederson, E. (2008). Animal Health Perspectives, 4(2): 3-4.

Olde Riekerink, R.G.M., Barkema, H.W., Kelton, D.F. and Scholl, D.T. (2008). J. Dairy Sci., 91(4): 1366–1377.

Oliveira, A.A., Mota, R.A., Perira, G.C., Langoni, H., Souza, M.I., Navegantes, W.A. and Sa, M.E. (2001). Onderstepoort J. Vet, Res., 68(4): 275-279.

Oliver, S. P., Gillespie, B. E. and Jayarao, B. M. (1998). FEMS Microbiol Lett., 160(1): 69-73.

Oliviera, U.V., Galvao, G.S., Paixao, A.R.R. and Munhoz, A.D. (2010). Rev. Bras. Saúde Prod. An., 11(3): 630-640.

Orpin, P. (2000). In: Proc. British Mastitis Conf., pp. 14-21.

Østeras, O., Sølverød, L. and Reksen, O. (2006). J. Dairy Sci., 89(3): 1010-1023.

Osumi, T., Kishimoto, Y., Kano, R., Maruyama, H., Onozaki, M., Makimura, K., Ito, T., Matsubara, K. and Hasegawa, A. (2008). Vet. Microbiol., 131(3-4): 419-423.

Palanivel, K.M., Suresh, R.V., Jayakumar, R., Ganesan, P.I. and Dhanapalan, P. (2008). Indian J. Vet. Med., 28(1): 34-36.

Pankey, J.W., Nickerson, S.C., Boddie, R.L. and Hogan, J.S. (1985). J. Dairy Sci., 68: 2684-93.

Parker, K.I., Compton, C.W.R., Anniss, F.M., Heuer, C. and McDougall, S. (2008). J. Dairy Sci., 91(1): 169–181.

Patel., P.R., Raval, S.K., Rao, N, Mandali, G.C. and Jani, R.G. (2000). In: Proceeding of 1st round table conference on Mastitis, Izatnagar, Bareilly, U.P. (India). Pp. 45-52.

Patil, R.B., Bijwal, D.L. and Bannalikar, A.S. (2009). In: Compendium of 27th ISVM International summit and convention at Chennai, Tamilnadu, India.. p. 17.

Paul, M.W., Parthiban, M., Menaka, R. and Mahalinga Naianr, A. (2000). Indian J. Anim. Hlth., 39(2): 79-81.

Paulin-Curlee, G.G., Singer, R.S., Sreevatsan, Isaacson, S.R., Reneau, J., Foster, D. and Bey, R. (2007). J. Dairy Sci., 90(8): 3681-3689.

Peeler, E.J., Green, M.J., Fitzpatrick, J.L. and Green, L.E. (2003). Preventive Veterinary Medicine, 59: 169–180

Peer, F.U., Battacharya, H.K., Malik, H.U. and Ansari, M.M. (2007). In: Proc. of XXV Ann. Conv. Of ISVM, Pantnagar, Uttarakhand, India. P.26.

Phogat, S. and Dahiya, N. (2003). In: Proceeding of 4th Round table conference on mastitis, Palampur, H.P. (India), 14-15 April, pp. 185-191.

Piccinini, R.E., Binda, L. and Zecconi, A. (2003). In: Proc. of 42nd NMC Annual Meeting, pp. 396-397.

Piepers, S., de Meulemeester, L., de Kruijff, A., Opsomer, G., Barkema, .W. and Vliegher, S.D. (2007). J. Dairy Res., 74(4): 478-483.

Pinho, L., Ferreira, J., Cabral, C., Lameira, R., Meireles, P., Vaz, F., Carvalheira, J. and Thompson, G. (2008). In: Lam, T.J.G.M. (2008). Mastitis control from science to practice. 1st edn., Wageningen Academic Publisher, The Netherlands. pp. 47-53.

Pisoni, G., Locatelli, C., Alborali, L., Rosignoli, C., Allodi, S., Riccaboni, P., Grieco, V. and Moroni, P. (2008). J. Dairy Sci., 91:136-139.

Pitkala, A., Haveri, M., Payorala, S., Myllys, V. and Honkanen-Buzalski, T. (2004). J. Dairy Sci., 87(8):2433–2441

Pouden, W.D., Amberson, J.M. and Jager, R.F. (1952). Am. J. Vet. Res., 13(4): 121-128.

Prabhakar, S.K., Singh, K.B. and Joshi, D.V. (1995). Buffalo Bulletin, 14(3): 63-67.

Prasad, B. (2000). In: Proceeding of Round Table Conference on Mastitis, No. 1., Izatnagar, Bareilly, U.P. (India). Pp. 16-22.

Quinlan, J.F. and McNicholl, V.J. (1993). Vet. Rec., 156: 376-380.

Quinn, P.J., Carter, M.E., Markey, B.K. and Carter, G.R. (1994). In: Clinical Veterinary Microbiology. Wolfe, Spain.

Radostits, O.M., Gay, C.C., Blood, D.C. and Hinchcliff, K.W. (2000). Mastitis. In: Veterinary Medicine, 9th ed., W.B. Saunders Company Ltd., London, pp. 603-687.

Rahman, H. and Baxi, K.K. (1982). Indian Vet. Med. J., 6(6): 78-82.

Rajala-Schultz, P.J., Smith, K.L., Hogan, J.S. et al. (2004). Vet. Microbiol. 102(1-2): 33-42.

Rajeev, N.K., Isloor, S., Rathnamma, D. and Shridhar, N.B. (2009). Indian Vet. J., 86(9): 883-885.

Rajendran, T., George, S.K., Harshan, H.M. and Antony, P. (2006). Vet. World, 4(12): 357-360.

Ramachandraiah, K., Sudharsan Kumar, K. and Sreemannarayana, O. (1990). Indian Vet. J., 67(2): 103-106.

Ramani Pushpa, R.N., Thangavel, K. and Anandkumar, P. (2010). Indian Vet. J., 87(2): 187-188.

Ranjan, R., Gupta, M.K., Singh, S. and Kumar, S. (2010). Vet. World, 3(1): 17-20.

Ranjan, R., Swarup, D. and Ram Naresh (2003). In: Proc. 4th Round Table Conf. on mastitis, Palampur, H.P. (India), 14-15 April, pp. 165-170.

Ray, D.K., Bhattacharyya, U.K., Chowdhury, B., Dasgupta, P. and Bhattacharyya, A.K. (1989). Indian J. Anim. Health. 28: 50-55.

Reed, D.E., Langpap, T.J. and Anson, M.A. (1977). Am. J. Vet. Res. 38: 1631-1634.

Reetha, T.L., Babu, M., Pugazhenthi, T.R. and Rajeswar, J.J. (2006). Tamilnadu J. Vet. & Anim. Sci., 2(4): 140-141.

Reksen, O., Sølverød, L., Branscum, A. J. and Østeras, O. (2006). J. Dairy Sci., 89(8):2928–2937.

Resende, D.F., Glenn, K., Cullor, J.S. and and Bruno, R.G.S. (2009). J. Anim. Sci., Vol. 87, E-Suppl. 2/J. Dairy Sci. Vol. 92, E-Suppl. 1 (Abstract). P.200.

Richard, G. M., Olde, R., Herman, W.B., Stefan, V., Doris, E. P., Randy, T. D. and Gregory, P. K. (2006). Can. Vet J., 47 (6):567-572.

Richards, J.L., McDonald, J.S., Fichtner, R.E. and Anderson, A.J. (1980). Am. J. Vet. Res., 41: 1991-1994.

Roberson, J.R., Warnick, L.D. and Moore, G. (2004). J. Dairy Sci., 87: 583-592.

Roberts, N.H. (1990). Vet. Rec., 127: 191.

Ross, R.G., Balakrishnan, G. and Anbiah, S.V. (2001). Indian Vet. J., 78(11): 1066-1067.

Rusov, C., Milojevic, Z. and Stojanovic, L. (1994). Vet. Glasnik., 48: 303-308.

Sahay, S., Sinha, B.P. and Verma, S.P. (2007). Indian J. Vet. Med., 27(1): 29-30.

Sahoo, S.S., Sahoo, N. and Parida, G.S. (2009). Indian Vet. J., 86(12): 100-101.

Saini, S.S., Sharma, J.K. and Kwatra, M.S. (1992). Vet. Rec., 131: 152.

Saini, S.S., Sharma, J.K. and Kwatra, M.S. (1994). Prevalence of sub-clinical mastitis in rural Punjab. (cited from Indian J. Dairy Sci. abstr. 47: 103-106).

Sampimon, O.C., Olde Riekerink, R.G.M. and Lam, T.J.G.M. (2008). In: Lam, T.J.G.M. (2008). Mastitis control from science to practice. 1st edn., Wageningen Academic Publisher, The Netherlands. pp. 39-46.

Sampimon, O.C., Sol, J. and Kock, P.A. (2006). Tijdschr Diergeneeskd., 131(1): 2-4.

Santos, R.C. and Marin, J.M. (2005). Mycopathologia,159: 251–253.

Sargeant, J.M., Leslie, K.E., Shirley, J.E., Pulkrabek, B.J. and Lim, G.H. (2001). J. Dairy Sci., 84(9): 2018-2024.

Sarode, D.B. (2002). In: Proceeding of Round Table Conference on Mastitis, No. 3., Izatnagar, Bareilly, U.P. (India). Pp. 40-42.

Saxena, R.K., Dutta, G.N., Borah, P. and Buragohain, J. (1993). Indian Vet. J., 70(11): 1079-1080.

Scaccabarozzi, L., Turchetti, B. Buzzini, P., Pisoni, G., Bertocchi, L., Arrigoni, N., Boettcher, P., Bronzo, V. and Moroni, P. (2008). J. Dairy Sci., 91(9):3474–3477.

Schalm, O.W. and Lasmanis, J. (1968). J. Amer. Vet. Med. Ass., 153: 1688.

Schalm, O.W. and Mead, S.W. (1943). J. Dairy Sci., 26: 823.

Schalm, O.W., Caroll, E.J.and Jain, N.C. (1971). Bovine mastitis. Lea and Febiger, Philadelphia.

Sebastian, S.R. and Vijayakumar, K. (2002). In: Proceeding of 3rd round table conference on Mastitis, Izatnagar, Bareilly, U.P. (India). Pp. 120-125.

Seinhorst, J.W., Sol, J. and Vecht, U. (1991). Vet. Rec., 128: 54-56.

Seleim, R.S., Rashed, A.Y.M. and Fahmy, B.G.A. (2002). Vet. Medical J. Giza, 50(3): 405-418.

Selvaraj, P., Ramprabhu, R., Srinivasan, S.R., Suresh, R.V., Prathaban, S. and Dhanapalan, P. (2008). In: Proc. of XXVI Ann. Conv. Of ISVM, Ranchi, Jharkhand, India. P.44.

Senthilvelan, A., Balachandran, C. and Sundar, N. (2006). Indian Vet. J., 83(12): 1256-1257.

Seyoum, T., Ameni, G. and Ashenafi, M. (2003). Bull. Anim. Health & Prod. Africa., 51(4): 182-189.

Shahan, T. A. and Pore, R. S. (1991). Agents Chemother., 35:2434–2435.

Sharma, A, Dhingra, P.,Pander, B.L. and Kumar, R. (2006). Intl. J. Cow Sci., Vol. 2, Number 1.

Sharma, A. and Kapur, M.P. (2000). In: Proc. 1st Round Table Conf. on Mastitis, IVRI, Izatnagar, (India),18th –19th Feb., p.8-11.

Sharma, A. and Prasad, B. (2003). In: Proceeding of 4th Round Table Conf. on Mastitis, Palampur, H.P. (India), 14-15 April, pp. 2024-213.

Sharma, A. and Sindhu, N. (2007). Ital. J. Anim. Sci. 6(Suppl. 2): 965-967.

Sharma, A.K. and Prasad, B. (2002). In: Comp. XX ISVM Convention and National Symposium at Bikaner, Rajasthan (India). 14th –16th Feb., p. 93.

Sharma, D.K., Jallewar, P.K. and Sharma, K.K. (2010). Indian Vet. J., 87(4): 407.

Sharma, Neelesh (2003). M.V.Sc. Thesis, I.G.K.V.V., Raipur (C.G.), India.

Sharma, Neelesh (2008). Intl. J. Zoological Res., 4(1): 64-67.

Sharma, Neelesh, Gupta, S.K., Sharma, U. and Hussain, K. (2007). Buff. Bull., 26(2): 56-58.

Sharma, Neelesh, Maiti, S.K. and Sharma, K.K. (2007). Intl. J. Dairy Sci., 2(2): 145-151.

Shathele, M.S. (2009). Int. J. Dairy Sci., 4(2): 57-66.

Shitandi, A. and Kihumbu, G. (2004). J. Vet. Sci., 5(1): 5-9.

Shitandi, A., Anakalo, G., Galgalo, T. and Mwangi, M. (2004). Israel J. Vet. Med., 59(1/2): 20-23.

Shukla, S.K., Dixit, V.P., Thapiyal, D.C. and Kumar, A. (1998). Indian Vet. Med. J., 22: 261-264.

Shwimmer, A., Freed, M., Blum, S., Khatib, N., Weissblit, L., Friedman, S. and Elad, D. (2007). Zoonoses and Public Health, 54(9/10): 353-357.

Siegler, H.H., Marschang, F. and Morscher, H. (1984). Tierärztl. Umschau., 39: 602-604.

Siji, P.C. and Vijayakumar, K. (2007). Indian J. Vet. Med., 27(2): 131-132.

Singh, M., Ahmad, N., Sudhan, N.A. and Singh, R. (2000). Vet. Practitioner, 1(1): 61-66.

Singh, N., Sharma, V.K., Rajani, H.B. and Sinha, Y.R. (1982). Indian Vet. J., 59(9): 693-696.

Singh, P.J., Singh, K.B., Jand, S.K., Dhingra, P.N. and Nauriyal, D.C. (1994). Indian J. Dairy Sci., 47(9): 730-733.

Singh, R., Sharma, Neelesh, Soodan, J.S. and Sudhan, N.A. (2005). J. Res. SKUAST-J., 4(2): 223-224.

Slanetz, L.W. and Barley, C.H. (1953). J. Infect. Dis., 92: 139.

Smith K.L., Todhunter D.A. and Schoenberger P.S. (1985b). J. Dairy Sci., 68: 402-417.

Smith, K.L. and Hogan, J.S. (1995a). Proc. of 3rd IDF International Mastitis Seminar, Book-11, Session 6. Tel-Aviv, IL. Pp. 3-12.

Smith, K.L. and Hogan, J.S. (1995b). The importance of coagulase negative Staphylococci. News letter of the IDF, No. 142, mastitis news letter, 20. pp. 26-29.

Smith, K.L., Todhunter, D.A. and Schoenberger, P.S. (1985a). J. Dairy Sci., 68: 1531-1553.

Sori, H., Zerihun, A. and Abdich, S. (2005). J. Appl. Res. Vet. Med., 3(4): 332-338.

Stuart, P. and Harvey, P. (1951). Vet. Rec., 63: 881.

Sudhan, N.A., Singh, R., Singh, M and Soodan, J.S. (2005). Indian J. Anim. Res., 39(2): 127-130.

Sumathi, B.R., Veeregowda, B.M. and Gomes, R. (2008). Vet. World, 1(8): 237-238.

Szczubia³, M., D¹browski, R., Kankofer, M., Bochniarz, M. and Albera, E. (2008). Bull. Vet. Inst. Pulawy, 52: 391-395.

Taponen, S. and Pyorala, S. (2009). Vet. Microbiol., 134: 29–36.

Taponen, S., Simojoki, H., Haveri, M., Larsen, H.D. and Pyorala, S. (2006). Vet. Microbiol., 115: 199–207.

Teale, C.J., Kay, A.C.S. and Knight, D. (1990). Vet. Rec., 127: 243.

Tenhagen, B.A., Hansen, I., Reinecke, A. and Heuwieser, W. (2008). In: Lam, T.J.G.M. (2008). Mastitis control from science to practice. 1st edn., Wageningen Academic Publisher, The Netherlands. p. 63.

Tenhagen, B.A., Oster, G.K., Wallmann, J. and Heuwieser, W. (2006). J. Dairy Sci., 89(7):2542–2551.

Thakur, D.K., Sinha, O.P. and Jha, N.K. (2001). In: Compendium of XIX Anuual Convention of ISVM, Jammu, India. 9-11 April, p.15.

Tijare, D.B., Chaturvedi, V.K. and Srivastava, A.B. (2002). In: Comp. of 3rd round table conf. on mastitis, Nagpur (M.S.), India, pp. 14-17.

Tijare, D.B., Singh, A.K., Chaturvedi, V.K. and Dhanesar, N.S. (1999). Indian Vet. J., 76(10): 912-915.

Todhunter, D.A., Smith, K.L. and Hogan, J.S. (1995). J. Dairy Sci., 78: 2366-2374.

Todhunter, D.A., Smith, K.L., Hogan, J.S. and Schoenberger, P.S. (1991). Am. J. Vet. Res., 52: 184-188.

Trinidad, P., Nickerson, S.C. and Alley, T.K. (1990). J.Dairy Sci., 73(1): 107-114.

Tuteja, F.C., Sharma, Anshu, Kapur, M.P. (2003). Vet. Practitioner. 4(1): 19-21.

Tuteja, R.C., Kapur, M.P., Sharma, A. and Vinayaka, A.K. (1993). Indian Vet. J., 70(9): 787-791.

Tweyongyere, R. and Kasirye, F.N. (1998). Bull. Anim. Hlth. Prod. Africa., 46(2): 89-93.

Ueno, R., Urano, N. and Suzuki, M. (2003). Microbiol. Lett., 223:275–280.

USDA-AHPIS Info Sheet (2008). Prevalence of contagious mastitis pathogens on U.S. dairy operations, 2007. Info Sheet, Oct., 2008.

Vargas, A. C., Lazzari, A., Santurio, J. M., Alves, S. H., Ferreira, G., and Kreutz, L. C. (1998). Mycopathologia, 142:135–137.

Varma, S.K. and Dorairajan, N. (2006). Indian J. Vet. Med., 26(2): 137-138.

Vecht, U., Wisselink, H.J. and Defize, P.R. (1989). Neth. Milk Dairy J., 43: 425-435.

Vijayalakshmi, P. and Prathaban, S. (2007). Indian J. Vet. Med., 27(1): 49-51.

Vijayalakshmi, P., Prathaban, S., and Dhanapalan, P. (2001). Indian Vet. J., 78(1): 4-6.

Vimalraj, T.R., Kavith, N. and Dhanalakshmi, B. (2006). Indian Vet. J., 83(10): 1120-1121.

Viseslava, M. and Vera, K. (1989). Acta Vet.-Beogr., 39: 121-125.

Vishwakarma, P. (2008). Studies on prevalence, diagnosis, therapy and control of mastitis in buffaloes. M.V.Sc. Thesis, Indira Gandhi Agricultural University, Raipur, Chhattisgarh.

Waage, S., Mork, T., Roros, A., Aasland, D., Hunshamar, A. and Odegaard, S. (1999). J. Dairy Sci., 82(4): 712-719.

Wang, G.Y. and Niu, Z.X. (2009). J. Shandong Agri. Univ. (Natural Science Edition): 2009-04.

Ward, W.R., Hughes, J.W., Faull, W.B., Cripps, P.J., Sutherland, J.P. and Sutherst, J.E. (2002). Vet. Rec., 151: 199-206.

Wellenberg, G.J., van der Poel, W.H. and van Oirschot, J.T. (2002). Vet. Microbiol., 88: 27–45.

Wellenberg, G.J., Van der Poel, W.H.M., Van der Vorst, T.J.K., Van Valkengoed, P.H.R., Schukken, Y.H.,Wagenaar, F. and VanOirschot, J.T. (2000). Vet. Rec., 147: 222-225.

Wilesmith, J.W., Francis, P.G. and Wilson, C.D. (1986). Vet. Record, 118: 199-204.

Wilson, D.J., González, R.N. and Das, H.H. (1997). J. Dairy Sci., 80(10): 2592-2598.

Yathiraj, S., Bhat, M.N., Deepti, B.R., Upendra, H.U. and Murlidhara, A. (2007). In: Proc. of XXV Ann. Conv. Of ISVM, Pantnagar, Uttarakhand, India. P.26.

Yeo, G. and Choi, W.P. (1982). Korean J. Vet. Res., 22: 121–124.

Zadoks, R.N. and Fitzpatrick, J.L. (2009). Irish Vet. J., 62(59): 59-70.

Zadoks, R.N., Allore, H.G., Barkema, H.W., Sampimon, O.C., Wellenberg, G.J., Grohn, Y.T. and Schukken, Y.H. (2001). J. Dairy Sci., 84: 2649-2663.

Zadoks, R.N., and J. L. Fitzpatrick, J.L. (2009). Changing trends in mastitis. Ir. Vet. J. 62(Suppl.): 59–70.

Zdragas, A., Tsakos, P. and Anatoliotis, K. (2004). J. Hellenic Vet. Medical Soc., 55(2): 113-119.

Zhang, Y., Jia, X.F., Ya, M.S., Siqinqimuge, Narisu, Liu, B.Z., Suyila,Ying, C., Gao, X.S. and Liu, Q.Y. (2009). China Anim. Husb. & Vet. Med., 2009-07.

Zhang, Z.W., Wu, G.J., Liu, F.H., Ma, S.Y., Li, H.R. and Li, N. (2002). J. Beijing Agri. College, 2002-2004.

□□□

CHAPTER

8

Epidemiology

Definition

Mastitis is defined as an inflammation of the parenchyma of the mammary gland. The International Dairy federation (1999) has recommended definitions and further classification into severe, moderate or mild clinical mastitis and sub-clinical mastitis. Severe and moderate clinical mastitis usually need antibiotic therapy and should be treated in the interest of animal welfare, while therapy decision for mild clinical mastitis and sub-clinical mastitis should be based more on economic evaluation (Osteras, 2006). Various definitions of epidemiology are available in different resources. Houe *et al.* (2004) translate epidemiology literally as the study (*logos*) of what is upon (*epi*) the population (*demos*). Epidemiology has traditionally been defined as the study of occurrence and distribution of diseases in population as well as the study of factors that influence disease occurrence (Osteras, 2006). The general aims of epidemiology are (Osteras, 2006):-

1. To describe the health status in the population.
2. To explain the etiology of disease by determining factors that causes the specific disease.
3. To predict the number of disease incidents and the distribution of health status within population and,

4. To control the distribution of disease in the population by prevention of new occurrences, eradication of existing cases and otherwise improving the health status.

It is important that epidemiologists strive to identify exposures and evaluate their associations with various outcomes of interest (e.g. health, welfare, productivity) so as to improve the lives of animals and their keepers. From this definition we also see that animal welfare and economics are included in epidemiology (Osteras, 2006). The two epidemiological tools are used in order to quantify udder health are "*prevalence*" and "*incidence*". Prevalence measures the amount of mastitis prevailing at a given point of time, and incidence measures the rate of new cases of mastitis over a period of time.

A general epidemiologic formula that defines prevalence can be used to help prioritize preventive measures:

Prevalence = Incidence × Duration

Table 8.1 : Two-by-two table for the relationship between breed and clinical mastitis.

	Clinical mastitis		No Clinical mastitis		
Crossbred cow	A	9	B	4	13
Zebu (Local)	C	23	D	26	49
		32		30	62

The formula for simple chi-square analysis for a 2 X 2 table is as follows:

$$\frac{(AD - BC)^2 N}{(A + B)(A + C)(B + D)(C + D)}$$

For the data shown in table 8.1, the chi-square analysis result equals 2.04 and is calculated as follows:

$$\frac{(9 \times 26 - 4 \times 23)^2 \times 62}{(9 + 4)(9 + 23)(4 + 26)(23 + 26)}$$

To reach a P value of 0.05, the chi-square value must be 3.84 for a 2 × 2 table; for a P value of 0.10, the chi-square value must be 2.70. For this example, the P value was 0.15. The strength of the relationship can be determined by odds ratios. The formula for calculating an odds ratio is-

$$\text{Odd ratio} = \frac{A \times D}{B \times C}$$

For the data above, the odds ratio = 2.54 ([9 × 26]/[4 × 23]).

This formula indicates that the amount of clinical mastitis a herd experiences is determined by the rate that new infections develop and the duration of infection. On many farms, control methods are focused on limiting duration. Duration is influenced by type of organism, accuracy of detection, treatment efficacy, vaccine use, culling, and death. For many pathogens, treatment efficacy is limited, the biology of the organism is such that duration of infection is long, and culling is the only remaining option. Focusing on the new infection rate (incidence) is often more rewarding and results in longer-term benefits.

Some important facts to be considered for epidemiological study

1. Record keeping

Records play an important part in monitoring the incidence and severity of disease. In fact, mastitis is one of the diseases where detailed analysis of the data can be used to help in control. Such analysis can prove invaluable when investigating herd problems due to a high incidence of clinical mastitis or a high somatic cell count. However, in India the recording system of mastitis data is very poor. It is very important aspect of dairy farming which play the role in exact calculation of economic losses due to mastitis and in the strategies for prevention and control of mastitis. The following data should be recorded for mastitis:-

- Total number of animals at the farm
- Number of animals in milking
- Animal identification number
- Age, lactation number and stage of lactation
- Type of milking and hygienic practices
- Date of occurrence
- Quarter(s) infected
- Treatments given and details of treatment including cost.
- Bacteriology and antibiotic sensitivity results (if available).

A case of mastitis is defined as one quarter affected once. Hence, a cow with mastitis in all four quarters counts as four cases of mastitis (Edmondson and Blowey, 1998). If a treated quarter clears up but mastitis recurs seven or more days after the remission of clinical signs, this is defined as a *new case of mastitis*. If mastitis recurs in the same quarter within seven days of the remission of clinical signs, this is defined as a *continuing case of mastitis*.

Mastitis cases can be recorded in a variety of ways (see Format-1 and 2). Ideally, any subsequent cases of mastitis in a cow should be recorded alongside the first case so that problem animals can be readily identified. From the records shown in the format-1, it is immediately apparent that cow A-111 has had repeated cases of mastitis. Although exactly the same information is displayed in the format-2, it is not as obvious that cow A-111 is such a problem. Ideally, a cow's mastitis history should be recorded on the same card for all lactations. Records should be checked towards the end of lactation and cows with four or more cases of mastitis should be culled at this time (or earlier if they are persistent) (Edmondson and Blowey, 1998).

FORMAT-1

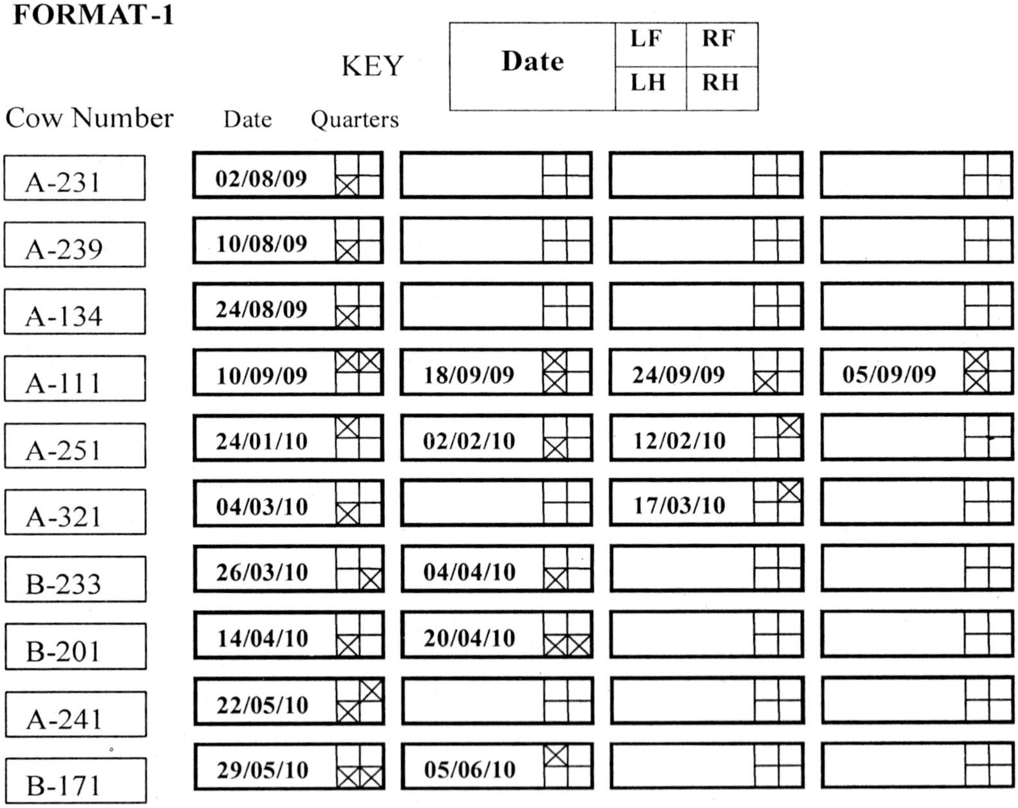

LF- Left fore, LH- Left hind, RF-Right fore, RH- Right hind

FORMAT-2

Cow Number	Date	Quarter(s)
A-231	02/08/09	LH
A-239	10/08/09	LH
A-134	24/08/09	LH
A-111	10/09/09	LF & RF

A-251	24/01/10	LF
A-321	04/03/10	LH
A-233	26/03/10	RH
B-201	14/04/10	LH
A-241	22/05/10	RF & LH
B-171	29/05/10	LH & RH

2. Mastitis rate

The mastitis rate is the number of cases of mastitis per 100 cows per year. It is an invaluable measure of the mastitis incidence as it allows comparisons to be made between herds irrespective of their size.

$$\text{Mastitis rate} = \frac{\text{Number of cases of mastitis per year X 100}}{\text{Total number of cows in the herd (Milking and dry)}}$$

A high mastitis rate indicates a high number of mastitis cases in the herd but does not identify what type of infection (i.e. contagious or environmental mastitis) is present.

3. Percentage of herd affected

The percentage of cows affected per year represents the number of milking cows that have had one or more cases of mastitis over a 12-month period.

$$\text{Percentage of herd affected} = \frac{\text{Number of affected with mastitis over a 12 months period X 100}}{\text{Total number of cows in the herd (milking and dry)}}$$

This data helps to give some indication of the type of mastitis present. For example, chronic recurring mastitis.

4. Recurrence rate

The recurrence rate is the percentage of quarters requiring one or more repeat treatments over a 12-month period. A repeat treatment refers to one or more cases of mastitis recurring in the same quarter.

$$\text{Recurrence rate} = \frac{\text{Number of mastitis cases requiring one or more repeat treatments X 1000}}{\text{Total number of mastitis cases}}$$

Risk Factors

Mastitis is a multifactorial disease, closely related to the production system and environment in which the cows and buffaloes are kept. Risk factors such as management practices (shed and udder hygiene, poor teat condition, poor environmental hygiene, sanitation, large herd size, use of hand wash cloth, improper teat dipping), host (breed, high yielder, udder immunity, teat lesions, genetic resistance) and diet (Cu, Co, Zn, Selenium and vitamin E deficiency) amongst others have been reported to be important in the prevalence and epidemiology of sub-clinical mastitis. To simplify understanding of the mastitis complexcity, it is useful to consider risk factors or disease determinants, which are broadly classified into three groups- host (cow or buffaloe), pathogen (micro-organisms) and environment (Figure 8.1). Evaluation of the relative importance of any single factor is difficult because it is usually impossible to observe the effect of factor apart from the effect of others, and because individual animals under apparently identical conditions differ in susceptibility (Plastridge, 1958).

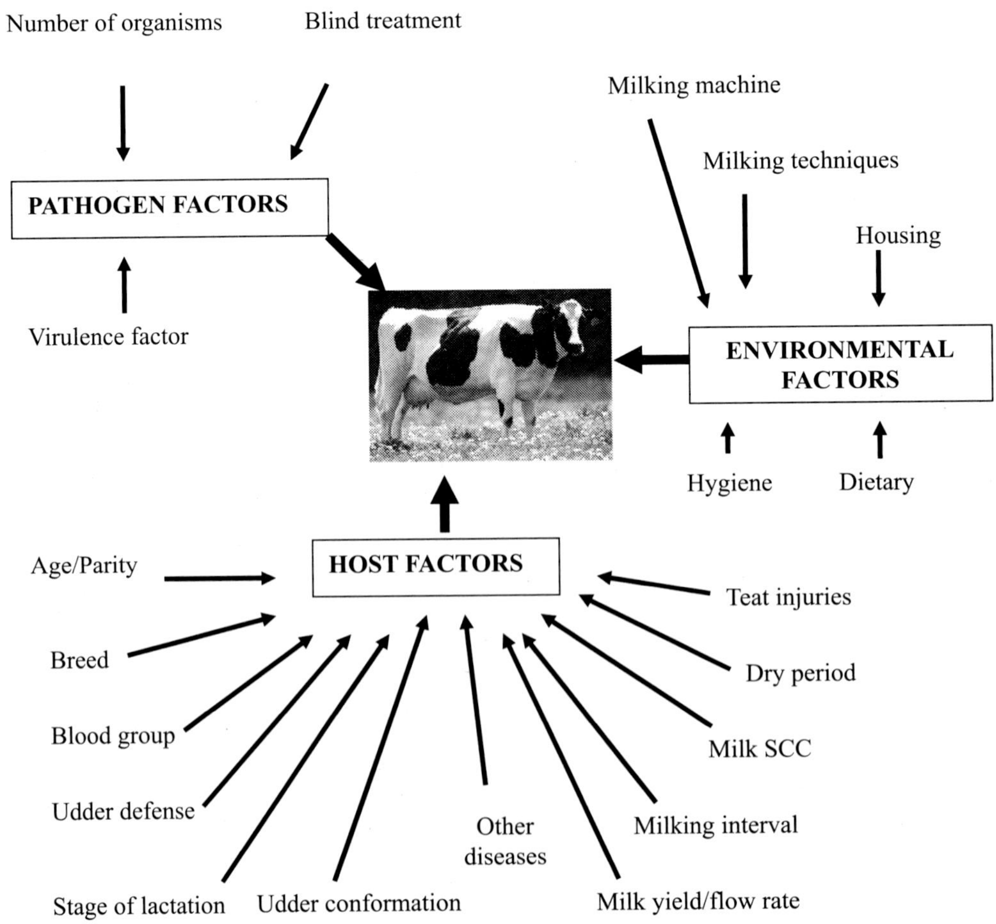

Figure 8.1 : Risk factors for mastitis.

The host is often seen as a passive element, although a certain number of studies have reported differences between animals where susceptibility to infections is concerned (Poutrel, 1982). Cows contract udder infection at different ages and at different stages of lactation cycle. Therefore, the host (cow or buffaloe) plays an active role in the development of mastitis.

Pathogens (micro-organisms) are directly responsible for the development of mastitis. More than 250 micro-organisms cause mastitis in dairy animals. However, Staphylococci and Streptococci occupies prime position (about 90% infections), other common mastitis pathogens are *E. coli, Pseudomonas, Corynebacterium, Klebsiella, Mycoplasma,* Yeast etc. Their habitats and route by which they reach the host are different; therefore control of mastitis is not an easy task.

The host environment influences both the numbers and types of organisms they are exposed to and their ability to resist these micro-organisms. Environmental factors like – climate, nutrition, housing, bedding, milking techniques, milking machine, mechanical injuries etc., influences the living conditions of bacteria the opportunity they are given to penetrate the streak canal and, to certain extent, the susceptibility of the animal. Numerous environmental conditions and dairy practices may serve to render the udder more susceptible to infection by bacterial agents. The environment of cow is rich in mammary pathogens and poses a constant threat to udder health. Streptococci and other infectious bacteria, in many instances, may fail to become established in the udder unless conditions are suitable for their development. Environmental factors or other influences that alter the susceptibility of the udder can be considered as *"predisposing"* or *"contributory"* causes of mastitis (Little and Plastridge, 1946). There are also some hereditary factors that may have a significant influence on the occurrence of mastitis. Infection of the mammary gland can occur during lactation or during the dry period, at any time of the year, in both housed or pastured cattle depends on various associated risk factors.

There are various risk factors which directly or indirectly affect or increase the susceptibility of cows and buffaloes to the intramammary infection (Figure 8.1).

1. Host risk factors

1.1 Age and parity

Incidence of infected quarters increases with the age (Sharma, 2003; Kumar and Sharma, 2002; Sharma and Prasad, 2002). Sharma *et al.* (2007) conducted a study on 500 lactating buffaloes of different age, parities and stage of lactation belonging to different organized or un-organized dairy farms,

Chhattisgarh State, India and found that the higher prevalence of sub-clinical mastitis (SCM) in buffaloes was recorded in 5 to 9 years old animals and in 3rd and 4th parities. Older cows (>10 years) are at more risk (44.6%), particularly for sub-clinical mastitis (38.6%), than younger cows (23.6%) in which clinical mastitis was predominant (Biffa *et al.*, 2005). Another report of Hogan and Smith (2000) that the primiparous and cows with 4 lactations had higher rates of intramammary infection (IMI) than the cows in the second and third lactations during the first month of lactation by environmental streptococci. An increase in age at first calving is also associated with increased risk of mastitis (Waage *et al.*, 1998). Increasing parity increased the risk of clinical mastitis in cows and buffaloes (Whist *et al.*, 2006; Kavitha *et al.*, 2009), although the reason for this association is not clear. However, McDonald (1968) reported that the teat canals lengthen and dilate with increase in lactational age. Plastridge *et al.* (1934) found that the rate of infection increased from 14 to 100%, and that the proportion of animals giving visibly abnormal milk intermittently increased from 8 to 86% from the 1st to 8th lactation. Cows with many calves (>7) have about 13-times greater risk (62.9%) of developing an udder infection than those with fewer (£3) calves (11.3%) (Biffa *et al.*, 2005). Hovi and Roderick (2000) have been reported that an increase in parity is significantly correlated with an increase in dry period clinical mastitis. The precise reason for these effects of age and stage are not known. Increasing disease with age is probably not due to increased intramammary susceptibility but to increasing ease of penetration of the teat canal by mastitis pathogens or accumulated previous infections. A greater predisposition to infection could be the consequence of a number of characteristics associated with age of lactation, in particular lengthening of teat, of more precisely of distance between udder and floor, lesions present on the teat and loss pf sphincter potency (Poutrel, 1982). Teat canals lengthen and dilate with increase in lactational age of cow (McDonald, 1968). After several lactations/parities the skin of the udder may become stretched and is less tightly applied to the underlying tissues. The suspensory apparatus which supports the udder becomes stretched, allowing it to become pendulous and more susceptible to injury, resulting mastitis. The teats become enlarged and it may eventually become difficult to attach the teat cups of the milking machine or for the calf to suckle (Jackson, 1996).

1.2 Breed

In many countries, the emphasis on improving dairy production has been to focus on breeds that have particularly high milk yields, especially Holstein, which is the most widespread dairy cattle breed, found in 128 countries worldwide (FAO, 2007). The Boran breed which is recognised for its relatively high milk yield compared to other cross-breeds, has been shown to be 3.4

times more likely to be affected by clinical and sub-clinical mastitis than the Tanzanian Shorthorn Zebu breed (Karimuribo *et al.*, 2006). Swedish Red and White Breed (SRB) are also having less incidence of mastitis than Swedish Friesian Breed (SLB) (Bendixen *et al.*, 1988). Increased risk of clinical mastitis in Friesian compared with Jersey and Ayrshire heifers (Compton *et al.*, 2007; Myllys and Rautala, 1995). In Southern Ehiopia, Biffa *et al.* (2005) reported that Holstein-Fresian cows are affected at a higher rate (56.5%) compared with local zebu (30.9%) and Jersey cows (28.9%). Sharma (2003) also found that Holstein-Fresian cows are at higher risk for mastitis than local zebu cows. These differences between breeds may be due to immune response to intramammary infection differs between breeds. Selection of crossbred dairy cattle on the basis of greater milk yield may therefore need to be combined with an improvement in control programmes for mastitis to ensure a sustainable industry (Zadoks and Fitzpatrick, 2009).

1.3 Species

The most of studies reported that cows are more vulnerable to intramammary infection than cows. The buffaloes are less susceptible to udder infections than cows, which may be possibly due to following reasons-

a) In buffaloes, teat orifice is tightly closed due to presence of well developed circular muscles.

b) The stratified squamous keratinized epithelium of streak canal lining is thicker in buffaloes than in cattle, which provides an extra resistance against penetration of pathogens through epithelium.

c) The stratum granulosum contained higher amount of keratohyalin granules in buffaloes than in cows. These keratohyaline granules may probably contribute in formation of large amount of keratin in lumen of streak canal.

d) In buffaloes keratin layers are thicker than in cows. Keratin helps in inhibition of bacterial penetration in streak canal by providing physical barrier.

e) Fissures in the keratin through which organisms can travel into teat cistern. These fissures are narrower and smaller in buffaloes than in cows.

1.4 Blood groups

A recent study was conducted on association of the M blood group system with bovine mastitis by Larsen *et al.* (2009) in Denmark. Associations of the 11 bovine blood group systems with mastitis were examined in Red Danish dairy cattle. A significant effect of the M blood group system on mastitis incidence was observed in the first and second lactation periods and a lower frequency of mastitis is found among animals lacking the *"M" factor* as compared to those having the M blood group factor. The significance of these results are discussed in view of the close relation between the M blood group system and the bovine lymphocyte antigens (BoLA), and the expected effect of eliminating the M gene from the breed is estimated. Among the remaining 10 blood group systems, the *"T" system* was the only system showing an overall effect on mastitis, and only in first and third lactation. However, the T system was inconsistent with regard to the effect of the T gene on the various mastitis diagnoses.

1.5 Stage of lactation

The incidence of mastitis is higher during just after parturition (first 2 months of lactation) and first 2-3 weeks of dry period (Figure 8.2) and Corbett (2009) suggests that the highest number of clinical mastitis cases occurs during the first week of lactation, and that the lactating cow is more likely to develop clinical mastitis during the first three months of lactation than the remainder of the lactating period. Fadlelmula *et al.* (2009) reported that the first month of lactation displayed the highest incidence of mastitis (62.7%), while the late stage of lactation showed the lowest incidence (11.2%) in Kingdom of Saudi Arabia. The high incidence of mastitis around calving is largely a consequence of high new infection rate in the dry period and a periparturient suppression of host defences. The neutrophils and lymphocyte function is diminished in the periparturient period. The onset of milk production imposes tremendous challenges to the mechanisms responsible for energy, protein, and mineral homeostasis in the cow. Negative energy, protein, mineral balance and/or oxidative stress associated with the onset of lactation may be partially responsible for the immunosuppression observed in periparturient dairy cattle. Sharma *et al.* (2011) reported that dairy cows seemed to have more oxidative stress and low antioxidant defense during early lactation or just after parturition than advanced pregnant cows, and this appears to be the reason for their increased susceptibility to production diseases (e.g. mastitis, metritis, retention of fetal membranes etc.) and other health problems. When the cow approaches the end of her gestation period, the calf secretes a high level of cortisol from its adrenal glands. This initiates the cascade of events that leads to parturition. However, cortisol is a highly immunosuppressive agent, and both the cow and the calf are immunosuppressed at the time of parturition. This is the major reason that fresh cows are more susceptible to new mastitis infections. Other factors are also responsible for high incidence of mastitis just after parturition e.g. onset of copious milk production can contribute to lower chemotactic response, inhibit phagocytosis and reduce leukocytic killing of phagocytosed bacteria by mammary gland neutrophils (MGN) during the immediate post partum period. In bovines, it is well documented that MGN have lower phagocytic and bactericidal activities (Kalorey, 2001). This is due to indiscriminate ingestion of milk constituents, degranulation and lower glucose metabolism. During early lactation environmental mastitis is more prevalent than contagious mastitis. For example, bacteria such as *Corynebacterium bovis* grow best in milk secreted in the middle of lactation, where as dry period secretion inhibits its growth. Sharma (2003) conducted a study on 550 lactating cows and 500 buffaloes and found that maximum rate of infection was recorded in early lactation stage (87.13% by Modified California Mastitis test) followed by late and mid lactation.

It is known that the growth of *E. coli* in the udder cistern is specially related with the period of lactation and parity of cows. *E. coli* mastitis with severe clinical symptoms is more frequently observed around calving and during early lactation in dairy cows, whereas symptoms are mild to moderate during mid and late lactation. Because of hormonal, metabolic and nutritional alterations associated with pregnancy, immune system is compromised around calving. The peri- and post-parturient metabolic changes, mainly the increased plasma levels of non-esterified fatty acids (NEFA) and â-hydroxy butyrate (BHB) impair their migration and phagocytic activity, enhancing the susceptibility of mammary gland to mastitis pathogens

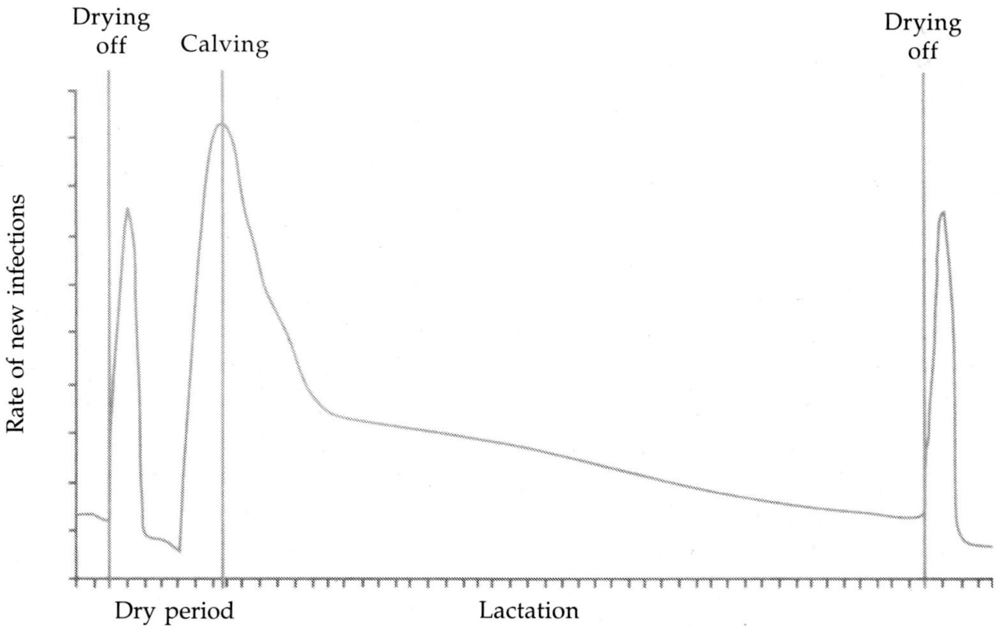

Figure 8.2 : A schematic illustration of the incidence of new intramammary infection during the lactation cycle. The peak in new infection rate, after drying off, is considerably higher in cows not receiving any form of dry cow therapy.

1.6 Dry period

A dry period or a stage of mammary involution is necessary during the lactation cycle of the dairy cow for optimal milk production in the ensuing lactation. Dry period, a short term of approximately two months, takes place during involution of old tissue and remodeling of new tissue in mammary gland. Bovine mammary involution is characterized by degeneration of the mammary alveolar structure and a loss of the majority of secretory epithelial cells (Wilde *et al.*, 1997). It is generally established that lactation should be terminated 45 to 60 days prior to parturition. Risk of new environmental *Streptococcal* infection is influenced by stage of lactation, parity, nutrition, and immunity, in addition to factors that increase teat end exposure. A study suggests that a longer dry period (>40 days) increased the risk of clinical mastitis (Peeler *et al.*, 2000). The rate of new infection is not constant across the dry period but is elevated during the two weeks following drying off and the two weeks prior to calving (Smith *et al.*, 1985) (Figure 8.2). Some studies said that the IMI rate is *2 to 12 times* higher during the dry period than at any other time during the lactation cycle of the cow (Vlieststra, 2003). Research showing that many cases of clinical mastitis in early lactation stem from infections originating through the dry period includes- 52% of clinical coliform mastitis, through the first 100 days of lactation, stemmed from a dry cow infection (Bradley and Green, 2000), 61% of all new gram-negative IMI occurred while dry (Todhunter *et al.*, 1991), 51% of all new environmental streptococci IMI occurred while dry (Todhunter *et al.*, 1995), 56% of clinical mastitis cases due to *Streptococcus uberis* originated in the dry period and 33% of clinical mastitis cases due to *Streptococcus dysgalactiae* originated in the dry period. (Bradley and Green, 2001).

The number of dry period infections increases with the age of the cow and in cows already infected in one or more quarters (Schalm *et al.*, 1971). Fast milkers may be involved more frequently. Increased susceptibility is due, in part, to changes in the teat canal, the primary defense barrier against bacterial penetration. Physical changes take place during this time that reduce resistance to infection: a) increased internal udder pressure due to milk stasis causes teat canal shortening and dilation allowing bacterial penetration (Nickerson, 1989); b) flushing of milk through the teat canal, which helps to remove colonized bacteria, is terminated; c) lack of keratin plug in the streak canal (Comalli *et al.*, 1984); 4) phagocytic and bactericidal activities diminishes (Paape *et al.*, 1992) and d) teat dipping and udder preparation are discontinued, allowing bacterial populations on teat skin to increase. Moreover, development of udder/teat edema may interfere with the sphincter muscle which functions to maintain tight closure of the teat canal. Resistance during the middle and late dry period was attributed to the keratin plug, which prevented multiplication and physical movement of bacteria (Nickerson, 1989). Several days are required following drying off for the plug to form, and it disappears 7 to 10 days before parturition.

In brief, for understanding and to know the exact time/stage of dry period susceptible to infection, it is important to differentiate the dry period into three phases, that is, involution, steady- state involution (involuted), and colostrogenesis (transition). During involution phase, the mammary gland is more susceptible to infection, mainly as a result of the cessation of milking and the slow transition to the involuted state. Upon cessation of milking, the flushing of bacteria from the streak canal ceases, teat dipping stops, and the streak canal becomes relatively compromised by the increased intramammary pressure following milk buildup. The slow transition to the involuted state delays the protective effects of lactoferrin and immunoglobulins while fat and casein levels remain high inhibiting leukocyte function. Clinical mastitis is rare during the mid non-lactating period, at which time the concentration of lactoferrin in mammary gland secretion remains at highest. In the fully involuted state, the mammary gland is considered very resistant to new infection due to higher activity/level of protective factors e.g. lactoferrin, immunoglobulin, enzymes and complete formation of keratin plug.

Lactoferrin is an iron chelating agent which inhibits the growth of enterobacterial organisms. This inhibition is mediated by lactoferrin's ability to reversibly bind iron, although available to some organisms (eg, *Streptococcus agalactiae*) the iron bound in lactoferrin is relatively unavailable to the Enterobacteriacae. The lactoferrin activity is enhanced in the dry gland by increased concentrations and a higher lactoferrin to citrate concentration (Sordill et al., 1987). Citrate competes with lactoferrin for iron-iron bound to citrate is available to the Enterobacteriacae. Lactoferrin is also immunomodulatory to leucocytes (Smith and Oliver, 1981), and can act synergistically with IgG1 against *E. coli* and *Klebsiella* spp (Oliver and Bushe (1987). Leucocyte concentration rises during the dry period (Jensen and Eberhart, 1981; McDonald and Anderson, 1981) and the mammary environment becomes more conducive to leucocyte function (Sordillo and Nickerson, 1988) as fat and casein concentrations in the mammary secretion drop. Immunoglobulin concentrations are also higher in the nonlactating gland (Eberhart, 1986).

During the transition to colostrogenesis, the mammary gland again becomes more susceptible to intramammary infection; as the levels of protective factors become diluted, the keratin plug breaks down and leucocyte function becomes impaired, coupled with the fact that antibiotic levels have dropped below the minimum inhibitory concentration (MIC) in cows that received antibiotic dry cow therapy (DCT) at drying off (Bradley and Green, 2004).

The importance of the dry period in control of environmental streptococcal IMI cannot be over emphasized (McDonald and Anderson, 1981; Todhunter *et al.*, 1995).

1.7 Milk yield and flow rate

Discussion is ongoing as to whether very high yielding cows have an increased risk of intramammary infection (Waage *et al.*, 1998; Suriyasathaporn *et al.*, 2000; Kornalijnslijper, 2003). High yielding cows are generally considered to be more susceptible to intramammary infection e.g. Holstein Frisian (HF), Jersey or HF and Jersey cross bred dairy cows are more susceptible to mastitis than Desi (Zebu) breeds of cows (Sharma, 2003) it might be due to more resistance to disease and they are low milk producer than cross bred cows. There is substantial evidence to suggest that high yielders are linked to high mastitis level (Sharma, 2003) and a genetic correlation between milk yield and clinical mastitis has been reported (Syvajarvi *et al.*, 1986). Kavitha *et al.* (2009) has also been reported that high milk yielding (4-7 lit.) buffaloes are more prone to mastitis when compared to low milk yielding buffaloes. In observational studies high producing herds typically showed higher rates of clinical mastitis (Sato *et al.*, 2008). A relationship between peak flow rate and mastitis has been found in several studies (Duda, 1995; Lacy-Hulbert and Hillerton, 1995; Dodenhof *et al.*, 1999; Rupp and Boichard, 1999). Cow with an increased milk flow and a yield of over 5.2 kg of milk during the first two minutes of milking are prone to mastitis. Miller *et al.* (1976) reported that cows with high milk yield have high milk flow rate and more susceptibility to mastitis. While some researchers have found no significant correlation between yield and incidence of infection and mastitis (Schmidt and Van Vleck, 1965; Smith and Schultze, 1970; Geer *et al.*, 1979). Relationships between milking characteristics and incidence of mammary infections remain, therefore much debated. Capuco *et al.* (1990) hypothesized that, as milk production increases, more keratin is lost during milking. Cows with higher milk yield often exhibit higher peak flow rates (Wagner and Ruegg, 2002; Inderwies *et al.*, 2003). Thelitis is a common complication of mastitis in heifers and often leads to a narrow and rigid teat canal, thereby altering the flow rate. In high yielding cows intramammary pressure is higher, probably due to larger vertical milk columns in the udder cisterns (Bruckmaier, personal communication). Quarter peak flow rate of >1.6 kg/min (compared to <0.8 kg/min) was associated with a *12 fold increase* in IMI (Grindal and Hillerton, 1991) and udder peak flow rate as well as mean flow rate of 3.5-4.0 kg/min was associated with the lowest IMI rate (Roth *et al.*, 1998). Higher flow rates and higher milk yield are associated with higher stretchability of the teat canal (Rathore and Sheldrake, 1977), and are caused by a combination of thinner teat walls and the fact that the teat canal is surrounded by a small volume of elastic tissue (rear versus front quarters, Ledu *et al.*, 1994). This may increase the penetrability of the teat canal. The increased volume of milk in the gland is thought to lower the concentration of the protective factors found in milk (Paape *et al.*, 1992). It is perhaps therefore not surprising to find that an increase in milk yield at drying off is positively associated with an increase in new intramammary infection. The funnel shape teats produced more milk than cylindrical shape teats (Prajapati *et al.*, 1995). However, effect of teat shape was not significant on milk flow rate (Tilki *et al.*, 2005). They also reported a significant negative correlation of milking time with milk flow rate. It can be said that milk flow rate increased with milk yield and extended milking time.

1.8 Milking interval

The dairy cow and buffaloes becomes adjusted to regular feeding and milking at fixed period's interval. Hence, deviations from the regular schedules are not conducive to complete emptying of the udder, since some cows and buffaloes may hold up their milk. The influence of an irregular interval between morning and evening milking (<12 or >12 hours/day) on the prevalence of mastitis may have been the consequence of an enhanced chance for bacteria to colonize teat ends and streak canals during the longer milking intervals (Doherr *et al.*, 2007). The number of quarters with milk leaking is well known to increase with prolonged intervals between milkings. Leaking of milk has a significant effect on the occurrence of clinical mastitis (Schukken *et al.*, 1991; Elbers *et al.*, 1998) which is assumed to result in enhanced frequency of sub-clinical mastitis. If these practices are continued at irregular intervals throughout a lactation period, the physiological effect on the secretory tissue and secretion may enhance the multiplication of the bacteria existing in the udder and may also provide a favourable environment for new bacterial visitations when they occur (Little and Plastrdge, 1946). Therefore, it is suggested that milking should be done at fixed time interval to reduce the incidence of mastitis.

1.9 Udder defense and Milk factors

There are a number of mechanisms employed by the cow in order to prevent infection. To prevent bacteria entering the teat canal, there is a sphincter muscle that surrounds the canal and ensures that it is closed between milkings. In addition, the teat canal produces antimicrobial substances, to act against any bacteria that enter the duct. Humoral and cellular factors inhibiting bacterial growth are in normal milk and in greater concentration in mastitic milk (Jain, 1979). Cell-free normal milk possesses a variable degree of growth inhibitory activity for *Streptococci*, *Staphylococci*, and *Coliform* organisms (Schalm *et al.*, 1971). Lactoferrin is bacteriostatic in vitro for a variety of bacteria because of its iron-chelating ability which makes iron non-available for bacterial growth. However, this line of defence is of a lesser importance during streptococcal infections, due to their relatively low requirement for iron during growth. Lactoferrin is low in normal milk, and in higher concentrations in dry secretion and mastitic milk. Thus, it is conjectured to play a role in protecting the mammary gland from infections during dry period and in controlling bacterial growth during mastitis (Harmon *et al.*, 1975). The presence of other substances such as immunoglobins, lysozymes and lactoperoxidase inhibit the proliferation of pathogens within the udder. The decrease in concentration of inhibitory substances in the udder during the periparturient period is thought to enable bacteria to proliferate and cause mastitis. A potent bactericidal system for *Coliform* organisms consists of antibody and complement and is in serum, milk, and colostrum (Schalm, *et al.*, 1971). The concentration or activity of this system in milk is dependent upon the degree of vascular permeability of the udder, i.e., the activity increases with the severity of mastitis (Jain, 1979). If bacteria do manage to enter the gland, the number of leukocytes, particularly neutrophils, massively increases within the milk. Their main role at this site is to engulf and kill invading pathogens (Jain, 1976). However, cells from milk seem to be less efficient phagocytes because of their i) reduced glycogen content which is thought to provide energy for phagocytosis, ii) surface coating of milk casein which seems to inhibit phagocytosis, and iii) ingestion of milk fat globules which makes the neutrophils less accommodative for bacteria (Jain, 1979; Paape and Wergin, 1977). Normal milk opsonizes bacteria for easy phagocytosis, and mastitic milk is superior in this respect because of its content of serum opsonins. The main function of immunoglobulins in secretions of the bovine mammary gland is opsonization of microorganisms for phagocytosis by leukocytes, but they also play a role as antitoxin (Nickerson, 1989). Immunoglobulins, mainly isotype IgG1, is selectively transferred into mammary secretions from blood; thus, it is the major isotype in mammary secretionsfor all stages of lactation. Bovine colostrum contains IgM antibodies and heat labile factor(s) which opsonize *E. coli* (Seto *at al.*, 1976). Mononuclear cells are generally numerous in milk from noninfected glands and in dry secretion. A part of the cells designated as *"epithelial cells"* in such secretions are macrophages (Jensen and Eberhart, 1975) and may, therefore, appear to provide another cellular barrier to infection. The milking process itself also reduces the level of bacterial colonisation in the mammary gland, due to the flushing action of the milk washing out any bacteria that are present. This is one reason why the gland is at a greater risk of infection during the dry period.

1.10 Milk somatic cells

Milk somatic cell count (SCC) is widely known to be an important risk factor for clinical mastitis (Suriyasathaporn *et al.*, 2000; Green *et al.*, 2007). It has been observed that low somatic cell counts (<100,000 cells/ml) are associated with increased incidence of toxic mastitis (Green *et al.*, 1996). There is continued debate as to whether a high somatic cell count (>200,000 cells/ml) is protective or simply an indication of the cows' ability to mount a rapid leucocyte response to infection. It is suggested that only a rapid and early neutrophilia within the milk will enable the infection to be overcome, otherwise clinical mastitis will develop. Normally, low bulk milk somatic cell count (BMSCC) in a herd is closely related to low individual SCC, indicating a low prevalence of sub-clinical mastitis. A decrease in BMSCC is associated with an increased risk for clinical mastitis in heifers (Waage *et al.*, 1998), but, in a study on summer mastitis (Hillerton *et al.*, 1995), increased risk is associated with a high BMSCC. Steeneveld *et al.* (2008) study indicates that SCC in the previous month and SCC in the previous lactation are significant cow-specific risk factors for an increased individual risk for clinical mastitis.

1.11. Udder conformation

Approximate averages of heritabilities are: udder depth- 0.25; udder support- 0.20; teat placement- 0.20; and udder quality- 0.10 (White, 1974). Norman *et al.* (1982) estimated heritabilities of 0.27 for visual udder depth and 0.12 for rear teat placement scores in Jerseys. Heritabilities of measured distance from udder floor to ground are 0.72 (Hebel et al., 1979), 0.38 (Shanks and Spahr, 1982), and 0.23 (Shanks and Spahr, 1982). Heritabilities of udder cleft are different as reported by various workers like 0.11 (Shaeffer, 1983), 0.09 (Seykora, 1983), and 0.12 (Thomas *et al.*, 1981). These heritabilities support genetic variation for udder conformation. Cows with poor conformation are *3.7 times* more likely to have mastitis than cows with good conformation (Jagoe, 2009). The same author has also been mentioned that the evidence from the study that cows with short teats, those with engorged udders at calving and those milked for the first time more than 12 hours after calving had a greater risk of *S. uberis* mastitis. Cows leaking milk before calving have *1.8 times* more likely to have mastitis due to *S. uberis*. A smooth muscle sphincter surrounds the teat canal holding it closed, thus preventing the leakage of milk and serving as the body's first line of defence against intra-mammary infection (IMI). After milking, this sphincter remains dilated for 1-2 hours, allowing bacteria to enter the teat canal (Sieber and Farnsworth, 1981; Neijenhuis *et al.*, 2000). Therefore teat-ends with a shape that allows the sphincter to remain dilated for longer periods are likely to predispose cows to IMI (Bhutto *et al.*, 2008). The various udder characteristics e.g. udder and teat size, low udders, udder depth, wide teats, large teats, flat teat ends, and fast milking speed are associated with increased risk for mastitis (Monardes *et al.*, 1990; Rogers *et al.*, 1991; Slettbakk *et al.*, 1995; Klaas *et al.*, 2004; Klaas *et al.*, 2005; Kamboj et al., 2008). Bjorck (1963) classifies udder as globular, trough shaped, bowl shaped and pendulous and further informed that pendulous udders are more prone for mastitis. A study was conducted on types of udders and teats in buffaloes by Khire *et al.* (1975) and reported that Murrah and Nagpuri buffaloes had 70% and 67.87% trough shaped udder. However, 83.33% Murrah buffaloes had cylindrical teats and 59.25% Nagpuri buffaloes had clinical teats. Khire *et al.* (1976) also studied on the type of udders and teats with relation to milk production in cows and found that Sahiwal cows showed higher proportion of trough shaped udders (63.72%) and cylindrical teats (51.96%), while, crossbred cows had higher percentage of globular udder and cylindrical teats.

Gajbhiye (1996) reported that the pendulous udders had highest incidence of mastitis (82%). The report of Gajbhiye (1996) is supported by the Kamboj *et al.* (2008), they also observed that highest (93.54%) incidence of sub-clinical mastitis was in pendulous shaped udder of cows followed by unbalanced (41.66%), goat type (33.33%), round (26.31%) and trough shaped udders (10.95%). Higher incidence of sub-clinical mastitis in pendulous udders may be attributed to nearness of teats to the ground and thus higher chances of injury to the udder in view of week suspensory ligaments in pendulous udders. Incidence of mastitis increases as the length of udder increased. The udders with lengths >65cm are significantly more affected (54.45%) than the udders with their lengths between 47 and 65cm (33.89%) and <47cm (5.26%) (Kanboj *et al.*, 2008). Kanboj *et al.* (2008) also found that udders are more sensitive to IMI those have width >76cm as compared to udders with their widths between 76 to 57cm or <57cm, and udders with circumference >110cm than the udders with circumference between 110 to 81cm or <81cm.

Teat-end shape varied from pointed to inverted, milk flow rate increased. Five classes of teat-end shape have been used by researchers to describe variation (Appleman, 1973): pointed, round, fiat, disk or plate shape, and inverted (also described as cone, concave, inverted funnel, and pocketed). Lojda *et al.* (1976) classified teat orifice location as either *central* or *eccentric*. Location of the teat canal orifice had no influence on incidence of sub-clinical mastitis. Using radiographic techniques, Appleman (1970) found teat ends that were disk or inverted had wider streak canals than those with pointed or round teat ends. Flat ends were intermediate. Inverted teat ends have advantages of eversion resistance and higher milk flow. Less pointed and more inverted teat-ends have been associated with increased susceptibility to mastitis as they retain milk which can act as a substrate for bacterial growth (Chrystal *et al.*, 2001) and have more dilated sphincters that facilitate bacterial invasion (Appleman, 1973). Milk is apt to stay at the bottom of the cone and serve as a substrate for multiplication of bacteria and find their way into the teat cistern. The larger diameter of streak canals associated with inverted teat ends also may allow bacteria easier access to the teat cistern and increase probability to intramammary infection. Majority of studies found that cows with inverted or disk-shaped teat ends had significantly higher incidences of mastitis than cows with round teat ends (Lojda *et al.*, 1976; Macha *et al.*, 1981; Seykora, 1983). Pointed teat ends may be subject to more irritation from longer milking times. Although Bakken (1981) found that prevalence of sub-clinical mastitis was higher for cows with inverted teat ends than for other shaped teats, the difference was not statistically significant (P>.05). The relationship between teat-end shape and mastitis may also differ for breeds and environments. Hindquarters of the udder have also been consistently found to have a higher incidence of clinical mastitis than forequarters (Sharma *et al.*, 2007). The hindquarters are more susceptible to infection through the higher probability of contamination with faeces because of their more caudo-ventral position.

It has been reported that cows with increased milk leakage, increased milk flow, asymmetric udders and flat/wide teat-ends were considered to be more susceptible to clinical mastitis (Slettbakk *et al.*, 1995). These characteristics may be important because they increase the chance of injury and exposure to pathogens from the cow's environment. However, increased mastitis associated with some or all of these udder characteristics may result from increased liner slips (Rogers and Spencer, 1991). Udder and teat morphology is very heritable (Seykora and McDaniel, 1986; Van Reden *et al.*, 1990) and could serve as a marker trait for selection to reduce mastitis in dairy cattle.

Kaiser (1975) found that cows with lighter skin pigmentation about the udders and teats appeared to be more susceptible to irritation of teat skin from harsh environment. However, Thomas *et al.* (1981) saw no relationship between pigmentation and teat soreness for suckled cows. Seykora (1983) computed the heritability of teat pigmentation 0.55, but pigmentation was not associated with somatic cell count.

1.12 Teat length and diameter

The size of teat has significant relationship with milk production (Tomer and Tomer, 1960). The correlations between teat length and clinical mastitis is high and high incidence for cows with long teats (Jong and Lansbergen, 1996). Hence, short teats are significantly superior for level of production and had less chances of mastitis (Hickman, 1964). While the findings of Rupp and Boichard (1999) and Boettcher *et al.* (1998) are not in support of Jong and Lansbergen (1996) reports. Heritabilities is 0.25 for teat length and 0.13 for teat wall thickness (Hebel *et al.*, 1979). Seykora (1983) reported heritabilities between 0.26 and 0.63 for teat size. A study involving German Black Pied cows showed heritabilities of 0.60 and 0.67 for teat length and width (Fiedler *et al.*, 1982). Size of teats has been associated with milking rate, injury, and mastitis infection (Seykora and McDaniel, 1985). Although Johansson and Malven (1960) found significant negative correlation between teat length and milk flow rate. The quarters with teat length <4cm have lower incidence of sub-clinical mastitis (17.39%) than quarters with teat lengths between 4 and 7cm (24.33%) or >7cm (28.12%) (Kamboj et al., 2008). Ovesen (1972) concluded that teat length influenced both average milk flow rate and yield on hand stripping. Cows with shorter teats milked faster and more completely. Teat diameter did not influence milking rate, but cows with teats of smaller diameter milked more completely, so there is no chance of retention of milk in teat and decrease the possibilities of intramammary infection. Rathore and Sheldrake (Rathore and Sheldrake, 1977) reported that the teats of larger diameter had larger orifices. Part of the correlation between teat orifice and mastitis may be due to older cows having both larger teats and more relaxed sphincter muscles (Appleman, 1970). Hickman (1964) reported incidence of mastitis increased proportionally to teat diameter. When teat thickness increases more than 5% (caliper measurement), teat duct microbial colonization is greater (Zecconi *et al.*, 1992).

1.13 Teat Shape

Teat shapes typically have been classified into three classes: funnel shaped, cylindrical, and bottle (Seykora and McDaniel, 1985). Cylindrical seems to be the most prevalent in dairy cows. Hickman (1964) found that cows with funnel-shaped teats had a significantly lower frequency of mastitis than those having cylindrically-shaped teats. Other researchers had also been reported that cows with cylindrical shape teats showed a higher incidence of mastitis (Prajapati *et al.*, 1995). It is hypothesized that the difference may be due to less teat cup crawl for cows with funnel-shaped teats. Funnel-shaped teats offered greater resistance to being drawn into the teat cup and appeared to milk out more completely Rathore (1977a). He also speculated that on cylindrical and bottle-shaped teats, the teat cups caused occlusion of the orifice between the gland sinus and teat sinus, causing a decrease and then complete stoppage of milk flow. This may cause traumatization of the teat-end orifice. Rathore (1977b) found that teat-end erosion was more frequent in cylindrical teats (22%) than funnel-shaped teats (7%). Gajbhiye (1996) studied the udder and teat shape and its relation with udder health in 256 crossbred cows and reported that crossbred cows had higher incidence of globular udders (59.84%) and cylindrical teats (80.90%). Kamboj *et al.* (2008) found that quarters with cylindrical teats had significantly higher (41.59%) incidence of sub-clinical mastitis followed by conical (15.63%) and bottle shaped (13.18%) teats. Another study is also showed that higher incidence in cylindrical teats (25%) followed by funnel (10.95%) and bottle shaped teats (9.09%) in buffaloes

(Shinde *et al.,* 2002). Although, Lojda *et al.* (1976) found no significant relationship between teat shape and incidence of sub-clinical mastitis, while Bakken (1981) found funnel-shaped teats had slightly higher incidence of *Stapbylococcus aureus* mastitis.

1.14 Teat end sphincter

At the end of the teat is surrounded by sphincter composed of circular smooth muscle fibers which remains constricted and prevent leakage of milk until milking commence and entry of the organisms into the teat canal. The a- and b-receptors are present in the circular smooth muscles of the bovine teats. Activation of b-receptors provokes relaxation of the teat and opening of the streak canal. The number and ratio of both receptor types may differ in different animals. Roets *et al.* (1986) suggested that this receptor distribution in the bovine teat is, to a great extent, responsible for the differences in the rate of milking between cows. Milking characteristics are highly correlated with the $b_2 : a_2$ adrenoceptor density ratios in teat tissue. Fast milkers have a low $b_2 : a_2$ ratio. Teats with weak, relaxed or incompetent sphincters are termed as *"patent"* or *"leaky teats"*. Animals with leaky teats are milk out within 2 to 3 minutes but are more prone to mastitis (Heald, 1985). Whereas, cows having teats with tight sphincters or narrow diameter teat canals are called *"hard milkers"* because milk flow is very slow. The hard milking cow takes about more than 10 minutes to complete milk out. The smooth muscle sphincter surrounding the teat canal inhibits bacterial penetration (infection) by maintaining tight closure of teat orifice. Loss of muscle tone increases susceptibility to mastitis.

The sphincter muscle surrounding the teat duct is tightly closed between milkings and impedes bacterial intrusion from the teat opening into the interior of the gland (Nickerson, 1994). During milking, the teat end sphincter is opening and closing about *60 times per minute*. At the end of milking, the muscles in the sphincter are fatigued, leaving the sphincter open for a period of time. Until the sphincter recovers and closes tightly (within 30-45 minutes), the mammary gland is at high risk for new infections if the teat end is place on bedding or in manure. Murphy (1944) observed that quarters having patent streak canals had greater likelihood of being infected. Redaelli *et al.* (1972) obtained a significant correlation of 0.10 between external diameter of the teat canal sphincter and *Streptococcus agalactiae* mastitis. The common route of mammary infections by the penetration of microorganisms through the teat canal with a few exceptions e.g. Tuberculous mastitis route is haematogenous. Hence the importance of the sphincter which ensures the closing of the end of the teat canal between milkings. The size of the streak canal and patency of the sphincter muscle are important in preventing invasion of bacteria into the teat cistern. Teat sphincter patency is usually estimated by the ease with which the quarter can be milked (Poutrel, 1982). A recommended animal husbandry practice is to prevent the cows from lying down until the teat canal has closed, to prevent bacterial penetration. By providing fresh feed after milking, the cows will remain standing to eat while the sphincter closes thus reducing the risk of infection (Kirk, 2000).

1.15 Teat injuries

Maintenance of healthy teat skin and teat-ends is a key part of any effective mastitis control program. Given that most mastitis-causing pathogens are thought to gain entry to the mammary gland through the streak canal, the presence and shape of teat-end lesions play an important role in the pathogenesis of the mastitis. Changes to teat tissue, particularly the skin of the barrel, teat-end, and teat canal may favor penetration of bacteria into the udder and increase the risk of new mastitis infections (Hamann *et al.*, 1994).

In India, cows and buffaloes are mainly reared in the poor hygienic environment by households except well organized dairy farms and used hand milking using calf suckling which may cause some injuries to the teat and cisterns membrane resulting increase the risk for mastitis. Calves may be vector of mastitis either by direct injury or by carrying infectious material to the teat orifice. Teat orifice and the teat itself may be injured by biting, squeezing or by abrading the skin. Cows with open udder/teat injuries are at far higher risk of acquiring udder infection (clinical -25.2%, sub-clinical - 43.6%) than those with no injuries (clinical - 5.4%, sub-clinical - 12.9%) (Biffa *et al.*, 2005). Udder tick infestation is another important factor that significantly affected prevalence of mastitis. The prevalence of mastitis is higher in cows with lesions and tick infestations on the skin, udders and teats than cows without lesions. Cows with open udder/teat injuries are at far higher risk of acquiring udder infection (clinical -25.2%, sub-clinical - 43.6%) than those with no injuries (clinical - 5.4%, sub-clinical - 12.9%) (Biffa *et al.*, 2005). They collected 2500 ticks from udders of mastitis cows, *Amblyoma variegatum* were the predominant species (53.0%) followed by *Amblyoma cohaerens* (29.0%), *Amblyoma gemma* (9.0%), *Rhipicephalus evertsi* (3.5%), *Rhipicephalus parvus* (2.9%) and *Boophilus decoloratus* (2.6%). Injuries caused by ticks are known to cause direct inflammatory reaction to the mammary gland, necrosis, and abscess formation, which may lead to udder damage and/or exposure to serious secondary infections. Also, Farnsworth (1995) found that teat-ends with severe erosions that were raw and ulcerated (broken skin) showed higher prevalence of mastitis. The presence of teat-end lesions within 5 days of calving is not associated with sub-clinical or clinical mastitis (Compton *et al.*, 2007). Insect damage to teats may be caused by blood-sucking flies (most commonly mosquitoes, midges, sand-flies, black flies or biting flies), nuisance flies or wasps. Damage to the teat skin, especially cuts and chaps, provides an ideal environment for the growth of mastitis organisms such as *S. aureus* and *S. dysgalactiae*. Therefore, they are a potential source of infection of deeper parts of the udder. The efficacy of post-milking teat disinfection may also be reduced, as the solution is unable to penetrate damaged skin. For these reasons, quarters with teat lesions are often associated with an increased incidence of clinical and sub-clinical mastitis. One of the commonest and most significant forms of damage is hyperkeratosis of the teat end by milking machine. This is characterized by a smooth or roughened ring of keratin, a dry creamy white tissue, surrounding the teat sphincter. Keratin acts like 'blotting paper', mopping up many bacteria present or trying to penetrate teat canal (Edmondson, 2001). All lesions are not damaged teat ends but may be normal teat-end morphology and to some degree genetic.

1.16 Previous exposure to mastitis

A greater probability of developing clinical mastitis is expected in cows that experienced clinical mastitis in the previous lactation and/or previously within the same lactation (Zadoks *et al.*, 2001; Berry and Meaney, 2005). If a cow have mastitis in the previous lactation, is 2.6 times more likely to have *S. uberis* mastitis this lactation (Jagoe, 2009). The increased susceptibility of cows infected in the preceding lactation, to new IMI at the subsequent calving, was identified by Browning *et al.* (1994). A positive association has been established between prepartum and postpartum intramammary infection e.g. quarter level prevalence of IMI was 18.5% precalving in heifers which was increased from 18.5% to 21.5% post calving or in subsequent lactation (Compton *et al.*, 2007; Aarestrup and Jensen, 1997). The probability of clinical mastitis occurring in cows that experienced at least one case of clinical mastitis in the previous lactation is 0.92 to 3.75 times that of a cow that experienced no clinical mastitis in the previous lactation (Berry and Meaney, 2005). Houben *et al.* (1993) reported that the risk of a cow developing clinical mastitis in the subsequent month of lactation is also a function of number of cases of clinical mastitis in the previous lactation, number of clinical cases in the previous months of the current lactation, and the occurrence of clinical mastitis in the current month. They found that the risk of contracting clinical mastitis is 4.8 times greater if the animal experienced clinical mastitis in the previous stage of lactation. Rowlands *et al.* (1986) reported that clinical mastitis occurred in 38% of cows that experienced clinical mastitis in the previous lactation, as opposed to 23% of those that had not. Cows with repeated episodes (>2) of udder infection are more affected by sub-clinical mastitis (42.7%) whereas those exposed only once are more affected by clinical mastitis (62.8%) (Biffa *et al.*, 2005).

1.17 Other diseases

Several epidemiological studies have demonstrated that there is an association between the development of metabolic disease and subsequent development of mastitis. The conditions that cause the animal to stay recumbent, such as lameness, hypocalcaemia or downer cow syndrome etc. It has been reported that peri-parturient diseases significantly increased the risk of mastitis (Rahman, 2009).

Dystocia and Retention of placenta

Dystocia and retention of placenta is associated with a high prevalence of mastitis (Bendixen *et al.*, 1988; Radostits *et al.*, 2000). The research findings of Emanuelson *et al.* (1993) and Peeler et al. (1994) have also been confirmed the positive association between the development of retained placenta and the incidence of mastitis. It is assumed that these two diseases are likely linked because both are due to immune suppression in affected cows. The suppressed immune system could also explain why the same cows are more susceptible to mastitis. Retained placenta probably does not cause mastitis but is symptomatic of a depressed immune system. Schukken *et al.* (1988) had also been suggested that the relationship between retained placenta and mastitis is mediated by the peripartum peripheral leucocyte activity.

Milk fever

Milk fever is a metabolic disorder usually occurs around calving time. The name milk fever is misleading since the cow does not have a fever. Although it is more properly termed periparturient hypocalcemia or periparturient paresis, as an elevated body temperature is not typically observed. It is an afebrile disease which typically is associated with parturition and beginning lactation (Sharma, 2011). Milk fever cows are at increased risk of developing mastitis. Dairy cows with milk fever are 8 times more likely to suffer from mastitis in the following lactation (Curtis *et al.*, 1983). Calcium is necessary for proper contraction of muscle. Severe hypocalcemia prevents skeletal muscle contraction to the point that the clinical syndrome known as "milk fever" occurs. The teat sphincter consists of smooth muscle (see chapter 4), which must contract if closure of the teat end is to occur. If low blood calcium reduces teat sphincter contraction, the teat canal may remain open inviting environmental pathogens to enter the mammary gland. Milk fever cows tend to spend more time lying down than normal healthy cow. Again this could increase teat end exposure to environmental organisms. Cows typically exhibit a 3-4 fold increase in plasma cortisol as part of the act of initiation of parturition. Hypocalcemia also acts as a stressor to the cow. It is also interesting to note that animals with sub-clinically hypocalcemic cows may have 5-7 fold increases in plasma cortisol on the day of calving and the typical milk fever cow may exhibit plasma cortisol concentrations that are 10–15 fold higher than pre-calving plasma cortisol concentration (Horst and Jorgensen, 1982). These higher levels of blood cortisol result in a more severe level of immunosuppression at the time of calving, making the animal much more susceptible to infectious diseases including mastitis (Corbett, 2009). More recent research has revealed that calcium is also an integral part of the immune system and is involved in intracellular signaling factors of white blood cells (Kimura *et al.*, 2006). It has been called the "second messenger" of the immune system, and the white blood cells of animals with hypocalcemia have a reduced ability to respond to invading pathogens (Corbett, 2009).

Ketosis

Ketosis is another metabolic disease that has an adverse effect on the immune system. Any time that the blood glucose level drops to a point where the necessary energy required for cell metabolism is not met, the body starts mobilizing fat stores for energy. This fat is metabolized into glucose in the liver. During this process, metabolites called *"ketone bodies"* are produced (Corbett, 2009). An associations between physiological changes in cows in the peripartum period, such as high serum ketone (BHBA) levels and negative energy balance, which are associated with depressed immune function and increased susceptibility to mastitis (Suriyasathaporn *et al.*, 2000). Ketone body particularly beta hydroxybutyric acid (BHBA) has an adverse effect on neutrophil function in several different ways (Grinberg *et al.*, 2008). Kremer *et al.* (1993) reported that cows in negative energy balance (with elevated BHBA) prior to experimental infection of the mammary gland experienced more severe mastitis compared to cows with low blood BHBA concentrations, indicating that negative energy balance may predispose cows to severe infections. An epidemiological study found that high concentrations of plasma ketones or a loss of more than 0.5 body condition score units are significant risk factors for the development of udder edema, which then is a risk factor for the development of clinical mastitis (Compton *et al.*, 2007); however, they also found that low concentrations of non-esterified fatty acids (NEFA) is also associated with increased risk of mastitis. Hill *et al.* (1985) showed an association between accumulation of lipids in liver and increased length of bacterial shedding in cows with mastitis. A Dutch study showed that ketonemic cows had more severe mastitis than non-ketonemic cows (Kremer *et al.*, 1993). The cow can have an ongoing mastitis infection which depresses her appetite and thereby makes her prone to the secondary form of ketosis (Palmer Veterinary Clinic, 2004).

Udder edema

Udder edema is common and an important risk factor for mastitis (Compton *et al.*, 2007). The finding that udder edema in heifers increased clinical mastitis cases by 80% (Waage *et al.*, 2001). Heifers calving for the first time are more likely to develop udder edema and this often leads to mastitis (Kirk, 2009). It has been suggested that edema of the udder may predispose to mastitis (Jackson, 1996). A possible explanation for the association between edema and mastitis is that the condition impairs milk removal (Waage *et al.*, 2001) with a reduction in the physical flushing effect, which results in sufficiently increased pathogen numbers to result in clinical mastitis. As calving approaches, the blood supply to the udder increases. Venous return and lymphatic drainage of the udder may be partially occluded by the bulk of the enlarging udder itself and by changes associated with the growth of the fetus. At this time the skin of the udder may become edematous.

Brucellosis

The infection of udder with *Brucella abortus* is not only alters the character of the secretion but results in histopathological changes in the secretary tissue which stimulate a low grade mastitis. Gill (1933) claimed that *Br. abortus* infection paves the way for streptococcal mastitis and that the incidence of streptococcal infections is much more prevalent in herds that harbor *Br. abortus* infection. However, *Br. abortus* infected cows may be susceptible to bacterial infection only when the damage to the udderis severe enough to allow the components of blood to pass into the udder in sufficient amounts to change the character of the secretion (Little and Plastridge, 1946).

Foot and Mouth disease (FMD)

The viraemia is an important systemic sign in foot and mouth disease (FMD). Following a few days of viraemia, the virus appears in the milk and saliva for upto 24 hours before the appearance of vesicle in the mouth. Mammary gland is another tissue in which persistence may take place, the FMD virus living in this tissue for 3 - 7 weeks. Vesicle may occur on the teats and when the teat orifice is involved, severe mastitis often follows (Sharma, 2008). The FMD virus replicates in the secretary epithelium of bovine mammary gland.

Other viral diseases

Many other viral infections also cause lesions on the udder and teats and increase the susceptibility to development of mastitis e.g. Bovine viral papillomatosis, cow pox, pseudo cow pox, buffalo pox, bovine herpes mamillitis and Vesicular stomatitis may increase the risk for mastitis. Srimannarayana and Ramachandraiah (1999) reported that 70% of buffalo pox affected buffaloes developed mastitis.

2. Pathogen risk factors

2.1 Number of organisms and its virulence factor

The incidence of intramammary infections seems to be related to the number of organisms on the teat skin and teat end (McDonald, 1977). Streptococci and Staphylococci are in high numbers on teat skin; hence, they are the cause of most intramammary infections. Adherence of bacteria commonly associated with mastitis to epithelial cells of different regions of the mammary gland (Jain, 1979). Adherence of many pathogens generally paralleled their prevalence as cause of mastitis. For example, *S. aureus and S. Agalactiae* adhered best while *E. coli* and *Klebsiella* spp. adhered poorly. Strains of *S. agalactiae, S. uberis* and *S. dysagalactiae* varied in their ability to adhere, and, hence, their *virulence* was related to adherence, i.e., those adhering well were pathogenic. The pathogenicity of *S. aureus* depends on the combined action of more than 40 different extracellular toxins, enzymes and cell surface proteins. *S. aureus* virulence factors comprise structural components, secretory products and mechanisms that contribute to the ability of the bacteria to survive in the host cause mastitis. The protein is believed to have antiphagocytic activity especially during the later stage of intramammary infection (Forsgren *et al.*, 1983). *S. aureus* secreted or produces different exotoxins and enzymes that destroy tissue and protect bacteria from host immune response. *S. aureus* isolated from bovine mastitis express a, b, g and d hemolytic toxins (Bramley *et al.*, 1989). *Corynebacterium bovis* adhered to squamous epithelium around the teat canal and not to the ductular epithelium. Menzies *et al.* (2003) had been reported that the risk of a cow developing *E. coli* mastitis was *23 times higher* if it had received parenteral calcium. Coliform bacteria do not appear to colonize inside the mammary gland, but multiply in the secretion without attachment to epithelial surfaces. Once coliforms enter the mammary gland, they often multiply rapidly or may remain dormant for several days.

2.2 Presence of minor pathogens

The quarters that harbor minor pathogens are less susceptible to new infections by major pathogens than uninfected quarters, a phenomenon that is possibly related to the protective effect of the cell response triggered by the minor pathogens. Several studies have reported that infection by the minor pathogens *Corynebacterium bovis* and the coagulase negative Staphylococci can prevent subsequent infection with the major pathogens (Doane *et al.*, 1987). On the other hand, Pankey *et al.* (1985) reported that C. *bovis*-infected quarters challenged by immersing in broth cultures of *Staphylococcus aureus* or *Streptococcus agalactiae* were *8.5-fold more susceptible* to *S. agalactiae* infection but 50% more resistant to *S. aureus* infection. Hogan *et al.* (1988) looked at rates of environmental *Streptococcal* intramammary infection (IMI) in quarters either infected with *C. bovis* or uninfected during periods of low and high prevalence of *C. bovis* infection. Challenge was by natural exposure. Rate of environmental Streptococcal IMI was *3.9 times greater* in *C. bovis*-infected quarters than in uninfected quarters. These studies strongly suggest that C. bovis-infected quarters represent a significant risk factor for environmental *Streptococcal* infections. Several studies have demonstrated that the presence of *C. bovis* at drying off increases the risk (Pankey *et al.*, 1985; Berry and Hillerton, 2002) of new IMI during the dry period, it may be due to the keratinolytic properties (Funke *et al.*, 1997). However, other authors have found *C. bovis* to be protective during the dry period (Huxley *et al.*, 2003), and also that the early acquisition of a new *C. bovis* IMI in the late dry period offers significant protection against clinical mastitis in the subsequent lactation (Green *et al.*, 2002). The role of minor pathogens might be linked to somatic cell count levels as they may stimulate a small cellular response in the udder, or it may be that their protective role could arise from *'competitive exclusion'*. The presence of a bacteriocin known to be inhibitory to *S. aureus* was shown to reduce the incidence of infection during the dry period when used alone and in combination with a dry period internal teat sealant (Twomey *et al.*, 2000). The whole story of teat closure and the possible involvement of *C. bovis* is complex, and is an area in need of further research.

2.3 Blind treatment

Nickerson (1989) pithy a note on role of intramammary infusion during dries period on chances of occurrence of mastitis. However, dry cow therapy reduces the incidence of occurrence of new cases of IMI at the time of calving. Awareness of protective tissues of the teat end becomes very important when administering intramammary therapy at drying off. Bacteria often colonize teat duct keratin, remaining there for months, and may require some form of mechanical assistance to penetrate into cisternal areas. Recommended procedures for treatment of mastitis include insertion of the syringe canula fully into the teat orifice to expel contents into the quarter. Full insertion of the canula could force keratin against the interior teat wall, creating a larger than normal opening and stretching the sphincter muscle, thereby enhancing bacterial penetration. Full insertion also may push bacteria colonizing teat canal keratin into the teat cistern. Because secretion is not removed during the non-lactating period, bacteria are not flushed out and have a better chance of establishing infection. The intramammary infusion products are not equally effective against all pathogens, and susceptibility to new IMI varies across the dry period; therefore, therapy is not effective against environmental pathogens that cause new IMI during the prepartum period (Smith and Todhunter, 1982). Blind treatment can destroy/kill the helpful minor pathogens e.g. *Corynebacterium bovis*. Mostly in field conditions, field veterinarians are using blind treatment in mastitis cases owing to lack of antibiotic sensitivity facility. This blind or indiscriminate use of drugs causes the drug resistance and also responsible for human health hazards, as drug residue in milk. Blind treatment also reduce the percentage of cure, because if the mammary infection is fungal, while field veterinarian or practitioner is treating with antibiotics effective against only Gram positive or Gram negative bacteria. In this situation affected quarter will not cure and increase the severity and complexity of the infection.

3. Environmental Risk Factors

3.1. Climate / season / heat stress

The two important factors of heat stress namely temperature (heat) and humidity directly responsible for the occurrence of mastitis. Temperature and humidity are related to intramammary infection, occurrence of clinical mastitis and milk somatic cell count. Exposure of animals to high temperature can increase the stress of the animal and alter the immune functions and udder health (Johnson and Vanjonack, 1975). The incorrect ventilation and high temperature and relative humidity enhance the multiplication of various bacteria on the skin (and in the litter). Heat and humidity may increase the pathogen load in the environment (field or housing) (Godden et al., 2003), resulting in a greater incidence of mastitis in warm weather. Shathele (2009) reported that, the incidence of mastitis decreased with increasing ambient temperature, but increased with decreasing ambient temperature. Heat stress depresses leukocyte responses in vitro (Elvinger *et al.*, 1991) and migration of leukocytes into the mammary gland (Elvinger *et al.*, 1992). However Paape *et al.* (1972) did not observe any increase in the somatic cell count (SCC) due to thermal stress. Similarly, Batra *et al.* (1977) did not find any seasonal relationship associated with clinical mastitis. In addition, evidence suggests that some of the seasonal changes in the levels of mastitis may result from a decrease in resistance of the cow's immune system, and the endocrine system (prolactin and cortisol) may be involved (Dahl, 2004). Light and temperature both increase prolactin levels. There is a relationship between lower prepartum concentrations of prolactin and higher health and performance in the next lactation (Dahl, 2004). Breed differences in tolerance to heat stress are also evident (Keister et al., 2002), with milk production and reproductive efficiency being less depressed in Jersey than Holstein cattle and Zebu (local) cattle are also have more heat tolering capability than the cross bred cows. There are few studies on the effects of cold stress on mammary gland immunity, but it is well recognized that cold condition can cause damages to the teat skin, especially when the teats are wet after milking and teat dipping. Shathele

(2009) reported that incidence of mastitis was higher in cold months i.e. highest during January and February and lowest during May and June months. Similarly, Pyorala *et al.* (1992) also reported that lactating cows are more often affected by bacterial mastitis in winter. On the other hand, Faull *et al.* (1983) observed in England that *E. coli* clinical mastitis was higher in summer months than cold months of the year. In India, the prevalence mastitis is high in summer and rainy months and less in winter months. While Palaivel et al. (2008) reported that occurrence of mastitis was highest during summer season (53.80%) followed by winter (41.30%) and rainy season (37.50%) in Chennai, Tamilnadu. The occurrence of mastitis in different seasons depends on the agro-climatic conditions of particular region. In India, lot of variations in the agro-climatic conditions in different states. The results of Dhakal *et al.* (2007) showed that 37.3% of buffaloes had clinical mastitis during the summer season followed by the autumn season (31.7%) and minimum (7.83%) during spring season (February, March and April) in Nepal. Healthy teat skin is coated with a protective mantle of fatty acids that slow the growth of bacterial pathogens. In cold, wet and windy conditions, the skin of machine-milked teats often becomes scaly, irritated or chapped (broken) and the protective surface coating may be removed – allowing colonisation of pathogens such as *S. aureus*. Cold, wet or muddy conditions also induce hardening or thickening of teat skin. All these factors will increase the risk for infections.

3.2 Housing system

Housing of cows was positively associated with an increase in new IMI to all major pathogens, *S. uberis*, coagulase positive Staphylococci, *E. coli* and other environmental organisms. Housing facilities and management practices on farms contribute to the contamination of environments and the exposure of teats to the environmental pathogens (Smith and Hogan, 1993). Housing has been previously identified as a risk factor for clinical mastitis and is thought to be related to an increase in exposure to environmental pathogens (Barkema *et al.*, 1999). Poorly designed facilities can contribute to increased incidence of environmental mastitis. In all housing systems, high stocking density, dirty bedding or ground, poor ventilation and high humidity are important risk factors (Figure 8.3).

Poor house design where ventilation and drainage are inadequate and thereby provide a favourable, humid environment for proliferation of bacteria. High levels of pathogen exposure during periods of heightened susceptibility lead to increased herd mastitis and these conditions frequently come together during the dry period (Smith and Hogan, 2009). Management risk factors include overcrowding, inadequate removal of slurry, infrequent replacement of dry bedding, use of rubber mats, inadequate training of young stock to use cubicles, extended or continuous housing of the herd and housing at or near the start of the calving period. Organic bedding materials can contain large numbers of both the coliform bacteria and the environmental streptococci and are a significant source of teat end contamination in the environments of dairy cows (Hogan and Smith, 1992). Organic bedding materials retain moisture and act as a food source for bacteria. Seasonal effects on bacterial numbers occur in most herds with significantly higher numbers in summer compared to winter. Wood products such as sawdust are known to promote coliform mastitis while straw bedding is a good source of the environmental streptococci. The housing of cows on sand yards as compared to straw yards was associated with a decrease in new IMI to *S. uberis*. Sand is the ideal bedding for dairy cows, is inorganic and does not support the growth of the environmental pathogens (Smith and Hogan, 2009). A study in India is also found that the incidence of mastitis is less on sand flooring than concrete, and that when soil was used as the bedding material, the incidence was high (Kavitha *et al.*, 2009). Pastured cows are generally thought to be at reduced risk for environmental mastitis when compared to cows in confinement housing (Smith and Hogan, 2009). In all housing systems, high stocking density, dirty bedding or ground, and high humidity are important risk factors.

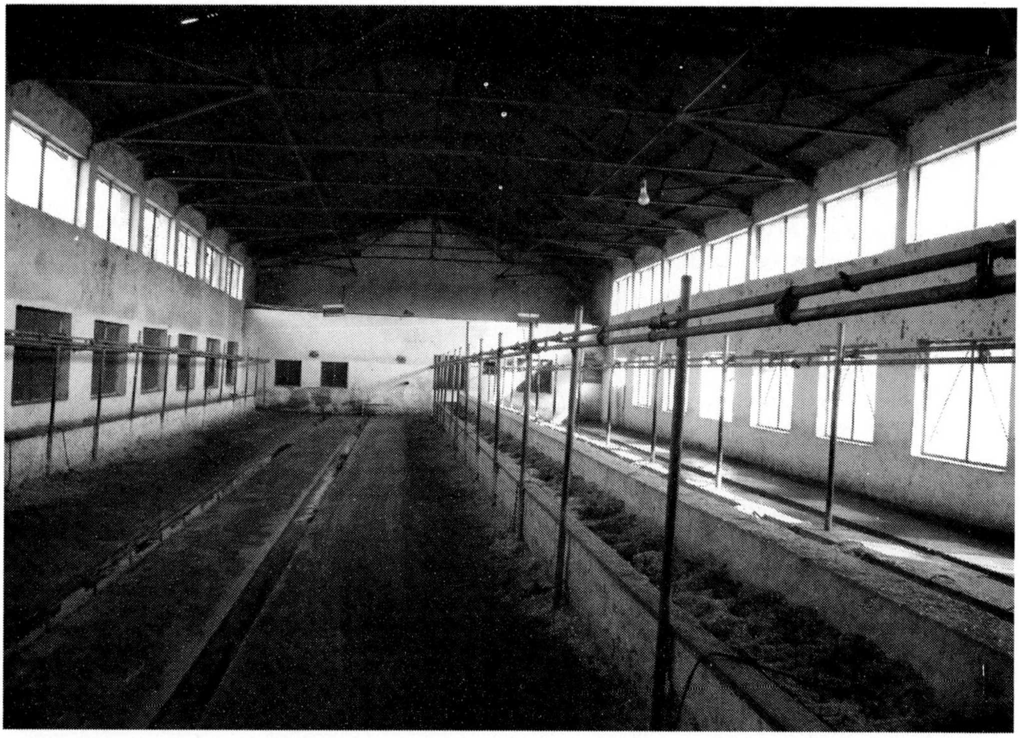

Figure 8.3: Good ventilation of housing is an essential component for minimizing proliferation of opportunistic organisms.

The faulty construction of barns and paddocks may contribute to injury of the udder and teat and thus predispose these parts to infection. Poorly constructed manure gutters, short and narrows stalls, and stalls without partitions predispose the udders and teats to injury, especially when cows can tread on one another's teats. When cows are lying down, the pressure of the uppermost leg on the distended udder may cause a relaxation of the sphincter of the teat duct, allowing milk to trickle through and moisten the teat orifice. Thus, if the teat end comes in contact with dirty bedding, manure gutters, or dirty floors, bacteria may be sucked up into the opening of the teat duct as soon as the pressure is released (Little and Plastridge, 1946). Housing and poor hygiene are associated with a higher risk for both clinical (Barkema *et al.,* 1999) and sub-clinical mastitis (Ekman, 1998).

3.3 Milking hygiene/Udder hygiene

Most of the pathogen transmits during milking via milker's hand, contaminated bedding and contact of teats with rear legs, tail switch, flies and wallowing in the contaminated water. Milking hygiene reduce the pathogenic organisms from inhabiting the immediate environment or skin of the animals and minimizing their spread during milking process. The practice of regular teat dipping is not much more common at house hold level in India. Therefore, prevalence of mastitis in cows and buffaloes is more at unorganized dairy farms as compared to organized dairy farms. Udder hygiene significantly associated with the risk of environmental pathogen intramammary infection in cows (Schreiner and Ruegg, 2003; Compton *et al.,* 2007). The presence of mastitis pathogens on teat ends is associated with the increased risk of IMI. Moisture, mud, and manure present in the environment of the cow are the primary sources of exposure for environmental mastitis pathogens, and hygiene scores of cows provide visible evidence of exposure to these potential sources. The use of high concentrate diets associated with looser feces and reduction in cow and facility cleanliness. Several studies have identified relationships between cow cleanliness and measures of milk quality (Reneau *et al.,* 2003; Schreiner and Ruegg, 2003). Unhygienic practices during the milking process can also provide an opportunity for environmental pathogens to gain access to the udder as does improper disinfection of the milk plant.

3.4 Milking machine

Milking machines are used more than most other pieces of equipment on the dairy farm and yet their function, maintenance and potential contribution to mastitis incidents are poorly understood by many farmers. Milking machines can influence the incidence of mastitis in one of the five ways (Edmondson, 2001): a) by acting as a fomite, b) by causing damage to the teat canal, c) by generating impact forces for reverse pressure gradients, c) colonization of the teat canal and, d) as a result of over/under milking. If there is poor pulsation and milk flow rates are reduced, the shear forces may not remove the excess keratin as effectively, leading to a build up in bacterial colonization of the teat canal. The bacteria may continue to grow up into the teat sinus and results in a new infection (Edmondson, 2001). The risk of new IMI by contagious as well as environmental pathogens such as *Streptococcus uberis* is increased by machine-induced changes such as greater degree of openness of the teat canal orifice after milking (Mein *et al.*, 2001). *Corynebacterium bovis* is a commensal of the teat canal. If it found in large numbers, this indicates a problem either with post-milking teat disinfection or the milking machine. It has been shown that poor liner wall movement, as a consequence of pulsation failure, can double the rate of new infection and also lead to an increase in petechial haemorrhaging of the teat (Mein *et al.*, 1983). Teat cup liner slips during milking have been implicated as a cause of new infections of the bovine udder (Spencer, 1989). It is thought that liner slips lead to new infections because they cause an abrupt loss of milking vacuum that may move pathogens located at the teat opening or within the streak canal into the teat cistern (Rogers and Spencer, 1991).

Mechanical forces during machine milking may induce changes in teat-end tissue. The white ring around the teat orifice is callus and is induced by milking. Teat end callosity (TEC) is a teat condition state that influences the resistance of the teat canal. Callus results from hyperkeratosis or hypertrophy of the corneous layer or *stratum corneum* of the skin (Neijenhuis, 2004). Teat-end callosity builds up until approximately 4 months of lactation and decreases thereafter (Neijenhuis *et al.*, 2000). Cow factors like teat-end shape, teat position, teat length, milk yield, stage of lactation, and parity are associated with the degree of TEC (Bakken, 1981; Graf, 1982; Neijenhuis *et al.*, 2000; Rathore, 1977; Sieber and Farnsworth, 1981). Severe teat-end lesions (erosions or scabs) are positively associated with the prevalence of sub-clinical mastitis (Sieber and Farnsworth, 1981; Jackson, 1970). Clinical mastitis cows had more TEC than their healthy herd mates, particularly when clinical mastitis occurred between the second and fifth months of lactation. Clinical *Escherichia coli* mastitis in the second or third month of lactation occurred in cows with less TEC than in cows with clinical mastitis caused by other pathogens (Neijenhuis *et al.*, 2001). The level of teat end callocity thickness (TECT) was higher in the clinical mastitis quarter than in the lateral healthy quarter within a cow, before and particularly during and after occurrence of clinical mastitis (Neijenhuis *et al.*, 2001). An increase in the risk of intramammary infection (IMI) is observed when thickness and/or roughness of TEC increase. This is caused by less tightly closed teat canals after milking, a too high turnover of keratin, or the harbouring of pathogens in TEC (Neijenhuis, 2004). The higher risk of IMI in teats without a callosity ring may be caused by a decreased rate of keratin regeneration in the teat canal. Increase in teat end callocity thickness and teat end callocity roughness can be used as an early warning signal for increased risk of clinical mastitis (Neijenhuis, 2004).

3.5 Milking techniques

Different types of milking methods (e.g. Stripping, knuckling, full hand method, machine milking etc.) are practiced by dairy farmers to milk out the animal. The milking procedure is one of the most important risk factors for both clinical mastitis and high SCC (Barkema *et al.*, 1999). Malfunctioning machine milking, knuckling and stripping method of milking can induce damage to the teat tissue increasing the risk for intramammary infections. The incidence of clinical and sub-clinical mastitis is high in buffaloes those are milked by knuckling method rather than stripping on comparison with the full-hand method (Kavitha *et al.*, 2009). Incomplete milking out is also an important risk factor. It is found that the act of milking on a dry teat, whether due to improper stimulation of the cow or over milking, increased severity of teat-end lesions (Sieber *et al.*, 1980). The milking routine is also very important. It is important to identify the cows during milking, which have mastitis. Mastitis cows should be milked last, or separately, to avoid spread of bacteria among animals. Try to avoid any type of stress during milking i.e. milking should be done in calm environment. Because stress can lead to milk retention by inhibiting oxytocin-mediated reflexes (Johansson, 2000). New environment, new milkers, painful milking technique and pain due to udder oedema are factors, which can be stressful for the animal. Inhibition of milk-let-down can cause sub-clinical mastitis to become clinical and will affect milk production.

It has been suggested that overmilking may increase the risk of intramammary infection. Dodd *et al.* (1950) found that the new infection rate increased almost 4 fold after cows were overmilked by 5 minutes. The overmilking for 5 minutes over a four months period caused teat sinus injury and loss of teat keratin. Hillerton *et al.* (1999) also demonstrated that the longer cows are overmilked, the greater the level of teat congestion, while overmilking has been demonstrated in several experiments to increase the level of teat orifice erosion. Undermilking may likewise have an influence on mastitis particularly on *S. agalactiae* infections because remaining milk in the udder acts as better growth media for bacterial growth and they multiply and increase in number between milkings.

3.6 Dietary factors

Nutrition can have significant effects on the cow's immune system, thereby affecting infection rate and severity of mastitis. The immune system has high requirements for specific nutrients and when these nutrients are not provided

in adequate amounts, immune function may suffer (Weiss, 2009). Work of the past 10 years has clearly demonstrated that diets of dairy cows can influence the resistance of cows to intramammary infection (Smith and Hogan, 1993). Specific components of diets that have been shown to be important are vitamins E, A, and β-carotene and the trace minerals selenium, copper, and zinc. Evidence clearly shows that vitamin E and selenium influence phagocytic cell function, and cows fed diets deficient in either component are at greater risk of environmental streptococcal mastitis (Smith *et al.*, 1984). The risk of low blood and tissue concentrations of vitamin E and selenium appears to be greatest around calving, a period of known high susceptibility to environmental streptococci (Smith and Hogan, 2009). Vitamin E and selenium improved udder health, and the effect of dietary supplementation is most evident at calving and in early lactation (Sharma and Maiti, 2005). Deficiencies in vitamin E and selenium lead to autooxidative damage to plasma membranes and elements of the cytoskeleton, resulting in impaired phagocytic cell function, a condition that would predispose cows to mastitis. Supplemental vitamin E and/or Se has been shown to reduced prevalence and severity of mastitis (Sharma and Maiti, 2005; Smith *et al.*, 1997). Conversely, a study conducted on commercial farms in Sweden found no reduction in clinical mastitis or SCC in early lactation when cows were supplemented with approximately 2200 IU of vitamin E/day (Waller *et al.*, 2007). The positive effect of Se supplementation on clinical mastitis is probably mediated via effects of Se on neutrophils and other immune cells. Vitamin C (ascorbic acid) is probably the most important water soluble antioxidant in mammals. Most forms of vitamin C are extensively degraded in the rumen, but cows can synthesize vitamin C and it is not considered an essential nutrient for cattle. The concentration of ascorbic acid is high in neutrophils and increases as much as 30-fold when the neutrophil is stimulated (Weiss, 2009).

Similarly, deficiencies in vitamin A and β-carotene are associated with increased incidence of mastitis. Low concentrations of plasma vitamin A (<80 μg/dl) and β-carotene (<200 μg/dl) are associated with severity of mastitis (Chew *et al.*, 1982). Chew and Johnston (1985) supplemented 60 Holstein cows with vitamin A and β-carotene starting at 30 d prepartum, continuing for 10 weeks postpartum, and found that supplementation reduced milk SCC during the subsequent lactation. It has been suggested that these nutrients may reduce the incidence and severity of mastitis by their influence on the bovine immune system. Deficiencies in these substances may lead to impairment of the mammary epithelial integrity, resulting in invasion of pathogens, as well as altered immunoglobulin transport and neutrophil migration into milk (Nickerson, 1989). Some studies have found positive effects on neutrophil and lymphocyte function when cows are supplemented with approximately 70,000 IU/day of vitamin A or 300 to 600 mg of β-carotene

(Michal *et al.*, 1994), but in a clinical study similar treatments had no effect on mammary gland health (Oldham *et al.*, 1991). Jukola *et al.* (1996) suggested that plasma concentrations of b-carotene in dairy cows should be >3 mg/L to optimize udder health.

Keratin is act as a physical barrier and have bactericidal properties, hence when it lost or decrease in the teat canal resulting increased the risk for development mastitis. Zinc is required for keratin formation. Cows receiving supplemental zinc methionine had significantly ($P<0.03$) more teat canal keratin (Spain *et al.*, 2005). Organic forms of zinc appear to be better absorbed and retained by the animal (O'Rourke, 2009). Scaletti *et al.* (2003) carried out a study in first lactation heifers to assess a potential role for dietary copper (Cu) in enhancing resistance to E. coli mastitis. They concluded that copper supplementation reduced the severity of clinical signs during experimental *E. coli* mastitis but that the duration of mastitis was unaffected. Currently available data suggest that diets should contain about 20 ppm of copper (assuming no antagonists) and 50 to 60 ppm of Zn. It has also been stated that overfeeding may cause mastitis (Little and Plastridge, 1946).

Source of Infection and Transmission

The detail knowledge of source of mastitogens and its transmission is very important for the effective prevention and control methods of mastitis. In general the mastitis pathogens may be physically transmitted from cow to cow or from one quarter to other quarters in the same animal. Cow-to-cow spread can occur through contaminated milk remaining on the liner during milking, while quarter-to-quarter spread can result from back flow of milk up the liner. Spreading mainly occurs during udder massage, udder washing and milking. Udder pathogens are also transported passively by milkers hands and udder towels. Transmission is also possible by *"milk-robber"* calves (buccal carriage) and may be important for staphylococci and streptococcus mastitis. Penetration of the udder by organisms is performed via the teat duct. In cases of systemic infections, haematogenous colonization is frequent (Tuberculosis, brucellosis and mycoplasmosis). It has been shown that *S. aureus* organisms are capable of spreading to the next 6 to 8 cows milked via a contaminated liner (Grindal and Bramley, 1989). While this may not necessarily result in infection- as the organisms may not invade the teat canal and should be killed by post milking teat disinfection. The risk of transmission is increased if the liners are worn, as bacteria adhere more easily to their roughened surface. Mycoplasma species infection can also be spread from cow-to-cow via the liner. Mycoplasma infections is more challenging because of variable shedding of the organism in milk. Current data suggest that a significant number of new outbreaks may occur via internal or animal-to-animal transmission of

Mycoplasma by asymptomatic carriers within the herd (Fox *et al.*, 2005). On-farm transmission may furthermore be maintained through aerosols from animals with respiratory Mycoplasma infection. Some states in the United States, such as Louisiana, have introduced a statewide control program for Mycoplasma mastitis in dairy herds (Owens and Nipper, 2008). But in India there is no any such type of control programme at state level or national level for mycoplasma mastitis. After the first case was identified in Louisiana in September 2002, a monitoring program was started.

Broadly, the micro-organisms causing bovine mastitis can be partly classified into two groups: contagious and environmental.

Contagious mastitis

Contagious mastitis results when bacteria are transferred from an infected mammary gland to a healthy one by different means. The udder and teats are the reservoir of infection. Transmission occurs during the milking process or udder preparation by contaminated hands, udder cloths and liners. Infection establishes on the surface of the teat and teat canal. Bacteria may then penetrate the mammary gland. Most infections are sub-clinical and result in raised cell counts. Control measures include post-milking teat disinfection, dry cow therapy and culling. Contagious bacteria include *S. aureus*, coagulase negative *Staphs*, *S. agalactiae* and *S. dysgalactiae*. If a herd somatic cell count is over 200,000/ml then this indicates that there is a problem with contagious mastitis. Careful application of control measures based upon teat disinfection and dry-cow antibiotic therapy will eradicate *S. agalactiae* over the course of one to two years provided infected animals are not introduced into the herd. *S. agalactiae* can also be eliminated through the use of *'blitz'* intramammary treatment during lactation and these bacteria are very sensitive to any of the penicillin antibiotics. In some herds, poor elimination rates of staphylococcal infection by therapy will require the heavy culling of chronically infected animals to achieve rapid progress. Mycoplasma spp. also come under this category, but these organisms are capable of colonizing and persisting in alternate host sites e.g skin, respiratory and genitourinary tracts. Nevertheless, the most important mode of transmission of these organisms involves the cow-to-cow transfer of bacteria-laden milk.

Environmental mastitis

The environment is a reservoir of infection. Environmental mastitis results when bacteria with reservoirs of infection distinct from the mammary gland (i.e. the environment) gain entrance to the mammary gland and cause mastitis. Infections are transmitted onto teats between milkings or during udder preparation. Contaminated bedding, water, fecal material, or fomites may all harbor and nurture bacterial populations capable of causing disease if introduced into the gland. Organisms are forced up through the teat canal during the milking process or after milking if cows are allowed to lie down immediately following milking. Most infections cause clinical mastitis. Sub-clinical infections are less common with *E. coli,* but frequently occur with *S. uberis.* Environmental mastitis is controlled through good environmental management, adequate accommodation for cows, a good milking routine, an efficient milking machine, good udder preparation, pre-milking teat disinfection and vaccination against coliform mastitis. Environmental organisms include *E. coli, S. uberis* (straw bedding), *Klebsiella* spp. (sawdust and shavings) and *Bacillus* spp. Although there is potential for interquarter transfer at milking time it appears not to be the predominant infection mechanism. Post-milking teat disinfection does not prevent infection. Antibiotic therapy has some beneficial effects on coliform mastitis prevention but does reduce the rate of new dry-period infection with *S. uberis.*

Status of bovine mastitis in India and world wide

Surveys of the prevalence of mastitis in most countries, irrespective of the cause, show a comparable figure of 50% among dairy cows and a quarter infection rate of 25% (Radostits *et al.,* 2000). Sub-clinical mastitis is believed to be more prevalent than clinical mastitis in most countries (Schukken *et al.,* 1995). The prevalence of sub-clinical mastitis on farms could range from 19 to 78% (Tuteja *et al.,* 1993).

Asia

India

In India, the teat dipping as a preventive measure is not regularly practiced by dairy farmers; hence, it is essential to educate the farmers regarding the economic losses, risk factors of mastitis and its prevention and control methods to reduce the economic losses due to mastitis. In 1988, Pathak and Sharma had been reported that incidence of clinical mastitis in buffaloes ranges from 8% to 40%. The average incidence of clinical mastitis in India has been calculated to be 1 to 10% (Prabhakar, 1986; Kumar, 1990) whereas the incidence of sub-clinical mastitis has been reported to vary from 10-50% in cows and 5-20% in buffaloes (Kumar, 1988; Singh, 1991). A technical report of Indian Council of Agricultural Research 1960-1961 indicates the incidence of mastitis in 267 animals in Bangalore was 24.8% and 21-2% in cows and buffaloes respectively and in 516 animals in Uttar Pradesh was 40-5% and 27% in cows and buffaloes respectively (Anon, 1963).

Studies conducted in different states of India reflect high incidence of the disease all over India for the past seven decades when the first record of the disease (mastitis) was made by Land in 1926. Higher incidence of mastitis in India may be due to lack of awareness and timely detection in absence of visible signs of abnormal milk, unhygienic milking practices and delay and incomplete treatment of clinical and chronic mastitis. Besides the persistence intramammary infection in non-lactating dry period or due to new infection getting access during colostrogenesis with dilatation of teat canal leads to such higher incidences of mastitis.

Jammu & Kashmir

Sharma (2009) reported prevalence of sub-clinical and clinical mastitis 42.18% and 10.93% respectively in dairy cows in Jammu. In a study on the prevalence of bovine mastitis in Kashmir valley conducted in the year 2006-2007 a prevalence rate of 34.0 and 15.4% was recorded under organized and un-organized farming conditions, respectively. Higher incidence of disease was observed during winter (18.8%) followed by summer (16.0%). The cows in 6-8 year age-group and early stage of lactation were found to have higher susceptibility to mastitis (Zahoor and Malik, 2009).

Himachal Pradesh

Pal *et al.* (1989) observed an overall incidence of SCM to be 23.08% on quarter basis in cows. The study conducted by Sharma *et al.* (1993) at an organized dairy farm, Palampur, Himachal Pradesh, showed 20.00, 5.12 and 2.82% of quarters positive for sub-clinical, acute and sub-acute mastitis respectively. The infection rate was 26.38, 24.30, 25.69 and 23.61% for LF, LH, RF and RH quarters respectively. The mastitis incidence was found highest during 3rd lactation. While in the study of Mandial *et al.* (1999), the prevalence of mastitis was about double (86.8%). Sharma (2000) reported 6.36% and 11.37% prevalence of mastitis in cows and buffaloes respectively. Katoch *et al.* (2003) have been reported 48.51% prevalence of mastitis in cattle.

Punjab

Bansal *et al.* (1990) reported 41.79% and 37.07% prevalence of clinical mastitis in cattle and buffaloes respectively. Saini *et al.* (1994) recorded the incidence of SCM among cross-bred cows in 4.87% quarters and 17.33% animals. They further observed that the incidence of SCM tended to increase with lactation number and was maximum in hind quarters. Singh and Singh (1994) claimed average incidence of SCM and clinical mastitis to be 43.90% and 6.40% respectively in cows, with 54.40% quarters affected in mastitis animals. Singh *et al.* (1994) studied the incidence of SCM in machine-milked cows on 8 farms in Punjab and reported it was 49.29 and 23.09% on animal and quarter basis respectively. Two-quarter infections were also noted more prevalent (50.00%) than one (34.29%), three (11.43) and four (4.29%) quarters.

The occurrence of infection was found to be higher in hind than in fore quarters and maximum in LH (29.23%), and the least in LF (20.00%). Bansal *et al.* (1995) had been reported prevalence of SCM 48.70% and 11.32% in cows and buffaloes respectively.

Haryana

Tuteja *et al.* (1993) examined 178 apparently healthy cows for mastitis and observed that 78.10% were found to be culturally positive and 53.90% were having SCC >5,000,00 per ml of milk. On the basis of infected quarters, 42.20% were found culturally positive. Of these 19.70% and 22.50% were having 'sub-clinical' and 'latent' mastitis respectively as per International Dairy Federation (IDF) criteria while 7.7% of quarters were having 'non-specific' mastitis. Sharma and Kapur (2000) reported 36.36% and 22.73% prevalence of sub-clinical mastitis on animal and quarter basis respectively, in buffaloes. Kumar and Sharma (2002) studied milk samples from 1253 quarters of cows and buffaloes in Hissar, and nearby areas during 1998-2000. Out of 142 cows and 415 buffaloes 59.86% and 66.27% respectively, were found culturally positive, whereas quarter-wise prevalence found to be 52.75% and 50.59% respectively. Both in cows and buffaloes single quarter and rear quarter involvement was maximum. Majority of cases occurred during third lactation, between 5 and 7 years of age. Maximum number of cases occurred during September, October and November, and during first three months of lactation. In a study 688 quarter milk samples were examined, 22.77% positive for sub-clinical mastitis by electrical conductivity test, while on cultural examination 13.22% samples were positive (Saxena *et al.*, 2001). Tuteja *et. al.* (2003) while examining 108 apparently healthy buffaloes of a single herd for mastitis reported 66.67% were found to be culturally positive and 41.67% were having somatic cell count (SCC) more than 500000 per ml of milk. On the basis of infected quarters, 36.43% were culturally positive. Of these 9.76 and 26.67% were having 'sub-clinical' and 'latent' infection, while 7.38% of the quarters were having non-specific mastitis. Sharma *et al.* (2006) had been reported 36.69% and 16.78% prevalence of sub-clinical mastitis at cow and quarter level, respectively (Sahiwal and Jersey) by cultural examination.

Samanta *et al.* (2006) carried out a study on 272 crossbred cows (66 Karan Swiss and 206 Karan Fries). The results indicated an overall incidence rate of 52.57% in the herd. The overall SCM incidences in Karan Swiss and Karan Fries breed groups were 53.03 and 52.43%, respectively. The breed difference was insignificant. The effect of stage of lactation, parity, level of milk production and teat tip to floor distance on the incidence of sub-clinical mastitis infection was significant ($P<0.05$). Incidence was higher in the late stage of lactation, later parities, low milk yield categories and groups having low teat tip to floor distance, regardless of the genetic group of the cows. Somatic cell count and the pH of the milk had a very high positive association with the SCM infection. The quarter-wise rate of infection in Karan Swiss varied between 30.30 (LF) and 38.46% (RH). In Karan Fries crosses, the quarter-wise infection rate varied between 26.70 (LF) and 33.33% (RF). In Karan Swiss crossbreds, a total of 34.73% quarters were affected by SCM, of which 12.98% were mildly affected, 11.07% were moderately affected and 10.69% were severely affected. The corresponding figures in the case of Karan Fries were 9.50, 10.97 and 8.26%, with a total infection rate of 28.73% of the quarters. The pH values of milk from healthy, mildy, moderately and severely affected quarters were 6.65, 6.84, 6.87 and 7.00, respectively, in Karan Swiss crossbreds. The corresponding figures in the case of Karan Fries crosses averaged 6.67, 6.80, 6.86 and 6.98, respectively.

Kamboj *et al.* (2008) reported 34.59% incidence of sub-clinical mastitis in crossbred dairy cows with hind quarters (29.24%) than the fore quarters (20.75%). A recent report of Khate and Yadav (2010) reported overall occurrence of mastitis in Sahiwal and Murrah was 26.43 and 18.91%, respectively. The incidence was the highest in 6th and above parity (41.66%), and lowest in the first parity (20.94%) in Sahiwal cows, whereas in Murrah buffaloes, the highest and the lowest incidence was in fifth (25.92%) and sixth and above parity (8.57%), respectively.

Rajasthan

Bhatnagar and Mehrotra (1969) collected 258 milk samples and found 37.98% prevalence of mastitis by MCMT. A study on 300 milk samples showed 60.25% prevalence in cows and 39.00% in quarters by cultural examination, and highest prevalence was found in 6th lactation on quarter basis and 3rd lactation on animal basis (Chahar *et al.*, 2005). Sharma *et al.* (2010) have been reported 60% prevalence of sub-clinical mastitis by cultural examination.

Uttar Pradesh

Sharma and Rai (1977) studied the epidemiological pattern of SCM in 242 cows and 134 buffaloes from organized herds in Uttar Pradesh. Out of these, 71 cows (29.34%) and 28 buffaloes (20.89%) were found positive to SCM. The quarter-wise distribution for cases of SCM in cows was 27 (20.93%) left fore, 35 (27.13%) left hind, 28 (21.70%) right fore and 39 (30.29%) right hind from 129 affected quarters. Out of 71 quarters, one-quarter incidence was in 59.15% in cows whereas of 28 quarters from buffaloes, one quarter involvement was 75.00%, two quarters 14.29%, three quarters 3.56% and four quarters 7.14%. It was also revealed that the incidence of SCM in cows was higher (29.34%) than in buffaloes (20.89%). Sharma (1978) reported that the incidence of clinical mastitis to be 8.15% and 4.84% in cows and buffaloes respectively, while incidence of SCM was 29% in cows and 21% in buffaloes in Western Uttar Pradesh with maximal prevalence in 5 to 9 years old animals. He observed 'blood in milk', of seven cows, which usually occurred after calving, and was not thought to be due to mastitis as rapid recovery occurred after parenteral administration of an antihistaminic. Parai *et al.* (1992) reported that herd and quarter incidence of SCM was 19.34% (259 of 1339 cows) and 9.95% (527 out of 2296 quarters) respectively, in cross-bred and exotic animals. Shukla *et al.* (1997) studied the incidence of mastitis among 154 animals (597 quarters) representating 78 cross-bred (302 quarters), 36 Sahiwal cows (145 quarters) and 40 Murrah buffaloes (155 quarters) in and around Pantnagar in Uttar Pradesh. The incidence figures revealed that fore quarters were more affected (49.05%) than hind quarters (35.91%) in case of cows; in buffaloes, the reverse was true. Further, the left quarters had higher prevalence (44.04%) than right quarters (33.33%). Mukherjee and Das (2002) reported 15.12% quarter-wise prevalence of bovine sub-clinical mastitis. De and Mukharjee (2009) have been reported the overall prevalence of clinical mastitis and sub-clinical mastitis were 15.18% and 42.93% respectively during the month of July and August. Kumar *et al.* (2010) reported 83% prevalence of bovine mastitis in Mathura.

Uttarakhand

Nauriyal (1996) reported overall incidence of clinical and sub-clinical mastitis in cows to be 74.56% and 74.10% respectively. Overall quarter infection rate among was 55.46 per cent. Pachauri *et al.* (2001) found overall prevalence of sub-clinical and clinical mastitis 74.10% and 3.15% respectively in cows. They also observed overall quarter infection rate in cows is 55.43%. The rear quarter showed greater involvement with the percentage of involvement being 52.43%. Lactation wise, the animals in their 3rd lactation were mostly affected. Singh *et al.* (2003) reported 30.68% incidence of clinical mastitis in buffaloes. Study of Nauriyal and Pachauri (2003) on 127 cross-bred cows and 21 Murrah buffaloes at the University farm of G B Pant University of Agriculture and Technology, Pantnagar revealed that the frequency of sub-clinical intramammary infection stood at 74.01% and 33.33% among cows and buffaloes respectively. The quarter-wise incidence of SCM was 47.04 and 17.50% in case of cows and buffaloes respectively with involvement of single quarter at a greater rate. Patel and Nauriyal (2003) tested a total of 46 cross-bred cows maintained at Livestock Research Station, Gujarat Agricultural University, Anand. From the view point of milk production in the current lactation, the cows included in the study were divided in to five categories viz. 1000 to 1500 kg, 1501 to 2000 kg, 2001 to 2500 kg, 2501 to 3000 kg and above 3000 kg. The infected cows in their respective groups were 100, 68.40, 81.80, 66.60 and 71.42% with an average of 73.91%. An epidemiological investigation on the prevalence of mastitis was made on 154 animals composed of 78 crossbred and 36 Sahiwal cows and 40 Murrah buffaloes. Of the 154 animals screened, 64.93% were found to have mastitis. Of these, 8.44% were affected clinically and 56.50% sub-clinically. Higher prevalence was recorded in cows compared to buffaloes (70.17 vs. 50%). The prevalence of clinical and sub-clinical mastitis in crossbred and Sahiwal cows and Murrah buffaloes was 8.97 and 67.94%, 8.33 and 47.22% and 7.50 and 42.50%, respectively (Shukla *et al.*, 2005). Total 225 lactating crossbreds were examined physically and clinically, and milk samples were subjected to different indirect mastitis tests. Of them, 42 (18.67%) animals were diagnosed as suffering from per acute/acute (12), sub acute (9), chronic (7) and sub-clinical (14) mastitis (Singh *et al.*, 2008). Sood *et al.* (2008) found 28.18% and 10% CMT positive milk samples and confirmed sub-clinical and clinical mastitis respectively in cows.

Madhya Pradesh

Shukla (1980) reported incidence of SCM in Malwa region of Madhya Pradesh to be 96.45% in bovines and 55.84% on over all quarter basis. Shukla and Supekar (1982) reported the incidence of SCM in cross breds on quarter basis as 22.56, 25.12, 24.10 and 28.20% in LH, LF, RH and RF quarters respectively. Shukla and Supekar (1986) reported 47.50% incidence of SCM in Gir cows. Incidence of SCM in Malvi (Desi) animals was 56.00% and quarter wise figures were 24.28, 25.71, 29.26 and 20.71% for LH, LF, RH and RF quarters respectively. The incidence of SCM in cows of Mhow region was recorded by Ali *et al.* (1989) as 44.80% on quarter and 78.10% on animal basis. The figures of incidence were 74.30%, 88.37% and 45.45% in cross-bred, Gir and Malvi cows respectively. In the same year Bajpai et al. (1989) had also reported 62.33% prevalence of sub-clinical mastitis in buffaloes. Devi *et al.* (1997) observed the incidence of SCM in Malwa region of Madhya Pradesh as 86.87, 75.00%, 57.35, 75.00 and 80.00% in Jersey, HF, Malvi, Sahiwal and Gir animals respectively. Tijare et al. (1999) reported 70.37% prevalence of sub-clinical mastitis by electrical conductivity test in Jabalpur. Tiwari *et al.* (2000) reported that the overall incidence of mastitis in cows was 53.54% (166 out of 310) in Malwa region of Madhya Pradesh. Taking into consideration the total number of lactating quarters tested, the affected quarters incidence was 25.12% (300 out of 1194). The blind teats were 3.70% (46 out of 1240). Out of 300 positive samples, 68 were CMT (trace), 120 (+), 74 (+ +) and 24 (+ + +). Fourteen (14) samples were beyond the limit of CMT (+ + +), therefore these have been graded as (+ + + +). While considering the cases of SCM in relation to the lactation, it was observed that the maximum incidence occurred during third and fifth lactations followed by 1st, 4th and 6th lactations.

In other lactations incidence of mastitis was lower. Tiwari and Sisodia (2000) studied a total of 400 lactating cows including 346 cross-breds, 33 Gir and 21 Malvi at different stages of lactation, parities and ages. The milk samples subjected to MDS and CMT revealed normal reaction in 1185 (76.90%) samples, mild to moderate reaction in 287 (18.62%) and 311 (20.18%), and advanced (severe) SCM in 67 (4.3%) and 45 (2.92%) quarter samples respectively. On overall basis, both MDS and CMT detected 356 (23.10%) quarters positive for SCM. Ghose *et al.* (2003) while screening 272 cows for SCM by CMT found 130 (47.79%) cows positive. The incidence rate of SCM in left fore, right fore, left hind and right hind quarters was 22.67, 19.24, 23.30 and 23.46% respectively. The incidence was more in rear quarters than the fore quarters and in the single quarter (51.53%) than the multiple quarters. Shukla *et al.* (2003) screened a total of 1243 cows (Gir, Sahiwal and Malvi) in the Department of Veterinary Medicine, Veterinary College, Mhow (M.P.). Out of 1243, 893 (71.84%) cows were found positive for SCM while quarter-wise incidence was reported to be 3146/3747 (83.96%). Das and Joseph (2005) collected 102 milk samples from clinical cases of mastitis in buffalo from Jabalpur region and found 84.31% prevalence of mastitis by cultural examination.

Chhattisgarh

Maiti et al. (2003) have been reported the incidence of sub-clinical mastitis in cow 70.37% and 43.06% animal-wise and quarter-wise respectively and also reported the animal-wise and quarter-wise incidence of sub-clinical mastitis was 54.17% and 26.59% respectively in buffaloes. Sharma et al. (2004) carried out a study on 155 Murrah buffaloes in Rajnandgoan district and found 70.32% incidence of sub-clinical mastitis, while quarter-wise incidence was 43.53% and blind teats were 1.45%. Presence study also revealed the somewhat higher incidence of sub-clinical mastitis in hind quarters than fore quarters. Sharma *et al.* (2007) conducted a study on 2000 quarters milk samples of 500 lactating buffaloes in Durg district of Chhattisgarh state and found 68.60% and 42% animal and quarter-wise prevalence of sub-clinical mastitis by modified California mastitis test (MCMT). The prevalence was highest during 3rd and 4th lactation and at 3 to 9 years of age. Single quarters and hind quarters involvement was maximum. Vishwakarma (2008) reported an average 7.90 and 41.07% prevalence of clinical and sub-clinical mastitis in buffaloes respectively in Durg and Rajnandgoan districts of the state.

Gujarat

Patel *et al.* (2000) reported 30.43% and 13.44% prevalence of sub-clinical mastitis and clinical mastitis respectively in cows. They also found that highest prevalence was in monsoon (37.02%) followed by summer (27.42%) and winter season (26.04%). Verma and Nauriyal (2009) reported the 58.76% overall prevalence of mastitis in cows with 78.50%, 63.63% and 38.88% in triple cross, Kankrej and HF cows respectively. While quarter-wise prevalence was 31.42%. Among infected quarters, greater involvement of rear quarters (53.72%) was noted with left rear quarters contributing higher share. Maximum number of cows (38.60%) exhibiting intramammary infection were found to be in their 2nd lactation (38.60%) and the infection rate was greater in late lactation stage.

Bihar

Sahay *et al.* (2002) examined a total of 110 lactating cows (440 quarters) and reported that 49 cows (71 quarters) were found positive for SCM. Animal wise and quarter wise incidence of SCM was found to be 44.54% and 16.13% respectively.

Jharkhand

Munda et al. (2007) reported 32.40% and 22.22% incidence of sub-clinical mastitis in cows and buffaloes respectively from Ranchi district. Ranjan et al. (2010) found 72.63% prevalence of bovine mastitis by cultural examination.

West Bengal

Roy *et al.* (1989) from a survey of 292 Jersey × Haryana, 114 Brown Swiss × Haryana and 242 HF × Haryana cross-bred cows in hot, humid tropical conditions of West Bengal reported that the incidence of SCM was highest (62.80%) in HF × Haryana, followed by Brown Swiss × Haryana (44.73%) and Jersey × Haryana (31.85%) cross-breds. The incidence of SCM was also found highest in 3rd lactation in Brown Swiss × Haryana and HF × Haryana crosses, and in 2nd lactation in Jersey × Haryana cross-bred cows. Chandra *et al.* (1989) find out 56.76% and 29.84% prevalence of SCM at cow and quarter level respectively, in cross-bred cows in organized farms and rural areas in and around Calcutta. Roy *et al.* (1993) based on investigations among 292 Jersey × Haryana (J × H), 114 Brown Swiss × Haryana and 242 HF × Haryana cross-bred cows recorded the total number of animals affected with mastitis in first, second and third lactations as 68 (10.49%), 112 (17.28%) and 116 (17.90%) respectively. Banerjee *et al.* (2002) reported 28.12% prevalence of mastitis in cows.

Orissa

Behera *et al.* (2008) found 41% prevalence of sub-clinical mastitis in dairy cows on quarter basis. Sahoo *et al.* (2009) reported 35.79% prevalence of mastitis in dairy cows on the basis of cultural isolation.

Assam

Saxena *et al.* (1993) reported that out of 50 cows tested in Assam, 32 (64.00%) were affected with SCM. Among the 191 quarters examined by them 9 were blind and 74 (38.75%) were infected. The LF was most frequently (31.08%) involved. The highest incidence (34.75%) was noted during 2nd lactation, and the cows in early-lactation got most frequently (78.13%) affected. Saharia *et al.* (1997) reported that 39 (47.56%) cows out of 82, and 34 (55.74%) out of 61 were positive for sub-clinical mastitis under pucca and wooden floor housing respectively. The incidence of sub-clinical mastitis with one teat involvement was maximum followed by two, three and four. The LH quarters were found to be most frequently involved followed in succession by LF, RH and RF ones. Buragohain and Dutta (1998) from a study of 50 lactating cows, reported that 28 (56%) cows were found positive for sub-clinical mastitis. Buragohain and Dutta (2000) reported that cows in their 3rd lactation showed the highest percentage of sub-clinical mastitis, followed by cows in their 4th and 2nd lactation. They found 74.87% and 3.74% overall prevalence of sub-clinical and clinical mastitis respectively, in dairy cows. Prasad et al. (2001) carried out a study in the hillocks of Meghalaya nearby the Khanapara and found 35.45% and 61.32% prevalence of sub-clinical mastitis at quarter and cow level respectively. A study was carried out in dairy cattle during the period from August, 1998 to September, 1999 in the Khanapara region of Assam and Meghalaya and overall prevalence of sub-clinical mastitis was found to be 64.70% (Nath and Dutta, 2005). The same author in the year of 2007 also reported the incidence rates of sub-clinical mastitis 73.46 and 73.82% cow-wise and quarter-wise, respectively (Nath and Dutta, 2007).

Mizoram

Lalrintluanga *et al.* (2003) found that 37.50% of the cows and 11.65% of the udder quarters were positive for mastitis. Only 2.6% of the udder quarters were positive for clinical mastitis while the rest were positive for sub-clinical mastitis. Cows aged 4-6 years were the most commonly affected (51.1%). Mastitis incidence was higher during the early stage of the third lactation (36.60%), single quarter infection was recorded more frequently (63.44%) and the left hind quarters were more frequently affected (30.25%). Tiwari *et al.* (2008) found overall incidence of mastitis 22% at cow level and 10.03% at quarter level. The incidence of clinical mastitis was 8% and 14% sub-clinical mastitis.

Meghalaya

Prasad *et al.* (2001) reported 35.45% and 61.32% incidence of sub-clinical mastitis at quarter and cow level respectively, in the hillocks of Meghalaya. Lactation-wise, the highest incidence was observed during the 3rd lactation.

A small study on 98 lactating cows on the hillocks of Meghalaya by Nath and Dutta (2007), found the 73.46% incidence of sub-clinical mastitis on animal basis and 73.82% quarter-wise. The highest (37.50%) occurrence was in the animals of 3rd lactation followed by 4th (20.83%) and 2nd lactation (15.27%).

Sikkim

Dubal *et al.* (2010) have been reported the 24.63% prevalence of sub-clinical mastitis in cattle.

Maharashtra

Kalorey *et al.* (1983) observed SCM in 59.20% cows with higher incidence in 2nd and 3rd lactation (4 to 6 years old). Infection of all the four quarters was common (31.00%) in cows. However, later study in Maharashtra showed 20.72% prevalence of bovine SCM (Dhote *et al.*, 1999). Dangore *et al.* (2000) applied MCMT and WST on 349-quarter milk samples of 90 cross-bred dairy cows. The incidence of sub-clinical mastitis with MCMT and WST was 42.22% and 35.55% respectively on animal basis; whereas, 16.90% and 14.04% on quarter basis respectively. The individual quarter positive to MCMT was found to be LF-17 (28.81%), RF-8 (13.50%), LH-20 (33.90%) and RH-14 (23.70%). A study showed 17.14% quarter-wise incidence in buffaloes (Shinde et al., 2002). A study by Shrirame et al. (2002) found 36.60% and 36.90% quarters milk samples positive to CMT in cows and buffaloes respectively. On cultural examination of milk samples, 68.97% prevalence of mastitis was found in cows by Sarode (2002). Bhikane et al. (2002) reported 41.77% and 50% prevalence of clinical mastitis in cows and buffaloes respectively. The season-wise distribution of cases indicated highest incidence in winter season (51.47%) followed by rainy (30.88%) and summer (17.64%). Studies on sub-clinical mastitis in buffaloes showed 39.56% incidence, while quarter-wise incidence was 17.71%. Prevalence of sub-clinical mastitis was 39.16% in Murrah, 36.00% in Jaffarabadi and 66.67% in Mehasana breed of buffaloes. This study indicated that higher percentage of incidence was found in late lactation and advanced age. Prevalence of sub-clinical mastitis recorded were 22.22%, 35.71%, 39.29%, 33.33%, 53.84%, 44.44% and 66.66% in 1st, 2nd, 3rd, 4th, 5th and 6th lactations respectively. The highest incidence was noticed in 7th lactation and the lowest in 1st lactation. The percentage of incidence in respect of single, double, triple quarters and all quarters was 22.33, 9.78, 4.44 and 4.00 respectively. Higher incidence of sub-clinical mastitis in hind and left side quarter of udder was recorded. The incidence was lowest (7.23%) in right hind quarters (Gowardhan *et al.*, 2008). Bhoyar *et al.* (2009) conducted a study in Nagpur and found 55.55 and 31.94% prevalence of sub-clinical mastitis by modified California mastitis test in cows.

Andhra Pradesh

Babu *et al.* (1983) recorded 10.70% cases of SCM in Jersey cows at a large exotic cattle breeding farm, Banavasi, Kurnool district, Andhra Pradesh. The incidence was higher in fore teats than in hind teats, and also higher in the left quarters than right. Rao *et al.* (1989) reported 5.1% prevalence of bovine clinical mastitis in Andhra Pradesh. Ramachandraiah *et al.* (1990) conducted study on 80 pure Jersey cows, where 51 cows (63.70%) were found positive on CMT and cultural examination. The quarter wise incidence was equally distributed among the four quarters. The percentage incidence of SCM mastitis was maximum (56.80%) in single quarter, followed by three quarters (19.60%), two quarters (17.60%) and four quarters (5.90%). In the year 2002, Kumari and Gupta collected 81 milk samples and found 71 (87.65%) positive by California mastitis test. The prevalence of "allergic mastitis" is more in buffaloes than in cows and mostly seen within 30 days after calving. However, incidence has crossed 40% in the first 10 days after calving and highest cases occurred during winter (October to January) followed by rainy season (Sreedevi et al., 2002). The incidence in Andhra Pradesh is restricted to coastal area mainly Godavari and Krishna districts. Lakshmi Rani *et al.* (2008) found overall 58.95% incidence of mastitis in buffaloes. Of these 22.12% and 77.87% clinical and sub-clinical mastitis. The buffaloes aged 6 to 8 years (47.90%) and yielding milk greater than 5 liters/day were mostly affected. On observation of a total of 1,000 quarters of buffaloes by Kavitha *et al.* (2009), it was found that 31 quarters were clinically affected with mastitis, and 17 animals were affected with sub-clinical mastitis. Among the clinically infected quarters, the inflammation was distributed as- fore left quarters 14.2%, fore right quarters 9.8%, hind left quarters 10.7% and hind right quarters 12.5%. Whereas 7.03% of fore left quarters, 10.1% of fore right quarters, 10.93% of hind left quarters and 10.93% of hind right quarters showed sub-clinical mastitis, which indicated higher prevalence of clinical and sub-clinical mastitis on hind quarters.

Karnataka

Swamy and Krishnamurthy (1999) conducted a study in Bangalore and found 36.11% quarters milk samples were positive for California mastitis test. A recent report of Kumar *et al.* (2010) shown that the overall mastitis incidence was 9.28, 3.59 and 4.10% for crossbred cows, indigenous cows and buffaloes, respectively. The number of clinical mastitis cases differed significantly over different seasons, lactation and stage of lactation. Mastitis incidence was highest during the rainy season, followed by winter and summer. The prevalence of subclinical mastitis in and around Bangalore on screening 1102 milk samples was 29.94% based on electrical conductivity test of milk as well as White side test on quarter basis. The prevalence was different in relation to different quarters. The prevalence was increased as the lactation number increased. The incidence was highest in fifth lactation. Incidence of sub-clinical mastitis increased as length of lactation and milk yield (Stanikzai *et al.*, 2010).

Tamil Nadu

Data indicated an average incidence of mastitis in Tamil Nadu is 13.01% in cows and 7.30% in buffaloes. Thirunavukkarasu and Prabaharan (1998) reported that the overall rate of incidence of mastitis was 13.01% in cows in Tamil Nadu. A higher incidence of mastitis was observed in exotic pure-bred (13.51 and 16.85%) than cross-bred cows (13.23 and 12.50%) in government/ university and private farms respectively. The incidence of mastitis was found to be 17.82, 12.43, 9.21 and 7.10% in cows in 1st, 2nd, 3rd and beyond 3rd quarters of lactation respectively. Further, the 1st parity cows registered higher incidence (10.69%) than their 2nd parity counterparts (10.54%). The incidence of mastitis was more in rainy (15.05%) than summer (13.97%) and winter (9.57%) seasons in cows. Prevalence of mastitis was studied on 30 dairy farms in Tamil Nadu, India between 1993 and 1995. The average infection rate was 13.01% in cows and 7.30% in buffaloes (Thirunavukkarasu and Prabaharan, 1999). Paul *et al.* (2000) reported higher incidence of SCM and clinical mastitis in cows (25.78% and 13.01% respectively) than buffaloes (10.60% and 7.37% respectively) in and around Chennai. Incidence of mastitis in Tamil Nadu was found to be higher in exotic pure bred cows (15%) than that of crossbred cows (13.07%) (Dhanapalan, 2000). In a study of Reetha *et al.* (2006) incidence of mastitis was 70% in Jersey cross, 23.5% in Zebu and 6.5% in Holstein Fresian crossbred cows. Mastitis incidence was high (62.3%) in animals which have calved more than once and less than 3 calves. Cows in 1 to 3 months post calving suffered most (33.3 %), 4 to 6 months (23.3%), 7 to 9 months (6.7%), 10 to 12 months (16.7 %) and more than 12 months (20%). Left Fore quarter was affected in 33.3% cases, Right Fore quarter 13.3%, Left Hind quarter 10 % and Right Hind quarter 16.7% and more than one quarter was affected in 26.7% of cases. A survey was conducted by Palanivel *et al.* (2008) on 300 graded Murrah buffaloes in Chennai during the period April, 2002 to March, 2003, results revealed that the prevalence of sub-clinical and clinical mastitis was 28.3% and 16.3% respectively, while overall prevalence was 44.70%. The involvement of single quarter infection in the present study was 74.60% and high in right hind quarter (29.60%) in comparison to 19.00% in left hind, 16.40% in right fore and 9.70% in left fore quarters. They also reported that occurrence of mastitis was highest during summer season (53.80%) followed by winter (41.30%) and rainy (37.50%).

Kerala

Sebastian and Vijayakumar (2002) reported 37.74% occurrence of mastitis in cows on cultural examination. Rajendran *et al.* (2006) reported 74.04%

milk samples were positive for modified California mastitis test. Mastitis prevalence was highest in the left hind quarter (32, 40%), followed by the right hind (21, 26.3%), left fore (15, 18.7%) and right fore quarters (12, 15%). Siji and Vijayakumar (2007) was reported 34% quarter-wise prevalence of sub-clinical mastitis in dairy cows.

The difference in the prevalence of mastitis may be attributed to variation in the number of cases studied, the techniques followed, geographical variations and different husbandry practices followed in different states/ regions.

World Wide

Other Countries of Asia

Bangladesh

Nooruddin et al. (1997) reported 21.20% prevalence of clinical mastitis in cattle in Dhaka.Kader *et al.* (2002) screened 118 exotic and cross-bred cows for SCM. The overall prevalence of SCM was found to be 46.60% on bacteriological examination of milk. Rahman *et al.* (2009) reported that the overall prevalence of mastitis was 19.9% and 44.8% in dry and wet seasons, respectively. The prevalence of mild mastitis was 17.3% and 40.7%, whereas that of moderate mastitis was 2.6% and 4.1% in dry and wet seasons, respectively. Uddin *et al.* (2009) reported 25.5% prevalence of mastitis with 21 and 5% prevalence of sub-clinical and clinical mastitis respectively.

Iran

Ghazaei (2006) reported 48.75% prevalence of mastitis in cows in Ardabil state. Kheirabadi *et al.* (2008) reported 29.03% milk samples were positive to CMT (sub-clinical mastitis) in cows. The occurrence of sub-clinical mastitis was highest during spring months (34%) than summer (25%). A total of 1452 and 1020 quarter milk samples were taken from Holstein and Sarabi cows, respectively and tested by California mastitis test (CMT) and somatic cell count (SCC). They found 16.87 and 14.41% quarter milk samples were positive in Holstein and Sarabi cows, respectively by CMT. While SCC was positive in 29.69% and 31.13% samples, respectively in Sarabi and Holstein cows (Ferdowsi *et al.*, 2009).

Israel

A 4-year retrospective study was performed to determine the clinical, bacteriological and epidemiological aspects of acute clinical mastitis in seven Israeli dairy herds. A total of 1124 clinical mastitis cases were detected by abnormal changes in the milk and udder with concurrent decrease of at least

25% in daily milk production. A total of 1190 quarters were affected with clinical mastitis in 1089 cows. The rear quarters had a higher incidence risk (64.7% of quarter cases) than the front quarters. The annual herd-year-incidence varied from 4.2 to 126.8 cases/ 100/ cows/ year. The whole-lactation incidence risk (LIR) was 20.8 per 100 lactations (Shpigel *et al.,* 1998).

China

A survey was conducted by Fang *et al.* (1992) and found 16.58% quarter-wise prevalence of clinical mastitis and 38.4% prevalence of sub-clinical mastitis in cows respectively. Prevalence of clinical mastitis was higher (40%) in summer season. Liu *et al.* (2005) reported 36.5% prevalence of sub-clinical mastitis and 16.7% clinical mastitis in dairy cows from Xingjiang corps. Li *et al.* (2009) conducted a study on 3178 quarter milk samples from 846 lactating cows, Zhejiang Province, China. Out of which 459 cows (54.3%) were found Hangzhou mastitis test (HMT) positive and 890 quarters (28%) were found having sub-clinical mastitis.

Jordan

Hawari and Al-Dabbas (2008) Milk samples were collected from 220 lactating cows to determine the clinical and sub-clinical mastitis by white side test and confirmed by cultural tests. It was found that 138 quarters 15.7% had been diagnosed as clinical mastitis with definite gross pathological lesions and change in udder secretion, in addition to that 276 quarters 31.4% showed sub-clinical mastitis.

Nepal

Joshi and Joshi (1997) collected milk samples from 85 apparently healthy cows and 363 apparently healthy buffaloes were tested with sodium lauryle sulphate (SLS) test and whiteside test. The result of investigation showed that the prevalence of sub-clinical mastitis (SCM) in cows and buffaloes were 30.6% and 32.2% respectively. Higher prevalence of SCM was recorded in cows and buffaloes (46% and 39.6% respectively) in the mid hill area than the low and high hills. Similarly, stall fed animals were found to be more affected then the free grazing. Likewise the prevalence of SCM in cows and buffaloes was in increasing trend in the successive lactations. The prevalence of SCM was found significantly higher in cows and buffaloes without having a suckling calf than those with calves. Infection of one teat was found to be common in both species. Among the SCM affected animals, 15% cows and 3.4% buffaloes developed clinical mastitis in their subsequent lactation. Epidemiological investigation on clinical mastitis (CM) in cows and buffaloes was conducted during 1994-1995 in the western hills of Nepal to ascertain the incidence as well as factors involved. A total of 74 animals (18 cows and 56 buffaloes) suffering from mastitis were investigated. CM was found in 127 teats of the animals. Higher incidence of CM was found in the first lactation of animals (64.4%) particularly during monsoon (July-Sept) season (71.0%) and during the first week of first calving (78.1%), in animals without suckling calf (69.0%) and raised under stall-fed management system (86.3%) (Joshi *et al.*, 1998). Dhakal *et al.* (2007) had been studied on milk samples from 355 Murrah cross buffaloes and of these a total of 319 cases recorded at the mastitis laboratory of IAAS were analyzed for the prevalence of clinical mastitis during different seasons. The maximum number of cases of clinical mastitis was observed in the month of July (16%) followed by June (12.2%) and August (13.5%). Results show that 37.3% of buffaloes had clinical mastitis during the summer season followed by the autumn season (31.7%). The months from June to August have the highest rainfall in the study area, when the average temperature was 30°C. In this study, 62% of buffalo affected by sub-clinical mastitis and 64% of buffaloes with clinical mastitis had an infection in a single quarter. The highest incidence of clinical mastitis (43.6%) was also observed during the first month of parturition. Following parturition, there was a decreasing trend of mastitis cases. A greater (51.6%) incidence of clinical mastitis was found in animals during their 1st calving, with subsequent reduction in the 2nd calving. The occurrence of mastitis decreased as the number of calvings increased. The difference found among reports may be due to various factors such as breed, season and husbandry system (Moroni *et al.*, 2006).

Pakistan

Said and Abd-el-Malik (1968) reported a prevalence of 38.07% in buffaloes on the basis of Whiteside test and California Mastitis Test (CMT). Anwar and Chaudhry (1983) have reported a prevalence of 47.5% in buffaloes after using Strip Cup test, pH test and Whiteside test. Hashmi and Muneer (1981) used cultural examination and reported a figure of 44.9% for buffaloes. Rehman *et al.* (1983) reported, on the basis of direct, indirect and cultural examination, a prevalence of 59.2 and 36.8% of sub-clinical mastitis in cows and buffaloes, respectively. Hussain *et al.* (1984) documented a prevalence of 33% in cows and 8% in buffaloes on the basis of results of Whiteside test. Shah (1987) used Ciba-Geigy mastitis test and found that 34.48% buffaloes suffered from sub-clinical mastitis. Rehman (1995) study has shown that quarter-wise and animal-wise prevalence of mastitis as 64 and 30.5%, respectively in buffaloes. Herd-mate animals had shown higher prevalence of sub-clinical mastitis in buffaloes i.e.75% versus 44.44% in individually managed animals. Bachaya *et al.* (2005) have been reported 44.17% quarter-wise and animal-wise prevalence was 44% in cattle by Surf field mastitis test. Bachaya *et al.* (2005) also reported that overall quarter-wise prevalence 58.7% while animal-wise prevalence was 77.98% in buffaloes on the basis of Surf Field Mastitis Test. Chishty *et al.*

(2007) found the overall prevalence of mastitis was 47.58% in cattle and 60.27% in buffaloes. The prevalence of clinical and sub-clinical mastitis in cows was reported to be 16.72% and 30.80% respectively, and in boffaloes 21.08% and 39.10% respectively.

South Korea

Nam *et al.* (2010) reported 54.3 and 35.5% prevalence of udder infections on the basis of somatic cell counts (>200,000 cells/ml).

Kingdom of Saudi Arabia

Shathele (2009) studied during November, 1991 to October, 1992 and ound 16.5% annual incidence of clinical mastitis in dairy cows. Fadlelmula *et al.* (2009) carried out an epidemiological study in a Saudi Arabian dairy farm with a capacity of 11,200 dairy cows for a period of 60 days in winter. The disease incidence was 1.8 cases per 100 cows per month. The first month of lactation displayed the highest incidence of mastitis (62.7%), while the late stage of lactation showed the lowest incidence (11.2%). The disease incidence increased with increasing age and lactation number. Repeated occurrence of mastitis (chronic mastitis) was 65.1% among cows with a significant decrease in milk yield. The prevalence of mild and acute mastitis was the 59.7% and 40.3% respectively.

North America (U.S.A.)

Ohio

Crist *et al.* (1982) reported that prevalance of infection declined more rapidly in the intense group with 42, 28 and 24% of cows infected vs. 39, 25 and 30% in the intermediate and 56, 35 and 42% in the control group in 1977, 1978 and 1979. Those herds adopting a teat dipping and dry cow therapy program had infection prevalence of 41, 25 and 20% of cows; bulk tank Wiskosin mastitis test (WMT) scores of 15.5, 14.7 and 11.4; and daily milk production of 18.4, 18.4 and 17.5 kg/cow in 1977, 1978 and 1979. Miller and Dorn (1990) reported 37% annual prevalence of mastitis. Bartlett et al. (1992) estimated the clinical mastitis incidence ranged from 2.19 to 4.36% in cows.

Wisconsin

Sato *et al.* (2002) reported 42% prevalence of mastitis in and around Wiscosin. In a report from Wisconsin where herds were investigated due to mastitis problems, the clinical mastitis incidence reported was of 48.7 cases / 100 cows/year (Cook and Mentik, 2006).

Louisiana

Trinidad *et al.* (1990) demonstrated that the prevalence of IMIs in unbred heifers and heifers during different stages of pregnancy was very high. Unbred heifers had a higher percentage (86.7%) of infected mammary quarters compared with the overall mean for pregnant heifers (70%). Initial studies in Louisiana, USA to determine the prevalence of mastitis in breeding age dairy heifers demonstrated that intramammary infections were present in 97% of heifers and 75% of quarters (Nickerson, 2009).

California

Resende *et al.* (2009) used a total of 370,748 milk samples for cultural examination between January of 1999 and December of 2008, and found 64.2% samples positive by cultural isolation.

Mexico

Jarillo Cabera (1980) collected milk samples from 564 Holstein-Friesian cows in 5 intensive milk production units were tested by California mastitis test during a 2 month trial. The average prevalence of mastitis was 20.82% overall, ranging from 15 to 25%, but in 2 of the herds av. incidence was 57.39%, owing to low standards of hygiene. Mendezy Cazarin et al. (2000) carried out a study on small scale dairy farms in the Morelia-Querendaro valley in Michoacan. There were 88.8% of the farms with sub-clinical mastitis with over 20% of prevalence. Avila Tellez et al. (2002) reported the mean prevalence rate of sub-clinical mastitis was 57% and prevalence rate of clinical mastitis was 7% in hand milked cows. In machine milked cows, the prevalence rate was 33%, incidence rate of sub-clinical and clinical mastitis were 10 per one hundred weeks-cow (7 of 70) and 0.96 per one hundred weeks-cow (1 of 104), respectively. They concluded that the udder health was better in machine milked cows than hand milked cows.

Canada

The rate of clinical mastitis is precisely 28% in Quebec, 22% in Alberta and 36% in the Maritimes and in Ontario. Data also showed that the rate of clinical mastitis is generally higher in tie stall farms than in free stall farms (Mastitis-flash, 2009).

South America

Brazil

Beloti *et al.* (1997) reported 29% prevalence of mastitis in Holstein Friesian cows. Afonso *et al.* (1999) evaluated CMT in bovine mastitis in Brazil in 1964 mammary quarters (434 cows) and reported 19.67% quarter-wise positive infection with SCC being 365728 in negative milk samples, and 1238399 SCC in positive tested samples. Brito et al. (2009) has been reported 46.50% and 48.30% prevalence of sub-clinical mastitis during dry and rainy season, respectively in dairy cows. Oliviera *et al.* (2010) reported 39.57% prevalence of mastitis in cows and 90% of the farms analyzed had at least one positive animal. Martins *et al.* (2010) reported 5.8 and 65% prevalence of clinical and sub-clinical mastitis in cows. These findings indicate that the status of mastitis become double from 1997 (29%) to 2010 (65%). While Oliveira *et al.* (2010) reported 6.6% prevalence of sub-clinical mastitis and 1.3% prevalence of clinical mastitis.

Uruguay

Uruguay is a major milk producer and exporter of dairy products in South America with 1423.5 million litres of milk being produced annually. The prevalence of subclinical mastitis was found to be high. On a cow-basis it was 58.1% and on a quarter-basis 32.5% (Ahlner and Axelsson, 2002). Gianneechini *et al.* (2002) reported 1.2% prevalence of clinical mastitis while subclinical mastitis was prevalent 52.4% on a cow basis and 26.7% on an udder quarter basis. Ahlner (2003) also reported 42.2 and 21.8% prevalence of sub-clinical mastitis on cow-basis and on a quarter-basis respectively.

Europe

Rupp and Boichard (1999) reported 12.60% occurrence of clinical mastitis in first lactating cows in France, while previous study of Biochard and Rupp (1997) reported the 20% overall frequency for complete lactations of all parities in the same herds. Reports form different parts of Europe are as- 10.9 % in Finland (Luttinen and Juga, 1997) and 11.1% in Sweden (Emanuelson *et al.*, 1988) for a lactation period from -10 to 150 days and 21% in Denmark for -10 to 180 days (Lund *et al.*, 1994). The higher frequency (26.3%) that was reported by Heringstad *et al.* (1997) corresponded to all clinical mastitis cases during the entire first lactation.

Sweden

Funke (1988) carriedout a study on Swedish Red-and-White and Swedish Friesian cows in 1985-1986, the prevalence of infectious mastitis was 27 and 34% respectively. Hemilton *et al.* (2006) reported 26 and 14.7% prevalence of subclinical and clinical mastitis respectively, in cows.

Italy

Pozzi (1998) reported the prevalence of udder infection was 30.47%, representing 1508 infected quarters. Values ranged from 24.7% in the Islands to 42.5% in Southern Italy. There was a higher incidence of environmental pathogens in early lactation. Incidence of contagious pathogens increase later. Moretti *et al.* (1998) found 29.7% positive milk samples by cultural isolation. Ferguson *et al.* (2007) reported 35.4% prevalence of intramammary infection by cultural examination of milk from Ragusa, Italy. Pagni *et al.* (2008) reported 41.43% prevalence of mastits in dairy cow. The prevalence of mastitis declined from > 25% in 2001 to 13% observed in 2007-2008 (Zecconi *et al.,* 2009).

France

Brochart *et al.* (1984) reported 22.2% incidence of mastitis. Robert *et al.* (2006) reported 12.8% quarter-wise prevalence of mastitis in cows.

Germany

Tenhagen *et al.* (2006) reported 26.4% prevalence of mastitis by cultutral examination. Cedeno *et al.* (2010) reported 53.13% prevalence of mastitis by CMT.

Norway

Bakken (1981) reported average prevalence rate of subclinical mastitis was 31% of the cows and 11.6% of quarters. Almost 50% of the cases were non specific mastitis. Osteras and Lund (1988) has been reported 47.9%prevalence of mastitis in cows. In 1997, Steras reported 44.6% prevalence of mastitis.

Turkey

Beytut *et al.* (2002) studied on 950 cows brought to the two local abbatoirs and found 11.02% incidence of mastitis by using CMT. They also carried out a pathological examination in udder lobes and reported that gross lesions were comprised of small nodular structures on both the wall of cisterna and parenchyma (45 lobes), abscesses covered by fibrous capsules on the cisterna and parenchyma (33 lobes), parenchymal fibrosis (9 lobes), necrotic masses covered by thick fibrous capsules in the cisterna (4 lobes), single or coalesced nodules the size of chickpea on the wall of cisterna and parenchyma (7 lobes), and haemorrhage and oedema (4 lobes). Dependent upon the lesions observed by histopathological examination of the lobes, mastitis was classified as acute mastitis and galactophoritis catarhalis (7 lobes), chronic mastitis and galactophoritis catarhalis (43 lobes), mastitis apestomatosa (33 lobes), nonpurulent interstitial mastitis (12 lobes), mastitis actinomycotica (8 lobes), acute mastitis gravis (5 lobes), chronic mastitis (4 lobes) and haemorrhagic mastitis (4 lobes). Ergun *et al.* (2004) reported 71.9% prevalence of mastitis in cows by CMT. Bastan *et al.* (2008) also reported similar prevalence (72.67%) of mastitis in cows.

Poland

Kotowski (1991) examined 632 Polish Black-and-White Lowland cows on 3 large scale farms in 1989-1990, clinical mastitis was diagnosed in 81, incidence ranging from 7.6 to 17.2% on individual farms. Primiparous cows were more affected than multiparous ones. Klossowska *et al.* (1996) have reported 48% prevalence of bovine mastitis on 10 farms in Poland. The prevalence of mastitis on individual farms ranged from 23 to 89%. Clinical and subclinical mastitis was diagnosed in 10.3% and 17.2% respectively. Borkowska and Rozycka (1999) examined 292 cows (1164 quarters) maintained on 32 individual farms using the CMT and result showed 107 samples were positive. Inflammation of mammary glands was more prevalent in older cows than in heifers and in second-lactation cows. Incidence of mastitis was higher in the summer and in cows with udder conformation defects.

Finland

The total incidence of clinical mastitis in Finland and other Scandinavian countries has been reported to be higher (10-30%; Syvajarvi *et al.*, 1986). The prevalence of mastitis on cow basis decreased from 47.8% in 1988 to 37.8% in 1995 (Myllys *et al.*, 1998). The prevalence of mastitis in Finland has been decreased from 38% in 1995 to 31% in 2001 (Pitkala *et al.*, 2004).

U.K.

The incidence of mastitis in U.K. has been reduced from an estimated 120 cases per 100 cows/year in 1960 (Dodd and Neave, 1970; Wilson and Kingwill, 1975) to the current level of 35-45 cases per 100 cows/year (Kossaibati *et al.*, 1998; Wilesmith *et al.*, 1986). Esslemont and Kossaibati (1996) recorded the mean incidence of mastitis to be 33.20% in HF herds in England. Data from 144 herds for the period 1994-1996 revealed an annual incidence of more than 43 quarter cases per 100 cows/year (Kossaibati *et al.*, 1998). A survey of DAISY (Dairy Information System) recorded herds in England and Wales reported the following parameters for clinical mastitis: 39.9 cases per 100 cows; 25.9% of cows affected and a recurrence rate of 18.3% (Kossaibati *et al.*, 1998). Another survey of English and Welsh dairy herds participating in an udder health programme found an average clinical incidence rate of 34 cases per 100 cows (Berry, 1998). The average reported incidence of clinical 22.8 cases per 100 cows/year, ranged from 0.6 to 147.1 in Great Britain (Peeler *et al.*, 1999).

Bradley and Green (2001) reported 41.6% incidence of mastitis in cows. A study on 482 British dairy herds, showed mean proportion of cows in the herd with clinical mastitis was 23.1% (range 0 to 80), with a mean of 1-50 quarter cases per cow. The mean incidence rate of clinical mastitis was 36.7

quarter cases per 100 cow years (range 0 to 208.2). Twelve per cent of the quarter cases showed systemic signs, including inappetence and severe lethargy. Over 22% of quarter cases occurred in the first seven days of lactation and over 50% occurred in the first 90 days of lactation. Cluster analysis indicated that the main difference between herds with a low and average incidence of mastitis was the proportion of clinical cases occurring in the first seven days of lactation, 14% compared with 44 %, respectively (Peeler *et al.*, 2002). Clinical cases range from the mild to the acute to the peracute. Approximately 60% of cases were considered 'mild' in one cohort study while the mortality in mastitis cases varied over a three year period from 0.3% to 0.6% (Wilesmith et al, 1986). In another study, mild, acute and per-acute cases were considered to occur in the approximate ratios of 70:29:1 (Blowey, 1986).

The Netherlands

Schukken *et al.* (1989) average annual incidence was 17.9 cases per 100 cows and ranged from none to 80 cases per 100 cows. Steeneveld et al. (2008) reported that the 11.04% positive for Gram positive and Gram negative organisms during 18 months study on mastitis. Sampimon et al. (2009) conducted a study in 12 Dutch provinces to know the status of mastitis. Quarter milk samples were collected from all 408 cows with a somatic cell count (SCC) =250000 cells/ml and 145 heifers with SCC=150000 cells/ml at the last milk test before the farm visit. Additionally, samples were collected from 519 (approximately 25%) of the remaining low-SCC cows and heifers with a SCC at the last milk test before the farm visit of <250 000 and <150 000 cells/ml, respectively. Bacterial growth occurred in 37.3% of milk samples of high-SCC cows and in 21.1% of low-SCC cows. Borne et al. (2010) carried out a study from July, 2004 to June, 2005 in primi- and multiparae cows in the Netherlands. Mean herd level sub-clinical mastitis prevalence was 12.8% in primi- and 27.1% in multiparae. Mean herd level clinical mastitis cases were observed 20.2 and 39.6 times per 100 cow-years at risk, respectively.

Switzerland

Roesch *et al.* (2007) carried out a study of sub-clinical mastitis on conventional and organic dairy farms and found cow level prevalences of sub-clinical mastitis were 35 and 40% in conventional and organics farms respectively, and quarter level prevalences were 15 in conventional and 18% in organic farms. This study indicates that the prevalence of sub-clinical mastitis was higher in organic dairy farms than conventional at quarter level.

Denmark

Dssing (1994) carriedout a study on 1012 dairy cows in 95 herds in West Jutland the prevalence of clinical mastitis in the dry period was 10.9%.

Byarugaba *et al.* (2008) reported 61.30% prevalence of CMT- positive cows, of which sub-clinical mastitis was 60.70%.

Oceania

New Zealand

The average cumulative incidence of clinical mastitis was 9.9% (range 0.9 - 21.4%) in 38 commercial New Zealand herds in early lactation (McDougall, 1998). A decreased prevalence of clinical mastitis was associated with an increased percentage of the herd treated with dry cow antibiotics. An increased prevalence of clinical mastitis was associated with both an increased percentage of cows treated in the previous season with lactating cow antibiotics and an increased percentage of heifers in the herd. In the year of 2004, the precalving prevalence of quarter intramammary infection with pathogen was 18.5% (Compton *et al.*, 2007).

Africa

In Africa, sub-clinical mastitis is a significant problem in dairy enterprises. In east Africa, the prevalence of sub-clinical mastitis, as defined by the California mastitis test (CMT), has been reported to range from 47 to 90 per cent of cows, and 28 to 33 per cent of quarters (Mulei 1999, Mungube 2001, Kivaria *et al.*, 2004).

Nigeria

Ameh *et al.* (1999) examined 5000 cows (in lactation and dry), within and around Maiduguri Borno State of Nigeria, of which 104 (2.10%) showed clinical mastitis involving 202 quarters. The survey revealed that majority of cases occurred in cows between 4 and 7 years of age, and that the incidence declined as the animals became older. The number of quarters affected were: LF, 49; RF, 45; LH, 51; RH, 57. With regards to the clinical state of mammary gland, the greatest numbers were of acute cases (25.00%), followed by sub acute (21.00%), chronic (19.00%) and gangrenous forms (3.00%). There was greater single quarter involvement, with hind quarters being more commonly affected. The increase in clinical mastitis with advancing age was entirely due to there being more infections among older cows.

Egypt

A study of Ahmed *et al.* (2008) revealed very low prevalence (9.69%) of sub-clinical mastitis in buffaloes by cultural examination. Osman et al. (2009) was detected mastitis in 34.12 and 9.64% quarter milk samples collected from cases of clinical mastitis in cows and buffaloes respectively.

Sudan

A study of Abdelrahim *et al.* (1989) reported 70.3% and 44.1% infection rates in cows and quarters, respectively in Sudan. Mohamed et al. (1993) reported 17.29% and 3.67% incidence of sub-clinical and clinical mastitis. This study is also supported by Ibtisam *et al.* (2006), they also reported that the incidence of sub-clinical mastitis is higher than clinical mastitis in cattle in Sudan and observed that higher prevalence of sub-clinical mastitis in the left fore quarters and lower incidence in left hind quarters. However, the pattern of clinical mastitis was opposite.

Ethiopia

In Ethiopia, livestock represents major national resource and form an integral part of agriculture production system. The country has a largest livestock population of any African country with estimated 35 million cattle. Cow represents the largest population of cattle production of the country, 42% of the total cattle heads are milking cows (Lakew *et al.*, 2009).

Yigezu (1990) indicated a mastitis prevalence of 44.6% in six different dairy sites, and 3.8% clinical and 40.8% of sub-clinical mastitis, respectively in the southern region of Ethiopia. Kerro (1997) in selected areas of southern Ethiopia reported a prevalence of mastitis to be 40.39% of which 41.93% clinical and 58.06% sub-clinical infection. Dagne and Abdicho (2001) reported a sub-clinical mastitis prevalence rate of 34.6%, 45.15% and 38.7% in Repi, Debre Zeit and Modjo, respectively.

A study on the management and economics of mastitis carried out by Mungube (2001) in dairy cows in the urban and periurban areas of Addis Ababa indicated an overall clinical mastitis prevalence of 6.6% cow and 2.8% quarter level. He also, indicated that out of the 51 farms studied at least a case of clinical mastitis was registered in 12 farms (24%) and the highest clinical mastitis prevalence was 27.3% in one large farm situated in the periurban production sub-system followed by 14% in another large farm while the highest prevalence in small-scale dairy farms was 33.3%. Workineh *et al.* (2002) reported, overall prevalence of mastitis in cows 38.2%. Biffa *et al.* (2005) carried out a study on 974 lactating cows in Southern Ethiopia and found that 34.9% cows had mastitis (11.9% clinical and 23.0% sub-clinical). A study from 109 households on 500 cross bred lactating cows, showed the prevalence of clinical mastitis at herd, cow and quarter levels was 8.3, 1.8 and 0.51% respectively, while that of sub-clinical mastitis was 54.7%, 22.3% and 10.1% respectively (Getahun *et al.*, 2008). Argaw and Tolosa (2008) were carried out a study in North Shoa Zone of the Oromia Regional state in central Ethiopia from March - April 2000. A cross section study was carried out on a total of 153 lactating cows for sub-clinical mastitis by using California Mstitis Test (CMT). Of all animal tested 137 (89.54 %) were found positive for mastitis. From 137 CMT positive animals, 122 were bacteriologically positive. The prevalence of sub-clinical mastitis 89.54% in cow and 63.1% quarters were recorded and the resulting quarter infection rate was 56.70%. Lakew *et al.* (2009) reported 26.5% and 38% prevalence of clinical and sub-clinical mastitis respectively, in cattle. A recent report indicated that prevalence of clinical mastitis on quarter level was 0.9% and prevalence of sub-clinical mastitis was 42.5% by CMT in cows (Abebe *et al.*, 2010). In another recent study a total of 107 cross bred milking cows were tested using California Mastitis Test. Prevalence of mastitis at cow level was 71.0% (76/107), out of which 22.4 and 48.6% were clinical and subclinical, respectively. The quarter level prevalence was 44.9%; from this the clinical and subclinical forms were 10.0% and 34.8%, respectively. Out of the 43 quarters with clinical cases, 31 had blind teats while 12 of them revealed active cases of mastitis. Samples from all 12 active clinical cases and 90.0% of the CMT positive subclinical quarters were found to be culture positive (Mekibib *et al.*, 2010).

A total of 300 lactating cows in Adama town, East Shoa, Ethiopia, were tested for mastitis using the CMT. One hundred and forty of the cows (46.7%) had mastitis, of which 10.0% (30/300) and 36.7% (110/300) showed clinical and sub-clinical mastitis, respectively. The quarter level prevalence was 29.0% (348/1200); from which the clinical form was 5.4% (65/1200) and the subclinical was 25.6% (283/1200). Of the 65 quarters with clinical cases, 18 had blind teats while 47 had active mastitis (Abera *et al.*, 2010).

Kenya

In the year of 1999, a report of Omore and associates suggests that prevalence of mastitis in cows varied from 43% to 80% in Kenya. In Kenya, the prevalence of sub-clinical mastitis, as defined by a positive bacteriological culture in smallholder dairy cows, was reported to be 63 per cent of cows and 21 per cent of quarters (Omore *et al.*, 1996). Shitandi *et al.* (2004) reported 19.6% prevalence of clinical mastitis at cow level and found right fore quarters are more affected.

Uganda

Byarugaba *et al.* (2008) reported 61.3% prevalence of mastitis in cows, of which 60.7% was sub-clinical mastitis.

Tanzania

Shem *et al.* (2001) reported incidence of sub-clinical and clinical mastitis as 62% and 4% respectively. They found that levels of infection were higher on smallholder dairy farms (75%) than on large scale farms (25%).

Kivaria *et al.* (2004) reported 3.8% and 90.30% prevalence of clinical and sub-clinical mastitis respectively in lactating cows by CMT during June to September, 2002 on smallholder dairy farms in Dar es Salaam region of Tanzania. While a previous study in Dar es Salaam region, reported the point prevalence of clinical mastitis was 27 and 70 cases per 100 cows for clinical and sub-clinical mastitis respectively (Kapaga *et al.*, 1995). These findings indicate that occurrence of clinical mastitis in Tanzania dairy cows is decreasing. Mdegela et al. (2005) reported 8.8% and 61.20% prevalence of clinical and sub-clinical mastitis in cattle. Karimuribo et al. (2006) have been reported 14.2% and 46.2% prevalence of clinical and sub-clinical mastitis in dairy cows.

A cross sectional study was carried out in the Iringa and Tanga regions of Tanzania between January to March, 1999 and reported mean prevalence of CMT-positive cows was 75.9 % and quarters was 46.2%, while prevalence of culture-positive cows was 43.8% and quarters wise 24.3% (Karimuribo *et al.*, 2008).

References

Aarestrup, F.M. and Jensen, N.E. (1997). J. Dairy Sci., 80: 307–312.

Abdelrahim, A.I., Shommein, A.I., Suliman, H.B. and Shaddad, S.A.I. (1989). Rev. Prod. Vet. Med. Trop. Countries. 42: 512-514.

Abebe, G., Ike, A.C., Siegmund-Schultze, M. Mané-Bielfeldt, A. and Zárate, A.V. (2010). Zoonoses and Public Health, 57(5): 367-374.

Abera, M., Demie, B., Aragaw, K., Regassa, F. and Regassa, A. (2010). J. Vet. Med. & Anim. Hlth., 2(3): 29-34.

Afonso-silva, J.A.B., Pereira, C.F., Mendonca, C.P., Vianni, M.C.T., Mendonca, C.P. and Vianni, M.C.E. (1999). Revista-Brasileria-Medicine-Veterinaria. 21(3):115-118.

Ahlner, S. (2003). Thesis, SLU Uppsala.

Ahlner, S. and Axelsson, A. (2002). Bulletin Minor Field Studies - International Office, Swedish University of Agricultural Sciences, No. 214. pp. 16.

Ahmed, W.M., Sherein, I., Abd Ei-Moez and Nabil, M. (2008). Global Veterinaria, 2(1): 41-45.

Ali, S.L., Supekar, P.G. and Shukla, P.C. (1989). Guj. Vet., 16 (2): 16-28.

Ameh, J.A., Edgbe-Nwiyi, T.N., Zaria, L.T. (1999). Vet. Ariv., 69(2): 87-95.

Anon (1963). Annual Technical Report of the Indian Council of Agricultural Research, India.1960-61. Pp. 157.

Anwar, M. and Chaudhry, A.Q. (1983). Pakistan Vet. J., 3: 142.

Appleman, R.A. (1973). J. Dairy Sci., 56: 411–423.

Appleman, R.D. (1970). Quantifying the genetic effects on the anatomy of the streak canal. In: Proc. VI Int. Conf. Cattle Dis., 104.

Argaw, K. and Tolosa, T. (2008). The Internet Journal of Veterinary Medicine., Volume 5 Number1.http://www.ispub.com/ostia/index.phpxmlFilePath=journals/ijvm/front.xml

Babu, Y.H. and Sudhakar, Srinivas, C.S. and Khan, M.A. (1983). Livestock Advisor, 8(4): 47-49.

Bachaya, H.A., Iqbal, Z., Jabbar, A., Abbas, R.Z. and Ali, R. (2005). Int. J. Agri. Biol., 7(6): 1034-1035.

Bachaya, H.A., Iqbal, Z., Muhammad, G., Yousaf, A. and Ali, H.M. (2005). Pakistan. Vet .J., 25: 134-136.

Bajpai, A.K., Supekar, P.G. and Shukla, P.C. (1989). Buffalo mastitis. In: Compendium of VIII Annual Convention of Indian Society for Veterinary Medicine, Izatnagar, India.

Bakken, G. (1981). Acta Agric. Scand., 31: 438-444.

Bakken, G. (1981). Acta Agriculturae Scandinavica, 31(3): 273-286.

Banerjee, K., Ray, J.P.; Sadhukhan, T., Das, R. and Chandra, S. (2002). Indian J. Anim. Hlth., 41(2): 109-112.

Bansal, B.K., Singh, K.B., Rohan, R., Joshi, D.V., Nauriyal, D.C. and Mohan, R. (1995). J. Res., 32(1): 79-81.

Bansal, B.K., Singh, M.B., Jand, S.K., Nauriyal, D.C. and Randhawa, S.S. (1990). Indian J. Dairy Sci., 43(3): 355-358.

Barkema, H.W., Schukken, Y.H., Lam, T.J.G.M., Beiboer, M.L., Benedictus, G. and Brand, A. (1999). J. Dairy Sci., 82:1643-1654.

Bartlett, P.C., Miller, G.Y., Lance, S.E. and Heider, L.E. (1992). Prev. Vet. Med., 12: 59-71.

Bas¸tan, A., Kaccar, C., Acar, D.B., Sahin, M. and Cengiz, M. (2008). Turkish J. Vet. Anim. Sci., 32(2): 119-121.

Batra, T.R., Nonnecke, B.J., Newlould, F.S.H. and Hacker, R.R. (1977). J. Dairy Sci., 60: 1169-1172.

Behera, S., Swain, R.K., Samantaray, D.P. and Dash, S.K. (2008). J. Pure and Appl. Microbiol., 2(2): 607-613.

Beloti, V., Muller, E.E., Friets, J.C.-de, Mettifogo, E., de-Freitag, J.C. (1997). Semina-Londrina. 18(1): 45-53.

Bendixen, P.H., Vilson, B., Ekesbo, I and Astrand, D.B. (1988). Prev. Vet. Med., 6: 17-25.

Berry, D.P. and Meaney, W.J. (2005). Irish J. Agric. Food Res., 44: 147–156.

Berry, E. and Hillerton, J.E. (2002). J. Dairy Sci., 85: 112–121.

Berry, E.A. (1998). In: Proc. British Mastitis Conf., Stoneleigh, October 7, 1998. pp. 78-79.

Beytut, E., Aydýn, F., Ozcan, K. and Gencc, O. (2002). Kafkas Üniversitesi Veteriner Fakültesi Dergisi, 8(2): 111-122.

Bhatnagar, R.N. and Mehrota, P.N. (1969). Indian Vet. J., 46: 106-111.

Bhikane, A.U., Anantwar, L.G., Yadav, G.U., Markandeya, N.M. and Deshmukh, Y.T. (2002). In: Proceeding of Round Table Conference on Mastitis, 4-5 Feb., 2002, Nagpur, M.S. (India). Pp. 133-134.

Bhoyar, A.R., Shende, C.V., Nalawade, N.A., Kakade, S.P., Salunkhe, M.S. and Karnewar, S.D. (2009). Green Farming, 2(10): 723-724.

Bhutto, A.L., Murray, R.D. and Zerai Woldehiwet, H.(2008). Udder shape and teat-end lesions as potential risk factors for high somatic. The Vet. J., (In press) doi:10.1016/j.tvjl.2008.08.024

Biffa, D., Debela, E. and Beyene, F. (2005). Intl. J. Appl. Res. Vet. Med., 3(3): 189-198.

Biochard, D. and Rupp, R. (1997). Interbull Bull. no. 15. Int. Bull Eval. Serv., Uppsala, Sweden. Pp. 54-60.

Bjorck, G.R. (1963). Zhivotnovodstov mosk, 27(15): 105-123.

Blowey, R.W. (1986). Vet. Rec, 119: 551-553.

Boettcher, P.J., Dekkers, J.C.M. and Kolstad, B.W. (1998). J. Dairy Sci., 81:1157–1168.

Borkowska, D. and Rozycka, G. (1999). Influence of some factors on udder health in cows bred on individual farms of Zamoœc´ voivodeship. Annales Universitatis Mariae Curie-Sklodowska. Sectio EE Zootechnica, 17: 31-38.

Borne, B.H.P., Schaik, G., Lam, T.J.G.M. and Nielen, M. (2010). Prev. Vet. Med., 96(1/2): 49-55.

Bradley, A.J. and Green, M.J. (2000). J.Dairy Sci., 83:1957.

Bradley, A.J. and Green, M.J. (2001). In: Proc of the 40th Annu. Meet. of the National Mastitis Council.

Bradley, A.J. and Green, M.J. (2001). Vet. Rec., 148: 683-686.

Bradley, A.J. and Green, M.J. (2004). Vet. Clin. Food Anim., 20: 547–568.

Bramley, A.J., Patel, A.H., O'Relly, M., Foster, R. and Foster, T.J. (1989). Infection and Immunity., 57: 481-512.

Brito, J.R.F., Souza, G.N., Rubialc, L., Faria, C.G. and Moraes, L.C.D. (2009). In: Proc. XIV International Soc. for Anim. Hygiene (ISAH) Cong, 19-23, July 2009, Vechta, Germany. Pp. 243-246.

Brochart, M., Barnouin, J. and Fayet, J.C. (1984). Bulletin des Groupements Techniques Vétérinaires, 5: 7-24.

Browning, J.W., Mein, G.A., Brightling, P. Nicholls, T.J. and Barton, M. (1994). Aust. Vet. J., 71: 179-181.

Buragohain, J. and Dutta, G.N. (1998). Indian Vet. J., 75(8): 736-737.

Buragohain, J. and Dutta, G.N. (2000). Intl. J. Anim. Sci., 15(2): 245-252.

Byarugaba, D.K., Nakavuma, J.L., Vaarst, M. and Laker, C. (2008). Livest. Res. Rural Develop., 20(1), 2008.

Capuco, A.V., Wood, D.L. Bright, S.A., Miller, R.H. and Bitman, J. (1990). J. Dairy Sci., 73: 1745-1750.

Cedeno, C.B., Alfaro, R.M., Cedeño, E.G., García, E.B., Domínguez, R.L., Vázquez, H.C. and Wolter, W. (2010). Etiological agents of the mastitis in dairy cows of the municipality of álvaro obregon michoacan. In: Proc. of XXVI World Buiatrics Cong., 14-18, Nov., Santiago de Chile, Chile.

Chahar, A., Gahlot, A.K. and Tanwar, R.K. (2005). Vet. Practitioner, 6(1): 84-87.

Chandra, A., Roy, C.R., Banerjee, F.K. and Guha, C. (1989). Indian Vet. J., 66(4): 277-282.

Chew, B.P. and Johnston, L.A. (1985). J. Dairy SCi., 08(Suppl. 1):191. (Abstr.)

Chew, B.P., Hollen, L.L., Hillers, J.K. and Herlugson, M.L. (1982). J. Dairy Sci., 65: 2111-2118.

Chrishty, M.A., Arshad, M., Avais, M., Hameed, S. and Ijaz, M. (2007). Buffalo Bull., 26(2): 50-55.

Chrystal, M.A., Seykora, A.J., Hansen, L.B., Freeman, A.E., Kelley, D.H. and Healey, M.H. (2001). J. Diary Sci., 84: 2549–2554.

Comalli, M.P., Eberhart, R.J., Griel Jr., L.C. and Rothenbacher, H. (1984). Am. J. Vet. Res., 45: 2236.

Compton, C. W. R., Heuer, C., Parker, K. and McDougall, S. (2007). J. Dairy Sci., 90(9): 4157–4170.

Compton, C.W.R., McDougall, S., Parker, K. and Heuer, C. (2007). J. Dairy Sci., 90: 4171-4180.

Cook, N.B. and Mentik, R. (2006). In: Proc. 45th Proc. 26th Annu. Mtg. Natl. Mastitis Counc., Orlando, FL. Pp. 234.

Corbett, R. (2009). In: Proc. NMC Annual Meeting, 2009. pp. 113-119.

Crist, W.L., Heider, L.E., Sears, P.M., Barr, H.L., Kowalski, J.J. and Schmidt, G.H. (1982). J. Dairy Sci., 65(5): 828-834.

Curtis, C.R., Erb, H.N., Sniffen, C.J., Smith, R.D., Powers, P.A., Smith, M.C., White, M.E., Hilman, R.B. and Pearson, E.J. (1983). J. Am. Vet. Med. Asso., 183: 559–561.

Dagne, A. and Abdicho, S. (2001). Tropical Animal Health and Product. 33, 511-519.

Dahl, G.E. (2004). New ideas in dry cow and transition management: Beyond nutrition. University of Illinois Extension. www.livestocktrail.uiuc.edu/dairynet/paperDisplay.cfm?ContentID=6758

Dangore, A.D., Bhalerao, D.P., Jagadish, S., Keskar, D.B. and Sharma, L.K. (2000). Indian Vet. J., 77(5): 380-381.

Das, P.K. and Joseph, E. (2005). Buffalo Bulletin 24 (1): 3-9.

De, U.K. and Mukherjee, R. (2009). Indian Vet. J., 86(8): 858-859.

Devi, B.K., Shukla, P.C. and Bagherwal, R.K. (1997). Indian J. Dairy Sci., 50(6): 477-478.

Dhakal, I.P., Dhakal, P., Koshihara, T. and Nagahata, H. (2007). J. Vet. Med. Sci., 69(12): 1241–1245.

Dhanapalan, P. (2000). In: Proceeding of Round Table Conference on Mastitis, 18-19 Feb., 2000, Izatnagar, U.P., India. Pp. 12-22.

Dhote, S.W., Kurkure, N.V., Kalorey, D.R. and Ganvir, P.T. (1999). Indian Vet. J., 76(3): 251-252.

Doane, R.M., Oliver, S.P., Walker, R.D. and Shull, E.P. (1987). Am. J. Vet. Res., 48: 749.

Dodd, F.H. and Neave, F.K. (1970). Nat. Inst. Res. Dairy. Bienn. Rev.: NIRD, Reading 21-60.

Dodd, F.H., Clough, P.A., Henriques, E. and Neave, F.K. (1950). J. Dairy Sci., 17: 107-111.

Dodenhoff, J., Sprengel, D., Duda, J. and Dempfle, L. (1999). Zuchtungskunde 71: 459-472.

Doherr, M.G., Roesch, M., Schaeren, W., Schallibaum, M. and Blum, J.W. (2007). Veterinarni Medicina, 52(11): 487–495.

Dssing, F. (1994). Dansk Veterinærtidsskrift, 77(8): 353-354, 356-359.

Dubal, Z.B., Rahman, H., Pal, P., Kumar, A. and Pradhan, K. (2010). Indian J. Anim. Sci., 80(12): 1163-1167.

Duda, J. (1995). Zuchtungskunde, 67: 467-476.

Eberhart, R.J. (1986). J. Dairy Sci., 69(6): 1721-1732.

Edmondson, P. (2001). In Practice, 3(March): 150-159.

Edmondson, P. and Blowey, R. (1998). In Practice, 6: 297-303.

Ekman, T. (1998). A study of dairy herds with constantly low or high bulk milk somatic cell countwith emphasis on management. PhD thesis, Swedish University of Agricultural Sciences, Uppsala, Sweden. pp.170.

Elbers, A.R., Miltenburg J.D., de Lange, D., Crauwels, A. P., Barkema, H.W. and Schukken Y.H. (1998). J. Dairy Sci., 81: 420–426.

Elvinger, F., Hansen, P.J. and Natzke, R.P. (1991). Am. J. Vet. Res., 52:1692–1698.

Elvinger, F., Natzke, R.P. and Hansen, P.J. (1992). J. Dairy Sci., 75: 449-62.

Emanuelson, J.L.F., Danell, B. and Philipsson, J. (1988). J. Dairy Sci., 71: 467–476.

Emanuelson, U., Oltenacu, P.A. and Grohn, Y.T. (1993). J. Dairy Sci., 76: 2765-72.

Ergun, Y., Aslantas, O., Dogruer, G. and Cantekin, Z. (2004). Veteriner Bilimleri Dergisi, 20(4): 25-28.

Esslemont, R.J. and Koshaibati, M.A. (1996). Vet. Rec., 139(20): 486-490.

Fadlelmula, A., Al Dughaym, A.M., Mohamed, G.E., Al Deib, M.K. and Al Zubaidy, A.J. (2009). Bulg. J. Vet. Med., 12(3): 199-206.

Fang, W., Jiang, C. and Liu, H. (1993). Prev. Vet. Med., 15: 169-180.

FAO (2007). State of the World's Farm Animal Genetic Resources [Online]. Available from: www.fao.org/Ag/AGAInfo/programmemes/en/genetics/documents/AH473e01.pdf [Accessed December 7 2008].

Farnsworth, R.J. (1995). Observations on teat lesions. In: Proc. Minnesota Dairy Health Conf., University of Minnesota: 28-33.

Faull, W.B., Walton, J.R., Barmley, A.J. and Hughes, J.W. (1983). Vet. Rec., 133: 415-425.

Ferdowsi, H., Adibmoradi, M., Asadi1, M., Rezakhani1, A. and Hasani1, A. (2009). In: Proc. XIV International Soc. for Anim. Hygiene (ISAH) Cong, 19-23, July 2009, Vechta, Germany. Pp. 215-218.

Ferguson, J.D., Azzaro, G., Gambina, M. and Licitra, G. (2007). J. Dairy Sci., 90(12): 5798–5813.

Fiedter, H., Breitenstein, K.G., Piur, S. and Herrendorfer, G. (1982). Arch. Tierz., 25(2): 87.

Forsgren, A., Ghetie, V., Lindmark, R. and Sjoquist, J. (1983). Protein A and its exploitation. In: Easmon CSF, Adlam, C. (Eds) Staphylococci and Staphylococcal infections, Vol. 2: The organisms in vivo and in vitro. 429-480, Academic Press, London.

Fox, L.K., Kirk, J.H. and Britten, A. (2005). Dis. Vet. Public Health 52:153–160.

Funke, G., von Graevenitz, A., Clarridge J.E. 3rd and Bernard, K.A. (1997). Clin. Microbiol. Rev., 10(1):125–159.

Funke, H. (1988). In: Proc. 6th Intl. Cong. on Animal Hygiene, 14-17 June, Skara, Sweden. Vol. 1, pp. 209-214.

Gajbhiye, A.R. (1996). M.V.Sc. Thesis, submitted to Dr. Panjabrao Deshmukh Krishi Vidyapeeth, Akola, India.

Geer, D.V.D., Grommers, F.J. and Van Houten, M. (1979). Vet_Q., 1: 204-2111.

Getahun, K., Kelay, B., Bekana, M. and Lobago, F. (2008). Trop. Anim. Hlth. Prod., 40(4): 261-268.

Ghazaei, C. (2006). J. Anim. Vet. Adva., 5 (4): 280-283.

Ghose, B., Sharda, R., Chhabra, D. and Sharma, V. (2003). Indian Vet. J., 80(6): 499-501.

Gianneechini, R., Concha, C., Rivero, R., Delucci, I. and Moreno López, J. (2002). Acta Vet. Scand., 43: 221-230.

Godden, S., Rapnicki, P., Stewart, S., Fetrow, J., Johnson, A., Bey, R. and Fransworth, R. (2003). J. Dairy Sci., 86: 3899-3911.

Gowardhan, A.P., Chavan, K.D. and Mote, M.G. (2008). Indian Vet. J., 85(6): 687-688.

Graf, R., (1982). Teat-end lesions caused by machine milking in cows. Thesis. Ludwig Maximilians Universität München, München, Germany.

Green, M.J., Bradley, A.J., Medley, G.F. and Browne, W.J. (2007). J. Dairy Sci., 90:3764–3776.

Green, M.J., Green, L.E. and Cripps, P.J. (1996). Vet. Record, 138: 305-306.

Green, M.J., Green, L.E., Medley, G.F., Schukken, Y.H. and Bradley, A.J. (2002). J. Dairy Sci., 85(10): 2589–2599.

Grinberg, N., Elazar, S., Rosenshine, I. and Shpigel, N.Y. (2008). Infection and Immunity. 76(6): 2802-2807.

Grindal, R.J. and Bramley, A.L.J. (1989). J. Dairy Res., 56: 683-690.

Grindal, R.J., and Hillerton, J.E. (1991). J. Dairy Res., 58: 263-268.

Hamann, J., Burvenich, C., Mayntz, M., Osteras, O. and Halder, W. (1994). Machine-induced changes in the status of the bovine teat tissue with respect to new infection risk. In "Teat Tissue Reactions to Machine Milking and New Infection Risk". Chapt 2 of IDF Bulletin 297, International Dairy Federation, Brussels, Belgium.

Harmon, R.J., Schanbacher, F.L., Ferguson, L.C. and Smith, K.L. (1975). Am. J. Vet. Res., 36:1001.

Hashmi, H.A. and Muneer, M.A. (1981). Pakistan Vet. J., 1: 164.

Hawari, A.D. and Al-Dabbas, F. (2008). Am. J. Anim. Vet. Sci., 3(1): 36-39.

Heald, C.W. (1985). Milk collection in lactation. B. L. Larson (ed.), Iowa State University press.

Hebel, P., Songen, W. and Beuing, R. (1979). Veterinaermed., 26: 667.

Hemilton, C., Emanuelson, U., Forslund, K., Hansson, I. and Ekman, T. (2006). Acta Veterinaria Scadinavica, 48:11.

Heringstad, B., Karlsen, A., Klemetsdal, G. and Ruane, J. (1997). In: Interbull Bull. no. 15. Int. Bull Eval. Serv., Uppsala, Sweden. Pp.45-49.

Hickman, G.C. (1964). J. Dairy Sci., 47: 777.

Hill, A.W., Reid, I.M. and Collins, R.A. (1985). Vet Rec., 117(21): 549-51.

Hillerton, J. E., Shearn, M.F.H. and West, J.G.H. (1995). In: Proc. 3rd Int. Dairy Fed. Int. Mastitis Sem., Tel Aviv, Israel. Int. Dairy Fed., Brussels, Belgium. Pp 88–89.

Hillerton, J.E., Pankey, J.W. and Pankey, P. (1999). In: Proc. on NMC annual meetings, 38: 202-203.

Hogan, J.S. and Smith, K.L. (1992). Creating a quality environment: bedding. In: Pro. National Mastitis Council. pp 201-203.

Hogan, J.S. and Smith, K.L. (2000). Research and reviews: Dairy. Special Circular. Ohio State University Bulletin-169-99.

Hogan, J.S., Smith, K.L., Todhunter, D.A. and Schoenberger, P.S. (1988). J. Dairy Sci., 71: 2520.

Horst, R.L. and Jorgensen, N.A. (1982). J. Dairy Sci., 65: 2332-2337.

Houben, E.H.P., Dijkhuizen, A.A., van Arendonk, J.A.M. and Huirne, R.B.M. (1993). J. Dairy Sci., 76: 2561–2578.

Hussain, M., Khalid, N. and Naeem, I. (1984). Pakistan Vet. J., 4: 161–164

Huxley, J.N., Green, M.J. and Bradley, A.J. (2003). Corynebacterium bovis – friend or foe? In: Proc. of British Mastitis Conference, Garstang, 2003.

Ibtisam, E.M., El Zubeir and El Owni, O.A.O. (2006). Res. J. Anim. Vet. Sci., 1(1): 25-29.

Inderwies, T., Riedl, J., Kiossis, E. and Bruckmaier, R.P. (2003). J. Dairy Res., 70: 289-292.

Jackson, P. (1996). In Practice, 2:76-80.

Jackson, V.I. (1970). Vet. Rec., 87: 2.

Jagoe, S. (2009). Mastitis at calving. From Diary news letter. Available at http// www.warrnamboolvet.com.au/pr01.htm

Jain, N.C. (1976). Theriogenology 6:153.

Jain, N.C. (1979). J. Dairy Sci., 52: 128-134.

Jarillo Cabrera, D. (1980). Veterinaria, Mexico, 11(1): 28-29.

Jensen, D.L. and Eberhart, R.J. (1981). Am. J. Vet. Res., 42: 743.

Jensen, D.L., and Eberhart, R.J. (1975). Am. J. Vet. Res., 36: 619.

Johansson, B. (2000). Effect of milking and feeding routines on milk production, hormone release and behaviour in dairy cattle. PhD thesis, Swedish University of Agricultural Sciences, Uppsala, Sweden. 46 pp.

Johansson, V.I., and Malven, P. (1960). Z. Tierz. Zuch tungsbiol., 74: 1.

Johnson, H.D. and Vanjonack W.J. (1975). J. Dairy Sci., 59: 1603-1617.

Jong, D.G. and Lansbergen, L. (1996). Udder health index:selection for mastitis resistance. Pages 42–47 *in* INTERBULL Bull. no. 12. Int. Bull Eval. Serv., Gembloux, Belgium.

Joshi, H.D. and Joshi, B.R. (1997). Veterinary Review. 12(1): 1-6.

Joshi, H.D., Joshi, B.R and Shrestha, H.K. (1998). Veterinary Review. 13: 12-15.

Jukola, E., Hakkarainen, J., Saloniemi, H. and Sankari, S. (1996). J. Dairy Sci., 79: 838-845.

Kader, M.A., Samad, M.A., Saha, S. and Taleb, M.A. (2002). Indian J. Dairy Sci., 55(4): 218-223.

Kaiser, A.G. (1975). Aust. J. Exp. Agric. Anita. Husb., 15: 17.

Kalorey, D.R. (2001). In: Compendium of 2nd Round Table Conference on mastitis, PAU, Ludhiana, India. pp. 81-86.

Kalorey, D.R., Purohit, J.H. and Dholkia, P.M. (1983). Indian J. Anim. Sci., 53(9): 961-963.

Kamboj, M.L., Singh, A. and Prasad, S. (2008). Indian Vet. J., 85(8): 846-848.

Kapaga.A.M., Weinhaupl, I. and Baumann, M.P.O. (1995). Risk indicators and Mastitis Prevalence in Dairy Cattle in The Region of Dar Er Salaam- Tanzania. Livestock Production & Diseases. In: Prco. 8th Conference, Institute of Tropical Veterinary Medicine. Berlin.Germany.

Karimuribo, E.D., Fitzpatrick, J.L., Bell, C.E., Swai, E.S., Kambarage, D.M., Ogden, N.H., Bryant, M.J. and French, N.P. (2006). Prev. Vet. Med., 74(1): 84-98.

Karimuribo, E.D., Fitzpatrick, J.L., Swai, E.S., Bell, C., Bryant, M.J., Ogden, N.H., Kambarage, D.M. and French, N.P. (2008). Vet. Record, 163: 16-21.

Katoch, R.C., Sharma, M., Verma, S., Chahota, R. and Dhar, P. (2003). In: Proceeding of Round Table Conference on Mastitis, 14-15 April., 2003, Palampur, H.P. (India). Pp. 195-134-203.

Kavitha, K.L., Rajesh, K., Suresh, K., Satheesh, K. and Syama Sundar, N. (2009). Buffalo Bull., 28(3): 134-137.

Keister, Z.O., Moss, K.D., Zhang, H.M., Teegerstrom, T., Edling, R.A., Collier, R.J. and Ax, R.L. (2002). J. Dairy Sci., 85: 3217-3224.

Kerro, O. (1997). A Study on bovine mastitis in some selected areas of Southern Ethiopia. Faculty of Veterinary Medicine, Addis Ababa University, DVM thesis.

Khate, K. and Yadav, B.R. (2010). Indian J. Anim. Sci., 80(5): 437-469.

Kheirabadi, P., Ebrahimi, A. and Barati, F. (2008). Indian Vet. J., 85(4): 375-377.

Khire, D.W., Thatte, V.R., Kadu, M.S. and Belorkar, P.M. (1975). Maharashtra Vet. I, 2: 25-28.

Khire, D.W., Thatte, V.R., Kadu, M.S. and Belorkar, P.M. (1976). J. Dairy Sci., 29(1): 67.

Kimura, K., Reinhardt, T.A. and Goff, J.P. (2006). J. Dairy Sci., 89: 2588-2595.

Kirk, J.H. (2000). Mastitis 101- The Basics. Fact Sheet and Information on Dairy Cattle, Veterinary Medicine Extension, University of California. http://www.vetmed.ucdavis.edu/vetext/INF-DA/INF-DA_MASTITIS101.HTML

Kirk, J.H. (2009). Effects of milk heifers prior to calving on udder health and production . Fact Sheet and Information on Dairy Cattle, Veterinary Medicine Extension, University of California http://www.vetmed.ucdavis.edu/vetext/INF-DA/Milk_Heifers.pdf. downloaded on Nov., 2009.

Kivaria, F.M., Noordhuizen, J.P.T.M.and Kapaga, A.M. (2004). Trop. Anim. Hlth Prod., 36(6): 581-592.

Klaas, I.C., Enevoldsen, C., Ersboll, A.K. and Tolle, U. (2005). J. Dairy Sci., 88: 128–136.

Klaas, I.C., Enevoldsen, C., Vaarst, M. and Houe, H. (2004). J. Dairy Sci., 87: 1217–1228.

K³ossowska, A., Malinowski, E. and Kuzma, R. (1996). Medycyna Weterynaryjna, 52(11): 700-702.

Kornalijnslijper, E. (2003). Health and welfare of high producing dairy cows. Thesis Utrecht University, Utrecht, The Netherlands.

Kossaibati, M.A., Hovi, M. and Esslemont, R.J. (1998). Vet. Record, 143: 649-653.

Kotowski, K. (1991). Medycyna Weterynaryjna, 47(12): 555-556.

Kremer, W.D.J., Noordhuizen-Stassen, E.N., Grommers, F.J., Schukken, Y.H., Heeringa, R., Brand, A. and Burvenich, C. (1993). J. Dairy Sci., 76: 3428-3436.

Kumar, A., Rahal, A., Dwivedi, S.K. and Gupta, M.K. (2010). Egyptian J. Dairy Sci., 38: 31-34.

Kumar, B. (1988). Studies on incidence, chemotherapy and control of mastitis in cattle and buffalo. M.V.Sc. thesis, Punjab Agricultural University, Ludhiana, India.

Kumar, G.S.N., Appannavar, M.M., Suranagi, M.D. and Kotresh, A. M. (2010). Karnataka J. Agric. Sci., 23 (2): 407-408.

Kumar, R. and Sharma, A. (2002). Indian J. Anim. Sci., 72(5): 361-363.

Kumar, S. (1990). Studies on mastitis in buffaloes with emphasis on resistance, chemotherapy and control. M.V.Sc. thesis, Punjab Agricultural University, Ludhiana, India.

Kumari, P.M. and Gupta, B.J.R. (2002). Indian Vet. J., 79(1): 89.

Lacy-Hulbert, S.J. and Hillerton, J.E. (1995). J. Dairy Res., 62: 395-404.

Lakew, M., Tolosa, T. and Tigre, W. (2009). Trop. Anim. Hlth. Prod., 41(7): 1525-1530.

Lakshmi Rani, N., Srinivas, M., Suresh, K. and Sreenu, Makkena (2008). Indian Vet. J., 85(12): 1350-1351.

Lalrintluanga, C., Ralte, E.L. and Hmarkunga (2003). Indian Vet. J., 80(9): 931-932.

Lam, T.J.G.M., Schukken, Y.H., Van Vliet, J.H., Grommers, F.J., Tielen, M.J.M. and Brand, A. (1997). Am. J. Vet. Res., 58: 17–22.

Larsen, B., Jensen, N.E, Madse, P., Nielsen, S.M., Klastrup, O. and Madsen, P.S. (2009). Animal Genetics, 16(3): 165-173.

Ledu, J., Delachevalerie, F.A., Taverna, M. and Dano, Y. (1994). Ann. Zootech., 43: 77-90.

Li, J.P., Zhou, H.J., Yuan, L., He, T. and Hu, S.H. (2009). J. Zhejiang University Sci. B., 10(10): 753-760.

Little, R.B. and Plastridge, W.N. (1946). Bovine mastitis. 1st edn., Mc Graw Hill book Comp. INC, New York.

Liu, W.J., Chen, C.F., Teng, W.J., Wu, J. and Ren, X.Y. (2005). Investigation on Mastitis Pathogens for Diary Cattle in Xinjiang. Ecology of Domestic Animal, 2005-04.

Lojda, L., Stavikova, M. and Matouskova, O. (1976). Acta. Vet. Brno., 45: 181.

Lund, T., Miglior, F., Dekkers, J.C.M. and Burnside, E.B. (1994). Livest. Prod. Sci., 39: 243–255.

Luttinen, A. and Juga, J. (1997). Interbull Bull. no. 15. Int. Bull Eval. Serv., Uppsala, Sweden. Pp. 78-83.

Macha, J., Manakova, K. and Masek, N. (1981). Acta Univ. Agric. Fac. Agron. 29: 203.

Maiti, S.K., Sharma, Neelesh and Awasthi, B.K. (2003). Vet. Practioner, 4(2): 90.

Mandial, R.K., Sood, P., Katoch, R.C. and Nagal, K.B. (1999). Indian Vet. J., 76(7): 650-652.

Martins, R.P., Silva, J.A.G., Nakazato, L., Dutra, V. and Filho, E.S.A. (2010). Prevalence and infectious etiology of bovine mastitis in the microregion of Cuiabá, MT, Brazil. Ci. Anim. Bras., Goiânia, 11(1): 181-187.

Mastitis-flash (2009). In the world of mastitis research-what's new? 2008-2009. Mastitis-flash, volume 3, No. 9, November, 2009. published by Canadian Mastitis Research Network (www.mastitisnetwork.org).

McDonald, J.S. (1968). Am. J. Vet. Res., 29: 1207-1210.

McDonald, J.S. (1977). J. Arner. Vet. Med. Ass., 170: 1157.

McDonald, J.S. and Anderson, A.J. (1981). Am. J. Vet. Res., 42(2): 229-231.

McDonald, J.S. and Anderson, A.J. (1981). Am. J. Vet. Res., 42: 465.

McDougall, S. (1998). N. Z. Vet. J., 46: 226–232.

Mdegela, R.H., Karimuribo, E., Kusiluka, L.J.M., Kabula, B., Manjurano, A., Kapaga, A.M. and Kambarage, D.M. (2005). Livestock Research for Rural Development, 17(11).

Mein, G.A., Brown, M.R. and Williams, D.M. (1983). J. Dairy Res., 50: 249-258.

Mein, G.A., Neijenhuis, F., Morgan, W.F., Reinemann, D.J., Hillerton, J.E., Baines, J.R., Ohnstad, I., Rasmussen, M.D., Timms, L., Britt, J.S., Farnsworth, R., Cook, N. and Hemling, T. (2001). In: Proc. 2nd Int. Symp. on mastitis and milk quality, Vancouver, BC, Canada: 347-351.

Mekibib, B., Furgasa, M., Abunna, F., Megersa, B. and Regassa, A. (2010). Vet. World, 3(9): 397- 403.

Mendez y Cazarin, M. D., Tzintzun Rasco, R. and Val Arreola, D. (2000). Livestock Research for Rural Development, 12(1): 1-10.

Menzies, F.D., Gordon, A.W. and McBride, S.H. (2003). An epidemiological study of bovine toxic mastitis. In: Proc. British Mastitis Conference, 2003, Garstang, p 1-13.

Michal, J.J., Heirman, L.R., Wong, T.S., Chew, B.P., Frigg, M. and Volker, L. (1994). J. Dairy Sci., 77: 1408-1421.

Miller, G.Y. and Dorn, C.R. (1990). Prev. Vet. Med., 8(2-3): 171-182.

Miller, R.H., Pearson, R.E., Wienland, B.T. and Fulton, L.A. (1976). J. Dairy Sci., 59: 957-964.

Mohamed, E., Ibtisam, E.G, and Elowni, O.A.O. (1993). A study on the incidence and etiology of bovine mastitis in Sudan. In: Proc. Second Sci. Cong., Egyptian Society for cattle diseases, 5-7 Dec. 1993, Assiut, Egypt. Pp. 326-336.

Monardes. H.G., Cue, R I. and Hayes, J.P. (1990). J. Dairy Sci., 73:1337.

Moretti, A., Pasquali, P., Mencaroni, G., Boncio, L. and Fioretti, D.P. (1998). J. Vet. Med. Series B, 45(3): 129-132.

Moroni, P., Rossi, C.S., Pisoni, G., Bronzo, V., Castiglioni, B. and Boettcher, P.J. (2006). J. Dairy Sci., 89: 998–1003.

Mukherjee, R. and Das, P.K. (2002). In: Proc. Round Table Conference on Mastitis, 4-5 Feb., 2002, Nagpur, M.S. (India). Pp. 36-39.

Mulei, C.M. (1999). J South Afric. Vet. Assoc., 70: 156-157.

Munda, V., Prasad, A., Tiwary, B.K. and Mahto, D. (2007). Vet. World., 5(12): 375-376.

Mungube, E.O. (2001). Management and economics of dairy cow mastitis in the urban and peri-urban areas of Addis Ababa (Addis Ababa milkshed). MSc Dissertation. Freie Universitat Berlin, Germany, and Faculty of Veterinary Medicine, Addis Ababa University, Ethiopia.

Murphy, J.M. (1944). Cornell Vet., 34: 64.

Myllys, V. and Rautala, H. (1995). J. Dairy Sci., 78:538–545.

Myllys, V., Asplund, K., Brofldt, E., Hirvela-Koski, V., Honkanen-Buzalski, T., Junttila, J., Kulkas, L., Myllykangas, O., Niskanen, M., Saloniemi, H., Sandholm, M. and Saranpaa, T. (1998). Acta Vet. Scand., 39(1): 119-126.

Nam, H.M., Kim, J.M., Lim, S.K., Jang, K.C. and Jung, S.C. (2010). Res. Vet. Sci., 88(3): 372-374.

Nath, A.K. and Dutta, J.B. (2007). Indian J. Vet. Med., 27(2): 117-118.

Nath, K. and Dutta, J.B. (2005). Intl. J. Cow Sci., 1(1): 63-65.

Nauriyal, D.S. (1996). Profile studies in bovine mastitis with special reference to therapeutic consideration of vitamin E and selenium. PhD. Thesis, G.B. Pant University of Agriculture and Technology, Pantnagar.

Nauriyal, D.S. and Pachauri, S.P. (2003). In: Comp. of XXI ISVM Convention and National Symposium at Anand, Gujarat, India. p. 100-101.

Neijenhuis, F. (2004). Teat condition in dairy cows. Dissertation Utrecht University, Faculty of Veterinary Medicine, Utrecht, The Netherlands.

Neijenhuis, F., Barkema, H.W., Hogeveen, H. and Noordhuizen, J.P.T.M.. (2000). J. Dairy Sci., 83: 2795-2804.

Neijenhuis, F., Barkema, H.W., Hogeveen, H. and Noordhuizen, J.P.T.M. (2001). J. Dairy Sci., 84(12): 2664 – 2672.

Nickerson, S.C. (1994). Agric. Pract. 15:8–18.

Nickerson, S.C. (2009). Vet. Microbiol., 134(1-2): 128-135.

Nooruddin, M., Ali, M.L. and Debnath, N.C. (1997). Bangladesh Veterinarian, 14: 43-47.

Norman, H.D., Power, R.L. and Moharnmad, W.A. (1982). J. Dairy Sci., 65(Suppl. 1): 93. (Abstr.).

O'Rourke, D. (2009). Irish Vet. J., 62: 15-20.

Oldham, E.R., Eberhart, R.J. and Muller, L.D. (1991).. J. Dairy Sci., 74: 3775-3781.

Oliveira, C.M.C., Sousa, M.G.S., Silva, N.S., Albernaz1, T.T., Campos, K.F., Mendonca, C.L. and Barbosa, J.D. (2010). Bovine mastitis prevalence and etiology in the rondon do para milk basin, para state, brazil. In: Proc. XXVI World Buiatrics Cong. Nov. 14-18, 2010, Santiago de Chile, Chile.

Oliver, S.P. and Bushe, T. ((1987). Am. J. Vet. Res., 48(12): 1669-1673.

Oliviera, U.V., Galvao, G.S., Paixao, A.R.R. and Munhoz, A.D. (2010). Rev. Bras. Saúde Prod. An., 11(3): 630-640.

Omore, A.O., McDermott, J.J., Arimi, S.M. and Kyule, M.N. (1999). Trop. Anim. Hlth. Prod., 31: 347-361.

Omore, A.O., Mcdermott, J.J., Arimi, S.M., Kyule, M.N. and Ouma, D. (1996). Prev. Vet. Med., 29: 77-89.

Osman, K.M., El-Enbaawy, M.I., Ezzeldeen, N.A. and Hussein, H.M.G. (2009). Revue Scientifique et Technique - Office International des Épizooties, 28(3): 975-986.

Osteras, O. (2006). Mastitis epidemiology practical approaches and applications. In: Proc. XXIV World Buiatrics Congress, Nice, France.

Osteras, O. and Lund, A. (1988). Prev. Vet. Med., 6: 79-90.

Ovesen, E. (1972). Anita. Prod., 15: 251.

Owens, W.E., and Nipper, W.A. (2008). Case study: Development of a *Mycoplasma* mastitis control program in Louisiana. Prof. Anim. Scientist on line http://findarticles.com/p/articles/mi_qa4035/is_200802/ai_n24393806 Accessed April 30, 2009.

Paape, M.J. and Wergin, W.P. (1977). J. Am. Vet. Med. Ass., 170:1214.

Paape, M.J., Miller, R.H., Young, M.D. and Peters, R.R. (1992). J. Dairy Sci., 75: 1849-1856.

Paape, M.J., Schultze, W.D., Miller, R.H. and Smith, J.W. (1972). J. Dairy Sci., 56: 84–91.

Pachauri, S.P.; Singh, S.V. and Nauriyal, D.S. (2001). Indian Vet. Med. J., 25(12): 317-321.

Pagni, E., Sgorbibini, M., Preziuso, G. and Bizzeti, M. (2008). Large Anim. Rev., 14: 161-164.

Pal, B., Verma, B.B. and Prasad, R.S. (1989). Indian Vet. J., 66(8): 785-787.

Palanivel, K.M., Suresh, R.V., Jayakumar, R., Ganesan, P.I. and Dhanapalan, P. (2008). Indian J. Vet. Med., 28(1): 34-36.

Pankey, J.W., Nickerson, S.C., Boddie, R.L. and Hogan, J.S. (1985). J. Dairy Sci., 68(10): 2684–2693.

Parai, T.P., Pandey, N.N. and Lal, S.B. (1992). Indian J. Vet. Med., 7(2): 146-147.

Patel, M.D. and Nauruyal, D.S. (2003). In: Comp. of XXI ISVM Convention and National Symposium on at Anand, Gujarat, India. p. 235.

Patel., P.R., Raval, S.K., Rao, N, Mandali, G.C. and Jani, R.G. (2000). In: Proc. Round Table Conference on Mastitis, 18-19 Feb., 2000, Izatnagar, Bareilly, U.P. (India). Pp. 45-52.

Pathak, N.N. and Sharma, M.C. (1988). Buffalo health management. In: A compendium of latest research information based on Indian studies. ICAR, New Delhi, pp. 160-161.

Paul, W.M., Parthiban, M., Menaka, R. and Nainar, A.M. (2000). Indian J. Anim. Hlth., 39(2): 79-81.

Peeler, E.J., Green, M.J., Fitzpatrick, J.L. and Green, L.E. (2002). Vet. Rec., 151: 170-176.

Peeler, E.J., Green, M.J., Fitzpatrick, J.L., Morgan, K.L. and Green, L.E. (2000). J. Dairy Sci., 83: 2464-2472.

Peeler, E.J., Green, M.J., Fitzpatrick, J.L., Morgan, K.L. and Green, L.E. (1999). In: Proc. of British Mastitis Conf., pp. 37-45.

Peeler, E.J., Otte, M.J. and Esslemont, R.J. (1994). Vet Rec., 134:129-32.

Pitkala, A., Haveri, M., Pyorala, S., Myllys, V. and Honkanen-Buzalski, T. (2004). J. Dairy Sci., 87: 2433-2441.

Plastridge, W.N. (1958). J. Dairy Sci., 41: 1141-1181.

Poutrel, B. (1982). Ann. Rech. Vet., 13(1): 85-99.

Pozzi, P. (1998). Obiettivi e Documenti Veterinari, 19(6): 30-33.

Prabhakar, S.K. (1986). Studies on clinical mastitis in cows and buffaloes. M.V.Sc. thesis, Punjab Agricultural University, Ludhiana, India.

Prajapati, K.B., Singh, D.V. and Patel, J.P. (1995). Indian J. Dairy Sci., 48: 255-258.

Prasad, H., Roychoudhury, R.K. and Patgiri, G. (2001). Indian Vet. J., 78(4): 316-318.

Pyorala, S., Somer, H.J. and Mero, M. (1992). Br. Vet. J., 148: 54-62.

Radostits, O.M., Gay, C.C., Blood, D.C. and Hinchcliff, K.W. (2000). Mastitis. In: Veterinary Medicine, 9th ed., W.B. Saunders Company Ltd., London, pp. 603-687.

Rahman, M.A., Bhuiyan, M.M.U., Kamal, M.M. and Shamsuddin, M. (2009). The Bangladesh Veterinarian, 26(2): 54-60.

Rajendran, T., George, S.K., Harshan, H.M. and Antony, P. (2006). Vet. World, 4(12): 357-360.

Ramachandraiah, K., Sudharsan Kumar, K. and Sreemannarayana, O. (1990). Indian Vet. J., 67(2): 103-106.

Ranjan, R., Gupta, M.K., Singh, S. and Kumar, S. (2010). Vet. World, 3(1): 17-20.

Rao, R., Choudhury, P.C. and Chetty, M.S. (1989). Indian J. Comp. Microbiol. Immunol & Infect. Dis., 10(1): 7-11.

Rathore, A.K. (1977). Br. Vet. J., 133: 258-262.

Rathore, A.K. (1977a). Br. Vet. J., 133: 454.

Rathore, A.K. (1977b). Br. Vet. J., 133: 258.

Rathore, A.K. and Sheldrake, R.F. (1977). Anim. Prod., 24: 215.

Redaelli, G., Ruffo, G., Alipmndi, L. and Veneroni, G. (1972). Dairy Sci. Abstr., 34: 766. (Atti Sco. Ital. Sci. Vet. 25:500.).

Reetha, T.L., Babu, M., Pugazhenthi, T.R. and Rajeswar, J.J. (2006). Tamilnadu J. Vet. Anim. Sci., 2(4): 140-141.

Rehman, F. (1995). Studies on I) Evaluation of surf field mastitis test for the detection of sub-clinical mastitis in buffaloes and cattles, II) Antibiotic susceptibility of pathogens. MSc Thesis, Univ. Agri. Faisalabad, Pakistan.

Rehman, H., Sambyal, D.S. and Baxi, K.K. (1983). J. Res. Punjab Agri. Univ. Ludhiana, India, 20: 208–212

Reneau, J.K., Saylor, A.J., Heinz, B.J., Bye, R.F. and Farnsworth, R.J. (2003). In: Proc. Natl. Masititis Conc., 42: 362-363.

Resende, D.F., Glenn, K., Cullor, J.S. and and Bruno, R.G.S. (2009). J. Anim. Sci. Vol. 87, E-Suppl. 2/J. Dairy Sci. Vol. 92, E-Suppl. 1 (Abstract). P.200.

Robert, A., Seegers, H. and Bareille, N. (2006). Vet. Res., 37(1): 25-48.

Roesch, M., Doherr, M.G., Scharen, W., Schallibaum, M. and Blum, J.W. (2007). J. Dairy Res., 74: 86-92.

Roets, E., Vandeputte-Van Messom, G. and Peeters, G. (1986). J. Dairy Sci., 69:3120-3130.

Rogers, G.W., Hargrove, G.L., Lawlor, T.J. and Ebersole, J.L. (1991). Correlations among linear type traits and somatic cell counts. J. Dairy Sci., 74: 1081.

Rogers, O.W. and Spencer, S.B. (1991). J. Dairy Sci., 74: 4189-4194.

Roth, S., Reinsch, N., Nieland, G. and Schallenberger, E. (1998). Zuchtungskunde 70: 242-260.

Rowlands, G.J., Lucey, S. and Russell, A.M. (1986). Prev. Vet. Med., 4: 222–231.

Roy, S.K., Pyne, A.K. and Maitra, D.N. (1993). Indian Vet. J., 70: 677-678.

Roy, S.K., Pyne, A.K., Mitra, D.N., Dattagupta, R. and Majumdar, S.C. (1989). Indian Vet. J., 66(9): 844-846.

Rupp, R. and Boichard, D. (1999). J. Dairy Sci., 82(10): 2198–2204.

Saharia, J., Saikia, S. and Dutta, G.N. (1997). Indian Vet. J., 74(5): 436-438.

Sahay, S., Sinha, B.P. and Verma, S.P. (2002). In: Proc. of Round Table Conference on Mastitis, 4-5 Feb., 2002, Nagpur, M.S. (India). Pp. 25-32.

Sahoo, S.S., Sahoo, N. and Parida, G.S. (2009). Indian Vet. J., 86(12): 100-101.

Said, A.H. and Abd-el-Malik, A.S. (1968). J. Vet. Sci. (United Arab Republic), 5: 171-181

Saini, S.S., Sharma, J.K. and Kwatra, M.S. (1994). Indian J. Dairy Sci., 47(2): 103-106.

Samanta, A, Prasad, S. and Ghos, C.P. (2006). Indian J. Dairy Sci., 59(1): 13-18.

Sampimon, O., Barkema, H.W., Berends, I., Sol, J. and Lam, T. (2009). J. Dairy Res., 76(2): 129-136.

Sarode, D.B. (2002). In: Proc. Round Table Conference on Mastitis, 4-5 Feb., 2002, Nagpur, M.S. (India). Pp. 40-42.

Sato, K., Bartlett, P., Ruegg, P., Kaneene, J., Robinson-Dunn, B., Downes, F.P. and Erskine, R. (2002). Dairy, Food and Environmental Sanitation. 22(3): 178-183.

Sato, K., Bartlett, P.C., Alban, L., Agger, J.F. and Houe, H. (2008). Acta Vet. Scand. 50: 4-11.

Saxena, R.K., Datta, G.N., Borah, P. and Buragohain, J. (1993). Indian Vet. J., 70(11): 1079-1080.

Saxena, V., Sharma, A., Manuja, B. and Kumar, A. (2001). In: Proc. Round Table Conference on Mastitis, 22-23 Feb., 2001, Ludhiana, Pb. (India). Pp. 113-116.

Scaletti, R.W., Trammell, D.S., Smith, B.A. and Harmon, R.J. (2003). J. Dairy Sci. 86, 1240–1249.

Schaeffer, L.R. (1983). Can. J. Anim. Sci., 63: 763.

Schalm, O.W., Caroll, E.J. and Jain, N.C. (1971). Bovine mastitis. Lea and Febiger, Philadelphia

Schmidt, G.H. and Van Vleck L.D. (1965). J. Dairy Sci., 48: 51-55.

Schreiner, D.A. and Ruegg, P.L. (2003). J. Dairy Sci., 86: 3460–3465.

Schukken, Y.H., Erb, H.N. and Smith, R.D. (1988). Prev. Vet. Med., 5: 181-190.

Schukken, Y.H., Grommers, F.J., Geer, D. van de and Brand, A. (1989). Vet. Rec., 125(3): 60-63.

Schukken, Y.H., Grommers, F.J., van der Geer, D., Erb, H.N. and Brand, A. (1991). J. Dairy Sci., 74: 826–832.

Schukken, Y.H., Lam, T.J. Nielen, M., Hogeveen, H., Barkema, W. and Grommers, F.J. (1995). Tijdschrift van Diergeneeskunde (in Dutch). 120: 208-213.

Sebastian, S.R. and Vijayakumar, K. (2002). In: Proc. Round Table Conference on Mastitis, 4-5 Feb., 2002, Nagpur, M.S. (India). Pp. 120-125.

Seto, A., Okabe, T., Sasaki, N. and Lto, Y. (1976). Am. J. Vet. Res., 37:635.

Seykora, A.J. (1983). Genetic parameters of udder and teat characteristics and their relationships to somatic cell counts. Ph.D. Dissertation., North Carolina State Univ., Raleigh.

Seykora, A.J. and McDaniel, B.T. (1985). J. Dairy Sci., 68(8): 2395.

Seykora, A.J. and McDaniel, B.T. (1986). J. Dairy Sci., 69: 2395.

Shah, A.H. (1987). Bovine sub-clinical mastitis due to Staphylococcus aureus and its treatment with cloxacillin, rifampicin and their combination. MSc Thesis. Univ. Agri. Faislabad, Pakistan.

Shanks, R.D. and Spahr, S.L. (1982). J. Dairy Sci., 65: 1771.

Sharma, A. (2009). Studies on prevalence, haematobiochemical and mineral alterations during mastitis in crossbred cattle and its therapeutic management. M.V.Sc. Thesis, SKUAST-Jammu, India.

Sharma, A. and Kapur, M.P. (2000). In: Proc. 1st Round Table Conference on Mastitis, IVRI, Izatnagar, (India), 18th –19th Feb., p.8-11.

Sharma, A., Dhingra, P., Pander, B.L. and Kumar, R. (2006). Intl. J. Cow Sci., 2(1).

Sharma, A.K. (2000). Studies on prevalence and therapeutics of mastitis in dairy animals. M.V.Sc. Thesis submitted to H.P.K.V., Palampur, India.

Sharma, A.K. and Prasad, B. (2002). In: Comp. XX ISVM Convention and National Symposium at Bikaner, Rajasthan (India). 14th –16th Feb., p. 93.

Sharma, D.K., Jallewar, P.K. and Sharma, K.K. (2010). Indian Vet. J., 87(4): 407.

Sharma, M., Katoch, R.C., Nagal, K.B. and Sambyal, D.S. (1993). Indian J. Dairy Sci., 46(1): 37-38.

Sharma, Neelesh (2003). Epidemiological investigation on sub-clinical mastitis in dairy animals: Role of vitamin-E and selenium supplementation on its control in cattle. M.V.Sc. Thesis, I.G.K.V.V., Raipur (C.G.), India.

Sharma, Neelesh (2008). Intl. J. Zoological Res., 4(1): 64-67.

Sharma, Neelesh (2011). Milk fever. In: Production diseases in dairy animals, (edited by Sharma, Neelesh, Singh, N.K. and Bacic, G. (2011)), 1st edn., Satish serial publication house, Delhi, India. Pp. 114-149.

Sharma, Neelesh and Maiti, S.K. (2005). Indian J. Vet. Med., 25(2): 76-79.

Sharma, Neelesh, Maiti, S.K. and Koley, K.M. (2004). Vet. Practioner, 5(2): 123-124.

Sharma, Neelesh, Maiti, S.K. and Sharma, K.K. (2007). Intl. J. Dairy Sci., 2(2): 145-151.

Sharma, Neelesh, Singh, N.K., Singh, O.P., Pandey, V., and Verma, P.K. (2011). Asian-Australasian J. Anim. Sci., 24(40): 479-484.

Sharma, S.D. (1978). Vet. Res. Bull., 1(2): 162-163.

Sharma, S.D. and Rai, P. (1977). Indian Vet. J., 54(6): 435-439.

Shathele, M.S. (2009). Int. J. Dairy Sci., 4(2): 57-66.

Shem, M.N., Malole, J.M.L., Machangu, R., Kurwijila, L.R. and Fujihara, T. (2001). Asian-Australian J. Anim. Sci., 14: 372-377.

Shinde, S.S., Kulkarni, G.B., Gangane, G.R., Degloorkar, N.M. and Murkunde, Y.V. (2002). In: Proc. Round Table Conference on Mastitis, 4-5 Feb., 2002, Nagpur, M.S. (India). Pp. 11-13.

Shitandi, A., Anakalo, G., Galgaio, T. and Mwangi, M. (2004). Israel J. Vet. Med., 59(1/2): 20-23.

Shpigel, N.Y., Winkler, M., Ziv, G. and Saran, A. (1998). Prev. Vet. Med., 35: 1-9.

Shrirame, K.R., Bhardwaj, S.S., Kalorey, D.R. and Harne, S.D. (2002). In: Proc. Round Table Conference on Mastitis, 4-5 Feb., 2002, Nagpur, M.S. (India). Pp. 18-22.

Shukla, P.C. (1980). A study to evaluate the relative sensitivity of some of the indirect diagnostic tests available for detection of sub-clinical cases of mastitis. M.V.Sc. & A.H. thesis, J.N.K.V.V., Jabalpur, M.P., India.

Shukla, P.C. and Supekar, P.G. (1982). Dairy Guide 4(8): 9-12.

Shukla, P.C. and Supekar, P.G. (1986). Livestock Advisor, (193): 47-49.

Shukla, P.C., Mehta, H. and Joshi, S.K. (2003). In: Comp. XXI ISVM Convention and National Symposium at Anand, Gujarat, India. p. 233.

Shukla, S.K., Dixit, V.P. and Chandra, R. (2005). Indian J. Vet. Med., 25(2): 118-120.

Shukla, S.K., Dixit, V.P., Thapli, D.C., Garg, S.K. and Kumar, A. (1997). Indian Vet. J., 74(11): 989-990.

Sieber, R.L. and Farnsworth, R.J. (1980). In: Proc. Natl. Mastitis Counc. Annu. Mtg. p.5.

Sieber, R.L. and Farnsworth, R.J. (1981). J. Am. Vet. Med. Assco., 178: 1263-1267

Siji, P.C. and Vijayakumar, K. (2007). Indian J. Vet. Med., 27(2): 131-132.

Singh, J.L., Dabas, Y.P.S., Singh, P.K., Shukla, S.K., Gupta, R.S., Garg, A. and Kumar, S. (2003). Intas Polivet, 4(2): 305-308.

Singh, J.L., Kumar, S., Verma, R.S., Singh, C.P. and Shivakumar, V. (2008). Indian J. Vet. Med., 28(2): 156-157.

Singh, P.J. (1991). Studies on mastitis at machine milked farms in Punjab. M.V.Sc. thesis, Punjab Agricultural University, Ludhiana, India.

Singh, P.J. and Singh, K.B. (1994). Indian J. Dairy Sci., 47(4): 265-272.

Singh, P.J., Singh, K.B., Jand, S.K., Dhingra, P.N. and Nauriyal, D.C. (1994). Indian J. Dairy Sci., 47(9): 730-733.

Slettbakk, T., Jørstad, A., Farver, T.B. and Holmes, J.C. (1995). Prev. Vet. Med., 24: 235–244.

Smith J.W. and Schultze W.D. (1970). Factors related to the level of natural resistance to udder infection. Proc. 6th Int Conf. on cattle diseases (Philadelphia USA), 38-43.

Smith, K.L. and Hogan, J.S. (1993). Management of cows from drying off to calving to maximize udder health. Accesses from http//www.veterinaria.uchile.cl/publicacion/congresoxi/.../bovi/14.doc, on 09/10/2009.

Smith, K.L. and Oliver, S.P. (1981). Lactoferrin: a component of non-specific defense of the involuting bovine mammary gland. In: Butler JE, editor. The ruminant immune system. New York: Plenum Press; p. 535.

Smith, K.L., and Hogan, J.S. (1993Vet. Clin. N. Am: Food Animal Pract., 9: 489-498.

Smith, K.L., and Todhunter, D.A. (1982). The physiology of mammary gland during the dry period and the relationship to infection. In: Proc. Annu. Mtg. Natl. Mastitis Counc., Inc., Arlington, VA., P. 87

Smith, K.L., Harrison, J.S., Hancock, D.D., Todhunter, D.A. and Conrad, H.R. (1984). J. Dairy Sci., 67: 1293.

Smith, K.L., Hogan, J.S. and Weiss, W.P. (1997). J. Anim. Sci., 75: 1659-1665.

Smith, K.L., Todhunter, D.A. and Schoenberger, P.S. (1985). J. Dairy. Sci., 68: 402.

Sood, R., Pachauri, S.P. and Nauriyal, D.S. (2008). Indian J. Vet. Med., 28(1): 17-19.

Sordillo, L.M. and Nickerson, S.C. (1988). Am. J. Vet. Res., 49: 1112.

Sordillo, L.M., Nickerson, S.C., Akers, R.M. and Oliver, S.P. (1987). Intl. J. Biochem., 19(12): 1165-1172.

Spain, J.N., Jones, C.A., Rapp, C. *et al.* (2005), The effect of complexed zinc on keratin synthesis in the teat canal and the establishment and severity of experimentally induced *E. coli* mastitis in dairy cows. In: Mastitis in dairy production: Current knowledge and future solutions. Hogeveen H (ed). P 948.

Spencer, S.B. (1989). J. Dairy Sci., 72: 1907.

Sreedevi, B., Malleswara Rao, U.V.N. and Reddy, T.V. (2002). In: Proc. Round Table Conference on Mastitis, 4-5 Feb., 2002, Nagpur, M.S. (India). Pp. 33-35.

Srimannarayana, O. and Ramachandraiah, K. (1999). Buffalo Bulletin, 18(1): 3-4.

Stanikzai1, P.M., Yathiraj, S, Shridhar, N.B., Ansar Kamran, C. and Narayana Bhat, M. (2010). In: Proc. XXVI World Buiatrics Cong., 14-18, Nov., Santiago de Chile, Chile.

Steeneveld, W., Hogeveen, H., Barkema, H.W., Broek, J. van den and Huirne, R.B.M. (2008). J. Dairy Sci., 91(4): 1391-1402.

Suriyasathaporn, W., Heuer, C., Noordhuizen-Stassen, E.N. and Schukken, Y.H. (2000). Vet. Res., 31:397–412.

Suriyasathaporn, W., Schukken, Y.H., Nielen, M. and Brand, A. (2000). J. Dairy Sci., 83: 1248-1255.

Swamy, M.C.M. and Krishnamurthy, G.V. (1998). Indian Vet. J., 75(2): 101-103.

Syvajarvi, J., Saloniemi, H. and Grohn, Y. (1986). Acta. Vet. Scand., 27: 223–234.

Tellez, A.S., Gutierrez Chavez, A.J., Sanchez Gomez, J.I. and Canizal Jimenez, E. (2002). Veterinaria México, 33(4): 387-394.

Tenhagen, B.A., Oster, G.K., Wallmann, J. and Heuwieser, W. (2006). J. Dairy Sci., 89(7): 2542–2551.

Thirunavukkarasu, M. and Prabaharan, R. (1998). Indian J. Anim. Prod. Mgmt., 14(2): 110-114.

Thirunavukkarasu, M. and Prabaharan, R. (1999). Cheiron, 28(3): 55-61.

Thomas, G.W., Spiker, S.A. and Mickan, F.J. (1981). Aust. J. Exp. Agric. Anita. Husb., 21: 5.

Tijare, D.B., Singh, A.K., Chaturvedi, V.K. and Dhanesar, N.S. (1999). Indian Vet. J., 76(10): 912-915.

Tilki, M., Colac, M. and Caglayan, S.I.T. (2005). Turk. J. Vet. Anim. Sci., 29: 275-278.

Tiwari, A. and Sisodia, R.S. (2000). Indian J. Vet. Med., 20(2): 80.

Tiwari, A., Sisodia, R.S. and Tiwari, G.P. (2000). In: Proc. Round Table Conf. on Mastitis held at Izatnagar (IAAVR), 18-19th Feb. 2000, p.23-37.

Tiwari, J.G., Chaudhari, S.P. and Tiwari, H.K. (2008). Indian Vet. J., 85(11): 1232.

Todhunter, D.A., Smith, K.L, Hogan, J.S. and Weiss, W.P. (1995). J. Dairy Sci., 78: 2366.

Todhunter, D.A., Smith, K.L., Hogan, J.S. and Schoenberger, P.S. (1991). Am. J. Vet. Res., 52: 184.

Tomer, N.S. and Tomer, S.P.S. (1060). Indian J. Dairy Sci., 26(1): 25.

Trinidad, P., Nickerson, S.C. and Alley, T.K. (1990). J. Dairy Sci., 73: 107-114.

Tuteja, F.C., Kapur, M.P., Sharma, Anshu and Vinayak, A.K. (1993). Indian Vet. J.,70 (9): 787-791.

Tuteja, F.C., Sharma, Anshu, Kapur, M.P. (2003). Vet. Practitioner. 4(1): 19-21.

Twomey, D.P., Wheelock, A.I., Flynn, J., Meaney, W.J., Hill, C. and Ross, R.P. (2000). J. Dairy Sci., 83: 1981-1988.

Uddin, M.A., Kamal, M.M. and Haque, M.E/ (2009). Bangladesh J. Dairy Sci., 7(2): 332-340.

VanRaden P.M., Jensen, E.L., Lawlor, T. and Funk, D.A. (1990). J. Dairy Sci., 73:191.

Verma, A.K. and Nauriyal, D.S. (2009). Indian J. Vet. Med., 29(1): 13-16.

Vishwakarma, P. (2008). Studies on Prevalence, Diagnosis, Therapy and Control of Mastitis in buffaloes. M.V.Sc. Thesis, Indira Gandhi Agricultural University, Raipur, Chhattisgarh state.

Waage, S., Ødegaard, S.A., Lund, A., Brattgjerd, S. and Rothe, T. (2001). J. Dairy Sci., 84:392–399.

Waage, S.S., Sviland, and Odegaard, S.A. (1998). J. Dairy Sci., 81: 1275-1284.

Wagner, A.M., and Ruegg, P.L. (2002). J. Dairy Sci., 85: 804-809.

Waller, K.P., Sandgren, C.H., Emanuelson, U. and Jensen, S.K. (2007). J. Dairy Sci., 90: 3640-3646.

Weiss, B. (2009). In: Proc. of NMC Regional Meeting. p 44-52.

Weiss, W.P. (2009). Nutritional influences on the prevalence and severity of mastitis in dairy cows. http://nmconline.org/articles/nutrition.pdf, downloaded on 31/10/2009.

Whist, A. C., Osteras, O. and Sølverød, L. (2006). J. Dairy Sci., 89: 4649–4659.

White, J.M. (1974). J. Dairy Sci., 57: 1267.

Wilde, J.C., Addey, V.C., Li, P. and Fering, G.D. (1997). Exp. Physiol., 82: 943-953.

Wilesmith, J.W., Francis, P.G. and Wilson, C.D. (1986). Vet. Rec., 118: 199-204.

Wilson, C.D. and Kingwill, R.G. (1975). A practical mastitis control routine. IDF Bull. International Dairy Federation, Brussels, 85: 422-438,

Workineh, S., Bayleyegn, M., Mekonnen, H. and Potgieter. L.N.D. (2002). Trop. Anim. Hlth. Prod., 34: 19-25.

Yigezu, S. (1990). Bovine mastitis in the Southern region of Ethiopia. Faculty of Veterinary Medicine, Addis Ababa University, Debre-Zeit, Ethiopia, DVM thesis.

Zadoks, R. N., Allore, H.G., Barkema, H.W., Sampimon, O.C., Wellenberg, G.J., Grohn, Y.T. and Schukken, Y.H. (2001). J. Dairy Sci., 84: 2649–2663.

Zadoks, R.N. and Fitzpatrick, J.L. (2009). Irish Vet. J., 62(Supl.): 59-70.

Zahoor, H. and Malik, H.U. (2009). Applied Biological Research, 11(1): 36-39.

Zecconi, A., Hamann, J., Bronzo, V. and Ruffo, G. (1992). J. Dairy Res., 59: 265-271.

Zecconi, A., Mazzilli, M. and Piccinini, R. (2009). In: Proc. European Buiatric Forum, Marseille, 1-3 Dec. 2009. p. 60.

□□□

CHAPTER

9

Pathogenesis

Inflammation of the udder tissue, known as "*mastitis*", has become one of the most costly and prevalent diseases affecting dairy cows worldwide. Mastitis is the body's defense against an injury caused to the udder tissue. Mastitis usually occurs primarily in response to intramammary bacterial infection, but also to intramammary mycoplasmal, fungal, or algal infections. Bovine mammary glands are exposed to diverse bacteria throughout lactation and in non-lactating periods. Mechanical trauma, thermal trauma, and chemical insult predispose the gland to intramammary infection. Trauma to the teat renders it more susceptible to bacterial invasion, colonization, and infection because of damage to keratin or mucous membranes lining the teat sinus. Occurrence of mastitis depends on the interaction of host, agent, and environmental factors. The severity of mastitis varies greatly and is determined by strain virulence, number of infecting organisms, season, immune status of the cow, parity and stage of lactation. The risk that a cow will develop mastitis is largely a function of pathogen load at the teat end and the cow's ability (udder immunity) to prevent a bacterial infection from becoming established in the mammary gland.

The teat end serves as the udder's first line of defense against infection. A smooth muscled sphincter, which surrounds the teat canal, functions to keep the teat canal closed, prevents milk from escaping, and prevents bacteria from entering the teat. The cells lining the teat canal produce keratin, a fibrous protein with lipid components (long chain fatty acids) that have bacteriostatic properties. Bacteria that pass this barrier and enter the teat cistern meet the second line of defense: phagocytic leukocytes. Phagocytes, consisting of neutrophils and macrophages, ingest and kill mastitis pathogens. Neutrophils exhibit directed migration toward chemical messengers produced by invading organisms, resulting in accumulation of neutrophils in the milk. The first pathological alteration in mastitis animals is the passage of serum-albumin into udder secretions due to increase vascular permeability irrespective of pathogen. In recent years, the quantitation of bovine serum albumin in milk by radial immunodiffusion test has been used diagnostically to assess the integrity of mammary epithelium and thus differentiating teat canal infection and mastitis.

Blood vessel endothelial cells, mammary epithelial cells, milk macrophages, and T and B lymphocytes of the peripheral immune system also play important roles in the local in?ammatory response, helping to recruit opsonizing antibodies and neutrophils from blood into milk for rapid phagocytic clearance of the opsonized pathogens. Indeed, it is clear that this in?ammatory response effectively deals with most intramammary pathogens on a regular basis because mammary quarters come into contact with mastitis-causing pathogens much more frequently than mastitis occurs. When the in?ammatory events that should lead to rapid antibody and neutrophil recruitment into the gland fail to occur or occur too slowly, however, health of the gland is put in jeopardy and animals develop clinical mastitis that can be acute and severe or more chronic in nature (Burton and Erskine, 2003).

Mastitis always causes a certain destruction of milk producing tissue which leads to a decrease in milk production. The decrease is affected by a number of factors, e.g. the cow's age and the potency of the inflammation (Hallen-Sandgren *et al.*, 1997). Sometimes the inflammation fails to eliminate the causal microbe and a degree of unreactivity "tolerance" is formed. This is what is called sub-clinical mastitis. We distinguish between this and clinical mastitis, in which there is detectable changes in either milk or udder.

There is increasing evidence that pathogens use various mechanisms to impinge upon cell death pathways. A number of pathogens are armed with an array of virulence determinants, which interact with key components of a host cell's death pathways or interfere with regulation of transcription factors monitoring cell survival. These virulence factors induce cell death by a variety of mechanisms, which include- 1) pore-forming toxins, which interact with the host cell membrane and permit the leakage of cellular components; 2) toxins that express their enzymatic activity in the host cytosol; 3) effector proteins delivered directly into host cells by a highly specialized type-III secretory system; 4) superantigens that target immune cells, and 5) other modulators of host cell death. Much progress has been made in understanding the role of apoptosis and necrosis in response to bacterial infection (Zhao and Lacasse, 2008).

A basic knowledge of mammary gland anatomy and physiology is necessary to understand how mastitis develops and how resistance mechanisms operate to reduce intramammary infections. The details anatomy of udder has already been discussed in chapter 4 of this book. The development of mastitis is more complex than this and can be most satisfactorily explained in terms of three stages: invasion, infection and inflammation. Of the three phases, prevention of the invasion phase offers the greatest potential for reducing the incidence of mastitis by good management, notably in the use of good hygienic procedures.

A. Invasion

The first step of the infection process is attachment of the microorganism to the exposed tissue cells within the different regions of the mammary gland. The ability of the mastitis-causing microorganisms to attach to the tissue lining in the mammary gland is directly related to their disease-producing potential. This is because the structure of the lining of the teat cistern is basically multi-layered, scale-like cells that have smooth surfaces. Such surfaces make attachment difficult and require the microorganisms to have special adhesion mechanisms. *S. aureus* and *S. agalactiae* possess this capability and are the most commonly encountered mastitis-causing bacteria associated with shallow penetration-type microbes.

Invasion is the stage at which mastitis causing pathogens move from the teat end to the milk inside the teat canal. Mastitis results once bacteria escape natural defense mechanism and pass through the teat duct and multiply in the udder. Organisms breach the teat duct in several ways. Between milkings, organisms may pass through the teat duct by multiplying inside the duct, or by physical movements resulting from pressure placed on the teat end as the cow moves about. During machine milking, organisms may be propelled into the teat duct or through the teat duct into the teat cistern via impacts against the teat end. Impacts are bacteria-laden droplets of milk that originate when air enters the milking system during liner slips (squawking). The potential for invasion is greatly increased by bacteria that reside in or colonize the teat duct. The practices of teat dipping in an effective germicide after each milking greatly reduces teat duct colonization (Nickerson, 1994).

There appear to be two ways in which bacteria commonly penetrate the teat canal (Blowey and Edmondson, 2010):

1) Growth through the canal- After transfer to the teat end, contagious organisms, especially *S. aureus* and *S. agalactiae*, have strong adhesive factors and begin their 'attack' on the udder by first establishing a colony at the teat end, i.e. they multiply. After colonising the teat end, bacteria literally grow up through the teat canal and move into the teat sinus.
2) Propulsion through the canal- Pathogens, particularly environmental bacteria such as *E. coli*, do not have adhesive properties and hence are often forced through the canal, usually with a reverse flow of milk, such as occurs with teat-end impacts. The exception to this is infections that develop during the dry period.

B. Infection

The infection occurs after bacteria gain entrance to the mammary gland via the teat canal (Figure 9.1). After bacteria overcome the anatomical defense, they must evade the cellular and humoral defense mechanisms of the mammary gland to establish disease. Infection is the stage in which the pathogens multiply rapidly and invade the mammary tissue. After invasion the pathogen population may be established in the teat canal and, with this as a base, a series of multiplications and extensions into mammary tissue may occur, with infection of mammary tissue occurring frequently or occasionally depending on its susceptibility.

In brief, the infection process involves the following five steps: (i) initial attachment to the host's cell tissue; (ii) adaptation to the new growth environment of the host; (iii) multiplication of the pathogen numbers; (iv) depression of the host's body defenses against the pathogen; and (v) the release of toxic materials by the pathogen that stimulates allergic reactions of the host. The ability of the pathogen to complete these steps varies from microorganism to microorganism. Hence the establishment of infection is varies from pathogen to pathogen and it depends on the adherence capability of pathogen. The adherence of bacteria to tissues lining the interior of the gland may enhance their ability to remain inside the gland, especially during lactation when the udder undergoes periodic flushing action during each milking. *S. agalactiae* and *S. aureus* appear to adhere well to tissues lining the milk collecting spaces. *E. coli* do not appear to adhere but multiply rapidly in quarters with low somatic cell counts (SCC) (Nickerson, 1994).

An inflammatory response is initiated when bacteria enter the mammary gland and this is the body's second line of defense (leukocytes). The main function of leukocyte is to engulf and destroy bacteria. If bacteria are eliminated by leukocytes, the infection is cleared; however, if bacteria persist, chronic inflammation follows. Bacteria appear initially to affect tissues lining the large milk collecting ducts and cisterns by inflicting damage to small areas of mammary tissues. Then bacteria enter small ducts and alveolar areas of the lower portions of the gland, probably by multiplication and via milk currents produced by cow movement. These bacteria multiply and produce toxins, enzymes, and cell-wall components which stimulate the production of numerous mediators of inflammation by inflammatory cells (Jones, 2009). The bacterial products and other irritants are that cause swelling and death of milk producing cells and leukocytes. If the infection is not eliminated, bacterial levels in the mammary gland eventually rise to a level at which they begin to damage the mammary epithelium.

C. Inflammation

Inflammation follows infection and represents the stage at which clinical changes occurs in both udder as well as in milk. In severe cases systemic signs may also occur. The inflammatory response is a complex series of physiological and biochemical vents, elicited by the host, that are a localized, protective response, to a variety of different stimuli such as trauma, infection, tissue damage or hypoxia (Fantone and Ward, 1999). The magnitude of the inflammatory response may be influenced by the causative pathogen, stage of lactation, age, immune status of the cow, genetics, and nutritional status. Abnormalities of the udder include marked swelling, redness, increased warmth and, in acute and per-acute stages, gangrene in some cases and abscess formation and atrophy of glands in chronic stages. In milk, the changes include presence of clots, blood, change of colour and consistency. The systemic effects are due to the mediators of inflammation.

Ultimately the udder injury activates an inflammatory response in the udder. The inflammation consists of three stages (Ahlner, 2003):

1. The acute transient phase

During the acute transient phase the local capillary circulation and the permeability of the capillaries increase as the endothelial cells contract. Inter-endothelial gaps are formed through which plasma and its proteins leak in the interstitium, causing udder edema. Fluids, blood clotting factors, and antibodies also leak into the affected area. Inflammation may be mild and go undetected (sub-clinical mastitis), or it may produce obvious clinical signs e.g. edema, redness, swelling, and abnormal secretions containing clots and red blood cells. Blood leukocytes begin to adhere to the endothelium. This leads to a change in the composition of the milk, e.g. the content of lactosis and casein is reduced while the content of saline is increased (Hallen-Sandgren *et al.*, 1997).

2. The sub-acute phase

During this phase cells migrate from the circulation to the infection site. These cells are leukocytes (lymphocytes, macrophages, neutrophils, eosinophils), but epithelial cells from the udder can also be found in the milk. After leukocytes cross blood vessels and move through udder tissues towards damaged tissue sites, they accumulate around alveoli, ducts, and cisterns before entering milk. During migration, the leukocytes may release enzymes that cause local destruction of milk producing cells. When a bacterial infection occurs, the amount of cells in the milk increases rapidly. The proportions are also changed from mainly lymphocytes and macrophages in a healthy udder, to over 95% neutrophiles in an infected udder. In addition, tissue debris, leukocytes, and blood clots occlude ducts draining area of secretory tissue. If bacteria are eliminated, inflammation subsides, clogged ducts are opened, and milk composition returned to normal in several days.

3. The chronic proliferative phase

Chronic proliferative phase is characterized by tissue degeneration, regeneration and formation of fibrotic tissue. If infection persists and ducts remain clogged, milk accumulates in alveoli, exerting pressure on milk producing cells. After destruction, alveolar structures are permanently replaced by scar tissue (fibrosis), leading to reduced milk yield in the current and subsequent lactation (Figure 9.2).

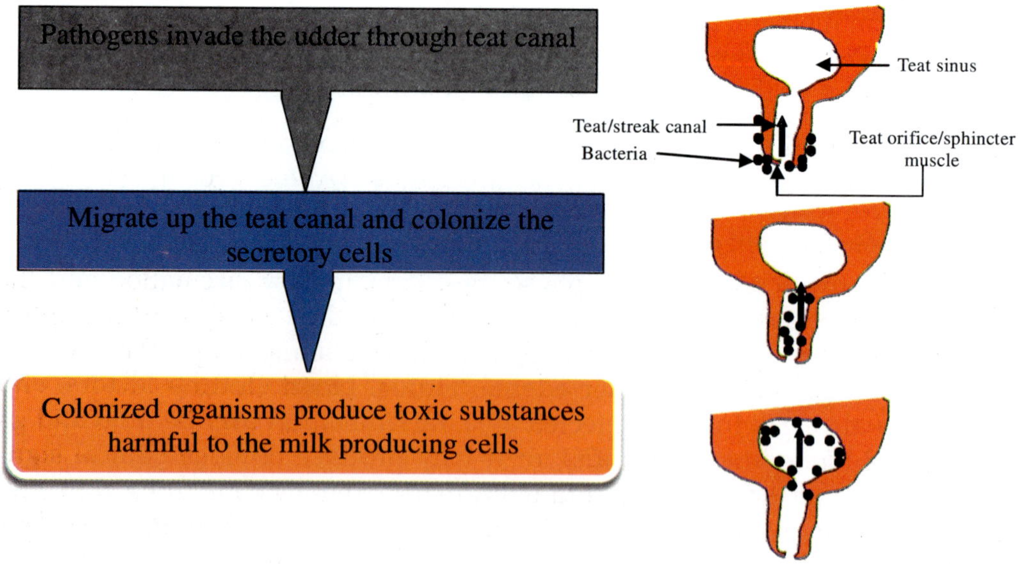

Figure 9.1 : How mastitis does develop?

Role of cytokines in the pathogenesis of mastitis

Following detection of pathogen invasion into the mammary gland, macrophages and epithelial cells release chemo-attractants. These agents trigger the migration of leukocytes, mainly polymorphonuclear cells (PMN), from the blood toward the mammary gland and increase their proportions from a basal level of 5 to 25% to approximately 90% of total cells in the milk. Macrophage and epithelial cells initiate the inflammatory response necessary to eliminate invading bacteria. These cells release chemoattractants for rapid recruitment of PMN to foci of infection. Initiation of the inflammatory reaction is caused by the production and release of tumor necrosis factor (TNF), interferons (INF), and interleukins (IL). These complex interactions result in accumulation of PMN in the mammary gland. Phagocytosis by PMN is the most effective defense against bacterial infection. Chemotactic factors released by infectious bacteria and other components of the immune system are the signals for neutrophil recruitment to sites of infection.

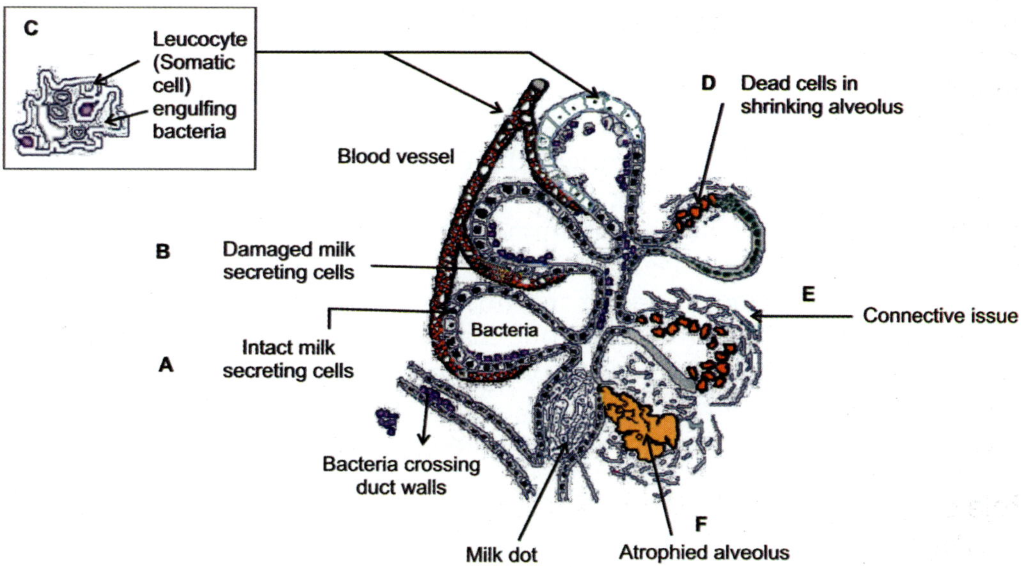

Figure 9.2 : Stepwise process of infection i.e. from infection to fibrosis.

In vitro studies have shown that mammary epithelial cells may participate in the immunoregulation during mastitis via cytokine production. These cells secrete IL-1 in response to LPS. IL-1β also appeared to be an important mediator for the release of IL-8 from mammary epithelial cells (Boudjellab *et al.,* 2000). When the proinflammatory cytokines (TNFα, IL-1) and other products of LPS-activated immune cells (mainly of macrophages) reach the central nervous system, these mediators initiate pyretic reaction and lead to marked changes in secretory pattern and/or serum level of numerous hormones. These cytokine-mediated neural and endocrine changes play key roles in the induction of systemic symptoms of mastitis, e.g. fever, lethargy, loss of appetite (anorexia) and many catabolic changes in energy (lipid, carbohydrate), protein and mineral metabolism. In more severe (usually Gram negative mastitis) cases simultaneous alterations are seen also in cardiovascular, pulmonary and gastrointestinal functions (hypotension, tachycardia, decreased cardiac output, respiratory distress, diarrhea), as well as in blood cell counts and blood coagulation system (Cullor, 1992; Sandholm *et al.*, 1995; Sordillo and Daley, 1995). These endotoxin- or cytokine-induced endocrine alterations may be dose-dependent and sometimes, also species-dependent (Huszenicza *et al.*, 2004). TNF-α and IL-1β were shown to affect tight junctions between the epithelial cells, lowering the trans-epithelial resistance (Royall *et al.*, 1989) and allowing exchange of inflammation metabolites and cells between the two blood-milk barrier compartments. Another action of IL-1 and TNF-α is to activate fibroblasts of the mammary gland, with subsequent IL-8 secretion (Lee *et al.*, 2003). TNF-α up-regulates PMN phagocytosis, adherence, chemotaxis, and release of reactive oxygen species. IL-8 is a PMN-specific chemoattractant and is produced in the response to inflammatory stimuli by a variety of cells. IL-8 induces PMN chemotaxis, respiratory burst, degranulation, and increased adherence to endothelial cells. IL-8 stimulated the transmigration of PMN through the endo-epithelial barrier in a dose-dependent manner suggesting that the production of IL-8 by mammary endothelial cells at the site of inflammation plays an important role in the recruitment of PMN into the infected gland (Lee and Zhao, 2000). In addition to the role in the pathogenesis of mastitis, cytokines initiate an increase in temperature and induction of metabolic changes, and prime or activate PMN. Cytokines can change the rate of bone marrow production and release of PMN. Cytokines also enhance PMN migration to the infection site, and increase PMN phagocytosis and respiratory burst (Sohn, 2005).

Role of enzymes and free radicals in the pathogenesis of mastitis

Polymorphonuclear leukocytes (PMNs) are the most important cellular elements of the antimicrobial self-defense mechanism. The main functions of PMNs are to engulf pathogens and destroy them via oxygen-dependent and oxygen-independent systems. At the same time, PMN can potentially harm the mammary gland. The exact mechanism by which PMN damage bovine epithelial cells during mastitis is still not fully understood. Neutrophils may promote tissue injury and disturb mammary function, via reactive oxygen metabolite generation (i.e., the respiratory burst) and granular enzyme release (i.e., degranulation) (Paape *et al.*, 2002).

Neutrophils promote tissue injury and disturbed mammary function via- a) reactive oxygen metabolite generation (the respiratory burst) and b) granular enzyme release (degranulation) (Paape and Capuco, 1997). The major free radicals found in biological systems are superoxide, hydrogen peroxide, hydroxyl radical, and fatty acid radicals. Hydrogen peroxide is found primarily in the cytosol of cells, and fatty acid radicals are found primarily in cell membranes. Superoxide and hydroxyl radicals can be found in both cell components. Because free radicals are extremely toxic to cells, the body has developed a sophisticated antioxidant system. Superoxide dismutase converts superoxide to hydrogen peroxide. Hydrogen peroxide is converted to water by the enzyme glutathione peroxidase. Those two enzymes effectively control most free radicals within the cytosol. Accordingly, the use of antioxidants to prevent oxidative stress has been studied in several types of inflammation (Sharma and Maiti, 2005). Peroxynitrite, produced during inflammation, has recently been implicated as a major cytotoxic agent. Peroxynitrite ($ONOO^-$) is the reaction product of superoxide ($O2^-$) and nitric oxide (NO). Pathological conditions such as activation of inflammatory cells induces tissues and phagocytic cells to produce superoxide and nitric oxide, leading to the formation of peroxynitrite.

The cytoplasm of mature bovine neutrophils contains many granules of varying size and Shape. One of the major characteristics of bovine neutrophils is the presence of three types of cytoplasrnic membrane bound vesicles or granules- specific/secondary granules, primary/azurophil granules and large tertiary granules. Bovine specific granules are released more readily than azurophil granules and have a higher enzymatic activity than azurophil granules.

Bovine neutrophils have been found to contain myeloperoxidase-1 (MPO-1), MPO-II, MPO-III, elastase, Pglucuronidase, α-galactosidase, β-galactosidase, acid phosphatase, α-mannosidase and N-acetyglucosaminidase.

Escherichia coli produces a number of proteinases, including collagenolytic enzymes, which contribute to the degradation of extracellular membrane (ECM) components. There is no doubt that these proteolytic activities contribute to the pathogenesis and necrosis of mammary epithelial cells. However, the degree to which they contribute is still unknown (Xhao and Lacasse, 2008).

The endotoxin-mediated cytokine (TNFα and IL-1) response increases the hypothalamic release of corticotrophin-releasing hormone that activates the pituitary-adrenal axis (Kakizaki *et al.*, 1999) and ultimately increased plasma cortisol level (Waldron *et al.*, 2003). LPS induced the mild to moderate elevations in circulating growth hormone (GH) concentrations, and a slower but marked reduction in plasma levels of insulin-like growth factor-I (IGF-I). (Elsasser *et al.* 1996; Nikolic *et al.*, 2003). The endotoxin-induced endocrine cascade also involves the glucoregulatory pancreatic hormones. Simultaneous with the TNFα and cortisol elevations, a significant but transient increase in insulin levels (Steiger *et al.*, 1999; Waldron *et al.*, 2003). The exact mechanism inducing these LPS-related alterations in the pancreatic endocrine function has not been fully understood. However, the effect of nitric oxide and cytokines

(TNFα), the early elevation of plasma cortisol and catecholamine levels, and the sympathetic neuroendocrine changes, have all been implicated in these LPS-related alterations in endocrine functions (Waldron *et al.*, 2003). It has been reported in LPS-treatment in cows, decline the plasma concentrations of thyroid hormones and lower T3/T4 ratio (Kahl *et al.*, 2000). In lactating cows simultaneous with these endotoxin-induced endocrine alterations, marked changes in plasma levels of certain energy-related metabolites were reported: concentrations of glucose tended to increase initially and subsequently declined; there was a tendency for increased non-esterified fatty acid (NEFA) levels, whereas plasma beta-hydroxy butyric acid (BHB) decreased linearly in dose dependent manner after LPS infusion (Waldron *et al.*, 2003).

Specific mastitis pathogenesis

Staphylococcal mastitis

Staphylococcus aureus (*S. aureus*) is one of the most important worldwide causes of mastitis in cattle. It is responsible for major financial losses in dairy farming and for the culling of many cows. Once cows become infected they pose significant problems. When infections have become established, they are difficult to remove and infected cows are a potential source of infection to other cows (Green and Bradley, 2004). The type of mastitis is produced by *S. aureus* ranges from sub-clinical to the per-acute life threatening form, one of

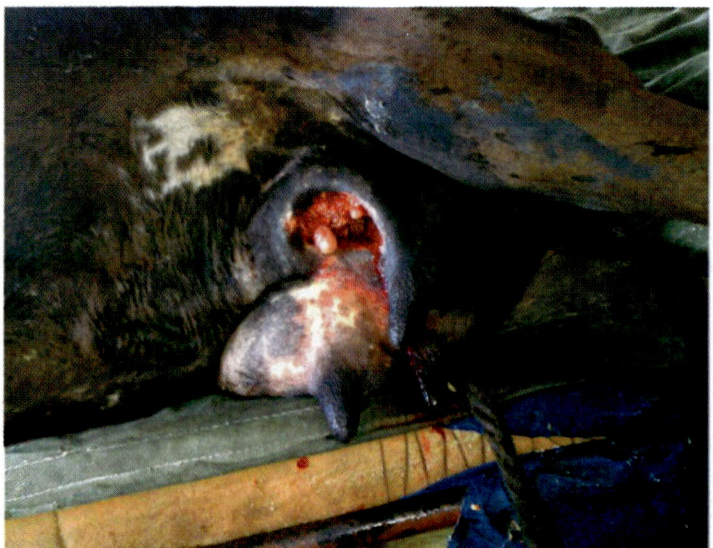

Figure 9.3: Burst abscess and sloughed right front quarter of a cow due to *S. aureus* (Gangrenous mastitis).

which is gangrenous mastitis (Figure 9.3). Gangrenous mastitis is caused by α-toxin that damages blood vessels, resulting in ischaemic coagulative necrosis of adjacent tissue. Gangrenous mastitis is characterized by a patchy blue discoloration, coldness of the affected tissue, and leaking of blood serum through the teat skin and sometimes eventually sloughs. Clinically infected quarters often show moderate swelling and visible signs of garget or chunks of milk, especially in forestrippings. Both chronic and sub-clinical mastitis lead to a gradual replacement of secretory tissue with fibrous tissue and a subsequent loss of milk production by the affected quarter.

The first stage of a *S. aureus* infection is the adhesion. The bacteria penetrates into the mammary gland and attaches itself to the gland tissue. To do so, at the beginning of its growth, it expresses proteins called '*adhesins*'. These proteins recognize the components of the gland, bind to them and allow *S. aureus* to attach. The bacteria can now multiply without running the risk of getting flushed out during milking. Once bacteria have reached sufficient numbers, they secrete virulence factors (toxins) that break down the gland tissue to extract nutrients and to migrate to other sites.

S. aureus is highly damaging to milk producing tissues due to the release of injurious toxins and enzymes. *S. aureus* produces α, β, γ and λ toxins, leukocidins, hemolysins, exfoliative toxins, enterotoxin, toxic shock syndrome toxin and coagulase. Of these, α-toxin appears to be the most toxic. It is particularly harmful to mammary tissues causing vasoconstriction, which leads to localized ischemia and cell necrosis. At this stage, the cow's immune system is already trying to fight the ongoing infection. Initially, bacteria damage the tissue lining cisterns, then move to the duct system and establish deep seated pockets of infection in the alveolar tissue.

The bacteria possess a wide array of virulence genes coding for factors that neutralize the cow's immune system. For instance, protein A and the capsule produced by *S. aureus* can elude the cow's antibodies and immune cells and prevent them from being effective. The bacteria also have mechanisms to guard against antibiotics. Indeed, *S. aureus* can produce a matrix called "biofilm" that can surround and protect bacteria. *S. aureus* is also able to penetrate inside mammary gland cells and hide from antibiotics and the cow's immune system (Parks *et al.*, 2004).

Persistent or difficult-to-treat infections may relate to the ability of this pathogen to form a slow-growing population termed "*small colony variants*" (SCVs) that can survive within professional and nonprofessional phagocytic cells and subsequently modulate immune responses (Sinha and Herrmann, 2005). Previously *S. aureus* has been viewed as an extracellular pathogen. However, its ability to survive intracellularly within polymorphonuclear leukocytes (Voyich *et al.*, 2005), and macrophages (Hebert *et al.*, 2000), as well as non-professional phagocytic cells, including cultured bovine aortic endothelial cells (BAEC) and a bovine mammary epithelial cell line (MAC-T) (Bayles *et al.*, 1998), has been established. Internalization of persistent strains of *S. aureus* within host cells has major consequences for host defense and antibiotic treatment (Brouillette *et al.*, 2004; van Belkum, 2006). In addition, the intracellular milieu appeared to favor the selection and/or survival of SCVs (Vesga *et al.*, 1996), which seem to survive within the host for long periods of time without triggering a cell mediated immune response (CMIR) (Atalla *et al.*, 2008).

Additionally, *S. aureus* can be induced to L-forms. It is thought that L-forms of *S. aureus* act as a transition stage to survive conditions such as disruption of bacterial cell wall synthesis by antibiotics that are deleterious to cellular integrity. Cell survival is possible due to lack of an organized cell wall in these *S. aureus* L-forms. L-forms provide *S. aureus* with benefits that include the ability to withstand antibiotic therapy, persist in the mammary gland, and re-emerge (flare-up) when conditions improve.

Streptococcal mastitis

The streptococcal species such as *S. uberis, S. agalactiae, S. dysgalactiae, S. epidemicus, S. bovis, S. equinus* have been implicated in bovine mastitis, although they are relatively infrequent (Leigh. 1999; Khan *et. al.*, 2003, Amosun *et al.*, 2010). *Streptococcus agalactiae* has been widely reported as an important pathogen of both animals and man. *Streptococcus agalactiae* is a gram positive bacterium which inhabits ducts and cisterns of the gland. This organism primarily infects the cisterns and the duct system of the lower portion of the udder. It causes an inflammation which blocks the ducts, leading to decreased milk production or produce agalactia, increased somatic cell count, and eventually to involution. If effective treatment is administered soon enough, and if the udder is properly stimulated and completely emptied during milking, the clots are removed and the affected area is restored. Streptococal mastitis may be sub-clinical or clinical. Cows infected by *S. agalactiae* often have more than one infected quarter. Fibrosis of inter-alveolar tissue occurs, which also leads to a loss of secretory function. *S. agalactiae* resides in the milk and on the surface of the milk channels but does not invade the tissue. Moreover, the bacteria spread rapidly within the udder and appear in the lumen of the milk ducts and secretory alveoli. It has been reported that *Streptococcus agalactiae* rarely cause severe illness, however, extensive scarring of a quarter may render it unproductive in subsequent lactation.

S. agalactiae has the ability to adhere to the mammary tissue of cows and the specific microenvironment of the bovine udder is necessary for the growth of the bacterium (Wagner and Dunny, 1984). The virulence of various strains is related to differences in their ability to adhere to the mammary epithelium (Jain, 1979).

Following entry through the teat canal, the organism attached and proliferates, and induces an influx of neutrophils into the secretory acini that is evident in 24 hours. This is followed by septal edema, vacuolation of secretory cells, necrosis of alveoli, and infiltration of septa by lymphocytes. As the disease progresses, there is hypertrophy of ductal epithelium, involution of glandular tissue, and early stage fibrosis. Streptococci are free and within alveolar epithelial cells and macrophages in the alveolar lumina, but are infrequent in neutrophils (Thomas *et al.*, 1994).

On the other hand, *S. uberis* is known worldwide as an environmental pathogen responsible for a high proportion of cases of clinical and subclinical mastitis in lactating cows and is also the predominant organism isolated from mammary gland during the non-lactating period (Bradley, 2002; Khan *et al.*, 2003). Resistance to phagocytosis and the bactericidal activity of neutrophils is a hallmark of *S. uberis* infection. Resistance to bactericidal activity of neutrophils may be due to the factors released by *S. uberis* as it replicates in milk.

Coliform mastitis

The only apparent prerequisite for a strain to cause mastitis is the ability to grow and multiply in mammary secretions. *E. coli* and *K. pneumoniae* are the species for which virulence factors have been most completely characterized (Hogan and Smith, 2003). *E. coli* is the most common Gram-negative mastitis causing bacteria. About 80% of coliform infection will result in clinical mastitis, and 10% will result in acute mastitis with a sudden onset of septic shock. The severity of bovine *E. coli* mastitis is mainly determined by cow factors rather than by the pathogenecity of the invading pathogen and management (Burvenich *et al.*, 2003). It is known that the growth of *E. coli* in the udder cistern is specially related with the period of lactation and parity of cows. *E. coli* mastitis with severe clinical symptoms is more frequently observed around calving and during early lactation in dairy cows, whereas symptoms are mild to moderate during mid and late lactation. Because of hormonal, metabolic and nutritional alterations associated with pregnancy, immune system is compromised around calving (Pezeshki *et al.*, 2010). Coliform mastitis is infrequent during mid or late dry period because secretions from fully involuted mammary glands do not readily support growth and multiplication of coliform bacteria (Oliver and Bushe, 1987). The limiting nutritional factor for many coliform bacteria in the dry mammary gland is iron (Smith and Schanbacher, 1976). Lactoferrin is an iron binding protein that increases in mammary secretion during involution and remains elevated until colostrogenesis. *Klebsiella pneumoniae* are more capable than most strains of *E. coli* to overcome the inhibitory effects of lactoferrin and infect involuted mammary glands (Todhunter *et al.*, 1990). Cow parity is another important physiological factor that influences the severity of clinical coliform mastitis (van Werven *et al.*, 1997; Vangroenweghe *et al.*, 2004). Clinical severe cases of coliform mastitis are mostly seen among multiparous cows rather than primiparous cows during early lactation (Pezeshki *et al.*, 2011).

The portal of entry for Gram-negative bacteria into the mammary gland is the teat canal. The manner that coliform bacteria traverse the teat canal is unknown, but probably involves an opportunistic entry into the gland whereby at least a portion of the canal is bypassed. Adherence of *E. coli* and *K. pneumonia* to epithelial tissue does not play a major role in the pathogenesis of bovine mastitis (Frost *et al.*, 1977; Opdebeeck *et al.*, 1988). Coliform bacteria do not appear to colonize inside the mammary gland, but multiply in the secretion without attachment to epithelial surfaces. The more rapidly that coliforms can adjust metabolically to mammary secretion, the more rapidly bacterial numbers increase and disease can occur. Therefore, the severity of clinical disease and peak coliform counts in mammary secretions are positively correlated (Hogan and Smith, 2003).

Once infection has occurred, the *E. coli* bacteria proliferate in great numbers, and die and lyse, endotoxin is released from the cell wall. This massive and sudden liberation of endotoxin results in a severe, life-threatening toxemia. The release of this endotoxin triggers a cascade of inflammatory responses resulting in acute swelling of the mammary gland and a marked increased in the number of neutrophils in the milk (Smith and Hogan, 1993). Tissue damage caused by coliform toxins can be found in the teat cistern, gland cistern, and large ducts within 1 hour after invasion. Initiation of the inflammatory reaction is caused by the production and release of tumor necrosis factor (TNF), interferons (INF), and interleukins (IL). These complex interactions result in accumulation of PMN in the mammary gland. Phagocytosis by PMN is the most effective defense against bacterial infection. Inflammation is centered in the ducts while the alveoli are filled with serous fluid and vacuolated desquamated epithelial cells, but leukocytes may be few or absent in the alveoli. If the course of the disease is prolonged, necrosis may be extensive. There is often severe edema of the subcutis. The supramammary lymph nodes draining the affected quarter often are enlarged and edematous, and necrotic foci may be disseminated widely in the nodes.

Gram-negative bacteria isolated from bovine intramammary infections possess a myriad of virulence factors. Endotoxin is the primary virulence factor of Gram-negative bacteria responsible for damage to the cow. Endotoxin refers to the lipopolysaccharide (LPS), which form the part of the outer layer of the Gram-negative bacterial cell wall. LPS comprises lipid-A, a lipopolysaccharide core and polysaccharide units (O-antigens) (Cullor 1996). Lipid-A is responsible for the toxic effects of LPS (Cullor 1996). LPS is considered to be a primary virulence factor of coliform mastitis and responsible for most pathophysiological reactions in coliform mastitis. LPS triggers formation of proinflammatory and inflammatory cytokines, produced predominantly by monocytes and macrophages (Persson Waller *et al.*, 2003). The cellular receptor for LPS is CD14, which mainly occurs on monocytes and macrophages, and to a lesser extent on neutrophils (Paape *et al.*, 2003). It facilitates recognition of LPS by the TLR4 receptor. Macrophages, dendritic cells and epithelial cells are expected to express TLR4 in the mammary gland (Werling *et al.*, 2006; Gonen *et al.*, 2007). Cytokines, such as tumor necrosis factor alpha (TNF-α), initiate the inflammatory response, which induces the acute phase response (APR) by activating the production of acute phase proteins (APP), such as serum amyloid-A (SAA), haptoglobin (Hp) and LPS-binding protein (LBP) (Soujala, 2010).

In fresh cows, coliform mastitis can become so severe that the life of the animal is threatened. In this severe form of the disease, bacterial toxin (endotoxin) from the infected mammary gland escapes into the blood stream causing cows to go off feed and to stop milking. It also causes inflammation to occur throughout the cow's body, leading to organ failure and shock. Because the onset of severe coliform mastitis is so rapid, there are no obvious clinical signs until after peak bacterial growth and endotoxin exposure have occurred. By that time, udder inflammation and shock are so massive as to leave few options for successful intervention. Thus, rapid death (or euthanasia) is a typical scenario for affected dairy cows. Chronic coliform mastitis develops when the initial inflammatory response and influx of somatic cells fail to eliminate all bacteria. This form of mastitis is characterized by periodic acute flare-ups, which may eventually be severe enough to destroy all bacteria. A unique feature of coliform infections is that, in the cows that recover, the udder tissue gradually returns to normal without fibrosis. In subsequent lactations the gland produces to its optimal capacity.

Mycoplasma mastitis

Several species of mycoplasma can infect cattle and buffalo, but *Mycoplasma bovis* is the most frequent cause of bovine mastitis. *M. californicum* and *M. bovigenitalium* are two other common causes. Mycoplasma mastitis is classified as a "contagious mastitis pathogen" because the infection can be spread from cow to cow during milking. *M. bovigenitalium* was the first species of mycoplasmas recognized as an agent of bovine mastitis (Stuart *et al.*, 1963). Clinical presentation in herds and cows is similar to *M. bovis*, although it has been reported that affected cows tend to recover over a period of a few weeks or months (Jasper, 1982). *"Mycoplasma mastitis should be suspected when cows are not responding to therapy or where multiple quarters are involved"*. Mycoplasma organisms are commonly found on the mucous membranes of the respiratory and urogenital tracts of healthy cows. However, stresses such as calving, extreme temperature variations, transportation, disease or external trauma may allow the organisms to enter other body tissues or directly into the mammary gland resulting in clinical mastitis. Thus, it is extremely important to realize that even though a dairy is not currently experiencing mycoplasmal mastitis, the organisms are more than likely present within the herd and the possibility of a mastitis outbreak always exists. Although infection probably occurs via the streak canal, the rapid spread of the disease to other quarters of the udder and occasionally from lungs or joints through the blood stream to the udder may occur. When *M. bovis* becomes established in the udder, it produces waste products and toxins. These byproducts elicit an inflammatory response in the mammary gland causing inflammation, edema and decreased milk production and ultimately "mastitis". Attachment of *M. bovis* to mucosal surfaces appears to be mediated by phase-variant surface proteins and multiple other surface proteins.

The important and first step of Mycoplasma infection is attachment to mammary epithelial cells. This attachment is mediated by variable surface lipoproteins (Vsps) on the outer face of the plasma membrane that are potent stimulants of the host immune response (Chambaud *et al.*, 1999). The Vsps are important factors in the inflammatory process, inducing the secretion of pro-inflammatory cytokines including tumor necrosis factor a, interleukin 1, and interleukin 6, and are probably also involved in leukocyte recruitment to the infected tissue (Razin *et al.*, 1998; Chambaud *et al.*, 1999). It has been reported that mycoplasmas are able to survive with little evidence of phagocytosis or inhibition growth in the presence of high concentrations of neutrophils in milk that are produced in response to IMI (Bennett and Jasper, 1978). Macroscopic and histologic changes observed in slaughtered cows that were infused intramammarily with *M. bovis* differed depending on the duration of infection.

Mycoplasma may persist for long-time (upto 13 months) in udder and some cows may become shedders of mycoplasmas without severe clinical signs being seen. The secretion from an affected quarter appears fairly normal in the early stages of infection, but if the milk is allowed to stand, a deposit of fine, flaky material settles out leaving a turbid, whey-like supernatant fluid. Leukocyte counts in the milk are usually very high, often over 20 million cells/ml. Clinical signs include a drop in milk production and the observance of severely abnormal stringy or granular thick secretion. In its most dramatic form, mycoplasma may infect all four quarters of a cow and milk production may completely stop, although cases that severe probably occur less than 20% of the time. Clinical Mycoplasma will be unlike acute coliform mastitis as there is little or no swelling in the gland and the cow usually does not appear toxic. Mycoplasma may sneak up on you as a milder case that may look like any other chronic or sub-clinical mastitis.

Summer mastitis

Aerobic-anaerobic mastitis, often termed "*summer mastitis*", is a suppurative infection (clinical mastitis) of the udder quarters of heifers and non-lactating cows. The infection is characterized by production of copious quantities of foul-smelling pus and a rapidly progressing course of hardening, tenderness, and eventual tissue destruction of the infected quarters. Most cases of aerobic-anaerobic mastitis occur during the summer pasture season and a fly, *Hydrotaea irritans,* is generally considered the vector. Microaerophilic *Actinomyces pyogenes* and anaerobic bacteria, especially *Peptostreptococcus indolicus* and *Fusobacterium necrophorum*, are the pathogens most often implicated in the bacterial etiology of summer mastitis. The most common aerobic isolates are *Streptococcus dysgalactiae* strains. Summer mastitis risk factors include lack of dry cow therapy, calving in the high risk period (autumn), teat damage and exposure to flies. Summer mastitis affects between 39% and 54% of herds every year in UK, with about 2.1 to 4.1 cases per affected herd (Berry, 1998). If you consider a cost per case of £270, there is considerable scope for putting in place insurance policies to prevent what could be a significant cost burden (Press release, 2006).

These bacteria may gain entrance through the wounds caused by the flies, but more often they are ordinary residents of the udder, having reached there the same way as the summer mastitis germ from the tonsils via the blood, or via the teat canal. A massive invasion of the mammary tissue via the teat canal results in large proportion of the gland being affected at one time. There is a severe systemic reaction and loss of function of the entire quarter. The secretion from the affected quarter is foul-smelling, attributable to the activities of the anaerobic *P. indolicus.* If the cow survives, the quarter becomes extremely indurated and abscesses develop, later rupturing through the floor of the udder, often at the base of a teat. Uncomplicated infections, with *A. pyogenes* alone, can also be serious with quarters so severely affected that there is a permanent loss of the quarter and sloughing can occur.

References

Ahlner, S. (2003). Prevalence of sub-clinical mastitis in Uruguay. Thesis, SLU Uppsala.

Amosun, E.A, Ajuwape, A.T.P. and Adetosoye, A.I. (2010). Afr. J. Biomed. Res., 13(1): 33-37.

Atalla, H., Gyles, C., Jacob, C.L., Moisan, H., Francois, M. and Mallard, B. (2008). Foodborne Pathogens and Disease, 5(6): 785-799.

Bayles, K.W., Wesson, C.A., Liou, L.E., Fox, L.K., Bohach, G.A. and Trumble. W.R. (1998). Infect. Immun., 66: 336-342.

Bennett, R.H. and Jasper, D.E. (1978). Vet. Microbiol., 2: 341-55.

Berry, E. (1998). Update on summer mastitis. In: Proc. British Mastitis Conference, Axient/ Institute for Animal Health, Milk Development Council/Novartis Animal Health. Pp.46-53.

Blowey, R. and Edmondson, P. (2010). Mastitis control in dairy herds. 2nd edn., CABI International, UK.

Boudjellab, N., Chan-Tang, H.S. and Zhao, X. (2000). Bovine interleukin-1 expression by cultured mammary epithelial cells (MAC-T) and its involvement in the release of MAC-T derived interleukin-8. In: Comp. Biochem. Physiol. A Mol. Integr. Physiol., 27: 191-199.

Bradley, A.J. (2002). Vet. J., 164: 116-128.

Brouillette, E., Grondin, G., Lefebvre, C., Talbot, B.G. and Malouin, F. (2004). Vet. Microbiol., 101: 253-262.

Burton, J.L. and Erskine, R.J. (2003). Vet. Clin. Food. Anim., 19: 1- 45.

Burvenich, C., Van Merris, V., Mehrzad, J., Diez-Fraile, A. and Duchateau, L. (2003). Vet. Res., 34(05): 521-564.

Chambaud, I., Wroblewski, H. and Blanchard, A. (1999). Trends. Microbiol., 7: 493-499.

Cullor, J. (1996). In: Comp. Cont. Ed. Food Anim., 18: 31-38.

Cullor, J.S. (1992). J. Am. Vet. Med. Assoc., 200: 1894-1902.

Elsasser, T.H., Richards, M., Collier, R. and Hartnell, G.F. (1996). Domest. Anim. Endocrinol., 13: 91-103.

Fantone, J.C. and Ward, P.A. (1999). Inflammation. In: Rubin E, Farber JL (eds.) Pathology 3rd ed. New York: Raven Press, 1999: 37-15.

Frost, A.J., Wanasingue, D.D. and Woolcock, J.B. (1977). Infect. Immun., 15: 245-253.

Gonen, E., Vallon-Eberhard, A., Elazar, S., Harmelin, A., Brenner, O., Rosenshine, I., Jung, S. and Shpigel, N. (2007). Cellular Microbiology, doi:10.1111/j.1462-5822.2007.00999.x.

Green, M. and Bradley, A. (2004). Clinical Forum - *Staphylococcus aureus* mastitis in cattle. UK-Vet, 9(4): 1-9.

Hallen-Sandgren, C., Svensson, C., Tivemo, M. and Emanuelson, U. (1997). Risk factor för juver inflammation (Sveriges lantbruksuniversitet, Fakta Husdjur nr 13). 4 s. Uppsala.

Hebert, A., Sayasith, K., Senechal, S., Dubreuil, P. and Lagace, J. (2000). FEMS Microbiol. Letter, 193: 57-62.

Hogan, J. and Smith, K.L. (2003). Vet. Res., 34: 507-519.

Huszenicza, G., Janosi, S., Gaspardy, A. and Kulcsar, M. (2004). Anim Reprod. Sci., 82-83: 389-400.

Jain, N.C. (1979). J Dairy Sci., 62: 128-134.

Jasper, D.E. (1982). J. Am. Vet. Med. Assoc., 81: 158-62.

Jones, G.M. (2009). Understanding the basics of mastitis. Virginia cooperative extension publication 404-233. Pp. 1-5, www.ext.vt.edu

Kahl, S., Elsasser, T.H. and Blum, J.W. (2000). Domest. Anim. Endocrinol., 18: 133-143.

Kakizaki, Y., Watanobe, H., Kohsaka, A. and Suda, T. (1999). Endocr. J., 46: 487-496.

Khan, I.U., Hassan, A.A., Abdulmawjood. A., Lanimler, C., Wolter, W. and Zschock, M. (2003). J. Vet. Sci., 4: 213-223.

Lee, J.W. and Zhao, X. (2000). Cell Biol. Int., 24: 889-895.

Lee, J.W., Paape, M.J., Elsasser, T.H. and Zhao, X. (2003). J. Dairy Sci., 86: 2282-2289.

Leigh, J.A. (1999). Vet. J., 157: 225-238.

Nickerson, S.C. (1994). In: Comp. dairy research report, Hill Farm Research Station, Lousiana State University, pp. 129-140.

Nikolic, J.A., Kulcsár, M., Katai, L., Nedic, O., Jánosi, Sz. and Huszenicza, Gy. (2003). J. Vet. Med. Assoc., 50: 22-29.

Oliver, S.P. and Bushe, T. (1987). Am. J. Vet. Res., 48: 1669-1673.

Opdebeeck, J.P., Frost, A.J. and O'Boyle, D. (1988). Vet. Microbiol., 16: 77-86.

Paape, M., Bannerman, D., Zhao, X. and Lee, J.W. (2003). Vet. Res., 34: 597-627.

Paape, M., Mehrzad, J., Zhao, X., Detilleux, J. and Burvenich, C. (2002). J. Mammary Gland Biol. Neoplasia, 7: 109-121.

Paape, M.J. and Capuco, A.V. (1997). J. Anim. Sci., 75: 556-565.

Parks, W.C., Wilson, C.L. and Lopez-Boado, Y.S. (2004). Nature. Rev. in Immun., 4: 617-629.

Persson Waller, K., Colditz, I.G., Lun, S. and Ostensson, K. (2003). Res Vet Sci., 74: 31-36.

Pezeshki, A., Capuco, A.V., De Spiegeleer, B., Peelman, L., Stevens, M., Collier, R.J. and Burvenich, C. (2010). J. Anim. Physiol. Anim. Nutr., 94: 27-30.

Pezeshki, A., Stordeur, P., Wallemacq, H., Schynts, F., Stevens, M., Boutet, P., Peelman, L.J., Spiegeleer, B.D., Duchateau, L., Bureau, F. and Burvenich, C. (2011). Vet. Res., 42: 15.

Press release (2006). Why gamble when it comes to summer mastitis? Intervet Schering-Plough Animal Health, UK. 27th May, 2006. http://www.intervet.co.uk/binaries/92_113774.pdf.

Razin, S., Yogev, D. and Naot, Y. (1998). Microbiol. Mol. Biol. Rev., 62: 1094-156.

Royall, J.A., Berkow, R.L., Beckman, J.S., Cunningham, M.K., Matalon, S. and Freeman, B.A. (1989). Am. J. Physiol., 257: L399-410.

Sandholm, M., Honkanen-Buzalski, T., Kaartinen, L. and Pyorala, S. (1995). The bovine udder and mastitis. University of Helsinki, Faculty of Veterinary Medicine, Helsinki, Finland.

Sharma, Neelesh and Maiti, S.K. (2005). Indian J. Vet. Med., 25(2): 76-79.

Sinha, B. and Herrmann, M. (2005). Thromb. Haemost., 94: 266-277.

Smith, K.L. and Hogan, J.S. (1993). Environmental mastitis. W.B. Saunders Company. pp. 489-498.

Smith, K.L. and Schanbacher, F.L. (1976). J. Am. Vet. Med. Assoc., 170: 1224-1227.

Sohn, E.J. (2005). The interelationship between CD14 and LPS during mastitis: release of soluble CD14 and cytokines by bovine PMN following activation with LPS. PhD dissertation, University of Maryland.

Sordillo, L. and Daley, M. (1995). In: Myers, M.J., Murtaugh, M.P. (Eds.), Cytokines in Animal Health and Disease. Marcel-Dekker, New York, pp. 389–419.

Soujala, L. (2010). Bovine mastitis caused by *Escherichia coli* – clinical, bacteriological and therapeutic aspects. PhD dissertation, University of Helsinki, Finland.

Steiger, M., Senn, M., Altreuther, G.,Werling, D., Sutter, F., Kreuzer,M. and Langhans, W. (1999). J. Anim. Sci., 77: 2523-2532.

Stuart, P., Davidson, I., Slavin, G., Edgson, F.A. and Howel, D. (1963). Vet. Rec., 75: 59-64

Thomas , L.H. , Haider, W., Hill, A.W. and Cook, R.S. (1994). Am. J. Vet. Res., 55: 1723-1728.

Todhunter, D.A., Smith, K.L. and Hogan, J.S. (1990). J. Dairy Sci. 73: 363-372.

van Belkum, A. (2006). Curr. Opin. Infect. Dis., 19: 339-344.

van Werven, T., Noordhuizen-Stassen, E.N., Daemen, A.J.J.M., Schukken, Y.H., Brand, A. and Burvenich, C. (1997). J. Dairy Sci., 80: 67-74.

Vangroenweghe, F., Duchateau, L. and Burvenich, C. (2004). J Dairy Sci., 87: 886-895.

Vesga, O., Groeschel, M.C., Otten, M.F., Brar, D.W., Vann, J.M. and Proctor, R.A. (1996). J. Infect. Dis., 173: 739-742.

Voyich, J.M., Braughton, K.R., Sturdevant, D.E., Whitney, A.R., Said-Salim, B., Porcella, S.F., Long, R.D., Dorward, D.W., Gardner, D.J., Kreiswirth, B.N., Musser, J.M. and DeLeo, F.R. (2005). J. Immunol., 175: 3907-3919.

Waldron, M.R., Nishida, T., Nonnecke, B.J. and Overton, T.R. (2003). J. Dairy Sci., 86: 3447-3459.

Wanger, A.R. and Dunny, G.M. (1984). J. Dairy Sci., 67: 2441-2445.

Werling, D., Piercy, J. and Coffey, T.J. (2006). Vet. Immunol. Immunopathol., 112: 2.

Zhao, X. and Lacasse, P. (2008). J. Anim. Sci., 86: 57-65.

□□□

CHAPTER

10

Clinical Signs

Mastitis is an inflammation of mammary gland, which is clinically associated with the changes in glandular tissue and milk, and severe cases also characterized by systemic involvement (i.e. affected animal show the systemic signs *e.g.* fever, high respiration and pulse rate, lack of appetite, dull, depress and sometimes recumbent). Clinical mastitis could be diagnosed on the basis of physical examination of udder and clinical signs for instance swelling in udder and changes in milk. But sub-clinical mastitis could not be diagnosed on the basis of only clinical signs. Prominent clinical signs of mastitis always stimulate the dairy farmer to consult the veterinary doctor as earliest as possible. Early detection and timely treatment of mastitis always increase the chances of recovery and reduce the financial losses.

Clinical cases range from the mild to the acute to the peracute. In another study, mild, acute and peracute cases were considered to occur in the approximate ratios of 70:29:1 (Blowey, 1986). Although Blowey (1986) suggests that 1% of clinical mastitis cases may be peracute, not all of these will result in death. The clinical findings should be used only as a guide because different pathogens can cause peracute, acute, gangrenous, chronic and sub-clinical forms of the disease, and clinical differentiation of the different causes of mastitis is difficult. The clinical findings in mastitis include abnormalities of secretion, abnormalities of the size; consistency and temperature of the mammary glands and frequently a systemic reaction. In other words, there are three categories of clinical mastitis: abnormal milk, abnormal gland and an abnormal cow (systemic disease) (Radostits *et al.*, 2006).

Mastitis is mainly divided into two category: clinical mastitis and sub-clinical mastitis on the basis of clinical signs. Clinical mastitis further subdivided into peracute mastitis, acute mastitis and chronic mastitis. Gangrenous mastitis is comes under the peracute or acute mastitis. Some clinicians classify the clinical mastitis as mild, moderate and severe (Figure 10.1).

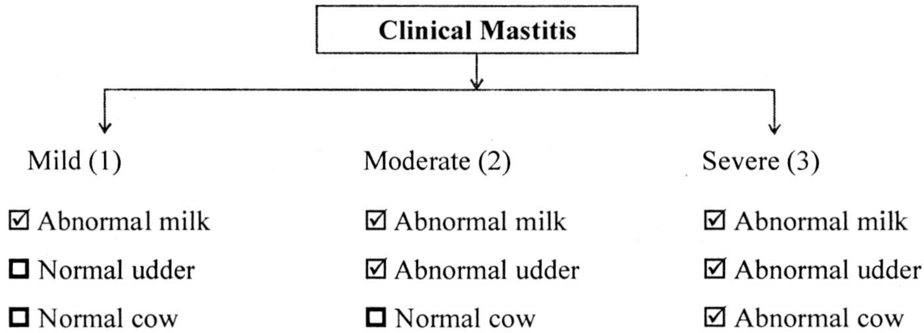

Figure 10.1: Classification of mastitis on the basis of severity of infection. [Note: 1. *Abnormal milk:* discoloration, watery, presence of flakes, clots and purulent material, 2. *Abnormal gland:* abnormal size (due to inflammatory swelling and fibrosis) and consistency of the mammary gland, 3. *Abnormal cow:* cow becomes abnormal due to systemic response including toxemia, fever, tachycardia, ruminal stasis, depression, anorexia and recumbency, depending on the severity of infection.]

Clinical mastitis

Clinical mastitis can present itself in a wide degree of severity of symptoms which can range from mild to moderate to severe. The degree of illness and the symptoms present will depend on many factors, such as the nutritional or immune status of the cow, which pathogen is responsible for the inflammation, and a range of environmental factors such as cleanliness, humidity and ambient temperature. Moderate to severe clinical cases can be very painful and unpleasant for the cow. Clinical mastitis is clinically characterized by grossly abnormal milk and evidence of varying degrees of udder inflammation (redness, heat, swelling, pain) resulting asymmetry of the udder (Figure 10.2), and systemic signs. The milk can vary from watery to purulent (consistency), greenish to yellowish in color (Figure 10.3), having a milk clots (garget), serum with clumps of fibrin and pus in the milk. Clinical mastitis can be further categorized into peracute mastitis, acute (gangrenous) mastitis and chronic mastitis.

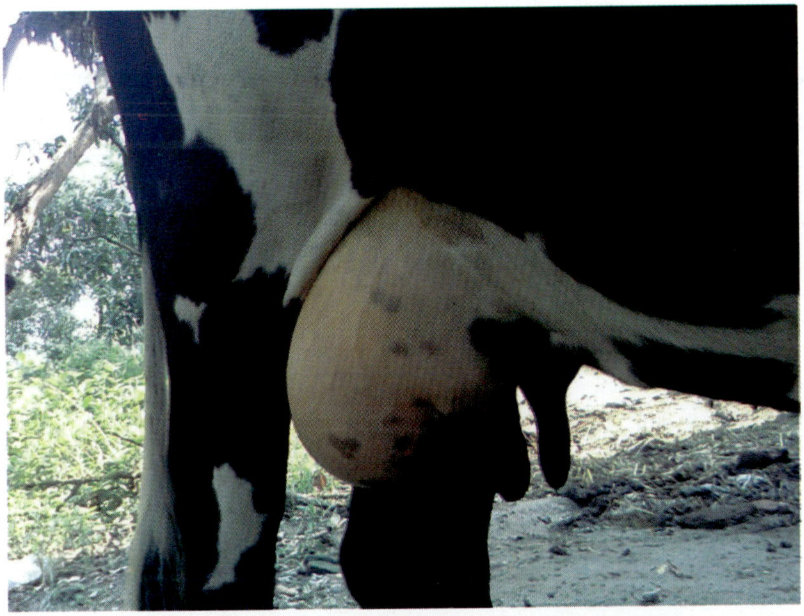

Figure 10.2: Asymmetry of the udder due to swelling in the right hind quarter.

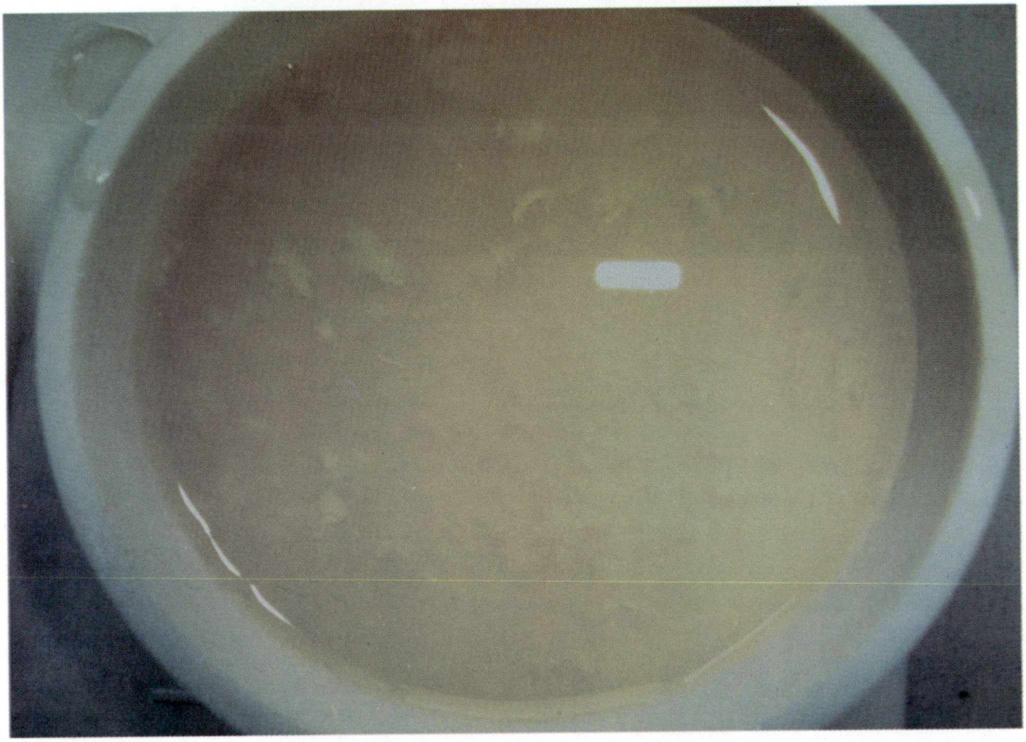

Figure 10.3: Yellow color of mastitis milk.

Mild clinical mastitis – only one symptom almost normal milk but with clots (Figure 10.4).

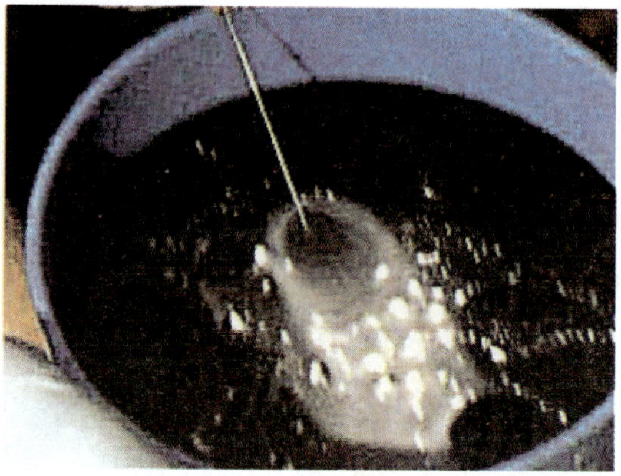

Figure 10.4: Clots in the milk. Source: Bacic (2009)

Moderate clinical mastitis– two symptoms, milk with clots and swelling of quarter or udder (Figure 10.5A, B).

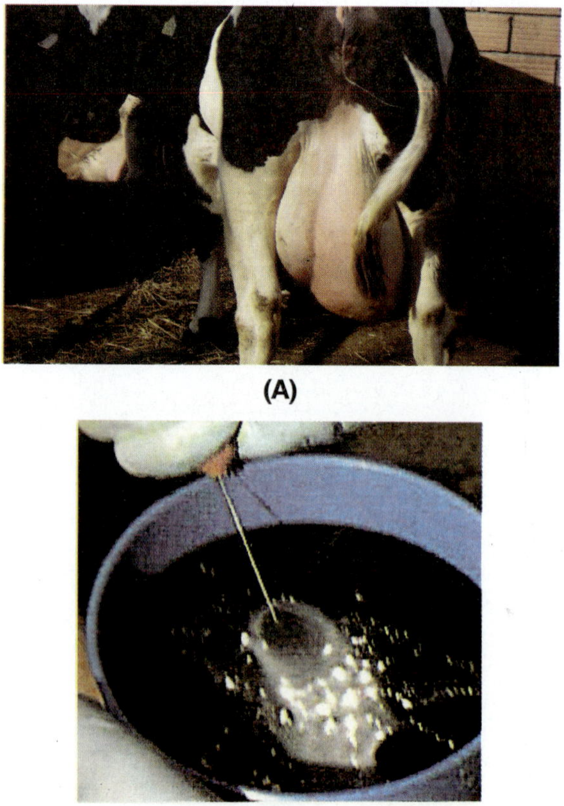

(A)

(B)

Figure 10.5: (A) Swelling in the left hind quarter, (B). Clots in the milk. Source: Bacic (2009)

Sub-acute mastitis

In sub-acute mastitis, the cardinal signs of mastitis are less pronounced, and there are no systemic signs.

Chronic mastitis

This form of mastitis may exhibit no clinical signs for prolonged intervals. In simple way, "long-term recurring persistent cases of the disease are termed "chronic". Events that are not well characterized may, from time to time, exacerbate the chronic infection, causing clinical signs of an acute infection. Frequently recurrence of mammary gland inflammation with watery milk is implicit as chronic mastitis. Somatic cell counts (SCC) are generally chronically elevated, with the mammary gland secretions periodically containing flakes, clots, or shreds of fibrin. Prolonged destruction of mammary gland alveoli and ducts with replacement by scar tissue results in reduced milk producing capabilities of the patient. In this form, quarter(s) becomes fibrosed and hard, and decrease or complete cessation of milk (agalactiae) due to permanent loss of milk secreting vesicles. In chronic mastitis, sometimes affected teat(s) becomes shrink (Figure 10.12) and in some cases the whole inner mass of affected quarter(s) become slough out (Figure 10.11). The bacteria commonly associated with this type of infections are coliforms, *S. agalactiae* and *S. aureus*.

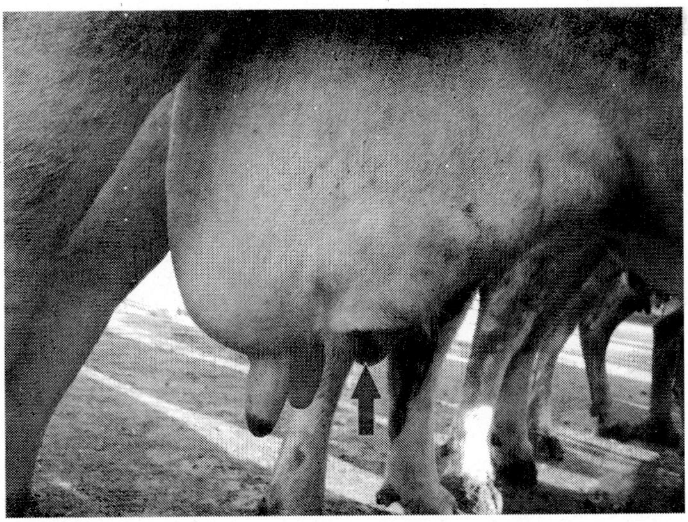

Figure 10.12: Shrinkage of right front teat (arrow) due to chronic mastitis.

Sub-clinical mastitis

Simply, sub-clinical mastitis is a type of mastitis which is characterized by the no visual changes in the quarter(s) and milk or the existence of inflammation in the absence of gross signs is referred to as sub-clinical mastitis.

Sub-clinical mastitis occurs when the mammary gland is infected and the number of somatic cell count is increased. In sub-clinical mastitis the milk appears grossly normal, and there is no visible sign of inflammation in the udder. With time, sub-clinical infections results in fibrosis of mammary tissue, a firmer and larger gland, and decreased milk production. Sub-clinical mastitis is most commonly associated with *S. aureus* and *S. agalactiae*.

Another Classification

Acute catarrhal mastitis

Acute catarrhal mastitis is characterized by a mild systemic response of short duration. This type of mastitis normally occurs in individual quarter. Milk may be bloodstained and contain flakes of inspissated pus. Gross glandular changes include, affected lobules are pale, firm and project above the cut surface. Flakes of purulent exudate are present in the cisterns and lactiferous ducts. Sometimes edema may be mild or pronounced.

Acute hemorrhagic mastitis

An acute hemorrhagic mastitis clinically characterized by marked swelling of the affected quarter(s) and by a severe systemic reaction which is often fatal. The small amount of mammary secretion that can be obtained consists of sero-sanguinous or fibrinous exudate. Gross glandular changes include the mammary tissue is intensely hyperemic and hemorrhagic with areas of necrosis. In this type cases gangrene may also occur.

Suppurative mastitis

Suppurative mastitis is usually caused by *Corynebacterium pyogenes* or *Pseudomonas aeruginosa* infection. This type of mastitis is characterized by multiple abscesses present in the affected quarter(s).

Granulomatous mastitis

Granulomatous mastitis is generally occurs due to infection with Mycobacterium, Nocardia, Cryptococcus, etc. and this is characterized by presence of nodular growths in affected quarter(s). This type of mastitis is normally a chronic type. Granulomatous inflammation progressively increased in severity and distribution with increasing duration of infection, it may be due to increases in total numbers of algae, of sporangia, and of empty degenerate algal forms. Granulomatous mastitis is mainly caused by S. *aureus*, it has the ability to invade more deeply into the interacinar tissue and establish themselves as persistent foci of infection (a granulomatous type reaction may be provoked).

Specific mastitis

Staphylococcal mastitis

To date, more than 50 staphylococcus species and subspecies have been characterized. The genus is divided into coagulase-positive staphylococci and coagulase-negative staphylococci (CNS) based on their ability to coagulate plasma (Pyorala and Taponen, 2009). The major pathogen, *Staphylococcus aureus*, is generally coagulasepositive although coagulase-negative strains of *S. aureus* do occur (Fox *et al.*, 1996). *S. aureus* is one of the most important worldwide causes of mastitis in cattle. It is responsible for major financial losses in dairy farming and for the culling of many cows. Various virulence factors of *S. aureus* have been compared with clinical characteristics of mastitis, but no specific virulence factor or combination of factors has been strongly associated with the severity of mastitis (Haveri *et al.*, 2008). Baselga *et al.* (1993) noted that the severity of ruminant mastitis decreased, but the bacterial capacity to colonize the mammary gland increased when the infection was caused by a mucoid (slime producer) rather than a non-mucoid *S. aureus* isolate.

S. aureus mastitis presents with varying degrees of severity- acute, sub-acute, chronic and sub-clinical, but it also may cause peracute mastitis and lead to gangrene of the quarters. The chronic and sub-clinical forms predominate and on a herd basis, are the most important.

Peracute *S. aureus* mastitis occurs usually in the first few days after calving and is highly fatal. There is a severe systemic reaction with high rise of temperature (106-107°F), tachycardia (100-120 beats/min), anorexia, profound depression, absence of ruminal movements and muscular weakness, often to the point of recumbency. The onset of the systemic and local reactions is sudden. The cow may be normal at one milking and recumbent and comatose at the next. The affected quarter is grossly swollen, hard and sore to touch, and causes severe lameness on the affected side (Radostits *et al.*, 2006). The acute/sub-acute form resembles other moderate cases of clinical mastitis but commonly develops into a chronic form. Clinically infected quarters often show severe swelling of the quarter(s) and visible changes in milk include purulent milk, garget or chunks of milk, especially in forestrippings. Extensive fibrosis and severe loss of function always result. Acute *S. aureus* infections generally develop late in the lactation or just prior to calving. However, the clinical symptoms (udder swelling or hardness, changes in appearance of milk) do not show up until calving or early in the next lactation.

Chronic and sub-clinical mastitis are often associated with fibrosis, abscessation and blocked ducts within the gland (Green and Bradley, 2004). It becomes difficult to successfully treat an infection because drugs are not able to penetrate to all infection sites and because the bacteria live inside the white blood cells. *S. aureus* produces an enzyme that inactivates most penicillin-based treatments, resulting in ineffective antibiotics. Bacterial toxins and toxic products are thought to be involved in the causation of mastitis and gangrene. The á-toxin is potentially the most damaging, because it causes vasoconstriction leading to ischemic necrosis of affected tissues and gangrene. Glands harboring nonpathogenic staphylococci (micrococci) commonly exhibit mild leukocytosis in milk without clinical mastitis. While coagulase negative staphylococci (CNS) usually cause sub-clinical or mild clinical mastitis, but they have also been reported to produce severe local and systemic signs (Jarp, 1991). Reports on the clinical characteristics of CNS mastitis are scant as CNS have been ignored in many studies on clinical mastitis. In heifers, quarters infected with "non-aureus staphylococci" exhibited leucocyte infiltration and a higher percentage of interalveolar stroma as compared with healthy controls, which can have deleterious effects on future milk production (Trinidad *et al.,* 1990).

Streptococcal mastitis

Approximately 50% of environmental streptococcal intramammary infections cause clinical mastitis during lactation. Streptococci have been known to be associated with bovine mastitis since 1900 and *S. uberis* was first clearly described in the 1920s and 1930s using biochemical and serological techniques. *S. uberis* mainly grows in residual and newly synthesized milk and the mastitis it causes can vary in its severity. *S. agalactiae* (commonly called "Strep ag") is a common cause of sub-clinical and mild to moderate clinical mastitis infections in dairy cows. With sub-clinical infections the cows have an elevated somatic cell count without abnormal milk. Cows infected by *S. agalactiae* often have more than one infected quarter. *S. agalagtiae* may exist as an acute clinical mastitis. Changes in milk include that the milk being easily coagulated and having alkaline pH and salted taste, and if the milk is left to stand for 24 hours, it separates into two layers, one lower formed by clots and leucocytes and one serous upper. Anatomical lesions primarily interest the walls of the galactophor sinus, suffering a noticeable induration on palpation. The duration of infection is shorter than staphylococci, primarily because of the better response to therapy. In *S. agalactiae* mastitis more than one quarter is usually involved but not uniformly. Most of the changes take place in the distal portion of the gland around the cisterns and larger ducts. In the acute stages, the glandular tissue is swollen and turgid and lobulations are distinct on the cut surfaces. Clinically characterized by fever (lasting for a day or two), is occasionally observed with the initial attack but the inflammation of the gland persists and the subsequent crises are usually of a relatively mild nature. The affected mammary tissue is grayish (whereas normal lactating tissue is more or less white in color). In the chronic stages, fibrosis becomes prominent. Clinical *S. dysgalactiae* mastitis can be acute with anorexia and pyrexia in addition to the local signs.

Coliform mastitis

The coliform species most commonly implicated in mastitis are *E. coli,* although other species including *Enterobacter aerogenes, Pseudomonas aeruginosa, Ent. oxytoca, K. pneumoniae* and *Citrobacter* spp. are also encountered. Infection is more common among housed cows and occurs particularly around calving. Sub-clinical infection is less common and peracute mastitis occurs frequently around calving. About 50% of these peracute infections die. Coliform mastitis may range in severity from fatal, peracute cases to sub-clinical infections detectable only on cultural examination. While the peracute forms attract much attention, such cases probably constitute only a small part of all coliform mastitis. Peracute form commonly occurs after parturition but may develop at any time during lactation. The characteristically sudden onset of the disease, i.e., normal at one milking and severely ill at the next, is due to rapid multiplication of bacteria followed by release and dissemination of endotoxin.

The pronounced signs during sudden onset or in peracute form are including complete anorexia, severe depression, fever (104-108°F), increased heart rate (100-120 beats/min), shivering and trembling, cold extremities, diarrhea, dehydration, depression, shivering, and rumen stasis. Within 6-8 hours after the onset of signs the cow may be recumbent and unable to stand. At that stage, the temperature may be normal or subnormal, all of which may superficially resemble parturient paresis. Inflammatory signs in the udder may be minimal at initial phase, and swelling may be detectable only after the udder is milked out and for this reason coliform mastitis may be missed on initial clinical examination. Later, the quarter is swollen and hard, and the teat may be thickened, edematous, and sensitive. Collateral edema extending over unaffected quarters may suggest that they also are involved. Milk becomes watery and yellowish in colour, contains clots and flakes, and milk yield is reduced drastically. Occasionally, acute coliform infection will result in complete cessation of milk production, but affected cows sometimes lactate normally in subsequent lactation. Decreased milk production during clinical coliform mastitis results both directly and indirectly from the local and systemic effects of endotoxin. Clinical mastitis causes decreased milk production, increased veterinary costs, and possible death or culling. Decreased milk production during clinical coliform mastitis results both directly and indirectly from the local and systemic effects of endotoxin. Clinical mastitis causes decreased milk production, increased veterinary costs, and possible death or culling. Signs of endotoxic shock may appear within a few hours of onset. At this time, the prognosis is guarded to poor. Recumbency, marked depression, progressive dehydration, diarrhea, and normal or below-normal rectal temperatures are associated with endotoxic shock.

Chronic mastitis is more characteristic of the *Ps. aeruginosa* infection with periodic acute flare-ups. The organism is persisted in a gland for as long as five lactations, but spontaneous recovery may occur. *Ps. aeruginosa* has a tendency to cause sudden outbreaks of clinical mastitis in several cows and buffaloes within a few days despite to apparent changes in management practices. In acute cases, there is a severe systemic reaction (fever 105-107°F), marked swelling of the udder and abnormal watery milk with flakes, clots, blood and the functioning gland is usually completely lost at the first attack. In addition, infected cows may show severe signs of toxaemia and many animals die despite aggressive treatment.

Summer mastitis

Summer mastitis is an acute mastitis typically occurring during the summer (July, August and September) in non lactating cattle, especially if warm and damp where the fly (*Hydrotoea irritans)* population is high usually close to wooded pastures. Summer mastitis has been reported from northern Europe, Japan, USA, Greece, Australia, Zimbabwe and Brazil. Regional variations occur in incidence and the classic area of occurrence is considered to be a sandy soil or low lying, wooded areas with poor drainage. The bacterium suspected to be mainly responsible, *Corynebacterium pyogenes* is a potent toxin and pus producing organism, occasionally found in the tissues, including the udder, of healthy animals.

The classic symptoms of summer mastitis are a hot, hard and swollen quarter, usually with a tense and enlarged teat. The affected cows are often lame because of the painful quarter and may develop swollen hocks. Some animals may abort (summer mastitis primarily affects pregnant cattle), and others give birth to a full-term but retarded and weakly calf (Blowey and Edmondson, 2010). Initially severe systemic signs including fever, inappetence, tachycardia, depression, mortality rate up to 50% (Radostits *et al.*, 2006). The milk of the affected quarter(s) may vary from cheese-like to whitish yellow, to thick reddish and dark clots and a typical rotten smell. Secretion from infected quarters initially watery with clots, later purulent. Then and only then you have typical summer mastitis. Neglected cases may die, especially if dry cows and pregnant heifers do not receive as much attention as they should.

Mycoplasma mastitis

There are several Mycoplasma species that can cause mastitis and they vary in their pathogenicity. *M. bovis, M. californicum,* and *M. bovigenitalium* are the most common. Characteristically, infection with *Mycoplasma* spp. leads to a mastitis, often involving multiple quarters, which is refractory to antibiotic treatment. The secretion may remain normal at the onset although a granular or flaky deposit is recognized on standing (Figure 13). In the later stages a purulent or thick secretion, without offensive smell is often reported. Swelling and firmness is common but after a few days the mammary gland may reduce in size. Response to treatment is very poor and the swollen udders become grossly atrophied. The classic clinical presentation is severe clinical mastitis in multiple quarters of multiple cows with minimal systemic signs of disease. Milk secretion is severely reduced. Swelling of the supramammary lymph nodes occurs and there may be pyrexia, transient malaise and arthritis. In lactating cows, there is a sudden onset of swelling of the udder, a sharp drop in milk production and grossly abnormal secretion in one or more quarters.

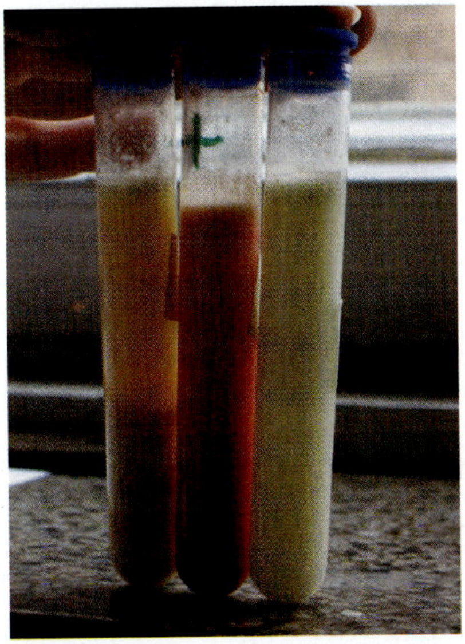

Figure 10.13 : Left and middle test tube – typical Mycoplasma infection abnormal milk secretion, watery with "sand like" sediment on the bottom of the tube. Right tube normal milk.

'In newly calved and housed animals the first signs are often tenderness in the quarter, which can be confused with excessive intramammary pressure, and local temperature. The milk will be discoloured, thick and creamy, rather than colostral, perhaps very clotted in a serous fluid, and frequently foul smelling. In addition to the extreme mastitis, in later stages pyrexia and lethargy develop. If the infection remains local there may be rupture of mammary abscesses to the exterior. More commonly, the animal becomes systemically ill with progressive lameness from the hind legs, swelling of joints and an elevated temperature (Hillerton, 2004).

Leptospira mastitis

The organism most involved is *Leptospira hardjo* and this is responsible for the so-called 'milk drop syndrome' and is also associated with abortion in affected herds. This is a herd syndrome in which the milk yield falls precipitately without there being any clinical evidence of disease, especially mastitis, or obvious deprivation of food or water. The characteristic milk drop appears initially as a mastitis, usually with the milk yield of all four quarters falling to zero within 24 hours. Pyrexia is common and the udder secretion is thickened or clotted and occasionally bloody. The udder remains flaccid and the condition usually resolves within seven to fourteen days (Edmondson and Bramley, 2004).

References

Bacic, G. (2009). Diagnostics and treatment of mastitis in cows, Veterinary College, Zagreb, pp. 20-34.

Baselga, R., Albizu, I., dela Cruz, M., del Cacho, E., Barberan, M. and Amorena, B. (1993).. Infect. Immun., 61: 4857-4862.

Blowey, R. and Edmondson, P. (2010). Mastitis control in dairy herds. 2nd edn., CABI International, UK.

Blowey, R.W. (1986). Vet. Rec, 119: 551-553.

Edmondson, P.W. and Bramley, A.J. (2004). Mastitis. In: Bovine mastitis: Diseases and husbandry of cattle (2004), edited by Andrew, A.H., Blowey, R.W., Boyd, H. and Eddy, R.G., 2nd ed., Blackwel publishing Co., pp. 326-336.

Fox, L.K., Besser, T.E. and Jackson, S.M. (1996). J. Am. Vet. Med. Assoc., 209: 1143–1146.

Green, M. and Bradley, A. (2004). Clinical Forum - *Staphylococcus aureus* mastitis in cattle. UK-Vet, 9(4): 1-9.

Haveri, M., Roslof, A., Rantala, L. and Pyorala, S. (2008). J. Appl. Microbiol., 103: 993-1000.

Hillerton, J.E. (2004). Summer mastitis. In: Bovine mastitis: Diseases and husbandry of cattle (2004), edited by Andrew, A.H., Blowey, R.W., Boyd, H. and Eddy, R.G., 2nd ed., Blackwel publishing Co., pp. 337-340.

Jarp, J. (1991). Vet. Microbiol., 27: 151-158.

Pyorala, S. and Taponen, S. (2009). Vet. Microbiol., 134: 3-8.

Radostits, O.M., Gay, C.C., Blood, D.C. and Hinchkliff, K.W. (2006). Veterinary Medicine. 10th edn. ELBS & Baillier Tindall.

Sharma, Neelesh, Gupta, S.K., Sharma, U. and Hussain, K. (2007). Buffalo Bull., 26(2): 56-58.

Trinidad, P., Nickerson, S.C. and Adkinson, R.W. (1990). J. Dairy Sci., 73: 639-647.

□□□

CHAPTER

11

Public Health Significance

In spite of improvements in dairy husbandry practices, the availability of a wider range of therapeutic agents, and the efforts of health and agriculture authorities toward control, bovine mastitis continues as a major problem in the dairy industry. Mastitis is the single disease that has the most significant impact on milk quality (LeJeune and Rajala-Schultz, 2009). The problem is twofold, encompassing both public health hazards to man and economic losses to the dairyman. When antibiotics and other chemotherapeutic substances are utilized for treating bovine disease such as mastitis, residues in the milk may lead to sensitization of persons and allergic manifestations in already sensitized individuals, while also rendering the manufacture of cultured dairy products such as cheese and yoghourt impossible or difficult. Penicillin is the main offender, but others are not without potential harm. Chronic mastitis in dairy cows, however, is becoming of increasing importance in spite of the ready availability of a variety of so-called *'wonder drugs'*.

The relationship between dairy cattle health and human health warrants mention. The dairy industry strives to produce milk and dairy foods that are safe and nutritious, and that are seen to be healthful and wholesome. The greatest risk of high SCC milk to human health is in the consumption of unpasteurized or improperly pasteurized milk (Oliver *et al.*, 2005). Viable pathogens and their toxins can be transferred from the milk of infected quarters directly to humans. A large and diverse group of human pathogens reside in the cow's environment including *Salmonella dublin, Campylobacter jejuni,* and *Listeria monocytogenes* (Oliver *et al.,* 2005). These microbes are often pathogens or normal flora of dairy cows. Evidence has been reported that *Mycobacterium avium* subsp. *paratuberculosis,* associated with Johnes in cattle and isolated from human patients with Crohn's disease, may survive some accepted milk pasteurization procedures. Although the possible association between shedding of the *Mycobacterium avium* subsp. *paratuberculosis* in milk and subsequent survival after pasteurization is compelling, the rate of shedding is low in infected cows and not related to an increase in SCC (Stabel, 2005). Surveys indicate that dairy producers and their families drinking milk produced on their own farms are among the demographic groups are at greatest risk to food borne diseases due to consumption of unpasteurized milk. Proper pasteurization of milk is very effective in preventing the transfer of viable pathogens from milk of infected mammary glands to humans. Pasteurization reduces the number of viable microorganisms, but often does not negate the effects of toxins produced by mastitis pathogens (Sharma *et al.,* 2011).

Infections that are naturally transmissible from vertebrate animals to humans and vice versa are classified as zoonoses (WHO, 2009). It has been estimated that about 61% of human infections are zoonotic (Taylor *et al.,* 2000). In the livestock sector, different farm animals naturally carry a wide range of zoonotic pathogens. In the dairy sector, zoonotic pathogens are normally present in dairy animals, raw milk, milk products, meat and the farm environment but are often difficult to diagnose. These zoonoses can be transmitted to humans in several ways that include consumption of infected raw milk and coming in contact with infected dairy animals, animal products and infected farm environments (Zinsstag *et al.,* 2007). However, most milk-borne zoonoses are mostly acquired through consumption of infected milk. Milk-borne zoonoses are of both public health and economic importance (Mosalagae *et al.,* 2011). Being a nutritional, balanced foodstuff, milk is a well-known medium that favours the growth of several microorganisms. Milk from a mastitis cow commonly contains the etiological agents, while milk from non-mastitic cows is known to be often contaminated from extraneous dirt or unclean processing water. The health hazards, posed by milk-borne zoonotic diseases such as Staphylococcal infection, Streptococcal infection, tuberculosis and brucellosis etc. and mastitis related enterotoxemia are well documented (Weinhaupl *et al.,* 2000; Shirima *et al.,* 2003; Kivaria *et al.,* 2006). Risks of milk borne zoonoses posed by the informal market are amplified by poor handling procedures on the market, the lack of quality standards and the fact that most consumers prefer raw milk. This situation is further compounded by the fact that many smallholder farmers blindly treat their mastitic cows with little or no consideration of antimicrobial withdrawal periods (Kivaria *et al.*, 2006). The profitability of the dairy industry is driven by both the quantity and the quality of the milk produced. Although milk has often been described in the popular media as *"nature's most perfect food,"* it cannot escape consumer scrutiny for quality and wholesomeness. As a result, many milk marketing and processing organizations have begun to penalize poor quality and give financial rewards for superior quality milk mostly in developed countries. Direct ingestion of bovine netrophils have the health concern. As the SCC increases, the percentage of cells those are neutrophils increases. In this strictest definition of the problem, any potential health risk of consuming milk with an elevated SCC would depend largely on the human health concerns of ingesting bovine neutrophils. Although the ingestion of large numbers of bovine neutrophils in milk may be objectionable, direct negative effects on the safety of humans have not been documented as a result of consuming dairy products made with milk having high SCC (Sharma *et al.*, 2011).

The public health concerns of bovine mastitis relate to the occurrence of both different mastitis pathogens and antibiotics residues in milk for human consumption. Early in this century, it was discovered that milk can transmit tuberculosis, brucellosis, diphtheria, scarlet fever, and Q fever to humans. Fortunately, over the decades, the threat of these diseases and the incidence of outbreaks involving milk and milk products have been greatly reduced due to improved sanitary of the milk production practices and pasteurization technique. However, a variety of microorganisms still contribute to illnesses and disease outbreaks. Raw (unpasteurized) milk has been found to participate in spreading out of illnesses caused by *Staphylococci spp., Streptococcal spp., E. coli, Mycobacterium bovis, Corynebacterium spp.* etc. (Hameed *et al.*, 2006). It is well known that mastitis caused by more than 250 organisms including bacteria, fungi, algae and virus, hence consumption of infected or mastitic raw milk carries more risk for human health. Varieties of micro-organisms that produce disease in man also inhabit the bovine udder and cause mastitis. Although certain streptococci and staphylococci are considered to be the primary infectious causes of mastitis, numerous other organisms have been shown to be involved. Detail etiological agents are discussed in etiology chapter (Chapter 7) of this book.

With severe clinical *mastitis*, abnormalities of milk are easily observed and milk is discarded by the producer. Such milk normally would not enter the food chain. But when milk of cows with sub-clinical *mastitis*, *i.e.* with no visible changes, is accidentally mixed into bulk milk, it enters food chain and can be dangerous to humans. Although pasteurization is likely to destroy all human pathogens, there is concern when raw milk is consumed or when pasteurization is incomplete or faulty (Hameed *et al.*, 2006).

Staphylococcus aureus is probably the most important species in this respect. In case of consumption of raw milk there can be a real hazard, the main threat being the fact that about 10% of mastitis staphylococci are known to be producers of enterotoxins. This toxin may be produced when *S. aureus* counts exceed 10^5cfu/ml (Whiting *et al.*, 1996). Therefore in view of the fact that 6.1 X 10^6 of *S. aureus* count per milliliter were observed in 6% milk samples, coupled with the heat stability of staphylococcal enterotoxins, this must be regarded as a public health hazard (Kivaria *et al.*, 2006). There are some important human health infections those transmitted from mastitic are discussed in detail.

1. Staphylococcal Infection

S. aureus is becoming as serious a problem in the veterinary as it is in the medical world. It causes bovine mastitis of a type most difficult to treat successfully and almost impossible to eliminate from a herd. *S. aureus* is a leading cause of community-acquired infections in humans and a cause of mastitis and skin diseases in milk producing animals (Klotz *et al.*, 2003; Lim *et al.*, 2004; Katsuda *et al.*, 2005). Staphylococcal food poisoning (staphylo-enterotoxicosis; staphyloenterotoxemia) is the name of the condition caused by the enterotoxins which some strains of *S. aureus* produce. Moreover, among food-borne intoxications, *S. aureus* is a major cause of gastroenteritis resulting from consumption of contaminated food products (Le Loir *et al.*, 2003; Bennett, 2005). Outbreaks of *S. aureus* food poisoning have been caused by the consumption of dairy products, including raw milk (Jorgensen *et al.*, 2005), low-fat milk and dried skimmed milk (Asao *et al.*, 2003) and cheeses (Rosec *et al.*, 1997). Milk from staphylococcal mastitis cows is chemically abnormal in composition (high in chloride and cells, low in lactose, casein and fat) but also contains an organism which is potentially pathogenic to Man who may become infected with such staphylococci.

Milk of infected animals is the main source of enterotoxigenic *S. aureus* of animal origin (Gilmour and Harvey, 1990). The genetic plasticity of *S. aureus* has facilitated the emergence of persistent and multidrug-resistant strains that have major impact on human and animal health (Foster, 2004). Persistent or difficult-to-treat infections may relate to the ability of this pathogen to form a slow-growing population termed "*small colony variants*" (SCVs) that can survive within professional and nonprofessional phagocytic cells and subsequently modulate immune responses (Alexander and Hudson, 2001; Sinha and Herrmann, 2005). Presence of *S. aureus* in milk due to the consumption of raw unpasteurized milk and ethnic cheese or due to postpasteurization contamination may present a public health hazard. This is mainly because many strains of bovine origin produce heat stable enterotoxins (Srinivasan *et al.*, 2006; Peles *et al.*, 2007), and may be a source of antibiotic resistance genes (Mathew *et al.*, 2007). Although SCVs associated with human diseases are resistant to a number of antimicrobial compounds the potential risk of bovine SCVs in the context of food safety and human health is unknown. Clinical SCVs are frequently isolated from humans with persistent and relapsing infection following antibiotic treatment (von Eiff *et al.*, 1997; Kahl *et al.*, 1998).

The presence of *S. aureus* in milk, however, presents an additional potential hazard to public health by virtue of the fact that, under favourable conditions, some strains produce a heat-stable enterotoxin during milk storage, which heat processing, such as pasteurization, sterilization and desiccation cannot inactivate. Ingestion of preformed toxin leads to an acute, albeit non-fatal, form of food poisoning within 2 - 3 hours. As little as 1.0 μg of enterotoxin A can be sufficient to produce food poisoning. S. aureus present in a food at levels of 10^6/g or more could be dangerous if conditions for enterotoxin production are favourable. Rapid and adequate cooling of milk all along the line is essential to control this hazard.

The enterotoxins are proteins with a disulphide bridge and are resistant to most proteolytic enzymes and are relatively heat tolerant. The optimum temperature for the production of enterotoxin is 35-40°C. *S, aureus* itself is destroyed by pasteurization and cooking but enterotoxin-A is destroyed only gradually at 100°C for 30 minutes and can survive short or light cooking. The bovine mammary gland can be a significant reservoir of enterotoxigenic strains of *S. aureus.* Two different types of toxin with super-antigen activity can be produced: enterotoxins and toxic shock syndrome toxin (TSST-1). The staphylococcal enterotoxins (SEs) have been divided into five serological types (SEA, SEB, SEC, SED, and SEE) on the basis of their antigenic properties (Dinges *et al.*, 2000). The strains producing the staphylococcal enterotoxin type C (SEC) have been widely isolated from *mastitis*-afflicted cows (Lee *et al.*, 1998, Cardoso *et al.*, 1999). The occurrence of other new types of SEs (SEG to SEJ) has been reported (Su and Wong, 1995; Munson *et al.*, 1998). Kenny *et al.* (1993) reported a significant correlation between the SEC and TSST-1 in *S. aureus* from mastitic milk. However, the relationship between these new SEs and bovine *mastitis* has not been sufficiently clarified. According to Hayakawa *et al.* (1998) the production of exfoliative toxins by *S. aureus* isolated from mastitic cow's milk or from bulk milk seems to be rare. The importance of pathogenity of toxin formation of *S. aureus* for udder remains unclear. However, the super-antigenic toxins might overstimulate or reduce the host immune response (Hameed *et al.*, 2006).

S. aureus most frequently causes diseases in humans in various suppurative (pus-forming) infections. It causes superficial skin lesions such as boils, styes and furunculosis; more serious infections such as pneumonia, mastitis, and urinary tract infections; and deep-seated infections such as osteomyelitis and endocarditis. The onset of symptoms in staphylococcal food poisoning is usually rapid and in many cases acute, depending on individual susceptibility to the toxin, the amount of contaminated food eaten, the amount of toxin in the food ingested, and the general health of the victim. The most common symptoms are nausea, vomiting, retching, abdominal cramping, and prostration. Some individuals may not always demonstrate all the symptoms associated with the illness. In more severe cases, headache, muscle cramping, and transient changes in blood pressure and pulse rate may occur. Recovery generally takes two days, however, it is not unusual for complete recovery to take three days and sometimes longer in severe cases.

2. Streptococcal Infection

Streptococcus agalactiae has been widely reported as an important pathogen of both animals and man (Keefe, 1997; Mosabi *et al.*, 1997; Ko, *et. al.*, 2001). *S. agalactiae* is an important bovine pathogen, especially as a cause of both clinical and sub-clinical mastitis in dairy cows.

In humans, *S. agalactiae* has been described as one of the most common factors of invasive infections in neonates, but it also causes invasive and non-invasive infections in adults (Schuchat, 2001). "Scarlet fever" is caused by certain strains of the group A streptococci bacteria (which also causes strep throat) and it is common to think of scarlet fever as *strep throat* with a rash. In simple words, the scarlet fever is that the streptococci originate in the throats of the milk handlers and through contamination gain access to the supply. Symptoms usually develop about 1 to 7 days (incubation period) after being exposed to someone with strep throat or scarlet fever. Scarlet fever is most common in children under 10 years old and begins with a fever and sore throat. Other symptoms can include vomiting, headache, chills and abdominal pain. Many children with this infection have a high fever initially, which may reach 103 to 104 degrees F. Without treatment, the fever may last 5 to 7 days, but usually quickly goes down within a day after starting antibiotic therapy.

This pathogen is also one of the leading causes of invasive infections in non-pregnant immunocompromised individuals and also causes bacteremia, septicaemia, meningitis, and pneumonia. Colonization of the rectum and vagina of pregnant women with group-B streptococcus (GBS) is correlated with GBS sepsis in newborn infants with early onset disease Occasionally, human carriers of group A streptococci may, however, infect the udders of cows, and subsequently numerous organisms are excreted in the milk, to cause serious and widespread epidemics of milk-borne septic sore throat and scarlet fever. *S. agalactiae* also causes neonatal septicemia in humans. Human infection is generally acquired from other human sources, although there may be some risk associated with direct exposure to infected animals or their products. Overall there is considerable homology between strains isolated from septicemic infants and mastitic cows (Wagner and Dunny, 1985). Although some surface antigens seem to be specific to the cow (Wagner and Dunny, 1987), *S. agalactiae* is now recognized to be part of the normal bacterial flora in the human throat, genitourinary tract and rectum (Mhalu, 1976).

3. *E. coli* infection

Escherichia coli (E. coli) are bacteria that normally live in the intestines of healthy people and animals, primarily cattle. Coliform mastitis particularly *E. coli* mastitis is more prevalent in bovine. *E. coli* infection may also transmitted to the human being through consumption of raw milk. The public health hazard of *E. coli* has been emphasized by many authors, because these bacteria have been implicated in human cases of gastroenteritis, epidemic diarrhoea in infants, sporadic diarrhoea in children as well as in cases of food poisoning. Enteropathogenic and enterotoxigenic *E. coli* have been identified as causes of human diarrhea for at least 50 years (Ryser, 1998). The most common clinical syndrome is diarrhea, nausea, abdominal cramping and fever. In contrast, enterohemorrhagic *E. coli* caused by O157:H7 is noteworthy because of the seriousness of the syndrome. Hemorrhagic colitis with severe abdominal pain may progress to hemolytic uremic syndrome (HUS) resulting in acute renal failure.

Within the bovine mastitis *E. coli* species, a specific verocytotoxigenic strain may cause haemorrhagic colitis, the most important one is the enteroheamorrhagic type E. coli O157:H7 (Leclerc *et al.*, 2002). Although, *E. Coli* O157:H7 has only rarely been associated with disease in cattle.

The symptoms of *E. coli* 0157:H7 infection in human are variable. Some individuals have no symptoms (asymptomatic). Others may have mild to severe diarrhea, which may contain blood. Abdominal cramps, nausea and vomiting may occur. Usually there is little or no fever present. A small number of patients develop complications, such as hemolytic-uremic syndrome (HUS). Hemorrhagic colitis with severe abdominal pain may progress to hemolytic uremic syndrome (HUS) resulting in acute renal failure. The elderly and children under 5 years of age are at greatest risk of developing a serious illness from *E. coli* 0157:H7 infection. Death due to *E. coli* 0157:H7 infection occurs infrequently, usually as a result of a complication of the infection. Crump *et al.* (2002) describe a large outbreak of *E. coli* O157:H7 infections that were directly transmitted from animals and their environment to people, largely children.

Control over stock remedies available to the farmer, constant vigilance over milk supplies, and advice to the milk producer have to some extent assisted in checking this problem. Awareness, teaching and training programmes for smallholder dairy farmers can improve disease control in animals and reduce the public health risk of milk-borne zoonoses.

4. Tuberculosis

Tuberculosis is important disease in humans and animals worldwide. The tubercle bacillus infects over 2 billion people or one third of the world's population and it is estimated that 1.5 to 2 million people die from tuberculosis each year (Tiruvulamala and Reichman, 2002). A total of 95% cases occur in people in developing countries.

The danger of milk-borne tuberculosis is mainly associated with tuberculous mastitis which is caused by *Mycobacterium bovis.* Mills (1898-99) recorded the first positive case of tuberculous mastitis (tuberculin positive) in a cow which later revealed typical tuberculous lesions in the lungs and udder. Its milk produced persistent diarrhoea in a European child and its own calf which died later. Presence of tubercle bacilli in milk sample was investigated in Bombay city, India by Joshi (1914), and out of 674 samples examined, he found acid fast bacilli in 7.6% (47) cases. The danger arising from tuberculous infection of the udder is too well known to necessitate discussion. It is safe to assume that it has been responsible for a large part of our human tuberculosis of bovine origin. *M. tuberculosis, M. bovis* and *M. avium* all the three species are capable of causing disease in humans although *M. tuberculosis* is by for the most common in humans with continues to be a major cause of morbidity and mortality throughout the world. Transmissions of tuberculosis in humans are mainly by inhalation and ingestion of raw milk or unpasteurized dairy products (Rahman and Samad, 2008). Rahman and Samad (2008) have been reported that 35.29% lactating cows, 20.0% non-lactating pregnant cows, 33.33% weaned calves and 20.0% unweaned calves showed positive reaction to bovine tuberculosis in Bangladesh. Recent report of Doran *et al.* (2009) describes an outbreak of tuberculosis affecting cattle and people on a dairy farm in southeastern Ireland following the consumption of milk from a seven-year-old cow with tuberculous mastitis. Bouzid *et al.* (2009) have been reported 8.22% prevalence of tuberculosis in dairy cattle in Algeria herds.

Tuberculosis in human may be pulmonary and systemic. The major clinical signs are coughing, chronic fever and gradual loss of body weight. Bovine tuberculosis is commonly transmitted in the peoples those are in close contact to the affected cows. Previous understanding of the origin of tuberculosis postulated that it began as a zoonosis at the time that humans domesticated and lived closely with cattle although molecular genetic studies have suggested that this may not have the case, and that human tuberculosis (*M. tuberculosis*) may have predated tuberculosis in animals (*M. bovis*) (Thoen *et al.*, 2009).

5. Brucellosis

Brucellosis is another disease of animals which has considerable direct and indirect public health implications and causing abortion and sterility in cattle. It reduces productivity and thus the amount of available meat and milk. Brucellosis is the most common zoonosis in the world, accounting for the annual occurrence of more than 500,000 cases (Pappas *et al.*, 2006). Dairy cows are frequently affected and excrete the organisms in their milk. Infection of the consumer may follow ingestion of milk and certain dairy products. The high rate of isolation of the *Brucella* from the udder and the supra mammary lymph nodes is reflected in the numbers excreted in milk which can vary from a few hundreds up to 200,000 organisms/ml of milk (Corbel, 1988). Thus, the milk is an important material to be processed for knowing the prevalence of brucellosis in particular area.

Brucellosis is caused by different species of *Brucella* and is an important disease of livestock species and wild animals, as well as a significant health hazard when they are in contact with human beings. *Brucella* contaminated milk presents a potential threat to the new born calves and human beings as it can spread through ingestion and causes infectious abortion and undulant fever. Dairy products prepared from unpasteurized milk such as soft cheeses, yoghurts, and ice-creams may contain high concentration of the bacteria and consumption of these is an important cause of brucellosis. It is the commonest mode of transmission in case of *B. melitensis* and *B. abortus* infections in general population. Those with a professional risk of acquiring infection include livestock producers, abattoir workers, shepherds, farmers, veterinarians, and laboratory personnel. Brucellosis is common in rural areas because farmers live in close contact with their animals and often consume fresh unpasteurized dairy products (Mantur and Amarnath, 2008).

In organized dairy farming, reproductive disorders, viz. infertility, retained placenta, abortions and endometritis, etc. are the main impediments to profitability (Chahota *et al.*, 2003). The rates of infection vary greatly from one country to another and between regions within a country. The highest prevalence is seen in dairy cattle. Bovine brucellosis is widespread in India and appears to be on the increase in recent times, perhaps due to increased trade and rapid movement of livestock (Renukaradhya *et al.*, 2002). In India, brucellosis was first recognized in 1942 and is now endemic throughout the country. Various studies in India revealed that brucellosis has been recognized, both by isolation and serological studies, as one of the most serious diseases among different livestock species as well as animal handlers in the past few decades (Kataria and Verma, 1969; Sharma *et al.*, 1979; Chakraborty and Kwatra, 1980; Manicham and Mohan, 1987; Katoch *et al.*, 1996; Verma *et al.*, 2000; Chahota *et al.*, 2003). Bouzid *et al.* (2009) have been reported 10.44% prevalence of brucellosis in dairy cattle in Algeria herds. It is still an uncontrolled serious public health problem in many developing countries including India. Brucellosis in India is yet a very common but often neglected disease (Mantur and Amarnath, 2008).

Human brucellosis is known for protean manifestations (Mantur *et al.*, 2006). However, the most common presenting symptom is fever. The symptoms and signs most commonly reported are fever, fatigue, malaise, chills, sweats, headaches, myalgia, arthralgia, and weight loss (Mantur *et al.*, 2007). Boiling of milk should be done as a general measure of food safety. Monitoring of brucellosis in animals and people should be a continuous undertaking.

6. Corynebacterium Infection

Within this group there is a lot of species that are part of normal flora of skin and mucous membranes of humans and animals. Under favourable conditions opportunistic infections are caused by these microorganisms in immunocompromised hosts. The most frequently isolated bacteria from this group are *C. bovis, C. pyogenes* and *C. ulerans*. Of these *C. bovis* is considered as contagious but less pathogenic to cow mammary gland. While *C. pyogenes* causes an acute suppurative mastitis (Summer mastitis) and *C. ulcerans* may cause sub-clinical mastitis in cows and buffaloes. Summer mastitis is associated with abscesses within the udder and milk losses in affected quarter, and may even lead to the death of the animal. Unpasteurized milk and raw dairy products derived from infected cows and direct contact with animals constitute potential sources of Corynebacterium infections in humans. *C. pyogenes* has been reported to cause ear infections, endocarditis, cystitis and Cutaneous abscesses as well. Human patients infected with *C. bovis* exhibited signs of septicaemia and purulent conjuctivits. Toxigenic *C. ulcerans* strains may cause pharyngeal infections mimicking classical diarrhea, ulcers and sinusitis in humans. Non-toxigenic strains cause pulmonary nodules and necrotizing granulomas (Andrzejczak and Malinowski, 2010).

References

Alexander, E.H. and Hudson, M.C. (2001). Appl. Microbiol. Biotechnol., 56: 361-366.

Andrzejczak, E. and Malinowski, E. (2010). Medycyna Wet., 66(11): 756-760.

Asao, T., Kumeda, Y., Kawai, T., Shibata, T., Oda, H., Haruki, K., Nakazawa, H. and Kozaki, S. (2003). Epidemiol. Infect., 130(1): 33-40.

Bennett, R.W. (2005). J. Food. Prot., 68(6): 1264-1270.

Bouzid, R., Laouabdia Sellami, N., Benkhelil, A., Hocine, A., Ouzrout, R. and Touati, K. (2009). African J. Agric. Res., 5(4): 316-321.

Cardoso, H.F.T., Silva, N., Sena, M.J. and Carmo, L.S. (1999). Letters in Applied Microbiology, 29: 345-349.

Chahota, R., Sharma, M., Katoch, R.C., Verma, S., Singh, M.M., Kapoor, V. and Asrani, R.K. (2003). Veterinarski Arhiv, 73: 95-102.

Chakraborty, A. and Kwatra, M.S. (1980). Indian J. Path. Microbiol., 23: 125-128.

Corbel, M. J. (1988). In: Fertility and Infertility in Veterinary Practice. Laing, J. A. (ed), 4th Edition. ELBS, Bailliere Tindall. pp. 189-221.

Crump, J.A., Sulka, A.C., Langer, A.J., Schaben, C., Crielly, A.S., Gage, R., Baysinger, M., Moll, M., Withers, G., Toney, D.M., Hunter, S.B., Hoekstra, R.M., Wong, S.K., Friffin, P.M. and Van Glider, T. J. (2002). N. Engl. J. Med., 347(8): 555-560.

Dinges, M.M., Orwin, P.M. and Schlievert, P.M. (2000). Clinical Microbiology Reviews, 13: 16-34.

Doran, P., Carson, J., Costello, E. and More, S.J. (2009). Irish Veterinary Journal, 62(6): 390-397.

Foster, T.J. (2004). J. Clin. Invest., 114: 1693-1696.

Gilmour, A. and Harvey, J. (1990). Society for Applied Bacteriology Symposium Series, 19: 147S-166S.

Hameed, K.G.A., Sender, G. and Korwin-Kossakowska, A. (2006). Animal Science Papers and Reports, 25 (2): 73-85

Hayakawa, Y., Hayashi, M., Shimano, T., Komae, H., Takeuchi, K., Endou, M., Igarashi, H., Hashimoto, N. and Takeuchi, S. (1998). J. Vet. Med. Sci., 60: 1281-1283.

Jörgensen, H.J., Mork, T. and Rorvik, L.M. (2005). J. Dairy. Sci., 88: 3810-3817.

Joshi, L.L. (1914). In: Proc 3rd All India, Sanit. Conf. Lucknow, 1914, Vol. I, pp. 126-128 (Suppl. to Indian J. Med. Res. 1914).

Kahl, B., Herrmann, M., Everding, A.S., Koch, H.G., Becker, K., Harms, E., Proctor, R.A. and Peters, G. (1998). J. Infect. Dis., 177: 1023-1029.

Kataria, R.S. and Verma, G.P. (1969). Indian Vet. J., 46: 15-16.

Katoch, R.C., Joshi., V.B., Sharma, M., Batta, M.K. and Nagal, K.B. (1996). Ind. J. Anim. Sci., 66: 1130-1131.

Katsuda, K., Hata, E., Kobayashi, H., Kohmoto, M., Kawashima, K., Tsunemitsu, H. and Eguchi, M. (2005). Vet. Microbiol., 105: 301-305.

Keefe, G.P. (1997). Can. Vet. J., 1(38): 429-437.

Kenny, K., Reiser, R.F., Bastida-Corcuera, F.D. and Norcross, N.L. (1993). J. Clin. Microbiol., 31: 706-707.

Kivaria, F.M., Noordhuizen, J.P.T.M. and Kapaya, A.M. (2006). Trop. Anim. Hlth. Prod., 38: 185-194.

Klotz, M., Opper, S., Heeg, K. and Zimmermann, S. (2003). J. Clin. Microbiol., 41(10): 4683-4687.

Ko, W.C., Lee, H.C., Wang, L.R., Lee, C.T., Liu, A.J. and Wu, J.J. (2001). Eur J. Clin. Microbiology Infect. Dis., 20: 334-339.

Le Loir, Y., Baron, F. and Gautier, M. (2003). Genet. Mol. Res., 2(1): 63-76.

Leclerc, V., Dufour, V., Lombard, B., Gauchard, F., Garin-Bastuji, B., Salvat, G., Brisabois, A., Poumeryrol, M., De-Buyser, M.L., Gnanou-Besse and N., Lahellec, C. (2002). Livest. Prod. Sci., 76: 195-202.

Lee, S.U., Quesnell, M., Fox, L.K., Yoon, J.W., Park, Y.H., Davis, W.C., Falk, D., Deobald, C.F. and Bohach, G.A. (1998). J. Food Protect., 61: 1384-1386.

LeJeune, J.T. and Rajala-Schultz, P.J. (2006). Unpasteurized Milk: A Continued Public Health Threat. Food Safety CID, 48(1): 93-100.

Lim, S., Joo, Y., Moon, J., Lee, A., Nam, H., Wee, S. and Kon, H. (2004). J. Vet. Med. Sci. 66(5): 581-584.

Manicham, R. and Mohan, M. (1987). Indian Vet. J., 64: 546-549.

Mantur, B. G., Amarnath, S.K. and Shinde, R.S. (2007). Indian J. Med. Microbiol., 25: 188–202.

Mantur, B.G. and Amarnath, S.K. (2008). J. Biosci., 33: 539-547.

Mantur, B.G., Biradar, M.S., Bidri, R.C., Mulimani, M.S., Veerappa, K.P., Patil, S.B. and Mangalgi, S.S., (2006). J. Med. Microbiol., 55: 897-903.

Mathew, A.G., Cissell, R. and Liamthong, S. (2007). Foodborne. Pathog. Dis., 4: 115-133.

Mhalu, F.S. (1976). J. Clin. Pathol., 29: 309-312.

Mills. B. (1898-99). Ann. Admn. Rep. Civil. Vet. Deptt. in India, 1898-99, P. 144.

Mosabi, J.M., Arimi, S.M. and Kangethe, E.K. (1997) Epidemiol. Infect., 118: 215-220.

Mosalagae, D., Pfukenyi, D.M. and Matope, G. (2011). Trop. Anim. Health Prod., 43: 733-739.

Munson, S.H., Tremaine, M.T., Betley, M.J. and Welch, R.A. (1998). Infection and Immunity, 66: 3337-3348.

Oliver, S.P., Jayarao, B.M. and Almeida, R.A. (2005). In: Proc. 44th National Mastitis Counc., Annual Meeting. Orlando, FL, pp. 3-27.

Pappas, G., Papadimitriou, P., Akritidis, N., Christou, L. and Tsianos, E.V. (2006). Lancet. Infect. Dis., 6: 91-99.

Peles, F., Wagner, M., Varga, L., Hein, I., Rieck, P., Gutser, K., Kereszturi, P., Kardos, G., Turcsanyi, I., Beri, B. and Szabo, A. (2007). Int. J. Food Microbiol., 118: 186-193.

Rahman, M.M. and Samad, M.A. (2008). Bangl. J. Vet. Med., 6 (2): 175-178.

Renukaradhya, G.J., Isloor, S. and Rajasekhar, M. (2002). Vet. Microbiol., 90: 183-195.

Rosec, J.P., Guiraud, J.P., Dalet, C. and Richard, N. (1997). Int. J. Food. Microbiol., 35(3): 213-221.

Ryser, E.T. (1998). In: Applied Dairy Microbiology. E.H. Marth and J. L. Steele, ed. Marcel Dekker, Inc. NY. Pp. 263-404

Schuchat, A. (2001). Clinical Infectious Diseases, 33: 751-756.

Sharma, Neelesh, Singh, N.K. and Bhadwal, M.S. (2011). Asian-Australasian J. Anim. Sci., 24(3): 429-438.

Sharma, V.D., Sethi, M.S., Yadav, M.P. and Dube, D.C. (1979). Int. J. Zoonoses, 6: 75-81.

Shirima, G.M., Kazwala, R.R. and Kambarage, D.M. (2003). Preventive Vet. Med., 57: 167-172.

Sinha, B. and Herrmann, M. (2005). Thromb. Haemost., 94: 266-277.

Srinivasan, V., Sawant, A.A., Gillespie, B.E., Headrick, S.J., Ceasaris, L. and Oliver, S.P. (2006). Foodborne Pathog. Dis., 3: 274-283.

Stabel, J.R. (2005). In: Proc. 44th NMC Annual Meeting. Orlando, FL, pp. 36-40.

Su Y.C. and Wong, A.C. (1995). Appl. & Environ. Microbiol., 61: 1438-1443.

Taylor, L.H., Ltham, S.M. and Wopolhouse, M.E. (2000). Transactions of Royal London Society of Biological Sciences, 356: 983-989.

Thoen, C.O., LoBue, P.A., Enarson, D.A., Kaneene, J.B. and deKantor, I.N. (2009). Veterinaria Italiana, 45(1): 135-181.

Tiruvulamala, P. and Reichman, L.B. (2002). Annu. Rev. Public Health. 23: 403-426.

Verma, S., Katoch, R.C., Sharma, M. and Nigam, P. (2000). Vet. Arhiv., 70: 75-82.

von Eiff, C., Peters, G. and Becker, K. (2006). Injury, 37(Suppl 2): S26–S33.

Wanger, A.R. and Dunny, G.M. (1985). Res. Vet. Sci., 38: 202-208.

Wanger, A.R. and Dunny, G.M. (1987). Infect. Immun., 55: 1170-1175.

Weinhaupl, I., Schpf, K.C., Khaschabi, D., Kapaga, A.M. and Msami, H.M. (2000). Trop. Anim. Hlth. Prod., 32(3): 147-154.

Whiting, R.C., Sackitey, S., Calderone, S., Morely, K. and Philips, J.G. (1996). Intl. J. Food Microbiol., 31: 231-243.

WHO. (2009). Annual report. Zoonoses and veterinary public health. Brucellosis (WHO Document Production Services, Geneva, Switzerland).

Zinsstag, J., Schelling, E., Roth, F., Bonfoh, B., de Savigny, D. and Tanner, M. (2007). Emerging Infect. Dis., 13: 527-531.

□□□

CHAPTER

12

Diagnosis

Mastitis is a parenchymal inflammation of the mammary gland, which is caused by microorganisms, usually bacteria that invade the udder, multiply and produce toxins which are harmful to the mammary gland (Sharma *et al.*, 2006). It is characterized by physical, chemical and usually bacteriological changes in milk and pathological changes in glandular tissues. Mastitis is one of the most important deadly diseases of milch animals is responsible for heavy economic losses and also causes the changes in glandular tissues affecting quality and quantity of the milk (Sharma *et al.*, 2007). It is a global as it adversely affects animal health, quality of milk and economics of milk production and every country including developed ones suffer huge financial losses (Sharma *et al.*, 2007).

Diagnosis of clinical mastitis is based on the local and systemic reactions and changes in milk (e.g. off color, watery, bloody appearance and presence of flakes, clots and pus). While diagnosis of sub clinical mastitis is more problematic since the milk appears normal but usually has an elevated somatic cell count. Early diagnosis of mastitis is vital because changes in the udder tissue take place much earlier than they become apparent. Various methods based on physical and chemical changes of milk and cultural isolation of organisms are used for diagnosis of sub clinical mastitis. However, the diagnosis of mastitis according to the International Dairy Federation (IDF) recommendations is based on the somatic cell counts (SCC) and microbiological status of the quarter. Bacteriological culture of milk samples is the standard method for identifying mastitis. However, the logistic and financial considerations involved with sampling all fresh cows have precluded this technique from being widely adopted. Milk culture will identify the presence of mastitis pathogens but will not provide a measure of the degree of inflammation associated with the infection.

Unlike the clinical mastitis, in sub-clinical mastitis there is neither visual abnormalities in milk (like blood, clots, flakes *etc.*) nor in mammary gland (like swelling, hotness, cracks *etc.*). Therefore, knowledge of routine physical examination of udder and diagnostic screening tests for early detection (*i.e.* during sub-clinical form) of mastitis (Figure 12.1) and proper treatment of affected animal is one of the paramount importance in order to minimized losses encountered due to sub-clinical as well as clinical mastitis (Sharma *et al.*, 2009).

Physical examination of udder

The clinician's initial step in the detection of bovine mastitis is a careful physical examination of the udder. A physical examination may be defined as clinical examination of the mammary glands by visual observation and digital palpation. The digital palpation is determined by employing the fingers and thumbs of both hands. The results of the physical examination, when correlated with other observations, facilitate the clinician for a complete diagnosis. Physical examination of each gland must be made on the empty udder. The most opportune time, therefore, is immediately after milking when the hormone stimulation has ceased and the udder is completely relaxed.

Technique of physical examination

Any system of udder examination should begin with a uniform numbering of the individual quarter, so that all workers will be in accord. The one recommende and generally used as follows-

A convenient way to fix this system in the clinician (examiner's) mind is to consider that he is approaching the cow from the right side and numbering the quarters as he would read the lines of an illustration. Thus, the left of the udder corresponds to the first line and the right side to the second line.

Consequently, the development of more practical, precise, and cheaper methods to assess udder health on farms is needed. Systematic clinical examination of udder and teat characteristics is relatively inexpensive and may provide valuable information (Klaas *et al.*, 2004).

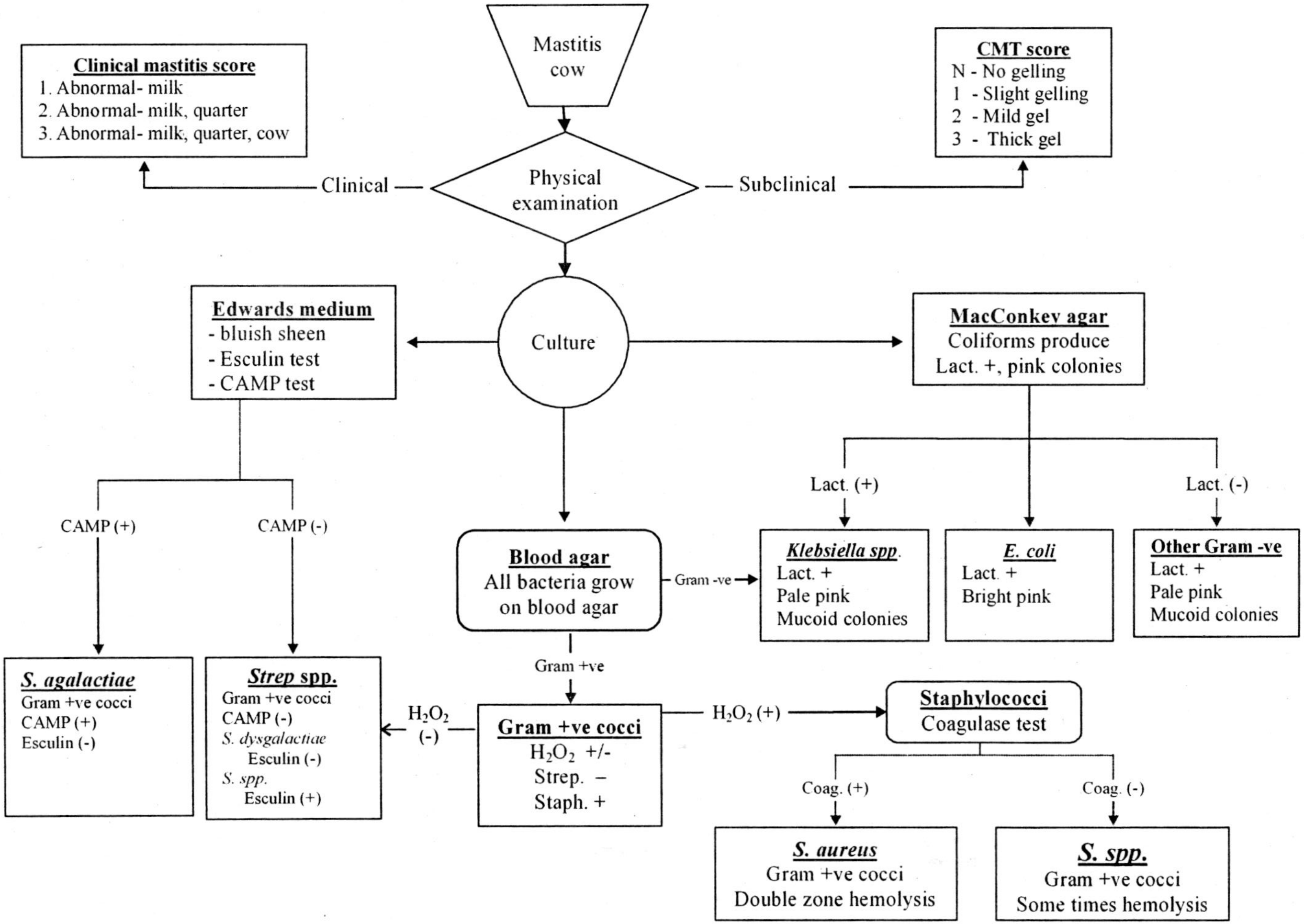

Figure 12.1 : Flow chart of complete examination for diagnosis of mastitis.

1. Visual observations/ Inspection

By this method clinician can observe so many undesirable features like udder symmetry (e.g. oat like, rounded, step shaped and pendulous udder) and, teat shape and placement which can help in the confirmatory diagnosis. Any abnormalities such as misplaced teats, supernumerary teats, extra openings in the side of the teats (teat fistulas), enlarged supramammary lymph glands, abscesses or boils, cow pox, cuts, lacerations, scars and chapped or cracked teats. The age of the animals should be kept in mind by clinician or examiner. This is important to consider because the normal elasticity of the glandular tissue in a young cow is firmer than that of the older animal, especially the heavy produce. A distinct induration in the gland of a young animal may have more pathological significance than a similar induration in the gland of an older cow. The size of the udder often increases gradually with each lactation, becoming heavier and more pendulant with age and production.

2. Visual observations combined with palpation

a) Examination of the surface of the udder

Any abnormalities observed on the surface of the udder and teats should be examined carefully, especially those which may have a direct or indirect influence on the infection of the udder. Stepped-on teats, bruises, cuts and many other conditions, depending on their location on the udder and teats, are factor that may be the indirect cause of mastitis.

During visual examination of udder the hygiene score should be recorded as a trouble shooting tool - to quantify hygiene on a farm, and as a monitor - to assess improvements in hygiene management (Table 12.1). *In scoring of udder-* observe the udder from the rear and the side if possible. The presence of visible manure near the teats is a risk factor for udder infection. Score 1 is no manure present. Score 2 is minor splashing of manure near the teats. Score 3 is distinct plaques of manure on the lower half of the udder and Score 4 is confluent plaques of manure encrusted on and around the teats. *In scoring of upper legs-* score 1 is no manure. Score 2 is minor splashing of manure. Score 3 is distinct plaques of manure with hair showing through, and Score 4 is confluent plaques of manure. *In scoring of upper legs-* score 1 is little or no manure above the coronary band. Score 2 is minor splashing above the coronary band. Score 3 is distinct plaques of manure above the coronary band, but with leg hair visible. Score 4 is a solid plaque of manure extending high up the leg.

Table 12.1: Criteria or scoring system for assessment of udder hygiene and rear body.

Score	1	2	3	4
Udder	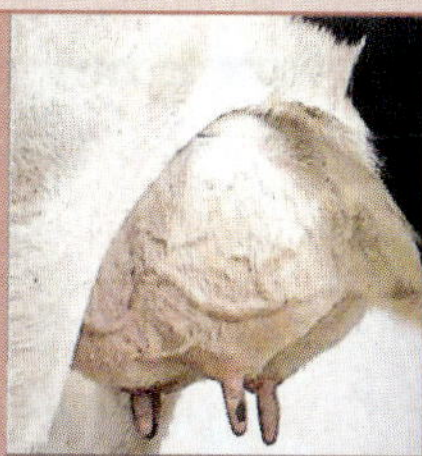 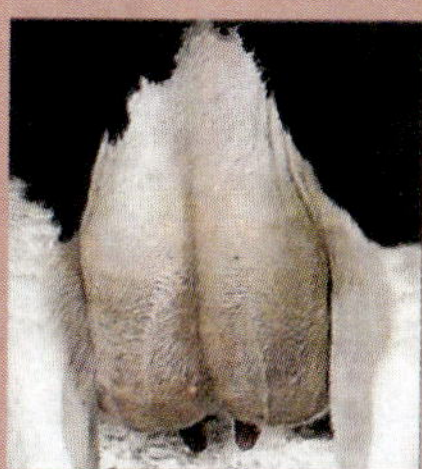	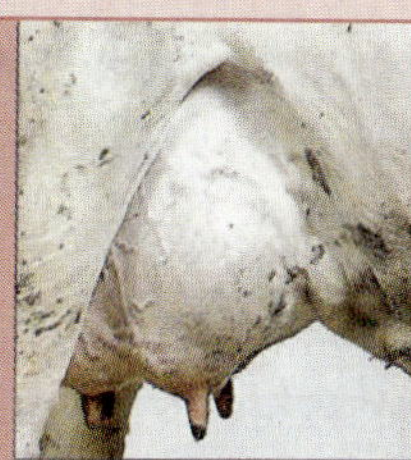 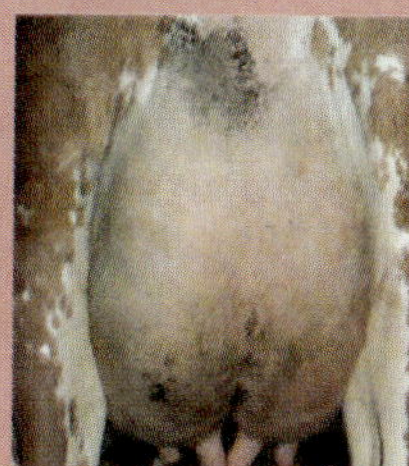	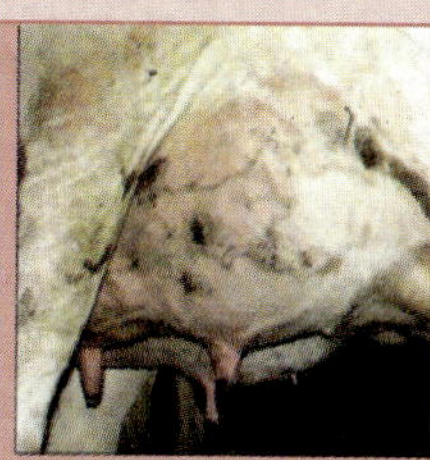 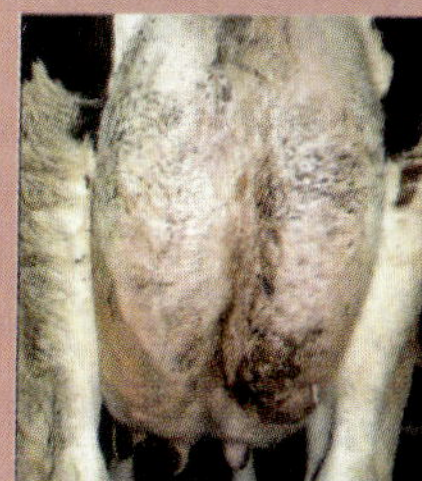	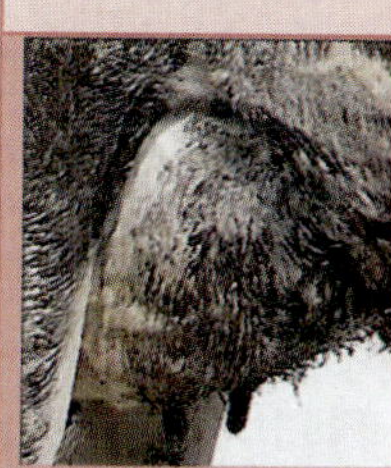 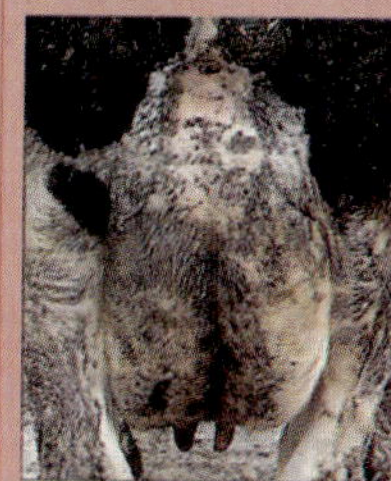
Upper leg	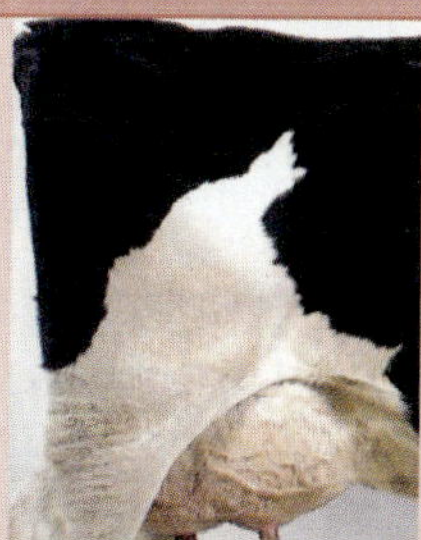	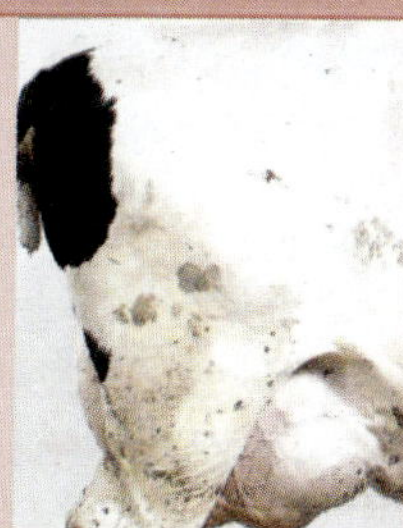	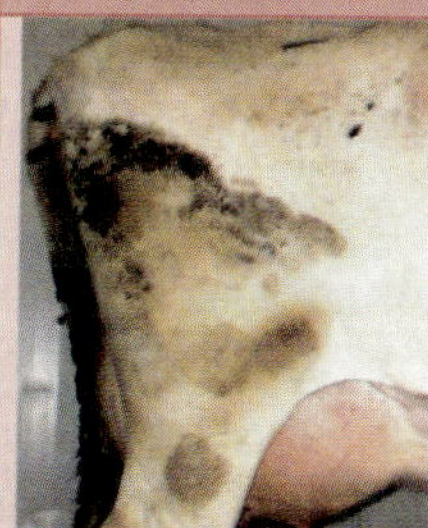	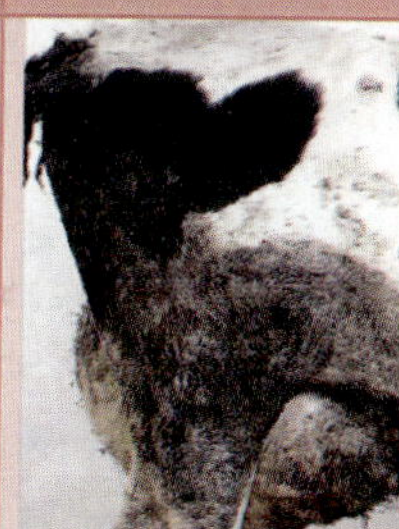
Lower leg	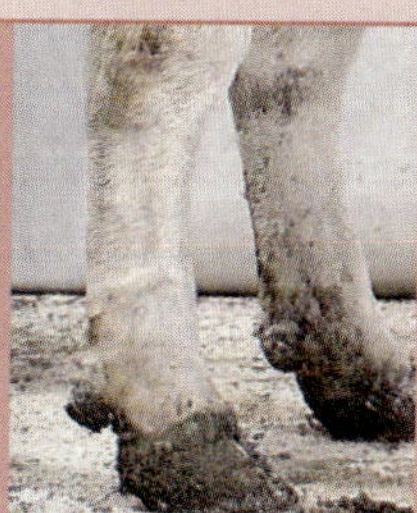	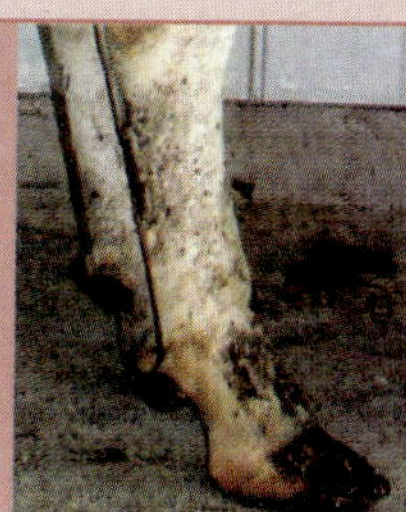	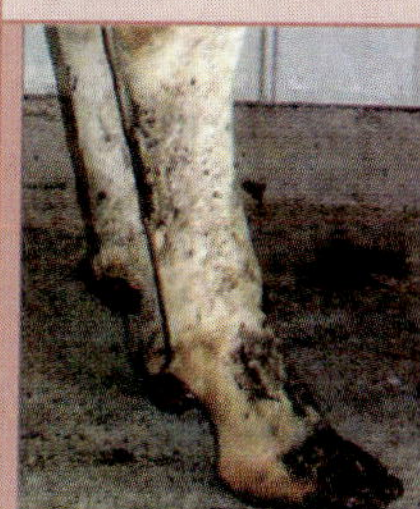	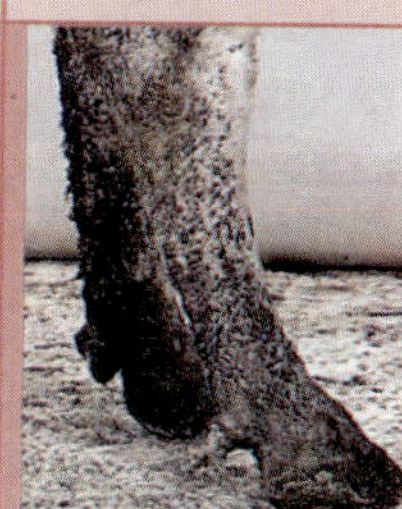

Healthy teat skin is coated with a protective mantel of fatty acids that are derived from the dermal layer and which retard the growth of bacterial pathogens . When exposed to cold, wet and windy conditions, the skin of machine-milked teats often becomes scaly, irritated or chapped (broken skin) and the protective surface coating may be removed, thereby allowing colonization of pathogens such as *Staphylococcus aureus* (Fox, 1995). Cold, wet or muddy conditions induce hardening or thickening of teat skin. Mud, as it dries, draws moisture from the skin with a consequent loss of elasticity of the teat skin.

Teats may vary in color within cow and within a herd according to breed and to breeding. Black teats obscure most changes in teat color induced by machine milking or any hypersensitivity in response to environmental factors or treatments. Black teats often appear to have drier skin since minor flaking is more obvious on a black than on a pink background. Teat skin condition scoring must take this into account. Most teats have some non-pigmented areas that should be the primary examination areas. Any part of the teat may be affected, so observations should include the whole barrel and orifice. The cow is the unit exposed to all variables likely to be tested, except in split udder trials (NMC, 2007).

On practical grounds, in making assessments during milking time it is acceptable to score only one fore and one hind teat, usually those closer to the observer. However, to ensure an appropriate sample of cows and teats are screened, use both sides of a milking parlor, or another method of examining left and right side teats equally. When assessing teat condition, record all lesions observed. Few lesions and no infections should be found if good husbandry is being applied. Identification of any lesions should be rare in routine teat condition monitoring in developed dairy industries (NMC, 2007).

Examine the teat orifice by turning the ends of the teats upward for a clear view. By gentle pressure note the ease of milking. To examine the teat duct and teat cistern, grasp the end of the teat with the fingers of the left hand, and pull down gently to stretch the teat. Then with the thumb and forefinger of the right hand examine the canal and cistern from the distal end (teat orifice) to the base of the udder. This will a comparison between teats. If one is thickened, cordy, or enlarged, this may mean that it is the site of an early infection. To examine the specific effects of the environment and teat treatments, it is best to observe teats prior to milking and teat cleaning.

During thorough examination of teats following parameters should be considered (Table. 12.2, Figure 12.2a,b,c) (NMC, 2007):

Table 12.2: Parameter, conditions and scores for teat skin.

Parameter	Condition	Score[#]
Colour	Normal and pink	N
	Red and irritated	R
Skin dryness	Smooth	N
	Slightly rough	SR
	Very rough	VR
Chaps	None	N
	Minor	M
	Severe/extensive	SE

Cutaneous damage	Suckling	S
	Insect	I
	Abrassions	A
	Cuts	C
	Sun burn	SB
	Frost bite	FB
Hyperkeratosis (Callocity)	Thickness - none	N
	- slight	ST
	- moderate	MT
	- thick	TT
	- extreme	ET
	Roughness - none	N
	- rough	R
	- very rough	VR

The letters used as a symbol is usually the first letter of the descriptor e.g. N = Normal.

3. Palpation of the Udder

Digital examination is an art, and its success depends upon correct instruction, practice and experience. First use *superficial palpation* of the entire surface of all quarters. The examination of the gland cistern and lower portion of the quarter is made by comparing the two rear quarters and by comparing the two front quarters, front and rear, conform in size and shape to each other. Abnormal lobulation or contour can see by this method. After superficial palpation, use *deep palpation*, grasp the quarters with both hands, and lift up for comparison of size, weight, elasticity, and consistency. It should be pointed out here that, in some cases of udder induration associated or not associated with udder infection, the cultural examination of the secretion from the affected quarters may fail to show the presence of microorganisms which would account for the alteration in the gland or secretion. Such changes may the result of a previous infection, age, overwork or may be due to some undetermined physiological reaction.

When mastitis has been present in a quarter for even a relatively short time, the character of the udder tissue becomes appreciably altered. The changes which are found on clinical examination of a diseased quarter may be either in the form of distinct firm nodules or diffuse thickening of the glandular tissue. The lesion in either case represents an invasion of the normal secreting tissue following inflammation of the gland. If the mastitis is only transient in nature, the proliferative process becomes static, but the indurations remain as a permanent record of the attack. Unfortunately, the majority of the cases of mastitis are caused by bacterial invasion, and as a rule the infection establishes itself permanently in the udder. In this event the disease tends to progress with varying degrees of rapidity from the original site of localization,

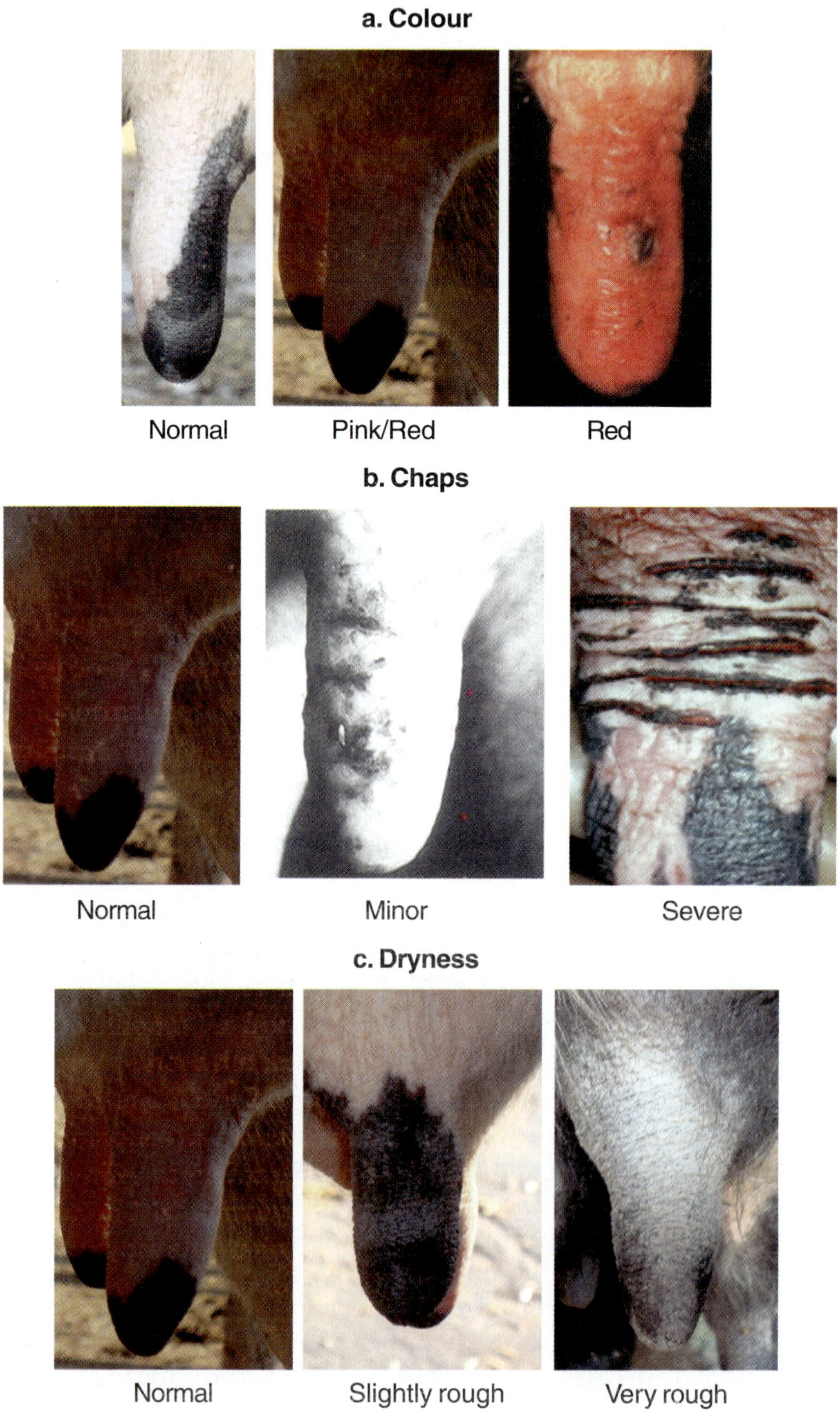

Figure 12.2 a,b,c : Examples of teat conditions.

usually the cistern, to the rest of the quarter. Induration of the glandular tissue accompanies this progression until in many cases there is practically a complete replacement of the secreting tissue by scar tissue.

On completion of the examination, the individual quarters are to be graded according to the degree of fibrosis, induration, or other abnormalities by the following cipher:

Code	Findings
N	No fibrosis. Normal pliability and elasticity of the glandular tissue i.e normal in all respects.
S	Fibrosis slight. A few slight diffuse indurations, or a single distinct induration, 1 to 2 inch in diameter.
D	Fibrosis distinct. Multiple slight diffuse indurations, or a single distinct induration, 2 to 3 inch in diameter.
M	Fibrosis marked. Multiple extensive indurations replacing most of the elastic glandular tissue, or a large single induration.
A	Atrophy
P	Patent teat sphincter.

With the use of the physical examination, it is possible to select the udders most suitable for specific therapy and to identify the cows in which the disease has advanced to such extent that slaughter is indicated. A careful physical examination is essential in any complete mastitis control programme and can not be ignored even though it does not provide the bacteriological information necessary for treatment and for prosecution of a complete mastitis-control programme based on bacteriological methods.

Examination of the milk

Before conduction of any mastitis test, the freshly drawn milk should be examined by necked for the visible abnormalities in the milk. In dry period milk changes to watery. Appearance of udder secretion in advanced cases of *chronic mastitis* is usually abnormal in appearance at irregular intervals. In case of *acute mastitis,* the secretion becomes grossly altered in the early stages of the disease. The visible abnormalities may be the presence of flakes or clots in the milk, or the milk may be thin or watery and at times yellow in color.

Over a period of years many tests have been developed for the diagnosis of mastitis. For convenience they may be divided into two groups, viz., (A) *Indirect Tests-* which depend upon the development of palpable lesions in the udder or changes in the composition of milk; and (B) *Direct or cultural test-* to determine the presence and identity of mastitis organisms in the milk,

A. Indirect Tests

Indirect tests are useful in determining the quality of milk, and in the absence of laboratory facilities those which are suitable for use in the field conditions may be helpful in detecting and eliminating some of the cows that are affected with chronic mastitis. Certain indirect tests, especially the leukocyte count, are needed to supplement cultural findings in the diagnosis of mastitis. Among the simplest tests, which do not require any complex laboratory equipment, are solutions containing detergents. "Detergents" decrease surface tension, change the structure and conductivity of cell membrane and nucleus, disturb osmotic balance, block oxidizing and stimulate proteolytic enzymes, and increase milk viscosity (Spakauskas *et al.*, 2006).

Subclinical mastitis in cows is diagnosed using superficial active agents (detergents) and indicators. The anion superficial active agents are the most useful for this purpose. The most commonly used superficial active agents of this group are those which, in solutions, dissociate into anions. For the production of tests, alkilsulphates, alkilsulphonates, alkilbensol-sulphonates, alkilarilsulphonates, and laurilsulphates are most often used. Modern mastitis tests allow for indirect determination of the number of somatic cells in milk (Spakauskas *et al.*, 2006). Several indirect tests are using to detect changes in the milk.

1. Strip cup test

It was Moak who first made use of strip cup test for the detection of visible particles of milk as a means for diagnosing of mastitis. This test is useful in field conditions for physical examination of milk. This test can be carried out by laymen at farm itself. In this test, enamel plate divided in four strip cups is used. The bottom of the plate is black colored so that it gives a good contrast to easily observe the milk flakes (Figure 12.3). The milk flakes can be seen by tilting the cups at an angle. This test is very useful in primary screening of animals for mastitis.

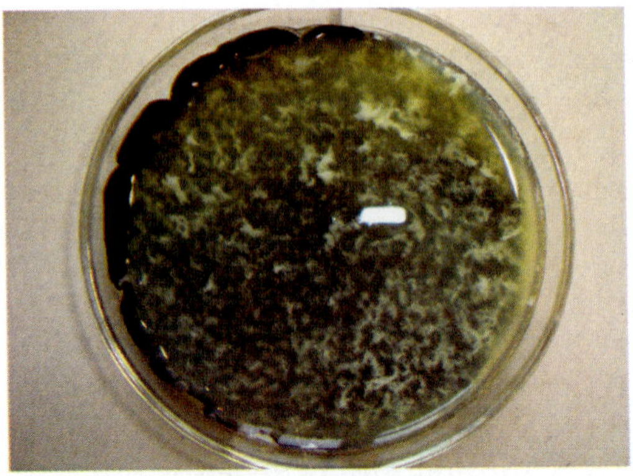

Figure 12.3: Strip cup test (clear flakes in mastitic milk).

2. Blackboard strip test

This test is also another type of strip cup test. This usually consists of some flat material with a smooth black surface, cut to fit at an angle lengthwise in a shallow basin, such as a small rectangular baking pan. As the streams of milk from each teat are milked on the sloping black surface, any pinpoint flakes, clots, or thick milk are revealed, just as with the strip cup test. Marked wateriness, much of which is not detectable by any other stable test, can easily be shown by the blackboard test. Lesser degree of wateriness can also be detected; but, while these are probably of significance in some cases, one should be cautious in their interpretation.

3. Somatic Cell Count (SCC)

Early diagnosis of subclinical mastitis with reliable tests facilitates successful treatment and control. One of the techniques used to monitor the level or occurrence of subclinical mastitis in herds or individual cows or quarters is to determine the SCC of milk samples. Somatic cells are indicators of both resistance and susceptibility of cows to mastitis. SCC is a useful predictor of intramammary infection (IMI), and therefore, an important component of milk under aspects of quality, hygiene and mastitis control. The SCC is commonly used as a measure of milk quality. Yet many producers fail to completely understand the implications of SCC for udder health or how high SCC can affect milk production and quality.

What are somatic cells?

The Canadian Oxford Dictionary defines the word *somatic* as: '*of or relating to the body*'. In the context of the mammary gland, somatic cells are products of the cow's body rather than cells, like bacteria, that are foreign. Somatic cells are mainly milk-secreting epithelial cells that have been shed from the lining of the gland, and white blood cells (leukocytes) that have entered the mammary gland in response to injury or infection (Dairyman's digest, 2009). As the inflammatory process develops in udder tissue the number of these cells (particularly leucocytes) in milk sharply increases. Due to inflammation response, white blood cells migrate from the peripheral circulation to the udder. The count of these cells may reach up to several millions in one milliliter of milk.

In simple language, somatic cells are simply animal body cells present at low levels in normal milk. The term milk somatic cells include neutrophils, macrophages, lymphocytes, erythrocytes and epithelial cells. Erythrocytes can be found at concentrations ranging from 0 to 1.51 X 10^6/ml (Paape and Weinland, 1988). The cells found in milk consist of about 75% leucocytes and about 25% epithelial cells. Leucocyte numbers increase in response to bacterial infection and tissue injury and stress. Studies identifying cell types in milk have shown that epithelial cells or the cells which produce milk are infrequently found in udder secretions, including those from the dry gland, and range from 0 to 7% of the cell population (Lee *et al.*, 1980). Thus, increases in SCC at the end of lactation are not due to sloughing epithelial cells. The epithelial cells are part of the normal body function and are shed, and renewed in normal body processes and increase as a result of injury or infection. The white blood cells serve as a defense mechanism to fight infection, and assist in repairing damaged tissue. During inflammation (mastitis) the major increase in SCC is due to the influx of neutrophils into the milk to fight infection. Over 90% of the cells present early in inflammation may be neutrophils. In other words, the white cells are attracted into milk. The measurement of the number of somatic cells in milk is known as a *somatic cell count* (Sharma *et al.*, 2011). As the count of these cells is the most liable to change, diagnostic tests of mastitis make possible diagnosis of mastitis in the early stage before clinical signs become apparent.

What are normal somatic cells?

In milk from normal uninfected lactating mammary glands the macrophage is the predominant cell type (35%), followed by neutrophils (26%), lymphocytes (24%) and epithelial cells (15%) (Miller *et al.*, 1991; Paape and Tucker, 1966). Lee *et al.* (1980) reported much lower values for neutrophils (3%) and epithelial cells (2%), and higher values for macrophages (79%). The normal composition of milk somatic cells varies with the type of secretion or lactation cycle (Table 12.3).

Table 12.3: Composition of somatic cells in different mammary secretions.

Type of mammary secretion	Milk somatic cells (%)			
	PMN	Macrophage	Lymphocytes	Epithelial cells
Milk	3	80	16	2
Colostrum	62	35	4	0
Dry gland secretion	3	89	7	1

Source: Sharma *et al.* (2011) PMN= Polymorphonuclear cells

Normally, in milk from a healthy mammary gland, the SCC is lower than 100000 cells/ml, while bacterial infection can cause it to increase to above 1000000 cells/ml (Bytyqi *et al.*, 2010). However, some studies stated that the normal SCC in milk is generally below 200000 cells/ml, but may be blow 100000 cells/ml in first lactation animals or in well managed herds. One study estimated that 50% of uninfected cows had SCC under 100000 cells/ml and 80% were under 200000 cells/ml (Eberhart *et al.*, 1979). Somatic cell count above 250000 to 300000 cells/ml is considered abnormal and nearly always is an indication of bacterial infection causing mastitis.

Eberhart *et al.* (1979) taken cell counts in composite samples from cows with all four quarters free of infection have been reported to average from 113000 to 251000 cells/ml depending on the cow's age. High levels of these cells in milk indicate abnormal, reduced quality milk that is caused by an intramammary bacterial infection. When large numbers accumulate they are visible as pus.

Counting technique

Accuracy of milk SCC is very important to most dairy farmers and to the dairy industry. Individual cow cell counts are commonly used as a management tool for aiding in decision making. More recently, automated devices for rapidly determining the SCC of milk samples have become available. On-going development in counting technology has resulted in the routine application of high capacity flow cytometric counters with much improved performance in advanced milk testing laboratories. The two most commonly used devices are the Coulter Milk Cell Counter, which counts particles as they flow through an electric field, and the Fossomatic which stains cells with a fluorescent dye and then counts the number of fluorescing particles. Both devices are capable of rapid determination of the SCC in large numbers of samples (Sharma *et al.*, 2011).

The direct microscopic method is inexpensive and most commonly used in India (Sharma, 2003) (Figure 12.4). The detail direct microscopic method has already been described by Schalm *et al.* (1971). Researchers and veterinarians need to pay careful attention to counting techniques and methodology when evaluating caprine SCC levels.

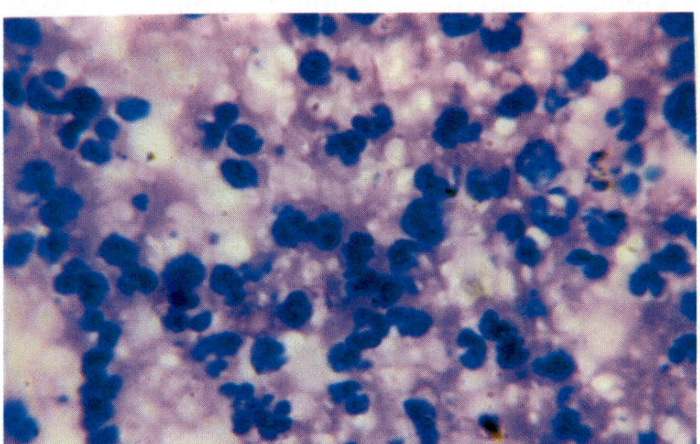

Figure 12.4: Somatic cells in milk smear under oil immersion (100X).

However, there is very little information on its specific application of these methods in ewe milk (Gonzalo *et al.*, 1993), which has a higher content of total solids than cow milk. Also, the presence of extracellular membranous matter, nuclear remains and cell fragments, described in ewe milk (Schalm *et al.*, 1971; Lee and Outteridge, 1981). When evaluating macrophages on a stained milk film, many will have a "foamy" cytoplasm. The direct microscopic method from methylene blue staining is best method for enumeration of ewe milk SCC (Gonzalo *et al.*, 2003).

The detail procedure of SCC in bovine is divided in following sub-headings-

Preparation of milk smear

The test milk sample should be thoroughly mixed by gentle shaking the vials and 10ml (0.01ml) of milk take on the pre drawn one square cm (1cm^2) marked area over a grease free clean glass slide (Figure 12.5). Milk spread uniformly over the measured area with a standard sterilized bacteriological platinum loop. The smear of milk for SCC must be prepared within one hour of its collection to minimize disintegration of leukocytes. The smear allows to dry at room temperature.

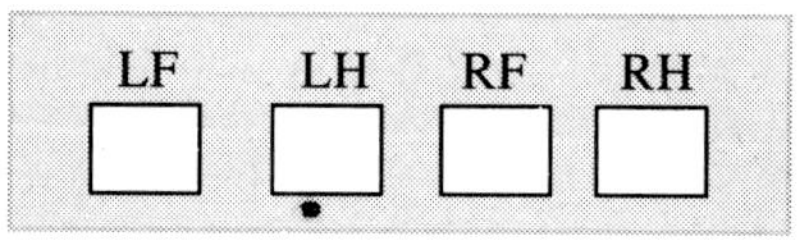

Figure 12.5: Glass slide with demarcated one square cm area (1cm^2).

Staining of milk smear

The prepared smears stain with the modified Newman's Lampert stain, by keeping the prepared slide in the staining solution for 1 to 2 minutes. After that gently wash the smears in tap water and dried. The dried stained smears examine under the oil immersion lens of the microscope.

Counting of cells

Count the cells in 30 different fields under oil immersion lens (100x) and repeat thrice per smear to assess average number of somatic cells in 30 fields and average number of the cells per field. The average number of cells is multiplied by the multiplication factor of the microscope to obtain the number of cells per ml of the milk.

Microscopic factor determination

Microscopic factor was determined in this study as described by Shukla (1980). The diameter of the field of 10x eyepiece was predetermined by using stage micrometer. The lowest division of micrometer scale was 0.01mm. Accordingly, the diameter was measured and obtained as 0.016cm. The area of the microscopic field was determined by the formula r^2. The calculations were made as under:

Diameter	=	0.016cm
Radius	=	0.008cm
Area (pr^2)	=	$3.14 \times (0.008)^2$
	=	0.000201
Microscopic factor	=	$100 \times 1/\text{Area}$
	=	$100 \times 1/0.000201$
	=	497512.43 or 497512

Interpretation of SCC

There often is confusion about somatic cell numbers and scores, how the numbers are computed, and their relevance to milk quality and food safety. Various methods are used to represent the number of somatic cells like means, linear score etc. However, in most reports somatic cell numbers are represented in the form of mean. References are made to arithmetic means and geometric means. What is the difference between these two types of means (Shook and Ruegg, 1999)? The two different methods may be used to calculate an "*average somatic cell count*" when multiple samples have been taken. For example, if the past three monthly cell counts were 600000, 400000 and 500000, the average would be calculated by arriving at a total and dividing by 3, (1500000/3=500000). This produces an "*arithmetic mean*" or average (Sharma *et al.*, 2011).

A different method, used in Europe and other locations, is used to calculate an average somatic cell count. It is termed the "*geometric mean*". The geometric mean calculation always produces a value somewhat less than the arithmetic mean for the same data set. For the data set used before (600000, 400000, 500000) the geometric mean would be calculated as approximately 493000. A single high count in a data set has a greater impact on the arithmetic mean than the geometric mean and one very high value is not as likely to trigger regulatory action using the geometric mean procedure (Ingalls, 2001).

Herd somatic cell numbers can be the result of testing individual cows and averaging the values or may be based on a bulk tank sample (BTSCC) that represents the whole herd. Bulk tank values are indicative of the status of the herd when all the milk produced is blended together in the bulk tank and then sampled. Bulk tank SCCs do not give you the udder health status of individual cows in your herd. A few high-SCC cows, for example could push your bulk tank count higher. That reduces the quality of milk in your tank but doesn't mean all your cows have mastitis. Similarly, a low BTSCC tells you most of your cows have low counts, but it doesn't tell you how many have very low SCC, or how low they might be? This is especially true for small herds when a high cell count cow can significantly influence the BTSCC. In a large herd this is less likely to happen because of the dilution effect. Individual cow cell counts are a good measure of the infection status of all cows in the herd (Sharma *et al.*, 2011).

Research has established a straight-line relationship between milk loss and the logarithm of the SCC. This value is referred to in Canada as *"Linear Score"* (LS); in the US it is *Somatic Cell Score* (SCS). The linear somatic cell count provides a more meaningful method of evaluating mastitis in herd. Linear somatic cell counts (SCC) help you: measure effects of subclinical mastitis on your herd; identify cows affected by subclinical mastitis; measure reduction in subclinical mastitis as improvements in management are made; and identify temporary or long-term problems that might otherwise be undetected. Each increase of 1 in score is associated with a doubling of cell counts (Table 12.4a, b). Linear scores are more informative than raw SCC in evaluating the udder health status of a cow or herd. High SCC test results for one or two cows have less influence on the herd average LS than on the herd average SCC. Another advantage of using LS rather than SCC to assess herd udder health status is that the herd average LS will be very close to the value the lowest 50% from the highest 50% of cows in the herd. In contrast, a few cows with very high SCC can inflate the herd average, distorting its interpretation as the average level of infection for the herd (Dairyman's digest, 2009). LS is also more useful that SCC in genetic selection programmes.

Table 12.4a: Somatic LS, SCC and milk production loss (Ingalls, 2001).

LS	SCC (1,000 cells/ml)		Milk yield loss (lbs/305 days)
	Mid Point	Range	
0	12.5	0-17	0
1	25	18-34	0
2	50	35-70	0
3*	100*	71-140	400
4	200	141-282	800
5	400	283-565	1200
6	800	566-1130	1600
7	1600	1131-2263	2000
8	3200	2263-4525	2400

Note: Production losses are assumed to start at 100000 cells/ml (LS of 3).

Table 12.4b: Milk production loss due to increased SCC

Somatic Cell Count (1000/ml)	Annual milk production (liters)
50	9000
100	8820
200	8640
400	8460
800	8280
1600	8100

There often is confusion about somatic cell numbers and scores, how the numbers are computed, and their relevance to milk quality and food safety. References are made to arithmetic means and geometric means. What is the difference between these two types of means? The two different methods may be used to calculate an "average somatic cell count" when multiple samples have been taken. For example, if the past three monthly cell counts were 800,000, 400,000 and 600,000, the average would be calculated by arriving at a total and dividing by 3, (1,800,000/3=600,000). This produces an arithmetic mean or average.

A different method is used to calculate an average somatic cell count. It is termed the "geometric mean". The practical definition of geometric mean is "the average of the logarithmic values of a data set, converted back to a base 10 number". The geometric mean calculation always produces a value somewhat less than the arithmetic mean for the same data set. For the data set SCC used before (800,000 cells/ml, 400,000 cells/ml, 600,000 cells/ml 200,000 cells/ml) the geometric mean would be calculated as approximately 500,000. A single high count in a data set has a greater impact on the arithmetic mean than the geometric mean and one very high value isn't as likely to trigger regulatory action using the geometric mean procedure.

e.g. SCC values at different time intervals.

800,000
400,000
600,000
200,000

Arithmetic mean = 500,000 cells/ml

Geometric mean = 442672.76 cells/ml

The hidden danger in routine SCC

The composite sampling is important to consider that high cell count milk from infected quarters be diluted with low cell count milk from uninfected quarters and vice versa. Always remember that infection occurs at the quarter level. A new infection in one quarter is diluted by clean milk from the other three uninfected quarters, limiting the impact on the overall SCC measure. Cows which become persistently infected in a single quarter may go undetected. This is particularly the case where the remaining quarters have low SCC levels. One quarter yielding milk at 2 million cells/ml mixed with equal volumes of milk from three quarters at 50000 cells/ml will have a commingled SCC reading in the region of 500000 cells/ml (Hanks and Biggs, 2005). Therefore, the dilution of high cell count milk from infected quarters with low cell count milk from uninfected quarters is an important consideration in the interpretation of composite sample cell counts. This dilution effect on SCC measures is causing delay in recognizing new infections. Consequently infections are frequently well established by the time that the SCC count reaches a level that is noticed as a problem by the farmer (Sharma *et al.*, 2011).

Factors Affecting Somatic Cell Count

Although the presence or absence of an intramammary bacterial infection is the prevailing factor influencing milk somatic cell count at the herd and individual level, variation in cell count may occur for a multitude of reasons. It is known that individual cow cell counts will vary with conditions other than an intra mammary infection. Several studies have confirmed commentaries that there is significant variation in both bulk milk and individual cow somatic cell counts between milking and between individual cows.

No evidence exists that SCC in normal secretion from uninfected quarters is significantly influenced (i.e. exceeds 200000 cells/ml) by parity, stage of lactation, or heat stress (Harmon, 1994). Many of the causes of somatic cell count variation are due to internal and external factors that should be taken into consideration when interpreting somatic cell counts to make decisions regarding your herd.

There is a normal (diurnal) variation in SCC with the fraction of milk collected throughout a milking and during the time between milkings (Dohoo and Meek, 1982). There is little evidence that any factor other than normal diurnal variation has a major influence on SCC in the absence of intramammary infection. In general, cell counts are highest in the strippings and lowest immediately before milking. The elevated SCC may persist for up to 4 hours after milking and then gradually decline. This difference in high and low SCC in strippings vs foremilk at milking time may vary from 4 to 70-fold in individual quarters (White and Rattray, 1965).

The ability to correctly interpret somatic cell counts depends on an understanding of the factors which may affect the number of somatic cells.

These factors may wield their influence at the quarter, cow or herd level. There are the following factors-

[a] Mammary gland infection level (Mastitis)

The most important factor affecting the somatic cell count of the milk from an individual quarter, and consequently the cow and the herd, is the infection status of the quarter (Dohoo and Meek, 1982). In comparison, other factors have only a minor effect (Shultz, 1977). The SCC increases with severity of infection (Sharma, 2003). Sharma (2003) conducted a study on 2161 milk samples of lactating cows and SCC value £100000 cells/ml considered as threshold or negative for California mastitis test (CMT). SCC values were classified into four groups as 1 - 3 (X10^5/ml), 3 - 9 (X10^5/ml), 9 - 27 (X10^5/ml) and 27 - 81 (X10^5/ml) or >81 (X10^5/ml) with respect to severity of intramammary infection as CMT score: trace, +, + + and + + + respectively. Out of 2161 milk samples, 844 had <100000 cells/ml of milk and the maximum samples (32.29%) had SCC between 3 - 9 (X10^5/ml).

One of the basic host responses to a bacterial infection is the infiltration of white blood cells from the blood into the udder. This is accomplished through the processes of diapedesis and chemotaxis. The degree and nature of the cellular response are likely to be proportional to the severity of the infection (O'Rourke and Blowey, 2004). A figure 12.6 is showing the relationship between SCC and udder infection status of cow.

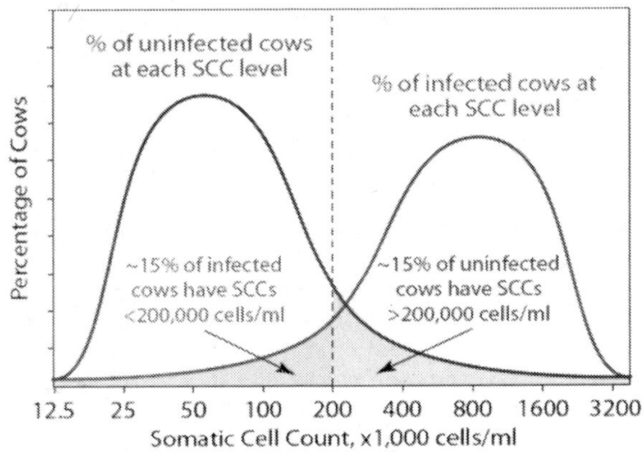

Figure 12.6: Relationship between SCC and udder infection status of cow. (Adopted from: Dairyman's Digest, Winter (2009).

The average number of composite (cow) milk SCC increases with increase in the number of quarters infected i.e. one to two quarters or one to three. An approximate doubling of the SCC has been reported with each additional quarter that was infected (Natzke *et al.*, 1972). Using a total and differential

SCC, the ability to correctly classify cows as infected or uninfected has risen from 77.9% to 92.7% as the number of quarters infected rose from one to four (Meek *et al.*, 1980). During inflammation (mastitis), the major increase in SCC is because of the influx of PMN into the milk. The proportion among various cell types in milk changes drastically during inflammation. The PMN increases with severity of mastitis and occasionally can approach 100% of the total somatic cells. In chronic mastitis, the number of mononuclear cells may increase (Schalm *et al.*, 1971).

[b] Stage of lactation

It is general observation by most of researchers that SCC increases with the progressing lactation (late lactation). Somatic cell counts have been found to be elevated immediately after calving (1st week), regardless of whether the cow is infected or not (Dohoo and Meek, 1982). This SCC elevation appears to be part of an animal innate immune system response in preparation of calving, to enhance the mammary gland defense mechanism at this critical calving time. The elevation in count has been variously reported to last for five days to two weeks and consequently elevated cell counts during the first two weeks of lactation must be interpreted with caution. During early and late lactation the percentage of neutrophils tends to increase while the percentage of lymphocytes decreases.

During involution of the gland neutrophils are the predominant cell type (60%) during the first 4 weeks after cessation of milking, followed by macrophages (25%), and lymphocytes (15%) (Miller *et al.*, 1990). During the first two weeks before parturition lymphocytes predominate (60%), followed by macrophages (30%) and neutrophils (10%) (McDonald and Anderson, 1981). At parturition SCC are usually higher than one million per ml, and decrease to 100000 cells/ml in the 7 to 10 days postpartum (Jensen and Eberhart, 1981). Throughout the remainder of the lactation, somatic cell counts have been reported to increase as the lactation progresses (Schultz, 1977), while some studies reported that no rise in SCC throughout lactation occurred (Natzke *et al.*, 1972; Eberhart *et al.*, 1979). As the milk volume decreases in the latter part of lactation, an apparent increase in cell numbers occurs from mere concentration of cells in a smaller volume of milk. Bodoh *et al.* (1976) found SCC at the end of lactation rose only after production had dropped below 4 kg/d, but the infection status of these cows was not determined. Feed or water deprivation results in dramatic decreases in milk production and proportional increases in SCC. This result can be interpreted as a dilution phenomenon.

The presence of high cell numbers in colostrum may be due to an excessive desquamation of epithelial cells in a small volume of milk in a gland resuming

functional activity after a dormant period (Schalm *et al.*, 1971). Whether or not there is a rise in the SCC of milk from uninfected cows immediately before drying off is debatable issue for future research.

[c] Age

Various researchers have reported that SCC increases with increasing age (Beckley and Johnson, 1966; Blackburn, 1966). This increase is primarily due to an increased prevalence of infection in older cows and is not due to any large increase due to *age per se*.

[d] Breed

Brolund (1985) has reported that variability in SCC within breed was greater than differences in SCC among breeds. The high producing cattle breeds such as Brown Swiss (423.31 X 10^3 cells/ml) and Black Holstein (310.36 X 10^3 cells/ml), seem to be more exposed to the higher presence of SCC/ml in milk. Other breeds, like Red Holstein (190.38 X 10^3 cells/ml), Simmental (214.60 X 10^3 cells/ml), Crosses (282.98 X 10^3 cells/ml) and Montbeliard (285.87 X 10^3 cells/ml) tend to have lower SCC counts (Bytyqi *et al.*, 2010). SCC in various breeds of cows in India (Singh, 2002) (Table 12.5).

Table 12.5: Mean normal values of SCC in milk of indigenous cross breed dairy cows.

Breed of cow	SCC (X 10^3 cells/ml)
Tharparker	1.26
Sahiwal	1.31
Karan Fries	1.61
Karan Swiss	1.54

Source: Singh, 2002.

[e] Parity

The level of SCC has been reported to be influenced by parity (Blackburn, 1966; Lindström *et al.*, 1981). There is little change in SCC of uninfected quarters as number of lactations increase (Sheldrake *et al.*,, 1983). In general, SCC increases with increasing the number of lactations (parities). Bartlett *et al.* (1990) reported that SCC increased in older cattle and/or at the end of lactation due to an increased prevalence of infection and permanent glandular damage from previous infections. Skrzypek *et al.* (2004) was found that the SCC increases with advanced parities. In the first parity, the SCC is lower than in all other parities in all the months of lactation. In a study conducted by Schepers *et al.* (1997), the natural log of SCC from uninfected quarters of first-parity cows was highest during the first part of the lactation because of

the relatively flat SCC curve, although the mean natural log of SCC in first-parity cows was lowest. Erdem *et al.* (2010) has also been shown significant effect of parity on SCC.

[f] Season

Somatic cell counts are generally lowest during the winter and highest during the summer season (Dohoo and Meek, 1982) which coincides with an increased incidence of clinical mastitis during the summer months (Hogan *et al.*, 1989; Khate and Yadav, 2010). While another study in Kosovo reported that the effect of month on SCC in raw milk shows a higher presence of SCC in December (469 X 10^3 cells/ml), followed by November (426.74 X 10^3 cells/ml), and October (401.14 X 10^3 cells/ml), respectively and During August, September, January, February and March, this number seems to be lower (125.06, 147.12, 297.55, 276.64 and 153.65 X 10^3 cells/ml) (Bytyqi *et al.*, 2010).

The elevated counts during summer are reported to persist after the temperature humidity index starts to decline and this phenomenon has been called the *"summer carry over"* effect (Wegner *et al.*, 1976). During summer season, the growth and number of environmental bacteria is increased in the bedding material of housed stock due to favorable temperature and humidity. Hogan *et al.* (1989) also support the association of rates of clinical mastitis with bacterial counts in bedding. These findings support the concept that temperature stress *per se* is not the cause of increased SCC, but the increased SCC is a result of greater exposure of teat ends to pathogens, resulting in more new infections and clinical cases during the summer months (Harmon, 1994).

[g] Stress

Stress is a physiological state which developed when increase in the level of free radicals due to stressors, stressors may be managemental, milking techniques, environmental and infectious organisms etc. Free radicals are chemicals that possessing an unpaired electron. Free radicals are very unstable and react quickly with other compounds, trying to capture the needed electron to gain stability. Physiological stressing conditions acting via the hypothalamic-pituitary-adrenal axis have been associated with a number of responses among them a blood neutrophylic leucocytosis in dairy cows. SCC levels usually are lowest in a clean, dry, comfortable environment. Smith *et al.* (1985) suggested that the stress of high temperatures and humidity could have increased the susceptibility to infection (Coliforms) as well as increased the numbers of pathogens to which cows were exposed. The increased incidence of clinical mastitis in the summer months is generally due to a warm and moist environment that increases pathogen exposure and numbers. Some

observations have suggested a positive relationship between the stresses of high summer environmental temperatures and high somatic cell count in milk (Nelson *et al.*, 1969). Over crowding of animals increase the stress and resulting increased SCC. Kay *et al.* (1977) reported that mixing of groups has increased the bulk tank SCC from approximately 175000 to a peak of 420000 cells/ml four days after mixing. Stresses of various types and estrus have been implicated in causing increases in SCC. While in other study, there is no increase in SCC associated with cows being in estrus (Forster *et al.*, 1967). Average values of SCC are higher in hand milked animals than machine milked cows (Dang and Anand, 2007).

[h] Teat injury

In dairy cows tramped teats are a common source of teat injury. However, beef cows generally have smaller udders and shorter teats, which decreases the risk of teat trampling. Multiple lacerations of varying depth and length may be seen in the skin of the udder and teats. Deep horizontal cracks may occur as a result of excessive sucking or biting by older calves or even older animals (Jackson, 1996). The likelihood of cows developing mastitis is 50% higher in injured than in non-injured cows (Modransky and Welker, 1993). Teat injury has been associated with high SCC in dairy cattle (Jorstad, *et al.*, 1989), and numerous studies have indicated a positive relationship between milk SCC and udder disease (Emanuelson *et al.*, 1988; Shook, 1989; Weller *et al.*, 1992). Irritated teats or an injury to the mammary gland may cause the SCC to rise, but not usually over about 300000 cells/ml.

[i] Diurnal / Day to day variation

The variation in the SCC level produced throughout the day and from one day to the next, in milk produced by individual quarter of animal. The SCC also varies during and between milking. In general, SCC are highest in the strippings and lowest immediately before milking. The elevated SCC may persist for up to 4 hours after milking and then gradually decline. This difference in high and low SCC varies from 4 to 70-fold for individual quarters (White and Rattray, 1965). Because correlation is high ($r = 0.86$) between SCC in foremilk and composite or bucket milk (Dohoo and Meek, 1982). Studies have shown that two consecutive milkings from the same cow fluctuates 30% from the average SCC and morning milkings have about 20% fewer somatic cells than those from the afternoon milkings.

Day to day variation in cell counts has been investigated in quarter, cow (composite) and herd (bulk tank) samples. SCC has small variation from day to day. Some studies estimate that the day to day variation in SCC can fluctuate to more than 40% without any of the circumstances of the herd changing.

[j] Sample transportation and preservation

It has been reported that the method of transportation and storage of milk samples, as well as the method used to count the somatic cells, all have an influence on the resultant counts (Dohoo and Meek, 1982). Gonzalo *et al.* (2003) used different milk preservatives e.g. potassium dichromate (100 mg/ 100 ml), azidiol (24 mg sodium azide/100 ml) and bronopol (50 mg/100 ml) and studied their effects on SCC. They found highest SCC values in without preservative milk samples (5.72 X 10^3 cells/ml), followed by milk preserved by bronopol (5.67 X 10^3 cells/ml), potassium dichromate (5.63 X 10^3 cells/ ml), and azidiol (5.62 X 10^3 cells/ml). These results showed a false overestimation of SCC in without preservative milk due to bacterial proliferation.

[k] Management

The many management factors plays most important role in the development of contagious disease like mastitis in dairy animals. Of these unhygienic conditions is more important, increase the chances of IMI and resulting increase in SCC. Other managemental factors are type of flooring, feeding, teat dipping, milking techniques etc. Herds with more clinical mastitis had more cows with stepped-on teats, and that leaked milk, and did not disinfect the maternity area. These herds also used post-milking teat dip, and had lower bulk milk SCC. Teat injuries and leakers commonly occur because of stall and platform design. Using post-milking teat dip appears to predispose some very low SCC herds to more clinical mastitis-in particular mastitis caused by *E. coli*. Current milking hygiene routines are specifically designed to prevent the spread of contagious mastitis bacteria like *S. aureus*. Some of these practices may not be as necessary for low-SCC herds that have eradicated contagious mastitis sources and can maintain that status (Sharma *et al.*, 2011).

4. California Mastitis Test (CMT)

California mastitis test is a simple, inexpensive and rapid screening test for mastitis. The test is based on the increase in number of leukocytes and alkalinity of the mastitis milk. These changes are due to inflammatory exudation and increased contents of basic salts during inflammation. The CMT uses 3 percent Tri-ethanolamine sulphate and bromocresol purple to react with the deoxyribonucleic acid in somatic cells, thus rupturing the cell walls and gelling the milk (Schalm *et al.*, 1971). The original Schalm reagent (Tri-ethanolamine sulphate and bromocresol purple) is not available in India. But recently B.V. Biologicals, India launched a CMT reagent kit along with plastic paddle by the name of CMT kit. The accuracy of this method is found to be 75.52% when bacterial culture considered as standard test (Sharma *et al.*, 2010a). This difference in accuracy may be due to change of CMT reagent.

Fresh, unrefrigerated milk can be tested using the CMT for upto 12 hours, reliable readings can be obtained from refrigerated milk for up to 36 hours. If stored milk is used, the milk sample must be thoroughly mixed prior to testing because somatic cells tend to segregate with the milk fat.

Test procedure

A plastic paddle with four chambers or shallow cups used to perform the test. About 3 ml of milk directly striped into the labeled cups, LF, LH, RF and RH, from the respective four quarters (Figure 12.7). To ensure equal quantity of milk in each cup, the paddle should be tilted slightly at an angle of 45° to allow overflow of excess of the milk samples, if any in any cup. Then approximately equal quantity of the test reagent (CMT reagent) adds to each cup. The mixture of the milk and reagent is shaken gently in a rotating manner of the paddle in the horizontal plane.

Immediately after mixing or reaction must be scored within 15 seconds of mixing because weak reactions will disappear after that time. Any reactions of trace (T) or higher indicates that the quarter has sub-clinical mastitis. The reaction is graded by intensity of gel formation (Figure 12.8 to 12.12) as detailed below:

CMT score	Description	Interpretation
N (Negative)	No change	Healthy quarter
T (Trace)	Slime formed which disappeared with continuous movement of paddle	Sub-clinical mastitis
1 (Weak)	Distinct slime, but no gel formation.	Sub-clinical mastitis
2 (Distinct positive)	Viscous with gel formation, which adhered to the margin.	Serious mastitis infection
3 (Strong positive)	The gel formation with convex projection, the gel did not dislodge after swirling movement of the paddle	Serious mastitis infection

CMT scores are directly related to average somatic cell counts (Table 12.6). Any reaction of T (trace) or higher indicates that the quarter has subclinical mastitis.

Table 12.6: Relationship between CMT score and SCC.

CMT Score	Somatic Cell Range	Interpretation
N (Negative)	0 - 200,000	Healthy Quarter
T (Trace	200,000 – 400,000	Subclinical Mastitis
1	400,000 – 1,200,000	Subclinical Mastitis
2	1,200,000 – 5,000,000	Serious Mastitis Infection
3	>5,000,000	Serious Mastitis Infection

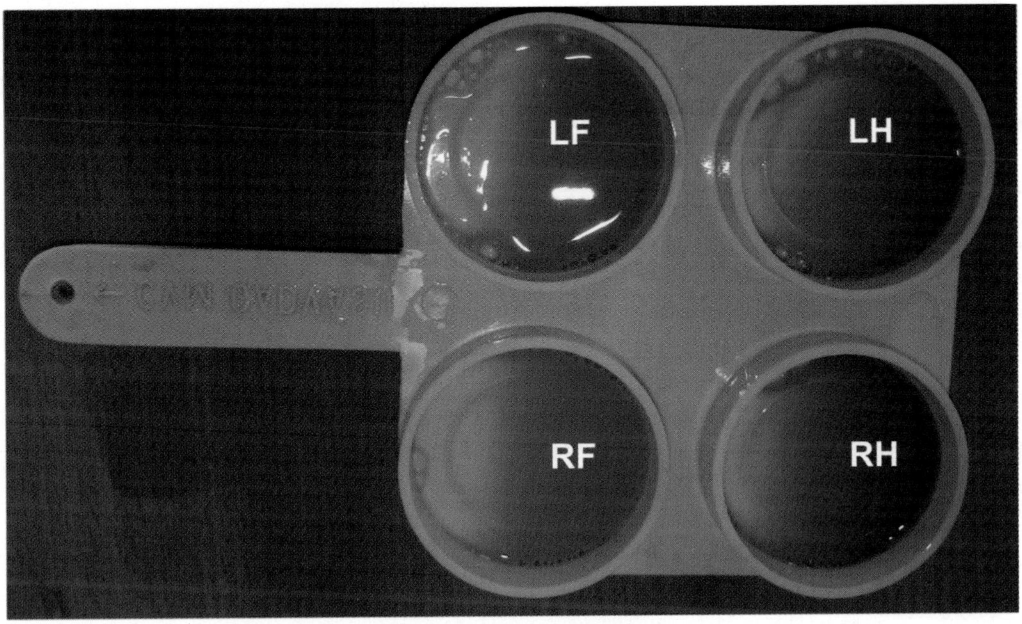

Figure 12.7: CMT test

CMT results-

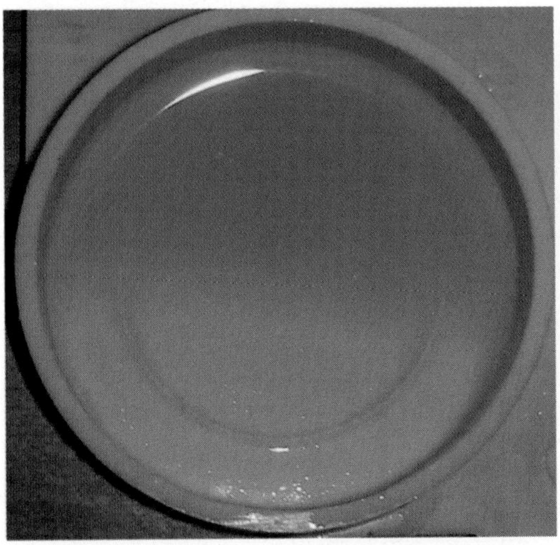

Figure 12.8: Showing CMT Negative

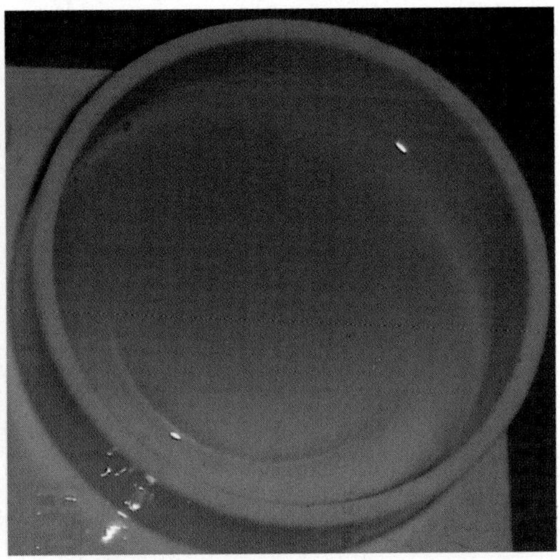

Figure 12.9: Showing CMT Trace

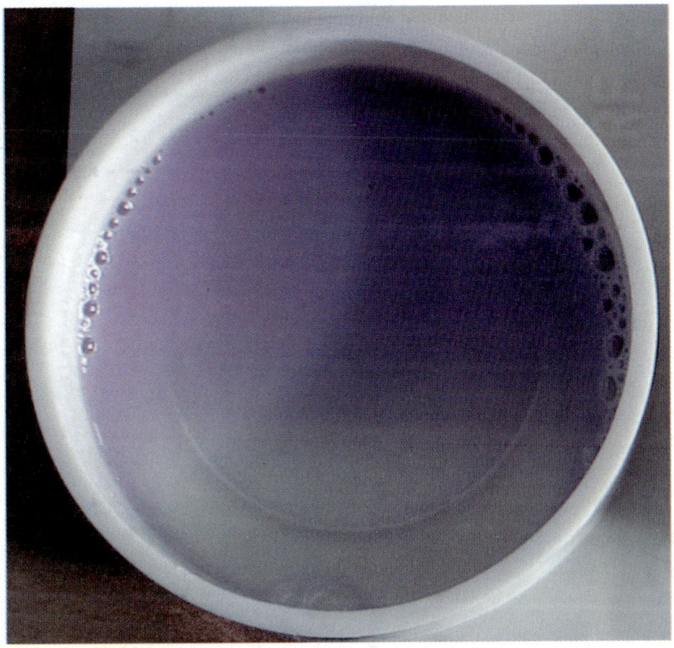

Figure 12.10: Showing CMT "+"

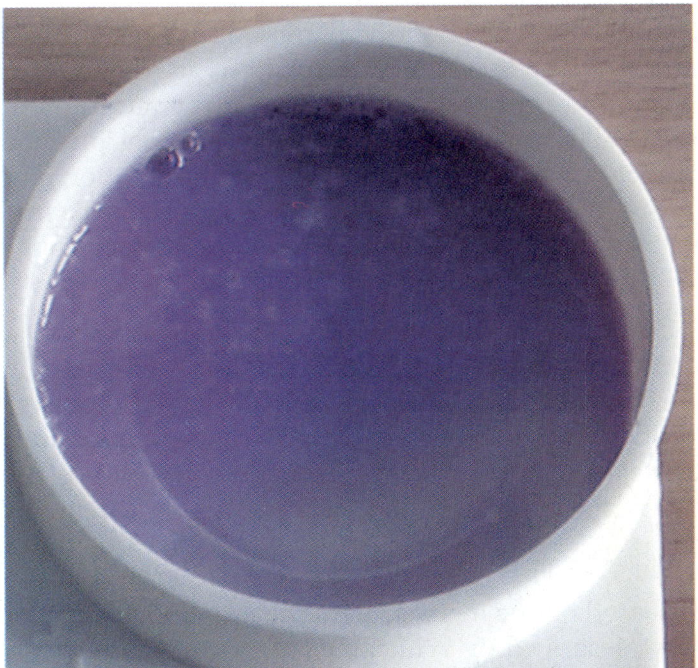

Figure 12.11: Showing CMT "+ +"

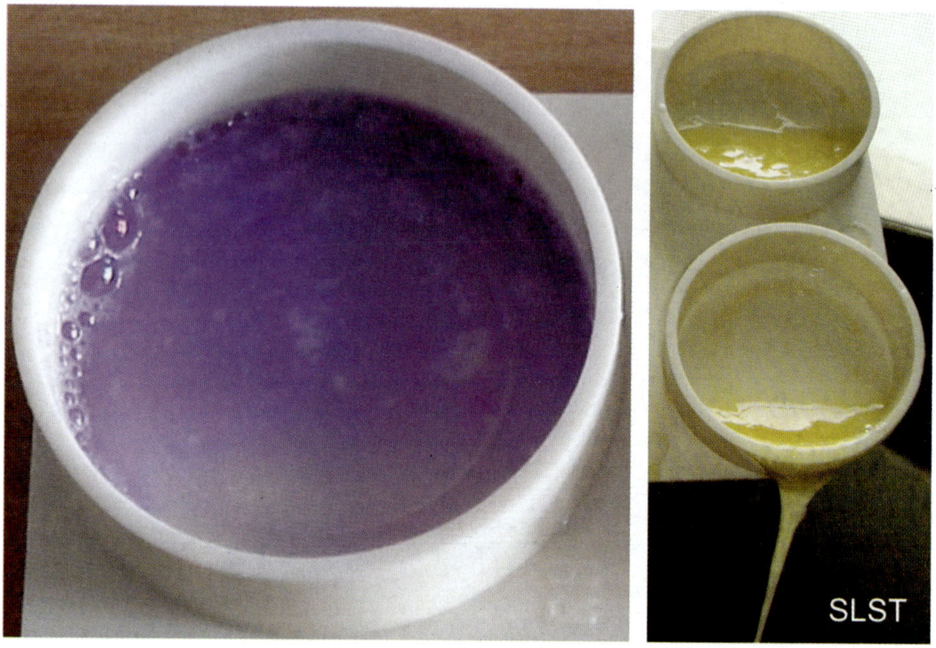

Figure 12.12: Showing CMT "+ + +"

5. Sodium Lauryl Sulphate Test (SLST)

This test is similar to CMT in principle as well as procedure. The difference is that in this test 3% sodium lauryl sulphate is used with instead of CMT reagent. This solution (test reagent) is prepared by adding 3 gm of sodium lauryl sulphate to 100 ml of distilled water. The suspension should be heated to 50°C so as to make a clear solution. The pH of the solution is adjusted to 8.0 by using HCL or NaOH as per the need. The accuracy of this method is found to be 88.66% (Sharma *et al.,* 2010b). Some workers mentioned this test as modified CMT.

Some precaution should be taken during the handling of sodium lauryl sulphate (SLS). A study at the University of Georgia Medical College, indicated that SLS penetrated into the eyes as well as brain, heart, liver, etc., and showed long-term retention in the tissues. It may also cause hair loss by attacking the follicle. Another extremely serious problem is the connection of SLS with nitrate contamination. Nitrates are potential cancer-causing carcinogenics.

6. White Side Test (WST)

The test is based on the increase in number of leukocytes in mastitis milk. The original test described by Whiteside (1939) was made by stirring 2 ml of normal NaOH into 10 ml of milk. The development of a "viscid mass" was regarded as positive.

The test was modified by Murphy and Hanson (1941), they added one drop of normal NaOH to five drops of milk on a glass slide and stirred the mixture for 20 seconds with a glass rod. Negative samples were entirely free of precipitate. The amount of precipitate formed was graded from slight to tick viscid mass and was considered to be indicative of the degree of irritation in the udder. They regarded this procedure as superior to the bromothymol blue test for use in the field as a presumptive test for chronic bovine mastitis.

Later on, this was further modified by Schalm *et al.* (1971), they use one drop of 4% NaOH to 5 drops of milk to be tested on a clean glass slide and mixed vigorously with a glass rod for 20 seconds. The results are graded on the basis of precipitation of milk:

Grading	Description
Mixture remains opaque and free of particles	(-) Negative
Fine dispersed particles on close inspection	(+/-) Trace
A definite thickening and mixture separates into a milky whey and white particles	(+) Distinct positive
Mixture thickens immediately and follows glass rod.	(+ +) Strong positive

Allore (1999) stated that the Whiteside (WST) and Modified Whiteside tests (MWST) use 4 per cent NaOH and 0.5 per cent alkyl arylsulfonate combined with 1.5 per cent NaOH, respectively, to react with deoxyribonucleic acid in the somatic cells to form sa;ts and produce a precipitate. The reaction is greatly reduced in cow's milk compared to buffalo's milk because of higher fat concentration and lipid size affect the sensitivity of the Whiteside test.

7. Surf Field Mastitis Test (SFMT)

This test was developed by Muhammad *et al.* (1995). This test is easy, cheap and enough sensitive to detect all cases of sub-clinical mastitis. The advantage of this test is that the readily available house hold surf (detergent) is used as reagent. The principle of this test is the reaction of somatic cells DNA with detergent (surf) and leads to the formation of gel of varying degree depending upon the number of somatic cells in the milk.

Procedure

1. 3% Surf solution- Dissolve 3 g of surf in 100 ml of clean tape water or 6 teaspoonfuls of house hold detergent, surf in 500 ml of clean tape water. The test solution is stable for 6 months at room temperature.
2. A plastic paddle with four receptacles for the respective quarters of an animal can be fabricated from locally available plastic or bakelite. When

this paddle is not at hand, suitable container such as tea cups or glass may be substituted.

3. Take equal quantity of 3% reagent and milk in the paddle or container. The mixture is swirled for about 1 minute and then examined visually for the presence of small floccules and gel. If floccules or gel is formed it indicates the positive for intramammary infection. In absence of any floccules or gel, sample is negative.

8. Mastest

A new test for subclinical mastitis in cows has been developed and tested in the Lithuanian Veterinary Institute (Spakauskas *et al.*, 1998). Mastest has upto 99.05% correlation with CMT (Spakauskas *et al.*, 2006). This test is more commonly used in Scandinavian countries.

Procedure

This test is very simple and easy to perform. The grading of severity of infections is also very easy and depends on the formation of gel. For the test take 2 ml of test solution in a special white plate and mixed with 2 ml (equal quantity) of milk sample. After turning a plate for 5-10 seconds, consistency and colour of the mixture is visually determined and indicate the severity of infection. According to changes in consistence and colour of the mixture, the reaction is estimate using the 5-point system.

Five (5)-point system

Point	Description
1	Consistency of mixture is homogenous, liquid, without visible changes
2	Insignificant fakes develop and disappear when the plate is rotated
3	Clots appear, the viscosity of the mixture increases
4	The mixture becomes viscous, while rotating the plate a clot can be seen which localizes; when the rotation ceases the mixture disperses on the bottom
5	The mixture becomes very viscous, a yolk-like clot is visible; when the content of the plate is poured out the clot extends and falls out

9. Modified Aulendorfer Mastitis Probe (MAMP) Test

This test can be effectively used to detect sub-clinical mastitis in cows but time consuming. The test involves the use of MAMP reagent, which contains sodium lauryl sulphate and urea. Milk samples are collected and added to equal volume of reagent, mixed thoroughly in a test tube and left undisturbed for 24 hours at room temperature. A positive reaction will be gelatinous product, which will be milky initially and later becomes flaky and begins to clear from bottom depending on the intensity of reaction.

10. Bromocresol Purple Test

Mastitis increases the alkalinity of milk. The pH of normal cow's milk lies in the range 6.5 to 6.8 but may exceed 7.0 in milks with high cell counts. During inflammation of the mammary gland, permeability of the blood capillaries increases, which allows alkaline blood constituents (sodium and bicarbonate ions) to enter the milk and consequently to increase milk pH. Indicator dyes such as bromocresol purple (BCP) and bromothymol blue (BTB) have been used for many years in mastitis diagnosis to detect pH changes in milk (Baker and Van Slyke, 1919; Fay *et al.*, 1938). Because of the influence of fat content on the color produced by BCP this dye largely has been replaced by BTB.

This test is a pH indicator test and east to perform. Take 2-3 drops of 0.9% bromocresol purple solution in a test tube and add 3 ml of freshly drawn milk. Normal milk appears as yellow (pale grayish purple) while mastitis milk will appear as blue or purple.

11. Bromothymol Blue (BTB) Test

This is pH indicator test, after adding the milk with bromothymol blue, develops the different colors due to changes in pH of milk. The normal pH of milk is 6.4 to 6.8 and isotonic with blood plasma. In mastitis, during late lactation and dry period, the concentration of lactose and casein in the milk is reduced whereas sodium chloride and sodium bicarbonate pass into the alveoli from plasma to maintain isotonicity. Therefore, during such situations milk become alkaline with greater amount of chlorides (Galdhar *et al.*, 2005). In 1920 Baker and Breed used bromothymol blue to detect changes in the pH value in milk. Subsequently, the test has been widely used in the diagnosis of mastitis.

However, it generally is accepted that the BTB indicator test is not particularly sensitive for detection of subclinical mastitis, and with the introduction of rapid cow side tests for cell count e.g., CMT, the pH approach has fallen into disfavor. The main disadvantage with indirect tests such as CMT is that assessment of results is based on the degree of gel formation in the milk, and, consequently, untrained personnel often have problems in distinguishing between the various scoring categories. The BTB test, however, is assessed on the basis of color changes that are observed more readily.

For this test BTB card test papers may be prepared from whatman filter paper No.1. the diagnostic card can be prepared by adding one drop of BTB test solution (bromothymol blue-1.6 g in 100 ml ethanol) at 4 different spots on the paper and indicates left fore (LF), left hind (LH), right fore (RF) and right hind (RH) (Figure 12.13). One drop of suspected milk has to be put directly on the indicator spot and observe the change of color may be scored as pale green indicates normal quarter and +, ++ and +++ (according to change in color from moderate green to dark blue green). The only disadvantage of this test is that cows in later stages of lactation may give false positive reaction.

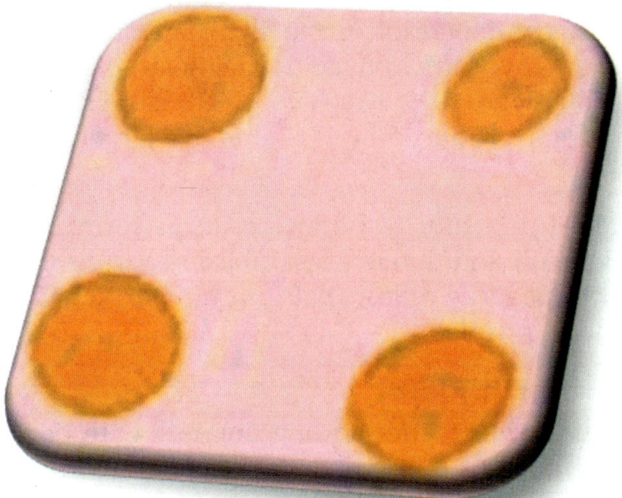

Figure 12.13: BTB card.

12. Mastrip Test

Mastrip is a cellulose based bromothymol blue strip impregnated with stabilized ions, marketed by Dabur Ayurvet Ltd., India for the detection of mastitis. One drop of milk is placed on the mastrip and reaction is read from the standard color matching strip. The colour reaction is graded as-

Grading	Description
-	No change in color (Yellow)
+	Light green
+ +	Dark green
+ + +	Bluish green

13. Electrical Conductivity Test (EC test)

Electrical conductivity (EC) of milk is determined by sodium, potassium, calcium, magnesium, chlorine, and other ions. Concentration of ions in secretion changes not only because of increased throughput of blood capillaries but also due to damaged active ion transport system. Secretory cells of mammary gland are distinguished by an active transport system when transporting Na^+ to the extracellular fluid and K^+ back into the cell. Na^+ and K^+ are transported from the secretory cells to milk in a passive manner. After disintegration of cells, ions contained in the extracellular fluid enter the alveolar chamber. Changes in ion concentration cause an increase in electrical conductivity. The change in electrical conductivity is one of the earliest manifestations associated with new infections making the early detection and recording of possible mastitis cases routine. Mastitic milk has a higher electrical conductivity than normal milk.

The greatest problem associated with this new technology is the sensitivity and specificity of electrical conductivity between herds. Recent advances in determining herd specific conductivity threshold levels have increased the value of this screening method in many herds. Milk conductivity is a screening test. A positive indication of increased electrical conductivity in a specific animal is an indication for further evaluation of that animal (temperature, udder examination, etc.) and not generally a signal for immediate treatment. Hand held conductivity meters are also available and may be useful for routine screening animals pre-milking. However, data on the diagnostic value of this method is contradictory (Spakauskas *et al.*, 2006). According to some authors (Hamann and Gyodi, 2000; Hillerton and Walton, 1991), EC of healthy cow milk is 4.0-5.5 milisenses (mS)/cm. When EC increases to 6.0 mS/cm or more, pathological processes in the udder tissue may be suspected.

Various factors may affect the electrical conductivity of milk. Electrical conductivity increases together with the temperature of a sample. Relationship with the temperature (15°C and 40°C) has been approximately linear, while increase coefficient has been 0.113 mS/cm (Nielen *et al.*, 1992). Electrical conductivity is also affected by other factors. Among such mastitis-related factors various authors indicate lactation stage, inter-herd differences, rutting, changes during milking, milk fat, various diseases, etc. When diagnosing mastitis it is important to note the udder quarter with the highest EC compared to other quarters.

14. Chloride Test

This test denotes presence of increased quantity of chloride in mastitis milk. In normal milk, chloride levels varies from 0.08 to 0.14%. There exists an inverse relationship between the concentration of lactose and sodium chloride which depends on the stage of lactation. Davis (1999) reported that in mastitis there is decreased amount of lactose and increased amount of sodium chloride to maintain the normal milk pressure hence during inflammation (mastitis) there is increase in the chloride content (>0.14%).

Solution

Solution A

Silver nitrate	- 1.34 g
Distilled water	- 1000 ml

Solution B

Potassium chromate	- 10 g
Distilled water	- 1000 ml

Take 1 ml of milk and add 5 ml silver nitrate solution (Solution A) followed by two drops of potassium chromate solution (Solution B). Observe for the change of color, development of yellow color indicates the chloride level >0.14%, i.e. quarter is positive for mastitis and appearance of brownish red color indicates chloride level <0.14% i.e. negative to mastitis (Figure 12.14). This test is more sensitive than the bromothymol test.

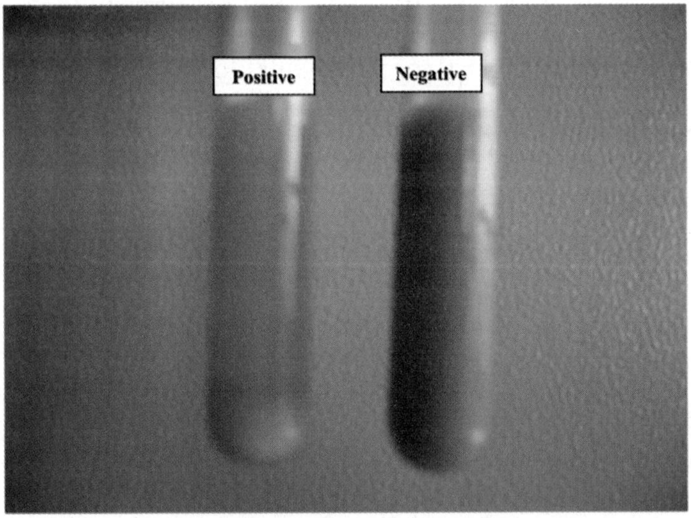

Figure 12.14: Chloride test.

Direct or Cultural Test

Milk culturing for mastitis causing pathogens can provide a great pact of valuable information for a dairy farmer. Designing a management strategy to reduce new cases and improve prognosis for cows already affected is aided by identifying the etiologic agents of mastitis. Knowledge of antibiotic susceptibility or resistance of mastitis pathogens is valuable to veterinarians and dairy producers. The identification of pathogens along with their anti-biogram results helps in developing therapy protocols for particular dairy farms.

The Gold Standard for mastitis investigations has been bacteriological examination of a milk sample, a process that takes in excess of 18 hours when the sample is in the lab, and often 48 hours, for several of the bacteria, to be confident of the results (Hillerton, 2003). Although, culturing is the "*gold standard*" for determining infection status, it is not perfectly sensitive and performance varies with bacteria. Culture data provides additional information that can be used with routine SCC to determine the source(s) of new infections as well as influence therapy decisions and appropriate use of antibiotics.

The value of the bacteriological examination of milk significantly depends upon the ability of the sampler to collect samples aseptically. Poor sampling will lead to contamination and often confusion as to the significance of the isolates (Buswell, 1995). It is of critical importance that milk samples are obtained as free of external contamination as possible.

Milk sample collection technique for cultural isolation

(a) Preparation of udder/teats

The critical keys to a useful laboratory is in proper training of cow handlers to collect appropriate samples and to carefully handle them so that over growth of contaminates does not occur. The teats must always be adequately disinfected prior to sample collection, with great emphasis paid to the teat orifice. The use of water should be discouraged as it simply provides a vehicle for contamination.

- Brush loose dirt, beddings, and hair from the underside of udder and teats.
- Grossly dirty teats and udder should be washed and dried thoroughly before proceeding with sample collect. When doing this, do the two teats on the far side of the cow first, followed by the two closest.
- Dipping teats in a good quality teat dip before collection can further reduce sample contamination. The teat dip should be thoroughly wiped from the teat with a paper towel, and the teats cleaned with 70% isopropyl alcohol. The teats must be dry before the sample is taken.

(b) Sample collection

Collecting a suitable sample is a crucial step in obtaining reliable culture results that can be interpreted and used to identify problems and monitor herd health. Milk samples for culture are collected at milking time after teat disinfection and just before the milking or milking machine is applied. The following steps should be kept in mind before sampling for culture:

- All milk sample collection vials should be properly sterilized. Label the tubes prior to sampling with date, name of farm/farmer, cow number, quarter etc.

- Discard a first few streams from the quarter in separate cup or bucket. First strippings should not be milked out on the floor.
- Using a sterile bottle, held almost horizontally to the floor to minimise the entrance of contamination into its mouth, a midstream sample should be taken.
- To collect individual quarter samples- begin sampling from the closest teat and move to the teats on the far side of the udder- reverse order from cleaning. When collecting a composite sample (milk from all quarters in the same vial) sample the teats closest to you first, followed by the two on the far side. This reduces the chance of contaminating the clean teats with your hands or arms reaching across under the cow before the samples are collected. The saying to remember the washing and sampling order is: *"wash towards (you), sample away"*.
- Remove the cap of the sample vial without touching the edges of the cap or the vial. Hold the cap in the same hand as the sample vial, facing downwards, while collecting the milk sample. Tilt the sampling vial while collecting the milk to reduce the chances of dust or dirt dropping from the udder into the vial. Maintain the vial at approximately a 45° angle while taking the milk sample.
- Collect adequate quantity of milk (10-15 ml) and, immediately replace and secure the cap and making sure the vial is tightly closed. Make sure milk entering the vial does not touch the fingers or hand. Sample vial should never be filled more than three-fourths full.
- All samples should be taken prior to antibiotic treatment.
- Just after collection refrigerate the samples on ice or in refrigerator and transport to lab. Sample that will be cultured at a later date (after 24 to 48 hours) should be immediately frozen.

If Mycoplasma mastitis is suspected a simple transport medium is the milk sample itself with ampicillin added at 5 mg/ml. the milk sample, in this case, is held at the ambient temperature to allow Mycoplasma groth during transportation. A second sample vial should be kept without the antibiotic, as a check for other mastitis causing pathogens.

Aseptic technique in sample collection for bacterial culturing is an absolute necessity. Not only are there organisms that are contaminants, but also these same organisms have the potential to cause the disease. Contamination is a major complication in identifying the causative agent of an intramammary infection. Contaminated samples may lead to misdiagnosis, increased work, confusion and frustration. Contaminants in a milk sample grow more quickly than pathogenic streptococci and staphylococci and interfere with the interpretation of results.

Culture media and inoculation of plates

Most of the mastitis causing bacteria grows on 5% calf or sheep blood agar. A MacConkey agar should be used for *Enterococcus faecalis* and any other Gram-negative bacteria that are able to grow on this medium. The EMB agar medium is the selective medium for *E. coli* bacteria. Edwards medium is highly selective medium for streptococci and also act as an indicator medium for hemolysis and for the hydrolysis of aesculin. A Sabouraud dextrose agar plate can be inoculated if a fungal infection is suspected. However, pathogens such as *Candida albicans* and *Aspergillus fumigatus* form colonies on blood agar at 37°C in 2-3 days, if there is little or no competition from faster growing bacteria (Quine *et al.*, 1994).

Mycoplasma bovis is the most common species of mycoplasma to cause mastitis in dairy cows. Mycoplasmas are fastidious organisms and most require specific growth factors, an isotonic medium and the absence of inhibitory substances for growth. The basic medium is a good quality beef infusion with supplements. Mycoplasma are difficult to culture. Although *M. bovis* belongs to the well growing mycoplasmas its isolation requires a specially equipped laboratory. There are more variants of suitable culture media for the isolation of *M. bovis* (Medium B, Hayflick's medium, Friis medium, etc.). These media usually contain a rich protein base (e.g. heart infusion), serum (horse and/or swine), yeast extract, glucose and/or pyruvate and selective agents (ampicillin, thallous acetate and amphotericin-B). After 3-5 days of incubation this organism forms typical fried-egg shape colonies (Figure 12.15). Films and spots production can also be observed.

Commonly bacteria are isolated and identified on the basis of morphological, cultural and biochemical characteristics (Table 12.7a, b). Briefly, 0.01ml of milk is streaked vertically across the diameter of an agar plate. The inoculum is then evenly spread over the entire surface of the plate by a back and forth motion at right angles to the central streak, using the same loop that is used for inoculation. Milk samples are plated on MacConkey agar to detect coliforms and Gram-negative bacteria, modified Edward media for streptococci and streptococci-like organisms, Vogel-Johnson agar for staphylococci, and modified Hayflick medium for Mycoplasma organisms.

Inoculated plates are incubated at 37°C for 36-48 hours. Mycoplasmal medium is incubated under modified atmospheric conditions. The plates were observed for bacterial growth after an incubation period of 24 and 48 hours. Bacterial colonies should be subjected to Gram's stain for identification of Gram negative and Gram positive micro-organisms. After tentative confirmation of type organisms, then subjected to different and specific biochemical tests for confirmation of species of micro-organisms.

The first step of identification of bacteria is Gram's stain. Taking a clean dry microscope slide and sterile saline, a single discrete colony is picked off from the culture using a straight wire. The organism is emulsified within a small drop of sterile saline on the slide to give an even suspension. This is allowed to air dry and the preparation is then fixed by passing through a Bunsen flame. The preparation is then submitted for Gram staining. The preparation is examined under an oil immersion objective. Organisms that retain the aniline dye after attempts to decolourise are termed Gram-positive while others, which are unable to retain the dye and then take up the counterstain, are defined as Gram-negative (Buswell, 1995).

Gram stain method

1. Clean the microscopic slide with 70% ethyl alcohol and it should make grease free.
2. Take 1-2 colonies of bacteria from culture plates and spread over the slide under sterilize condition or near the Bunsen flame.
3. After preparing the slide, it should be fixed by passing the slide quickly through the Bunsen flame, 2-3 times. Taking care not to overheat the smear. The reason for fixing the smears include killing the vegetative bacteria, rendering them permeable to the stain and ensuring that the material is firmly fixed to the slide.
4. The fixed smears placed on a staining rack over the sink.
5. Flood slide with a 0.5 per cent solution of crystal violet for 30 seconds.
6. Wash off in tap water and flood slide with Lugol's iodine for 30 seconds.
7. Rinse again in tap water and rapidly apply either acetone or alcohol for approximately 3-5 seconds to decolourise the preparation.
8. Wash off rapidly and counter stain with neutral red for 15 to 20 seconds.
9. Wash slide in water and gently blot dry.
10. Examine under oil immersion.

Table 12.7a : Important mastitis causing bacteria showing some of their main characteristics leading to a presumptive identification (Quinn *et al.*, 1994).

Bacteria	Gram reaction	Shape	Catalase	Oxi-dase	Haemolysis	Growth on Mac Conkey agar	Aesculin hydrolysis (Edwards medium)	CAMP test	Lance field group	Other characteristics and confirmatory tests
S. agalactiae	+	C	-	-	α, β, γ	-	-	+	B	CAMP test positive
S. dysgalactiae	+	C	-	-	α	-	-	-	C	Alpha-hemolytic, CAMP-negative
S. uberis	+	C	-	-	α, γ	-	+	-	-	Aesculin splitter, no growth on MacConkey agar
Enterococcus faecalis	+	C	-	-	α, γ	+	+	-	D	Pin-point red colonies on MacConkey agar, aesculin hydrolysis
S. pyogenes	+	C	-	-	β	-	-	-	A	Susceptible to bacitracin (0.04 unit disc)
S. pneumonia	+	C	-	-	α	-	±	-	-	Susceptible to optochin. Often mucoid.
S. equi subsp. zooepidermicus	+	C	-	-	β	-	-	-	C	Group C: trehalose -, sorbitol +, lactose +, and maltose +(-)
S. aureus	+	C	+	-	+	-				Golden-yellow pigment; double-zoned haemolysis; coagulase + and ferments maltose on purple agar base plus 1% maltose.
E. coli	-	R	+	-	±	+				'IMViC' test +/+/-/-, Metallic sheen on EMB agar. Occasionally mucoid, quite often haemolytic.
Klebsiella pneumonia	-	R	+	-	-	+				Mucoid colonies, non-motile
Eneterobacter aerogenes	-	R	+	-	-	+				Mucoid colonies, motile ('IMViC test -/-/+/+)
Serratia marcescens	-	R	+	-	-	+				Red pigment at 25°C, some strains at 37°C
Pseudomonas aeruginosa	-	R	+	+	±	+				Greenish-blue pigment, fruity smell
Actinomyces pyogenes	+	R	-	-	+	-				Small colonies, hazy haemolysis. Pits Loeffler serum slope.
Nocardia asteroids	+	F	+	-	±	-				Powdery white colonies, adherent to medium. MZN +. Requires 3-4 days inoculation. Growth on Sabouraud agar.
Pasteurella multocida	-	R	+	+	-	-				Colonies with sweetish smell, non-hemolytic, indole + and no growth on MacConkey agar.
P. haemolytica	-	R	v	+	+	+				No smell. Haemolyitc, indole - and red, pin-point colonies on MacConkey agar.
Bacillus cereus	+	R	+	-	+	-				Forms endospores. Wide zone of haemolysis. Large, flat, dry and granular colonies.

C = coccus, R = rod, F = filamentous, + = positive reaction, ± = most strains positive, v = strains vary, - = negative reaction, 'IMViC = indole, methyl red, Voges-Proskauer and citrate tests. MZN = modified Ziehl-Neelsen stain.

Table 12.7b : Morphological characteristic of important mastitis causing bacteria.

Bacteria	Morphological/colonies characteristics
Staphylococci	- The bacteria appear as small round cocci often occurring in small bunches (said to resemble grape-like clusters). - Growth on blood agar appears as small round convex colonies, approximately 2 to 3 mm in diameter (Figure 12.16). - The surface of the colony is shiny and can possess either golden yellow (hence the designation of *Staphylococcus aureus*) or white pigmentation. - Often, zones of either a- or b-haemolysis are found within the immediate vicinity of the culture.
Streptococci	- The streptococci appear as small round cocci, often in pairs (diplococci) or short chains. - On blood agar, cultures occur as small round translucent convex colonies, approximately 1 mm in diameter; these often appear white in reflected light (Figure 12.17). - The colonies are frequently surrounded by small zones of either a- or b- haemolysis. - On Edwards' medium, the organisms appear to give a bluish sheen in reflected light.
Actinomycetes	- The organisms appear as short, often beaded, Gram-positive rods, which may adopt a classical ***'Chinese-lettering'*** form. - After 18 to 24 hours' incubation, the appearance upon blood agar is that of a minute feathery growth. - Further incubation to 48 hours produces small white convex colonies, about 1 mm in diameter. These are often opalescent with a glistening surface. - Sometimes there is evidence of haemolysis.
Bacilli	- The bacilli produce large Gram-positive bacilli with rounded ends, which often possess large terminal or sub-terminal spores. - On blood agar, the growth appears as large, flat, irregularly shaped colonies with either shiny or matt surfaces. - *B. subtilis* is usually grey or white in colour, while *B. cereus* cultures often produce cream coloured pigmentation. - Growth of *B. cereus* and *B. subtilis* is inhibited upon MacConkey's agar.
E. coli	- Gram staining reveals short to medium sized Gram-negative rods. - On blood agar, the growth appears as round, shiny, convex grey-coloured colonies, approximately 3 to 4mm in diameter.

- The culture has a characteristic 'fruity' odour.
- Some strains can produce large clear zones of haemolysis surrounding the colonies.
- The organism grows well on MacConkey's agar with colonies fermenting lactose, as demonstrated by the characteristic pink/ red colouration (Figure 12.18).
- On EMB agar (selective media)- it show typical "metallic sheen" (Figure 12.19).

Klebsiella

- This bacteria appear as short Gram-negative bacilli often surrounded by a faintly stained red capsule on Gram staining.
- On blood agar, the colonies are usually grey coloured, with a mucoid appearance (Figure 12.20).
- A strong 'fruity' smell is again evident.
- Colonies can be somewhat irregular in size and glisten in appearance.
- On MacConkey's agar, colonies are pink/red in colour (denoting lactose fermentation), with a mucoid appearance.

Pseudomonas aeruginosa

- The organisms appear on Gram staining as short slender Gram-negative rods which can occur as parallel pairs or as short chains.
- On blood agar, colonies are raised and convex, often grey or dark green in colour and matt in consistency.
- Plates retained at room temperature produce a dark green pigment due to the production of pyocyanin.
- Growth on blood agar can often produce areas of clear haemolysis and any culture will have a characteristic pungent smell.
- Colonies on MacConkey's agar are non-lactose fermenting and sometimes produce a metallic sheen.

Nocardia asteroides

- This organism shows the white, powdery colonies, embedded in the agar after 3-4 days of incubation.
- Some strains are hemolytic.
- The colonies of *N. asteroides* have no smell, which differentiate them from *Streptomyces* spp., which have similar colonies but a pungent, earthy odour.
- Growth on Sabouraud dextrose agar: *N. asteroides* and some *Streptomyces* species have the unusual ability of being able to grow on Sabouraud agar, which is a selective medium for fungi.

Prototheca spp.

- *P. zopfii* and *P. wickerhamii* are achlorophyllic algae but they form bacterial like colonies on blood agar at 25-37°C, after 48-72 hours incubation. The colonies are small and grayish-white.
- They are best demonstrated in wet preparations or in smears stained by the Wright or Giemsa method.

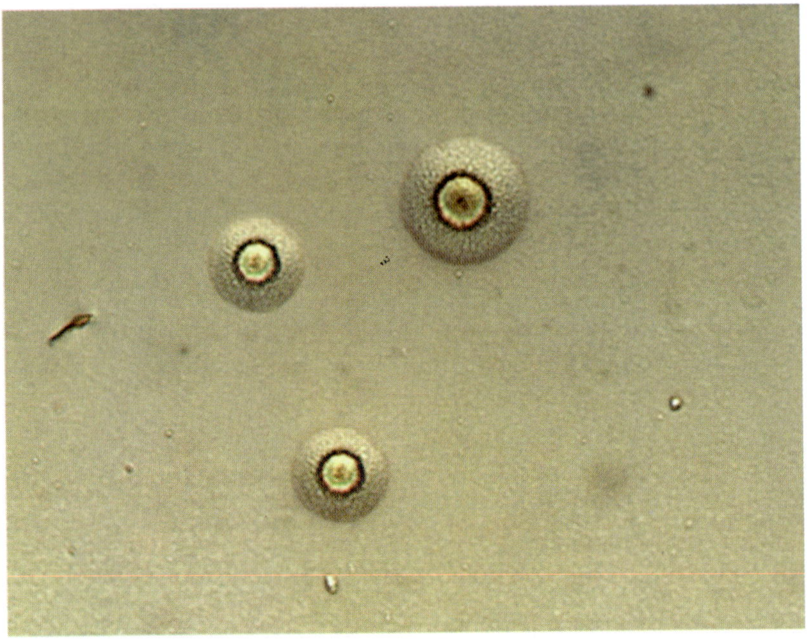

Figure 12.15: Colonies of mycoplasma on a special nutrient medium - a characteristic appearance as "*egg on the eye* ". (Courtesy of prof. Branka Sheol, Department of Microbiology and Infectious Diseases, Faculty of Veterinary Medicine, University of Zagreb)

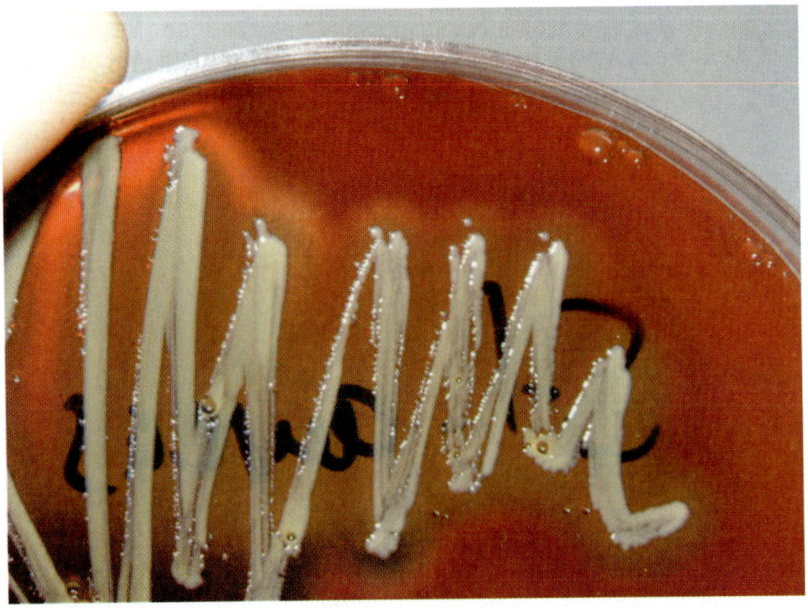

Figure 12.16: *S. aureus* bacteria on blood agar. (Courtesy of Dr. Miroslava Beniæ, CVI, Zagreb, Croatia)

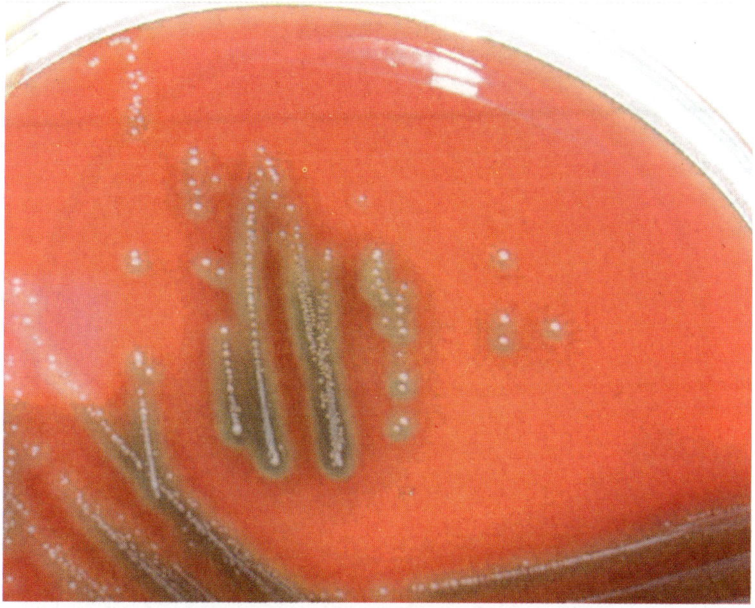

Figure 12.17: *S. dysgalactiae* bacteria on blood agar. (Courtesy of Dr. Miroslava Beniæ, CVI, Zagreb, Croatia)

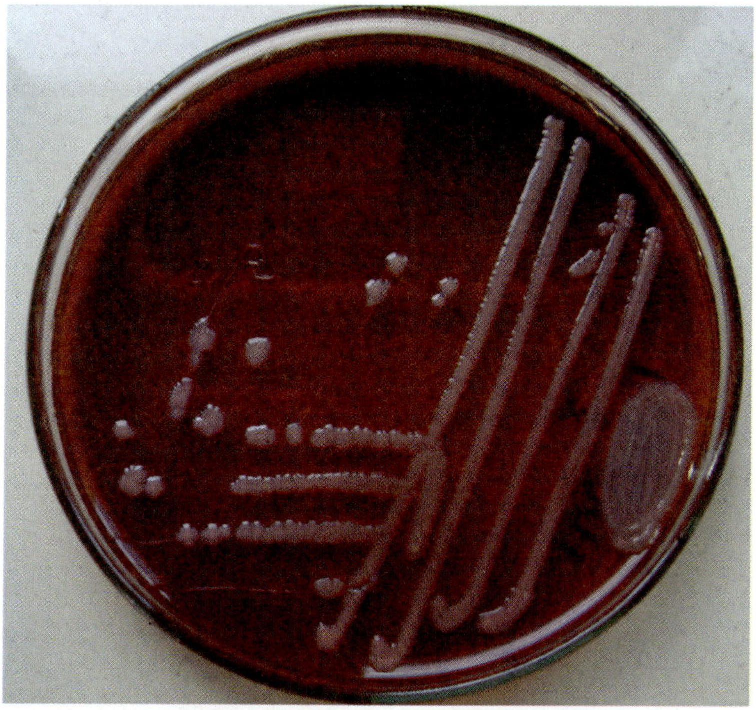

Figure 12.18: *E. coli* on Mc Conkey agar

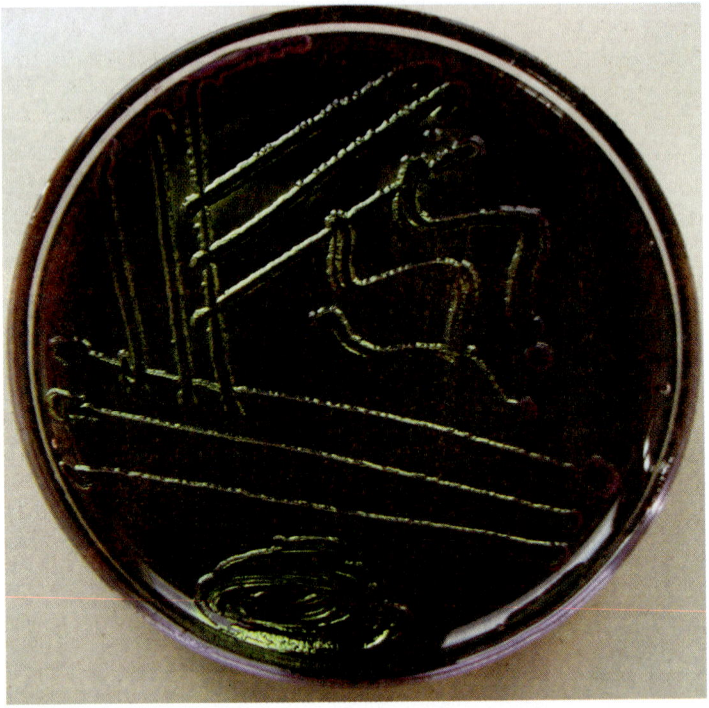

Figure 12.19: *E. coli* on EMB agar (metallic sheen).

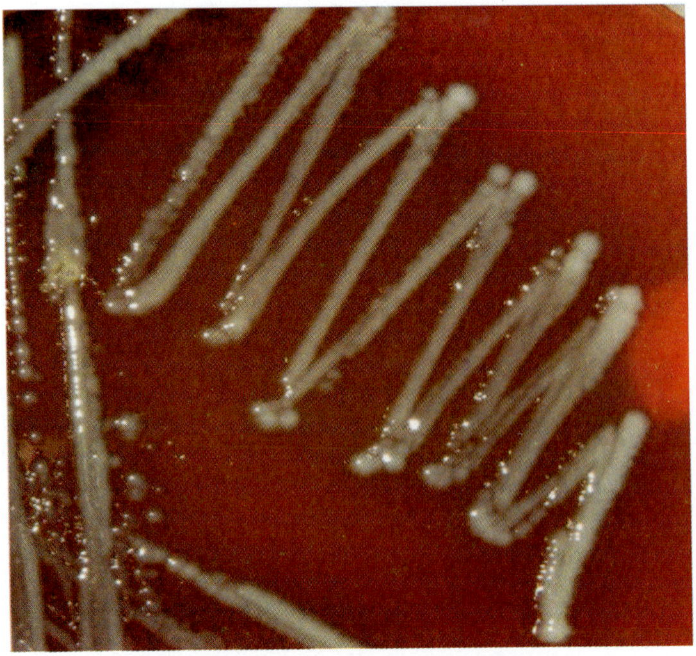

Figure 12.20: Klebsiella on blood agar.

Interpretation of cultural results and criteria of final diagnosis

The final interpretation after culture report is most important aspect in the management of mastitis and to reduce the economic losses due to treatment. *S. aureus, Streptococcus spp.* (environmental) and *S. dysgalactiae* are the most common pathogens found in both clinical and sub-clinical mastitis. In mastitis cases occurring at or near calving, *E. coli, Enterobacter spp* and other coliforms may be present. *Klebsiella spp* and *Serratia spp* can cause persistent mastitis symptoms. The most important thing is that the recovery of milk quality in quarters affected by these pathogens may not occur. If mastitis is caused by *Pseudomonas sp, Nocardia sp* and *Arcanobacter pyogenes,* such cases are incurable. Recovery of the former two pathogens from mastitis cases should indicate cull for slaughter of the affected cow especially if *Nocardia sp* are involved as these pathogens pose a potential human health risk. Mastitis due to Staphylococcus spp. and *Arcanobacter pyogenes* usually necessitates drying off affected quarter after treatment and reassessing damage to the quarter after subsequent calving. Recurrent cases of mastitis are usually due to chronic staphylococcal infection. The *S. aureus* is an intracellular organism, so in recurrent cases sampling should be done 2-3times at different time intervals.

After complete examination of mastitis case, both bacterial cultural findings and SCC should be considered for final decision. It gives more suitable and understandable interpretation of mastitis diagnosis (Table 12.8).

Table 12.8: Criteria for diagnosis of mastitis, based on cultural report and SCC of milk sample (IDF, 1971; Hamann, 2002).

Result from the milk sample		Diagnosis
Bacterial growth	**Inflammation (SCC >200000 cells/ml)**	
Yes	No	Latent infection[a] or Presence of bacterial growth[b]
No	Yes	Non-specific mastitis[a] Mastitis[b]
Yes	Yes	Mastitis

[a] International Dairy federation definition (1971)
[b] Alternative definition (National veterinary and Food Research Institute, Finland).

Other important facts

The prevalence of subclinical infection is difficult to ascertain, as this can only be determined by isolation of bacteria from the gland (Leigh, 1999). Many organisms present in the cow's environment can cause mastitis. When one of these organisms is isolated from mastitic milk the question arises as to whether it is the cause of the mastitis, or a contaminant (Jones, 1994). Bacteriology and cell counting are sometimes used together to determine the infection status of the mammary gland (Barkema *et al.*, 1997). However the interpretation of these combined results is not straightforward (Francis, 1993; Shoshani *et al.*, 2000). Francis (1993) present some of the possible reasons for contradictory results in table 12.9.

Table 12.9 : Possible reasons for inconsistent results using bacteriology and somatic cell counts Together (Francis, 1993).

High cell count and negative bacteriology	Low cell count and positive bacteriology
Small numbers of bacteria not being detected in the 10 ul aliquot cultured	Teat canal infections
Culture medium unsuitable for the causal agent	Sample contaminated during collection
Milk sample is bactericidal ("death in the post")	Long-standing subclinical infection
Physical or chemical damage to the udder	Contaminated sample bottle
Teat canal infections producing endotoxin which raises the cell count	

Reasons for negative culture results

Bacteriological culturing has been regarded as the most accurate method for detecting intramammary infection; however, reports indicate about 25-40% of milk samples from clinically affected quarters produce negative culture results. Reasons of undetected infection include-

1. At the time of sampling some bacteria may have left the gland or remained in numbers that are too low to be detected by culture.
2. The organisms may be shed intermittently or be walled off by clots in the gland e.g. *S. aureus*.
3. The organism may no longer be present and the clinical signs are due to by-products such as endotoxins e.g. *E. coli*.
4. Some infections are eliminated spontaneously by the leukocyte and other immune response mechanisms.
5. Antibiotics may have killed or suppressed organism numbers to unrecoverable levels.

6. Additionally Mycoplasma and other organisms that require selective culture media may have caused the infection, hence culturing on non-selective media yields negative results.
7. Storage may have reduced numbers of viable organisms to undetectable levels.

Kirk (2009) suggested some points to minimize the number of culture negative reports:

a) Train to milkers to detect clinical cases of mastitis. Let them know why it is important to collect milk samples at the very first instance of abnormal milk. This is particularly important in 2x milking herds.
b) To optimize the detection of contagious pathogens, particularly when attempting to detect sub-clinical infections in high somatic cell count cows, it is necessary to collect more than one milk sample for culture. The urgency of total detection will dictate whether 2, 3 or even 4 samples should be taken.
c) Deliver the milk samples to the laboratory soon (4–6 hours) after collection and keep them in crushed ice until they reach the laboratory.
d) If milk samples are to be frozen, try to limit the storage time in the freezer to less than one week.

Polymerase Chain Reaction (PCR)

Bacterial culture is a useful and effective tool for the detection of bacteria, but it does have some limitations. A low concentration of bacteria in the sample or selecting the incorrect culture media may lead to a "no growth" result. In some cases, additional cultures or tests must be performed to distinguish between two similar bacteria. Contamination of the milk sample at the farm1 is always a possibility and can lead to an incorrect diagnosis (4 to 20% of samples). Furthermore, the incubation time creates a waiting period and it may take a while before the results get to the farm. However, bacterial cultures are presently more affordable than PCR tests and are offered by all diagnostic laboratories across the country. PCR testing promises to overcome the limitations of bacterial cultures and will offer new avenues for research and for managing mastitis among herds. For the time being, bacterial cultures remain a readily available tool that is still relevant to on-farm udder health programs (CBMRN Fact sheet, 2008-09). Presently various PCR kits for mastitis diagnosis have been developed e.g. "Multiplex Real time PCR developed by University of Tenesse, US, PathoProof™ Mastitis PCR Assay from Finnzymes Oy, Finland etc.

References

Allore, H.G. (1999). Buffalo Bull., 18(4): 82-85.

Baker, J.C. and Breed, R.S. (1920). New York Agri. Expt. Sta. Tech. Bull., 80, pp. 239-155.

Baker, J.C., and Van Slyke, L.L. (1919). J. Biol. Chem., 40: 357.

Barkema, H.W., Van Der Schans, J., Schukken, Y.H., De Gee, A.L.W., Lam, T.J.G.M. and Benedictus, G. (1997). J. Dairy Sci., 80: 422-426.

Bartlett, P.C., Miller, G.Y., Anderson, C.R. and Kirk, J.H. (1990). J. Dairy Sci., 73: 2794–2800.

Beckley, M.S. and Johnson, T. (1966). J. Dairy Sci., 49: 746.

Bhikane, A.V. and Kawitkar, S.B. (2000). Hand book for Veterinary Clincian.Venkatesh Books. Udgir, India.

Blackburn, P.S. (1966). J. Dairy Res., 33: 193-198.

Bodoh, G.W., Battista, W.J., Schultze, L.H. and Johnston, R.P. (1976). J. Dairy Sci., 59: 1119.

Brolund, L. (1985). Kiel. Milchwirtsch. Forschungsber. 37: 286.

Buswell, J. (1995). In Practice. p. 426-432.

Bytyqi, H., Zaugg, U., Sherifi, K., Hamidi, A., Gjonbalaj, M., Muji, S. and Mehmeti, H. (2010). Veterinarski Archiv, 80(2): 173-183

CBMRN fact sheet(2008-09). In the world of mastitis research. What is new? www.mastitisnetwork.org, in the Toolbox section.

Dairyman's Digest (2009). What you should know about somatic cells. Winter issue.

Dang, A.K. and Anand, S.K. (2007). Livest. Res. Rural Develop., 19 (6).

Davis, L.G. (1999). Milk testing (The laboratory control of milk). Agrobotanical publishers, Bikaner, India.

Dohoo, I.R. and Meek, A.H. (1982). Can. Vet. J., 23(4): 119-125.

Dua, Kirti (2001). Indian Dairyman. 53: 41-48.

Eberhart, R.J., Gilmore, H.C., Hutchison, L.J. and Spencer, S.B. (1979). In: Proc. Nat. Mast. Coun., Inc., Arlington, VA. pp. 32-40.

Emanuelson, U., Danell, B.and Philipsson, J. (1988). J. Dairy. Sci., 71: 467-476.

Erdem, H., Atasever, S. and Kul, E. (2010). Asian J. Anim. Vet. Adv., 5(4): 253-259.

Fay, A.C., Cave, H.W. and Atkeson, F.W. (1938). Cornell Vet., 28: 40.

Forster, T.L., Ashworth, U.S. and Luedecke, L.O. (1967). J. Dairy Sci., 50: 675-682.

Fox, L.K. (1995). Colonization of Staphylococcus aureus on chapped teat skin. In: Proc. 3rd International Mastitis Seminar, Tel Aviv, Israel. pp II 6:51-55.

Francis, P. (1993). In Pract. 15: 288-290.

Galdhar, C.N., Chilgunde, S.N., Gaikwad, R.V., Smad, A. and Roy, S. (2005). J. Remount Vet. Corps, 44(3): 133-140.

Gonzalo, C., Baro, J.A., Carriedo, J.A. and San Primitivo, F. (1993). J. Dairy Sci., 76: 115-119.

Gonzalo, C., Martinez, J.R., Carriedo, J.A. and San Primitivo, F. (2003). J. Dairy Sci., 86: 138-145.

Hamann J. (2002). In: Proc. recent developments and perspectives in bovine medicine, XXII World Buiatrics Congress, Hannover,August 18–23, 2002, pp. 334–345.

Hamann, J. and Gyodi, P. (2000). Milchwissensch. 55: 303-307.

Hanks, J.D. and Biggs, A.M. (2005). In: Proc. British Mastitis Conf., Stoneleigh, pp. 65.

Harmon, R.J. (1994). J. Dairy Sci., 77: 2103-2112.

Hillerton, J.E. (2003). In: Proc. British Mastitis Conf., Garstang. PP. 55-61.

Hillerton, J.E. and Walton, A.W. (1991). Vet. Rec., 128: 513-515.

Hogan. J.S., Smith, K.L., Hoblet, K.H., Todhunter, D.A., Schoenberger. P.S., Hueston, W.D., Pritchard, D.E., Bowman, G.L., Heider, L.E., Brockett, B.L. and Conrad, H.R. (1989). J. Dairy Sci., 72: 250.

International Dairy Federation (1971). A monograph of bovine mastitis.

Jackson, P. (1996). In Pract., 18: 76-80.

Jones, T.O. (1994). Cattle Pract., 2: 55-57.

Jorstad, A., Farver, T.B. and Riemann, H. (1989). Acta Vet. Scand., 30: 239-245.

Kay, S.J., Collins, K.A., Anderson, J.C. and Grant, A.J. (1977). J. Dairy Res., 44: 589-593.

Khate, K. and Yadav, B.R. (2010). Indian J. Anim. Sci., 80(5): 467-69.

Kirk, J.H. (2009). http://www.vetmed.ucdavis.edu/vetext/INF-DA/No-growth.pdf

Klaas, I.C., Enevoldsen, C., Vaarst, M. and Houe, H. (2004). J. Dairy Sci., 87: 1217–1228.

Lee, C.S. and Outteridge, P.M. (1981). J. Dairy Res., 48: 225-237

Lee, C.S., Wooding, F.B.P. and Kemp, P. (1980). J. Dairy Res., 47: 39.

Leigh, J.A. (1999). *Streptococcus uberis*: Vet. J., 157: 225-238.

Lindström, U.B., Kenttämies, H., Arstila, J. and Tuovila, R. (1981). Acta Agric. Scand., 31: 199-203.

Marschke, R.J. and Kitchen, B.J. (1988). J. Dairy Sci., 68: 1263-1269.

McDonald, J.S. and Anderson, A.J. (1981). Am. J. Vet. Res., 42: 1366-1368.

Meek, A.H., Barnum, D.A. and Newbould, F.H.S. (1980). J. Food. Prot., 43: 10-14.

Miller, R.H. and Paape, M.J. (1985). In: Proc. Ann. Mtg. Natl. Mastitis Counc., p. 60.

Miller, R.H., Paape, M.J., Peters, R.R. and Young, M.D. (1990). J. Dairy Sci., 73(7): 1751-1755.

Miller, R.H., Pankey, J.W., Bright, S.A., Bitman, J., Wood, D.L. and Capuco, A.V. (1991). In: Proc. of the USDA, Agricultural Research Service.

Modransky, P. and Welker, B. (1993). Vet. Med., 88: 995-1000.

Mohammad, G, Athar, M, Shakoor, A, Khan, M.Z., Rehman, F and Ahmad, M.T. (1995). Pak. J. Food Sci., 5(3-4): 91-93.

Murphy, J.M. and Hanson, J.J. (1941). Cornell vet., 21: 47-55.

National Mastitis Council (2007). Guidelines for Evaluating Teat Skin Condition. In: Proc. National mastitis conf. on "A Global Organization for Mastitis Control and Milk Quality", July, 2007, 421 South Nine Mound Road, Verona, WI 53593 USA. (www.nmconline.org).

Natzke, R.P., Everett, R.W. and Postle, D.S. (1972). J. Milk Food. Technol., 35: 261-263.

Natzke, R.P., Everett, R.W., Guthrie, R.S., Keown, J.F., Meek, A.M., Merrill, W.G., Roberts, S.J. and Schmidt, G.H. (1972). J. Dairy Sci., 55: 1256-1260.

Nelson, F.E., Tranmal, H., Schuh, J.D., Wegner, T.N. and Stott, G.H. (1969). J. Dairy Sci., 52: 912. (Abstr.)

Nielen, M., Deluyker, H., Schukken, Y. and Brand, A. (1992). J. Dairy Sci., 75: 606-614.

O'Rourke, D.J. and blowey, R.W. (2004). Bulk milk testing and mastitis monitoring. In: Bovine Medicine:Diseases and Husbandry of Cattle, edited by Andrews, A.H., Blowey, R.W., Boyd, H. and Eddy, R.G. (2004), edn. 2nd, Blackwell Publishing Co., pp. 341-350.

Paape, M.J. and Tucker, H.A. (1966). J. Dairy Sci., 49: 265-267.

Paape, M.J. and Weinland, B.T. (1988). J. Dairy Sci., 71: 250-256.

Quinn, P.J., Carter, M.E., Morley, B. and Carter, G.R. (1994). California Mastitis Test (CMT). In: Clinical Veterinary Microbiology. 1st ed., Wolfe Publishing, London.

Radostits, O.M., Gay, C.C., Blood, D.C. and Hinchkliff, K.W. (2000). Veterinary Medicine. 9th edn. ELBS & Baillier Tindall. pp.563-618.

Schalm, O.W., Carrol, E.J. and Jain, N.C. (1971). Bovine Mastitis. Lea and Febiger, Philadelphia, U.S.A.

Schepers, A.J., Lam, T.J., Schukken, Y.H., Wilmink, J.B.M. and Hanekamp, W.J.A. (1997). J. Dairy Sci., 80: 1833-1840.

Schultz, L.H. (1977). J. Am. Vet. Med. Assoc., 170: 1244-1246.

Sharma, Neelesh (2003). Epidemiological investigation on subclinical mastitis in dairy animals: Role of vitamin E and selenium supplementation on its control. MVSc. Thesis, I.G.K.V.V., Raipur (C.G.) India.

Sharma, Neelesh, Gautam, A., Upadhyay, S.R., Hussain, K., Soodan, J.S. and Gupta, S.K. (2006). Ind. J. Field Veterinarian, 2: 73-76.

Sharma, Neelesh, Gupta, S.K., Sharma, U. and Hussain, K. (2007). Buffalo Bulletin, 26(2): 56-58.

Sharma, Neelesh, Maiti, S.K. and Sharma, K.K. (2007). International J. Dairy Sci., 2(2): 145-151.

Sharma, Neelesh, Maiti, S.K. and Sharma, R.K. (2010b). Indian J. Vet. Medicine, 30(1): 42-43.

Sharma, Neelesh, Pandey, V. and Sudhan, N.A. (2010a). Bulg. J. Vet. Med., 13(2): 98-103.

Sharma, Neelesh, Pandey, V. and Upadhyay, S.R. (2009). Indian Dairyman, 61(4): 21-27.

Sharma, Neelesh, Singh, N.K. and Bhadwal, M.S. (2011). Asian-Austra. J. Anim. Sci., 24(3): 429.

Sheldrake, R.F., Hoare, R.J.T. and McGregor, G.D. (1983). J. Dairy Sci., 66: 542-547.

Shook, G.E. (1989). J. Dairy Sci., 72: 1349-1362.

Shoshani, E., Leitner, G., Hanochi, B., Saran, A., Shpigel, N.Y. and Berman, A. (2000). J. Dairy Res., 67: 155-169.

Shukla, P.C. (1980). A study to evaluate the relative sensitivity of some of the indirect diagnostic tests available for detection of sub clinical cases of mastitis. M.V.Sc. & A.H. thesis, J.N.K.V.V., Jabalpur, M.P., India.

Singh, M. (2002). Somatic cell counts during lactation in bovines as a index of subclinical mastitis. In: Proc. all India dairy husbandry officers workshop NDRI, Karnal, 2002. pp. 64-77.

Skrzypek, R., Wójtowski, J. and Fahr, R.D. (2004). J. Vet. Med. A, 51: 127-131.

Smith, K.L., Todhunter, D.A. and Schoenberger, P.S. (1985). J. Dairy Sci., 68: 1531.

Spakauskas, V., Jodkonis, L., Matusevicius, A. and Stankevicius, A. (1998): Acta Veterinaria Baltica., 28-30.

Spakauskas, V., Klimiene, I. and Matusevicius, A. (2006). Vet. Arhiv., 76(2): 101-109.

Wegner, T.N., Schuh, J.D., Nelson, F.E. and Stott, G.H. (1976). J. Dairy Sci., 59: 949-956.

Weller, J.I., Saran, A. and Zeliger, Y. (1992). J. Dairy Sci., 75: 2532-2540.

White, F. and Rattray, E.A.S. (1965). J. Comp. Pathol., 75: 253.

Whiteside, W.H. (1939). Can. Pub. Health J., 30: 44.

❑❑❑

CHAPTER

13

Treatment

Mastitis denotes inflammation within the mammary gland, is one of the most important disease affecting quality and quantity of milk in high yielding dairy animals. It is caused by a diverse number of mastitis pathogens that can present many different clinical presentations to the dairy producers and veterinarians. These presentations range from *sub-clinical* mastitis to severe clinical mastitis. Despite world-wide efforts, mastitis has remained economically the most important disease in dairy cattle. It results in billions of dollars of lost milk production, production of lower quality milk, culled cows and treatment cost. Based on the effects on productivity, international trade, animal welfare and zoonotic risk, mastitis ranked highest, above all other infectious diseases of bovines such as foot and mouth disease, salmonellosis, paratuberculosis and bovine virus diarrhea (Wells *et al.*, 1998). Though, India is a leader of milk production countries, yet the challenge for early diagnosis, treatment, prevention and control of bovine mastitis continues to knock the door of veterinarians.

Approaches to therapy on farm have evolved considerably from the pre-antimicrobial era where symptomatic treatments such as massage, use of embrocations and "stripping out" were all that was available. The discovery of antimicrobials heralded a new era and hopes were that mastitis would be eliminated. However, for the last 60 years in the developed world, nearly half of all dairy animals contract mastitis at least once per lactation. Therefore, it is still true today that one of the most practical mastitis treatment decisions most dairy producers, milking personnel and veterinarians make is the choice of whether to use antibiotics at all to treat mastitis, which antibiotic if any, and the dose, route and duration of treatment.

Over the last few decades, efforts have been directed towards improving treatment efficacy, owing to the high frequency of clinical mastitis and the demand for high quality milk. Normally before going to treatment of mastitis, the question is arises that- why should I treat? In answer of this question, a common belief is that treatment will result in a benefit to the cow or herd (health, welfare gain) and ultimately benefit the dairy farmer.

Prevention of mastitis is the most effective strategy to control mastitis but effective treatment is necessary for production of high quality milk. Although, India has the top rank in milk production but milk quality is below expectations. Effective and economical mastitis control programmes rely on prevention rather than treatment. Treatment is required when a cow is obviously sick but in many instances, treatment of mastitis is voluntary. Many mild cases of clinical mastitis appear to resolve spontaneously and milk from cows with *sub-clinical* mastitis appears normal or may be sold. Research has shown that spontaneous recovery occurs in about 20 to 50 per cent of confirmed infections. Most spontaneous recoveries occurs in quarters with mild or recent infections and only rarely in the case of well established or chronic infections. It is likely that soon after an infection is established, changes in the cow's immune system take place in an attempt to eliminate the infecting microorganisms. Just after introduction of infecting organism, leukocyte numbers as well as their antimicrobial activity to become elevated, and with the help of antibodies locally produced in the udder, function to overcome the infection. Treatment of mild cases of clinical mastitis should be considered when the probability of cure is high, the rate of recurrence is expected to decrease with treatment and a financial benefit to the farm is expected.

Acute clinical mastitis affects dairy cows throughout the world and has a substantial impact on farm economics, milk quality and cow welfare. Dairy producers and veterinarians must make, clinical mastitis treatment decisions or recommendations on a frequent basis. Despite more than a century of research and tremendous amount of field experience, clinical mastitis remains a frustrating disease to treat. Some cows die, become agalactic, or fail to return to profitable milk production despite aggressive and expensive treatment. The outcome of clinical mastitis is influenced by a variety of factors, including the effectiveness of the cow's immune response, the severity of mastitis at the onset of treatment, the duration of infections at the onset of treatment, the causative pathogen, and the drug regimens and ancillary measures used.

Treatment of mastitis should be based on bacteriological diagnosis, clinical signs and take national and international prudent use guidelines into account. It is time to critically evaluate clinical mastitis treatment practices on dairy farms, identify reasons for treatment failures, and make biologically- plausible, evidence based treatment recommendations.

The treatment of mastitis can be highly effective in removing infection from quarter and returning the milk to normal composition. The best indicators of treatment efficacy are increased feed intake, improved milk production; additional milk marketed and reduced health or early culling rates. Treatment regimen will differ for mild, moderate and severe episodes of clinical mastitis, and for mastitis caused by different pathogens.

The objectives of therapy

The objectives of mastitis therapy have been summarized by International Dairy Federation (Hillerton, 1998):-

1. To cure clinical mastitis and ensure the most rapid limitation of pain and discomfort to the infected animal.
2. To eliminate infection, prevent recurrence of disease and limit spread of infection to uninfected quarters of the same animal and the rest of the herd.
3. To restore milk quality, making it free from bacteria and reducing the leukocyte content (SCC), as rapidly and completely as possible.
4. To minimize the impact of disease, and curative methods, on food production methods and consumer.
5. To maximize the durability and maintain the effectiveness of therapeutic method.

The basic tenet of all of this is that we have to treat mastitic cows rapidly and effectively to minimize suffering. The obligations of all involved in caring for animals, producing milk and consuming products must include the acceptance that treating mastitis is primarily a welfare issue, and that other matters must be secondary.

The term "*cure*" means disappearance of clinical signs, elimination of the infectious cause, or both of those plus returns to normal function and productivity. In other terms- mammary gland quarters that have an intramammary infection caused by a particular pathogen before but not have an intramammary infection caused by the same pathogen after treatment would be defined as "*cured*".

The complete cure is required a quick attention and use of appropriate drugs with sufficient dose and duration of therapy. Take the statement *"early treatment is crucial to get the best chance of success"*. Early can be taken as "at the first signs of abnormality". For clinical mastitis this would be visible changes e.g. swollen and hot quarter(s), clots or flaks in milk. For sub-clinical mastitis this would require laboratory tests e.g. California mastitis test positive, elevation of SCC, isolation of organism from milk. Early diagnosis and the prompt application of appropriate treatment will reduce the extent of mammary tissue damage and will increase the rate of recovery and the return of milk production to or approaching the original level. In 1987, Nocard and Mollerean pointed out that chronic bovine mastitis is an infectious disease caused by streptococci and attempted treatment by injecting a 4% solution of boric acid through intramammary route. Since that time, many different chemicals, both simple and complex, have been administered orally, subcutaneously, intravenously, and by direct infusion into the udder, as curative for the disease.

There are three areas of therapeutic mastitis control strategies:-

I. Treatment of acute clinical mastitis

II. Treatment of chronic and *sub-clinical* mastitis and,

III. Prophylaxis at drying off.

Although various measures and management practices can be effective, there is still a great need for efficient measures against *per-acute, acute* and *sub-clinical* mastitis. Currently these measures include antimicrobials, anti-inflammatory agents, and supportive therapy. Efficacious and economical treatment of mastitis is therefore an important component of livestock medicine. A major treatment breakthrough came in 1945 through the widespread use of penicillin, supplemented in later years by other antibiotics. Further advances since then have been through improved hygiene and management practices.

Antimicrobial Therapy

The microbial world is highly competitive as various microorganisms bid for the substrates that are required for survival, growth and the establishment of climax populations. The choice of a suitable anti-microbial agent is very difficult. Antibiotics are complex organic chemicals synthesized by microorganisms during their growth and which, in minute quantities, have a detrimental effect on other organisms. These chemical compounds are the metabolic products of bacteria and fungi. Most commonly, antibiotics are effective against bacteria but some have activity against viruses, rickettsia, mycoplasma, fungi and helminthes.

"Chemotherapy" can be defined as the use in the treatment of disease of pure chemicals that have a special antagonistic effect(s) on the organisms causing the disease. Antibiotics used in dairy cattle production primarily to treat or prevent disease and to a lesser extent to increase milk production or improve feed efficiency. Thus, antibiotic use in dairy production can be classified as *therapeutic* (treatment of an existing disease condition), *prophylactic* (administration during conditions of disease risk) or *sub-therapeutic* (administration for enhanced production) (McAllister *et al.*, 2001).

The first recorded use of antibiotic in dairy cattle was for the treatment of mastitis (Foley *et al.*, 1946) and this disease still accounts for the majority of antibiotic use in lactating dairy cattle. Despite the widespread use of antibiotics for over 60 years, mastitis is an extremely common disease in most dairy farms and consensus about the most efficient, safe, and economical treatment is still lacking. No antibiotic is completely effective at killing all target bacteria within the complex microbial communities that are frequently encountered within dairying.

There are some pros and cons of antibiotic therapy (Biggs, 2002).

The Pros

1. Increased chance of treatment success particularly with Gram positive organisms.
2. Reduced excretion of bacteria in milk and reduced spread within herd, which impacts on bulk milk somatic cell counts (BMSCC) and payment penalties.
3. More rapid resolution of clinical signs, more return of milk to bulk tank and avoidance of yield depression.
4. Improved milk quality.
5. Reduced chance of recurrence of infection.

The Cons

1. The cost of treatment (drugs).
2. Cost of milk discard especially significant in high yielding (fresh calved) cows.
3. Risk of contamination of milk supply.
4. Theoretical risk of increased antibiotic resistance.
5. Aspirations to magic bullet rather than husbandry and management to control mastitis.

6. May not significantly affect outcome especially in mild Gram negative infections.

The basic considerations before antibiotic therapy

Antimicrobial therapy is pivotal for its containment and recovery. Despite the wide spread use of these drugs, antimicrobial treatment of mastitis in general has been less effective than desirable. Generally, in the treatment of mastitis, practitioners select antibiotic depending upon availability, cost and occasionally by *in vitro* sensitivity testing, without considering the physiological properties, and pharmacokinetic of drug. The usual strategy during use of antimicrobial drugs in the treatment of mastitis is to select an appropriate antibiotic, which can achieve level in excess of the known minimum inhibitory concentration (MIC) and maintain it for an adequate period.

(1) The selection of antibiotic

The choice of a suitable antibiotic is very difficult task for veterinary practitioner. There are numerous factors to consider when selecting an antimicrobial agent, and the route (parenteral or intramammary) to use, for the treatment of mastitis. The site of infection needs to be located and the type of microbe established. Then the *in-vitro* antimicrobial sensitivity of the organism and the minimal inhibitory concentration need to be determined. The likely ability to penetrate the area, the action of the antibiotic in the local environment and the maintenance of an effective concentration at the area must be considered. The selection also has to include the possibility of any potential toxic side effects as well as meat and milk withholding times (Andrews, 2004). Once all these factors have been taken into consideration, the drug to be used, its dosage, route and frequency of administration can be determined.

Antimicrobial sensitivity testing

Although useful as a guideline for antimicrobial selection, *in-vitro* antibiotic testing does not guarantee the efficacy of an antibiotic *in-vivo*. In general, an organism sensitive *in-vitro* may be sensitive *in-vivo*, but one resistant *in-vitro* is also likely to be resistant *in-vivo*. Pre-treatment collection and examination of a milk sample is a particularly useful aid in selecting an anti-microbial for empirical treatment, which should commence at this time. Antibiotic resistance is the ability of bacteria to grow and multiply in the presence of an antibiotic. Resistance develops in bacteria with genes enabling them to produce proteins that protect against the effects of the antibiotic molecule.

Six methods have been used to determine the susceptibility of bovine mastitis pathogens to antimicrobial agents (Constable and Morin, 2003): (1)

broth dilution, (2) milk dilution, (3) agar dilution, (4) minimum bactericidal concentration (MBC) determination, (5) determination of killing kinetics, and (6) agar diffusion method. The first five methods are quantitative, whereas the agar diffusion method is qualitative. Because of issues related to cost and complexity of each testing procedure, the broth micro dilution method is the recommended *"gold standard"* method for *in-vitro* susceptibility testing, whereas agar diffusion provides a crude, inexpensive, and clinically practical method for determining *in-vitro* susceptibility.

Agar diffusion method is most commonly used for *in-vitro* testing including in India. This method is also known as "Kirby-Bauer method". The test procedure of this method has changed little since Bauer and associates standardized the method in 1966 (Bauer *et al.*, 1966; Anonymous, 1999). In brief, 3 to 10 representative bacterial colonies are selected from a blood agar plate and suspended in a fixed volume of sterile 0.9% NaCl to achieve the turbidity of a 0.5 McFarlane standard; the suspension is then spread evenly across the surface of an agar plate using a sterile cotton swab. Small circular discs of filter paper or tablets impregnated with antimicrobial agents are placed on the agar plate using flamed forceps or a special applicator and gently pressed down to ensure contact (Bauer *et al.*, 1966). The agar plate is selected based on the bacterial species being tested (for mastitis pathogens, Mueller-Hinton medium is used for susceptibility testing of *Streptococcus* spp. and *Corynebacterium* spp.) and is incubated at 37°C over night. During incubation, antibiotics dissolve from the filter paper or tablets into the surrounding agar and thereby inhibit bacterial growth. The diameter of the zone of inhibition is measured in millimeters (Figure 13.1) and categorized as sensitive (S), intermediate (I) and resistant (R) levels. Sensitive levels (S) imply an effective amount of drug can be obtained at the target tissue using normal label dosage (relative to the MIC of the bacterial agent), Intermediate (I) levels imply that MIC level can be reached at maximal dose ranges or in tissues where drugs may be physiologically accumulated, Resistant (R) levels imply that concentration of drug needed can not be reached reliability with normal dosage schemes or that the drug can not consistently reach the target tissue at sufficient MIC levels. The diameter of zone of inhibition is also correlated in some manner with the MIC for the bacteria (Anonymous, 2000).

Interpretative zone diameters differ for each antibiotic (Figure 13.1) because of differences in MIC and the diffusion and solubility of the antibiotic in Muller-Hinton medium. In other words, the antibiotic with the largest diameter for the zone of inhibition is not necessarily the antibiotic of choice for treating the mastitis episode (Bauer *et al.*, 1966). Isolation and antibiotic sensitivity test should be routinely taken up and appropriate treatment carried out. Even the same bacterial species isolated from different animals would be sensitive to different antibiotics. Sensitivity varies from the isolates made from the same animal at different times of mastitis attack (Tijare *et al.*, 2000). Hence, no accurate inference can be drawn from the past data, but can help to some extent for short period or till fresh result. Therefore routine isolation and sensitivity tests are necessary for excellent treatment results.

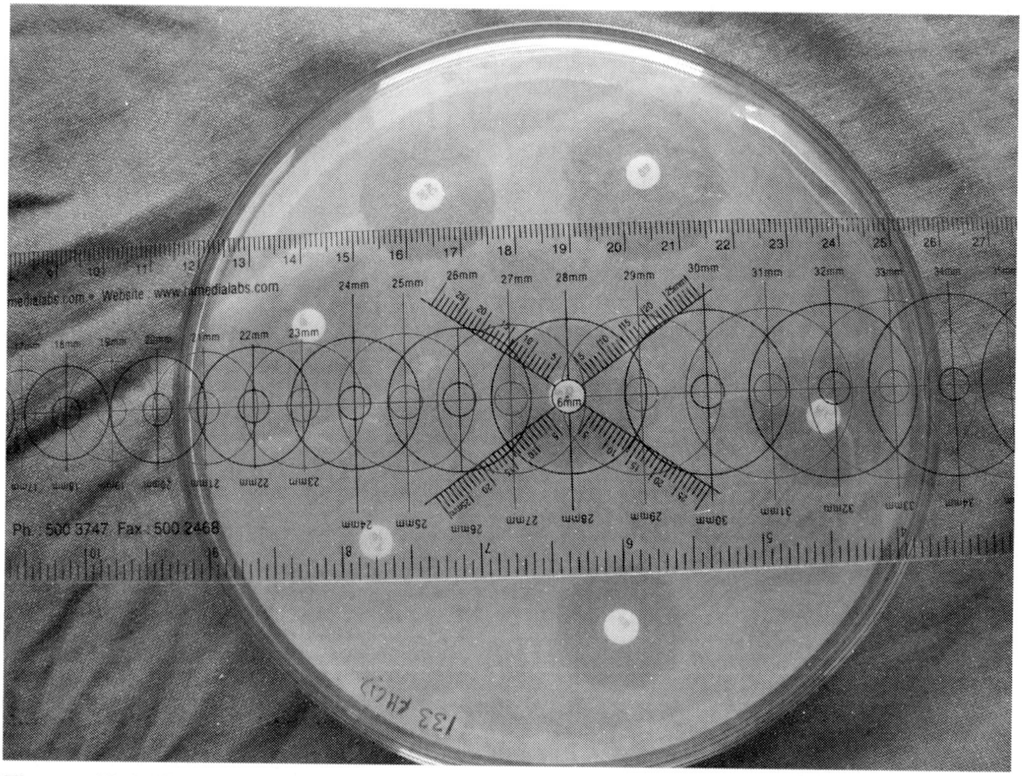

Figure 13.1: Photograph showing the antibiotic zone of inhibition and measuring the inhibition zone diameter with measuring scale.

There is need to be understood the basic concepts or terminology when interpreting the results of susceptibility testing. These terms are defined as:

[A] Minimum inhibitory concentration (MIC)

Minimum inhibitory concentration is the lowest antibiotic concentration (expressed in mg/ml or mg/ml) that under defined *in-vitro* conditions (usually on broth or on agar plates) prevents the growth of bacteria within a defined period of time (Anonymous, 2000). Statistics such as MIC_{50} and MIC_{90} are frequently used to summarize population data. The MIC_{50}, is the median MIC for all isolates and MIC_{90} is the MIC value that exceeds or equals the MIC for 90% of the isolates. In simple words, MIC_{50} means the lowest concentration of drug that inhibits growth of 50% of isolates and MIC_{90} means the lowest concentration of drug that inhibits growth of 90% of isolates. The data of MIC_{90} of various antibiotics for common mastitis pathogens are given in Table 13.1, 13.2 and 13.3. The data of MIC_{50} and MIC_{90} of some antibiotics for CNS at drying off and at calving is given in table 13.4. Selecting a substance with a low MIC value for the target pathogens is preferable, in particular if antimicrobials are used systemically (Prescott *et al.*, 2000).

Antimicrobials can be divided in *concentration-dependent* and *time-dependent* drugs. In first group (e.g. aminoglycosides and fluoroquinolones) concentration of several times of the MIC for the target organisms at the infection site increase the efficacy. In the later group (e.g. penicillins and macrolides) the efficacy depends on the time, during which the concentration exceeds MIC but high concentrations do not increase efficacy (Prescott *et al.*, 2000). The antimicrobial should preferably have bactericidal action, as phagocytosis is impaired in the mammary gland (Kehrli and Harp, 2001). An ideal drug for mastitis therapy should have a low MIC for mastitis pathogens.

[B] Break-point

Break points are specific MIC values used to assign bacteria to one of three categories- susceptible (sensitive), intermediate and resistant. The intermediate category indicates a MIC value that is close to the break point. The more important, the break points currently recommended for most antibiotics (Anonymous, 1999) are based on achievable serum and interstitial fluid concentrations in humans after oral or intravenous antibiotic administration. The relevance of these break points to achievable milk concentrations in lactating dairy cows after intramammary, subcutaneous, intramuscular or intravenous administration is dubious at best.

[C] Minimum bactericidal concentration (MBC)

MBC is the lowest concentration of an antibiotic that under defined laboratory conditions reduces by 99.99% (three log-reduction) the number of organisms in a medium containing a defined bacterial inoculum within a defined period of time.

Sensitivity pattern of some commonly used antibiotics against most common mastitis pathogens is given in table 13.5.

Table 13.1: Data of MIC_{90} (µg/ml) for *Staphylococcus aureus* from dairy cows.

Antibiotic	MIC_{90} (µg/ml) References								
	Jones *et al.* (1967)	DeOliveira *et al.* (2000)	Frankin & Rantzien, (1983)	Gentilini *et al.* (2000)	Watts and Salmon, (1997) β-lact (+)	Watts and Salmon, (1997) β-lact (-)	Owens *et al.* (1997)	Schaeren & Schaellibaum (1993)	Schaeren & Schaellibaum (1993)
Penicillin	>100	0.5	0.25	1.5	16.0	0.25	0.125	10.10#	33.30
Ampicillin	-	1.0	0.5	-	4.0	0.5	-	-	-
Cloxacillin	0.07	-	-	-	-	-	0.5	0.22	0.40
Oxacillin	-	1.0	0.25	0.5	1.0	0.25	-	-	-
Streptomycin	5.0	-	8.0	-	-	-	-	-	-
Tetracycline	0.6	-	2.0	-	-	-	-	-	-
Ceftiofur	-	1.0	-	-	1.0	1.0	2.0	-	-
Cephalothin*	-	1.0	-	0.75	0.5	0.25	0.25	1.21	-
Neomycin	-	2.0	8.0	-	-	-	-	0.39	0.55
Novobiocin	1.25	-	-	-	-	-	0.5	-	-
Pirlimycin	-	1.0	-	-	64.0	0.5	1.0	-	-
Erythromycin**	-	0.5	0.5	0.75	64.0	0.5	0.5	3.21	3.46

* or Cephapirin / Cefoperazone, ** or Spiramicin, # β-lactamse positive

Table 13.2: Data of MIC_{90} (µg/ml) for *Streptococcus uberis and Streptococcus dysgalactiae*[?] from dairy cows.

Antibiotic	MIC_{90} (µg/ml) References						
	Rossitto *et al.* (2002)	Salmon *et al.* (1998)	Owens *et al.* (1997)	Schaeren & Schaellibaum (1993)	Brown & Scasserra, (1990)	Schaeren & Schaellibaum (1987)	Schifferli *et al.* (1984)
Penicillin	0.25 (0.6)	2.0	0.125 (≤ 0.06)	0.11	≤ 1 (≤ 1)	0.25	0.07
Ampicillin	0.5 (0.6)	2.0	-	-	-	-	-
Cloxacillin	-	-	4 (0.5)	0.45	-	0.87	0.25
Oxacillin	1 (1)	16.0	-	-	-	-	-
Tetracycline	16 (16)	-	-	-	32 (8)	-	-
Ceftiofur	2 (0.25)	1.0	0.5 (1)	-	-	-	-
Cephalothin*	1 (1)	8.0	0.25 (0.25)	0.58	-	-	-
Gentamicin	-	-	-	3.33	-	3.13	-
Novobiocin	-	-	4 (2)	-	-	-	-
Pirlimycin	8(0.25)	4.0	-	-	-	-	-
Erythromycin**	8 (0.25)	4.0	1 (0.25)	0.34	256 (4)	0.16	0.27
Chloramphenicol	-	-	-	3.30	-	2.50	3.25

≤ Values listed are for *Streptococcus uberis* and in bracket for *Streptococcus dysgalactiae* respectively.
* or Cephapirin / Cefoperazone, ** or Spiramicin,

Table 13.3: Data of MIC_{90} (mg/ml) for Coliforms.

Antibiotic	References		
	Schaeren and Schaellibaum (1993)	Schaeren and Schaellibaum (1987)	Schifferli *et al.* (1984)
Penicillin	2.42	3.22	2.26
Streptomycin	-	-	3.51
Gentamicin	0.45	0.52	0.63
Neomycin	0.45	1.11	1.15
Tetracycline	-	-	1.81
Cefoperazone	0.48	-	-
Norfloxacin	≤0.07	-	-
Chloramphenicol	2.58	5.33	5.68
Cotrimoxazole	0.64	2.87	1.42

Table 13.4: Data of MIC_{50} and MIC_{90} (mg/ml) for CNS at drying-off and at calving.

Antibiotic	MIC_{50} (μg/ml)		MIC_{50} (μg/ml)		
	Dry-off	Calving*	Dry-off	Calving	
				Untreated	Treated
Ampicillin	≤ 0.12	≤ 0.12	0.5	0.5	0.5
Ceftiofur	≤ 0.5	≤ 0.5	1.0	1.0	1.0
Cephalothin	≤ 2.0	≤ 2.0	16.0	8.0	16.0
Erythromycin	≤ 0.25	≤ 0.25	>4.0	>4.0	>4.0
Oxacillin	≤ 2.0	≤ 2.0	4.0	≤ 2.0	4.0
Penicillin	≤ 0.12	≤ 0.12	1.0	0.5	1.0
Penicillin-novobiocin	≤ 1.0/2.0	≤ 1.0/2.0	4.0/8.0	2.0/4.0	4.0/8.0
Pirlimycin	≤ 0.5	≤ 0.5	2.0	4.0	4.0
Sulphadimethoxine	≤ 32	64	>256.0	>256.0	>256.0
Tetracycline	≤ 1.0	≤ 1.0	>8.0	>8.0	8.0

* At calving there were no differences in MIC_{50}'s between isolates from treated and untreated cows.

Table 13.5: Antibiotic sensitivities of selected bacteria isolated from clinical and sub-clinical bovine mastitis (reported as percent of isolates sensitive).

Antibiotic	Common pathogens					References
	Staphylococcus spp.	*Streptococcus* spp.	*E. coli*	*Corynebacterium* spp.	*Bacillus* spp.	
Enrofloxacin	20.34	25.00	25.00	22.22	-	Sharma *et al.* (2007)
	93.65[2]	83.33[3]	-	100.00	100.00	Sebastian and Vijayakumar (2002)
	100.00[2]	97.14[3]	100.00	100.00	-	
						Akhtar *et al.* (2003)
Cefotaxime	25.42	35.00	18.75	55.55	-	Sharma *et al.* (2007)
Penicillin G	23.73	R	-	-	R	Sarode (2002)
Ampicillin	16.95	R	00.00 (R)	00.00 (R)	-	Sharma *et al.* (2007)
	80.50[1], 68.80[2]	86.4[3], 83.30[4]	-	-	-	Baranski *et al.* (2008)
Teteracycline	20.34	15.00	12.50	22.22	-	Sharma *et al.* (2007)
	21.90[1], 6.20[2]	27.30[3], 5.50[4]	-	-	-	Baranski *et al.* (2008)
	75.00[2]	60.00[3]	90.00	50.00	-	
Gentamicin	13.56	10.00	31.25	R	-	Sharma *et al.* (2007)
	1.69	37.50	-	-	R	Sarode (2002)
	75.00[2]	71.42[3]	100.00	50.00	-	Akhtar *et al.* (2003)
Chloramphenicol	16.95	15.00	12.50	R	-	Sharma *et al.* (2007)
	32.73	50.00	-	-	100.00	Sarode (2002)
	93.65[2]	100.00[3]	100.00	-	100.00	Sebastian and Vijayakumar (2002)

R= Resistant, 1- CNS, 2- *Staphylococcus aureus*, 3- *Streptococcus agalactiea*, 4- *Streptococcus uberis*

The advent of antimicrobial drugs has resulted in the emergence of resistance to these drugs (Table 13.6). The sensitivity pattern is vary locally according to commonly and blind use of antibiotic. The use of antibiotics in therapeutic concentration results in an alteration of the microflora within the host (Andrews, 2004).

Table 13.6: Penicillinase (b-lactamase) active antibiotics.

Penicillins	Cloxacillin, Methicillin
Cephalosporins	Cephalexin, Cefoperazone, Cephalonium, Cephalothin. Cephaloridine,
Macrolids	Erythromycin, Oleandamycin, Spiramycin, Tylosin
Aminoglycosides	Gentamicin, Kanamycin, Amikacin, Neomycin
Fluoroquinolones	Enrofloxacin, Danofloxacin, Marbofloxacin
Nitrofurans	Nitrofurazone, Furazolidone, Nitrofurantoin
Others	Chloramphenicol, Bacitracin, Novobiocin, Licomycin, Sulphonamides, Trimethoprim.

Spontaneous mutation of organisms can occur it is probably only of limited importance in practice. However, transferable drug resistance is of significance. The main mechanism of development or transfer of resistance is through plasmids or transposons, is transferred to susceptible strains. Antibiotic sensitivity test results must be correlated with clinical and bacteriologic cure rates to confirm the validity of the assigned break points (Anonymous, 2000). *In-vitro* antimicrobial susceptibility test results have been suspected to be poorly correlated with treatment outcome for clinical mastitis by many investigators (Owens *et al.*, 1993; Pyorala and Pyorala, 1998; Pearson, 1964; Sandholm *et al.*, 1990) and the value of the agar diffusion method to guide mastitis treatment decisions has been questioned (Sandholm *et al.*, 1990). Myllys *et al.* (1992) concluded that "susceptibility testings in artificial media can not simulate what happens in mammary gland milk phase and as themselves can not predict the outcome of therapy".

(2) Clinical efficacy of antibiotics

In mastitis, it has been observed that the clinical efficacy of drug varies in response among herds and within herds due to the type of organisms involved, location of infection, degree of udder damage, physicochemical properties and kinetics of antibacterials employed for treatment, route of administration and sensitivity of udder pathogens.

The best antibiotic treatment regimen is simple; it must deliver the drug at a dose and site that will allow accumulation in the mammary gland [*pharmacokinetics*]. This requires identifying the pathogen and it's MIC [*sensitivity*] so that an effective drug concentration is maintained [*pharmacodynamics*] (Edmondson, 1989). The success of any antibacterial depends on achieving a drug concentration at the site of infection which is sufficient to inhibit the bacterial growth. Generally, we rely on culture sensitivity tests for the selection of anti-bacterials, but there are some doubts regarding *in-vitro* susceptibility tests and many consider they correlate poorly with the outcome of therapy *in-vivo* for bovine mastitis. This is in part due to the lack of pharmacokinetic data on the compatibility of drugs with milk, concentrations at the site of infection and interactions with endogenous inhibitors (Owens *et al.*, 1990a; Sandholm *et al.*, 1990). There are various factors which affect the efficacy of drug (antibiotic) in the treatment of mastitis.

(I) Targeting sites of antimicrobial therapy

In antibiotic therapy, the bacteria can be considered to be a receptor and the site of action may or may not be localized in a single compartment of the body (Garret, 1978). The pharmacological goal of antibacterial therapy is to attain effective concentrations of the drug at the site of the infection. Within the udder there are a number of sites where bacteria involved in mastitis may be found. When we consider the three sites we need to target within an udder the choice of antibiotic becomes important.

For bovine mastitis, there are three potential therapeutic targets, or pharmacological compartments (Erskine *et al.*, 2003):-

A. Mammary system
B. Parenchyma
C. Cow

(A) Mammary system

This is the most common targeted compartment, and consists of the milk and the epithelial lining of the ducts and alveoli of the mammary gland. The mastitis pathogens that typically reside in this compartment are generally non-invasive and are not believed to cause abscess formation in the parenchyma. The organisms reside in this compartment are *S. agalactiae*, *S. dysgalactiae*, CNS, *E. coli* and perhaps other Gram positive cocci of short duration (Table 13.7). *E. coli* is found in the milk with the clinical signs and udder damage being caused by the production of toxins. Thus, these organisms would be appropriately targeted via the intramammary route of therapy that attained effective concentrations in milk. However, there are some hitches to intramammary route of administration. Elimination of the drug from the milk compartment during routine milking, especially in animals that milk more than twice daily, may reduce concentrations in milk below effective levels when dose frequency remains according to product label instructions. Two exceptions to this are Pirlimycin and, most recently Ceftiofur. Available data suggests that effective concentrations of both can be maintained with once-a-day dosig despite milking three times per day (Erskine *et al.*, 2003).

Table 13.7: Where to target antibiotic therapy in mastitis due to different pathogens (Erskine *et al.*, 2003).

Mastitis pathogen	Pharmacological compartment		
	Milk/Ducts	Parenchyma	Cow
S. agalactiae	+ + +	– –	– –
Streptococcal spp.	+ + +	+	– –
S. aureus	+	+ + +	– –
Staphylococcal spp.	+ + +	– –	– –
Coliforms	+	– –	+ + +
Maycoplasma and other Gram positives	– –	– –	+ + +

(B) Parenchyma

This compartment comprises deep tissue of the mammary gland. The bacteria reside in this compartment are *S. aureus* and *S. uberis*. *S. aureus* is found inside macrophages in the milk and within udder tissue as well as potentially being engulfed by cells lining the teat and lactiferous sinuses during the early dry period. Fibrin cysts and microabscess formation interfere with distribution of intramammary infused drugs to the site of infection in the terminal alveoli. The *S. aureus* can grow a shaggy, slimy coat when in milk and avoid the attentions of patrolling white blood cells or macrophages.

(C) Cow

The cow/buffalo is the 3rd compartment for the mastitis therapy target. Recent studies have suggested that the primary target for treatment of severe coliform mastitis should be the 3rd compartment of mastitis therapy. Bacteremia can occur as a consequence of coliform mastitis and reported good results by parenteral therapy with Oxytetracycline and Ceftiofur (Wenz *et al.*, 2001a; Erskine *et al.*, 2002).

(II) Type of organisms involved

Even experienced veterinarians can not accurately predict the organism responsible for an episode of clinical mastitis on the basis of clinical signs. For higher efficacy of antibiotic, it is must to know the type of organism causing the mastitis at herd. There are various types of organisms (e.g. Bacteria, fungi, yeast, viruses etc.) are cause the intramammary infection. For details of individual mastitis causing organisms refer the etiology chapter of this book. A cow with a swollen mammary gland and clots in the milk might be infected with *S. uberis, E. coli, S. aureus, Mycoplasma bovis, Prototheca zopfi* or a number of other pathogens, the effectiveness of antibiotic treatment would vary markedly depending on the causing pathogen. Certain mastitis causing pathogens, such as Mycoplasma, Prototheca, Nocardia, Pseudomonas, and yeast are non-responsive or poorly responsive to antibiotics. Antibiotic therapy would be expected to fail and should be avoided in these cases. Hence, the importance of knowing the pathogens causing clinical mastitis in the herd. On the other hand, resolution of mastitis caused by *Streptococcus* spp. is enhanced when intramammary antibiotics are used, and antibiotic therapy should not be avoided in such cases.

In some herds, it is feasible to culture milk from all cows with clinical mastitis before initiating treatment; for mild episodes of clinical mastitis, waiting upto 24 hours for culture results before beginning treatment is unlikely to be detrimental to the outcome. In herds in which culturing each cow is not practical, it is still important to determine the pathogens most frequently responsible for clinical mastitis, so that appropriate treatment and prevention recommendation can be made (Morin, 2004a).

(III) Duration of therapy

The duration and time interval (gape between two subsequent injections) of antimicrobial treatment also play major role in the cure rate of clinical mastitis. In general terms, most antibiotic injections used for 3 to 5 days and for atleast one day after normality is reached. One reason for poor cure rate in mastitis therapy is probably the short duration of standard treatments. Unfortunately, many intramammary preparations have very short treatment lengths in the approved claims. Initially treatment protocols were treat once, repeat after 24 to 48 hours if no improvement was seen. Inter-treatment intervals were commonly 24 hours (once a day or every other milking) but more recently have tended to reduce to 12 hours (twice a day or every milking) (Biggs, 2002). It has been shown that experimental *S. uberis* infections treated every 12 hours had significantly better clinical cure and bacteriological cure rates than infections treated every 24 hours (Hillerton and Kliem, 2001).

Mastitis due to *S. aureus*, and probably also due to *S. uberis* benefits from a long duration of treatment (Milne *et al.*, 2000) (Table 13.8). Mastitis caused by *S. aureus* is the biggest challenge in mastitis therapy (Knight *et al.*, 2000). Some earlier studies have reported on better efficacy of a long treatment on *S. aureus* mastitis (Pyorala and Syvajarvi, 1988; Ziv and Storper, 1985), and recent studies have confirmed this efficacy (Pyorala and Pyorala, 1998; Deluyker *et al.*, 2005).

Table 13.8: Pathogen, natural duration of infection and cure rates.

Pathogen	Site of infection in udder	Natural duration of infection	Cure rates during Lactation	Reference
S. aureus	Microabscesses within secretory cells	Long	<35% (chronic infections) Upto 70% (new infections)	Sol *et al.* (1997), Owens *et al.* (1997)
S. agalactiae	Surface of secretory cells	Long	>90%	Erskine and Eberhart (1990)
S. dysgalaciae	Surface of secretory cells	Variable	>75%	Wilson *et al.* (1999)
Strep uberis	Surface of secretory cells, some invasive	Variable	>70%	Hillerton and Kliem (2002)
Coliforms (*E. coli, Klebsiella*)	Surface of secretory cells, sometimes bacteria in blood stream	Short	High rate (>85%) of spontaneous cure	Wilson *et al.* (1999)
CNS	Surface of secretory cells	Variable	High rate (>70%) of spontaneous cure	Wilson *et al.* (1999)
Mycoplasma bovis	Surface of secretory cells, bacteria in blood stream	Long	Very low rate of cure	

In shorter treatment course (and discarded milk less) helping to make this approach more attractive to the dairyman. This is likely to be as a result of practical experience of more and better cure rates with a quicker return to optimum milk quality when treatment frequency or duration is increased. This may reflect a change in emphasis in milk production from quantity to quality (Hillerton and Kliem, 2001).

(3) Pharmacological consideration in antibiotic therapy

Antimicrobials have been the class of drugs most often advocated in clinical practice and research as a therapy for mastitis (Erskine *et al.*, 1989). Bovine mammary gland is difficult target, due to pharmacokinetic and pharmacodynamic problems. Milk should not interfere with the activity of the drug; efficacy of macrolides, tetracyclines and trimethoprime-sulphonamides is reduced in milk. Our goal in selecting the best antimicrobial treatment regimen for mastitis is simple, administer the drug at a dose and site that will allow accumulation in the mammary gland (pharmacokinetics), and identify the pathogen and minimal inhibitory concentration (susceptibility) so that we can maintain effective drug concentrations (pharmacodynamics) (Erskine, 1998).

Despite long history of the use of antimicrobials to treat infections in dairy cows, knowledge of pharmacokinetics of many substances is still limited. Pharmacokinetic of an antimicrobial substance greatly affects its suitability for mastitis treatment. Penetration of a substance into milk when administered parenterally, or absorption and distribution throughout the udder when infused intramammarily depends on its main pharmacokinetic characteristics (Pyorala, 2006). These are lipid solubility, degree of ionization, extent of binding to serum and udder proteins, and the type of vehicle.

In addition to pharmacokinetics, attention should also be paid to pharmacodynamics, which studies the interaction between the bacteria and the drug, and should support pharmacokinetic studies in determining the optimum dosage of the antimicrobials. Very little is known about pharmacodynamics aspect of antimicrobials used in mastitis therapy, because these studies have appeared quite late in veterinary science (Pyorala, 2002). Susceptibility *in-vitro* for the antibiotic used is a pre-requisite for treatment of infections, but efficacy *in-vitro* does not guarantee efficacy *in-vivo*. Pharmacological studies have proven that udder is an extension of extravascular compartment and the extent of distribution of antibiotic largely determines the amount of drug which is to be administered to produce the desired concentration within therapeutic range (Srivastava, 2000).

The following general principles should apply for pharmacologic considerations of mastitis therapy (Erskine *et al.*, 2003):

1. The major factors that have the most influence on therapeutic regimens are the elimination half-life and MIC of the target pathogen for the drug.
2. Especially for antibacterial drugs that have relatively short half-life (<10–12 hours), it is probably better to increase frequency of dosing rather than amount of dose.
3. To attain effective time-dependent killing of microbes, initial therapy should be maintained without switching of antibacterial drugs unless susceptibility testing suggests otherwise.
4. When drugs are administered other than intravenously, a larger dose may be indicated; half-life may be extended, which may impact withholding periods and therapeutic regimens.

Although we have good knowledge regarding the pharmacokinetics of many parenteral antibiotics used to treat clinical mastitis, the majority of the pharmacokinetic data has been obtained in healthy cattle, and it has not been determined whether pharmacokinetic values in healthy cows are the same as those in cows with clinical mastitis. In addition, pharmacokinetic value for many of the intramammary antibiotics used to treat clinical mastitis are unknown and there is limited understanding of the pharmacodynamics of antibiotics in treating mastitis (Constable and Morin, 2003).

Blood-Milk barrier

Following parenteral administration, the therapeutic efficacy of antibiotic will depend mainly on its extent of penetration in udder tissue. Penetration depends on the degree of the pathological process. The location of the organism is also important, that is whether it is intracellular (e.g. *S. aureus*) or extracellular (e.g. *Streptococcus, E coli* etc).

Majority of antibiotics, investigated so far cross blood-milk barrier by passive diffusion and non-ionized fraction of drug is usually more lipid soluble, and easily penetrates through passive diffusion. Drug penetrates the barrier either by diffusion through the lipoprotein region of the membrane or by passing through the aqueous pores. Some antibiotics also enter through some specialized transport process. The ability of an antibiotic to cross biological membranes depends on many factors like- protein binding, lipid solubility, pH of the drug in relation to environmental pH, inflammatory exudates/ barrier of the site, molecular size and in some cases specific cellular transport mechanisms. Antibiotic is absorbed into the circulation, partly becoming bound to plasma protein. Binding varies e.g. from less than 50% with amoxicillin, streptomycin or oxytetracycline to more than 80% with cloxacillin or erythromycin (Andrews, 2004). The plasma protein binding of an antibiotic is an important index to assess the active fraction of drug present in blood and tissue compartments as only unbound or free drug is mainly available to show desired pharmacological action, and also for distribution and renal clearance (Kung *et al.*, 1993). Numerous studies have shown that the *in-vitro* antibacterial activity of an antibiotic in a sample containing plasma is indirectly proportional to the plasma protein level and fraction of antibiotic bound to plasma proteins (Altreuther, 1987). The extent of plasma protein binding of some drugs at therapeutic concentration is given in table 13.9.

Table 13.9: Plasma protein binding of drugs (%) in bovines.

Drug	Extent of binding
Sulphadiazine	24
Sulphisoxazole	76
Sulphadimethoxine	83
Benzyl Penicillin	48
Chloramphenicol	30
Lincomycin	34
Kanamycin	4
Sulphadimidine	55

Water soluble drugs are useful for extracellular organisms and where intracellular organisms have a high turnover rate, usually in the lysis of cells and release of organisms into fluid containing antibiotic.

Lipid solubility does have advantage for organisms that spend most of their time within cells or behind tissue barriers (Andrews, 2004). Both non-polar lipid soluble compounds and polar substances with sufficient lipid solubility passively diffuse through the predominately lipoidal barrier (Baggot, 1977). At a moderate level of milk production the ratio of the volume of blood circulating through the mammary gland to the volume of milk produced has been estimated to be 670:1; this provides ample opportunity for drugs to passively diffuse from the general circulation into milk. The rate of transfer is directly proportional to the concentration gradient across the blood-milk barrier and the lipid solubility of the drug. The milk to plasma equilibrium concentration ratio of total (non-ionized plus ionized) drug is determined by (i) the degree of ionization of the drug, which is pKa/pH dependent, in blood and milk. The proportion of drugs in non-ionized form depends on the dissociation constant (pKa) of the drug and the pH of medium in which it is dissolved, (ii) the charge on the ionized moiety and, (iii) the extent of binding of plasma proteins and milk macromolecules (O'Rourke and Baggot, 2004). It has been shown that only the lipid soluble, non-ionized moiety of a weak organic acid or base that is free (not bound to protein) in the plasma can diffuse through the cellular barriers and enter the milk (Rasmussen, 1966).

The distribution of antibiotics in the body is driven by the physico-chemical characteristics of the antimicrobials and the pH of various body compartments. Effectively the antimicrobials are divided into either acids or bases that accumulate in parts of the body with a complementary pH. Acidic antimicrobials accumulate in parts of the body with a pH above 7.0- the blood, while basic antimicrobials find their way into acidic sites such as tissues and bodily secretions such as tears and milk (Lawrence, 2002). In normal lactating cows (milk pH range 6.5-6.8), weak organic acids attain milk ultrafiltrate-to-plasma ultrafiltrate equilibrium concentration ratios less than 1; while weak organic bases attain milk ultrafiltrate-to-plasma ultrafiltrate equilibrium concentration ratios greater than 1 (Baggot, 2000). In brief, the agents that are predicted to reach the mammary gland more efficiently are *ionized, non-protein bound and lipid soluble.* The data for some important antibacterial drugs commonly used in the treatment with lipid solubility is given in table 13.10.

Table 13.10: Milk : Plasma concentration ratio for some antibiotics used in the treatment of mastitis (Srivastava, 2000).

Antibiotic	Lipid solubility	Concentration ratio between milk and plasma
Organic acids		
Penicillin	Low	0.13 - 0.26
Ampicillin	Low	0.24 - 0.30
Cephaloridine	Low	0.24 - 0.28
Sulphadimethoxine	Moderate	0.21
Sulphadiazine	Moderate	0.59
Weak Bases		
Tylosin	High	3.5
Erythromycin	Very high	8.7
Aminoglycosides	Low	0.5
Trimethoprim	High	2.9
Polymixin	Very low	0.3
Amphoteric		
Oxytetracycline	Moderate	0.75
Doxycycline	Moderate/High	1.53
Alcohol		
Chloramphenicol	High	1.00

The high concentration ratio attained by lipophilic organic bases (Macrolides, Licosamides and Trimethoprime) are attributed to the ion-trapping effect in acidic milk. Enrofloxacin and its active metabolite Ciprofloxacin formed by N-de-ethylation (a microsomal mediated oxidative reaction) in the liver, would be expected to attain concentrations in milk that would be expected to attain concentrations in milk that would be effective against Gram negative aerobic bacteria, in particular *E. coli* (O'Rourke and Baggot, 2004). When the pH of milk is weakly acidic (pH 6.4-6.8), antibiotic that are weak bases (Aminoglycosides, Trimethoprim, Macrolides, Polymyxin-B, Lincosamides) are thought to be preferentially concentrated in the mammary gland by ion-trapping. Milk from clinical mastitis cases can have a slightly alkaline pH (6.9 – 7.2) in the range of serum; thus antibiotics that are weak acids (Penicillins, Cephaloridine, Rifampin, Sulphonamides) may reach effective antibiotic concentrations in milk.

As a consequence the ion-trapping effect on lipophilic organic bases is reduced while the concentrations attained by weak organic acids are somewhat increased. The inflammatory reaction in udder tissues enhances the passage of penicillins into milk. The increased pH of milk does not affect eh concentrations attained by amphoteric drugs (Flouroquinolones, Tetracyclines, Rifampicin), but antimicrobial activity of these drugs is lower in milk than in extracellular fluid (O'Rourke and Baggot, 2004).

In general, choice of an antibiotic and the route of administration are dictated by antibiotic sensitivity, drug distribution, and the pharmacokinetics/ clearance of the active drug or compound (Ziv, 1980a). Generally, we rely on culture sensitivity tests for the selection of antibiotics, but many a times the sensitivity test do not truly predict the *in-vivo* efficacy of the anti-bacterial.

Route of administration

In the antibiotic therapy of mastitis, the most crucial question is the selection of route of administration. The first decision to be made is whether to treat a particular case systematically by parenteral injection or locally by intramammary infusion, or both. After the selection of the best anti-bacterial agent for the particular pathogen which is involved. Presently, two routes of administration i.e. intramammary and parenteral are being routinely used in the treatment of mastitis.

A general suggestion for antibiotic therapy of acute mastitis is to administer both parenteral and intramammary drugs initially if systemic signs are present depending on the severity of infection. Follow-up therapy is often restricted to the intramammary route if systemic signs have abated. Recently it has been pointed out that if parenteral administration of the drug achieves sufficient MIC at the site of injection for desirable period, intramammary infusion of the drug should be discouraged clinically. During intramammary administration, there is always a chance that infusion may cause additional infection and stress to udder tissues. Presently, parenteral administration i.e. intravenous (IV), intramuscular (IM) and subcutaneous (SC) routes are gaining significant importance in the treatment of mastitis in animals. The antibiotics which are quickly absorbed from the site of IM and SC injections, their duration for maintenance of antibacterial concentrations in milk mainly depends on their permeability through the blood-milk brrier, Vd(area), elimination half life and sensitivity to udder pathogens (Srivastava *et al.*, 2002). For effective therapy of mastitis antibiotics must be administered repeatedly for 5-7 days. Intramammary route is somewhat accepted route of choice in the treatment of *sub-clinical* mastitis. However, in acute clinical mastitis, where the udder parenchyma is swollen, and the milk duct system is either compressed or blocked by intramammary exudates, intramammary route may not be very effective and under such circumstances, parenteral route of administration should be preferred.

[1] Intramammary route (IMM)

Intramammary administration of antibiotic for the treatment of mastitis has developed as a preferred route used by bovine veterinary practitioners. This route of administration is appropriate when the therapeutic target includes the second compartment for pharmacologic consideration: the deep tissue of the mammary gland. However, the practical recommendations for the route of treatment are heterogeneous. In Northern Europe, the parenteral route is widely used to treat all types of mastitis, whereas, in other countries including India, it depends more on how the disease is presented, e.g. the parenteral route is often reserved for the treatment of severe clinical mastitis or chronic infections caused by *S. aureus* with bacteria located in the udder parenchyma (Serieys *et al.*, 2005).

The advantages of IMM route are high concentrations of antibiotics achieved in the milk compartment of the mammary gland, and low consumption of the antimicrobial substances as the drug is administered straight to the infection site. The absorption and distribution of individual antibiotic in udder after IMM administration vary from poor to good (Table 13.11). IMM preparations are used, often in combination with parenteral preparations (depending on severity of infection), to treat clinical mastitis and at the end of lactation to treat *sub-clinical* infection and prevent the establishment of new infections during the dry period (O'Rourke and Baggot, 2004).

Intramammary antibiotics are widely used in the treatment of clinical mastitis, but this route has some limitations or disadvantages. Disadvantages could be the uneven distribution of many substances throughout the udder, risk for contamination when infusing the drug via the teat canal, and possible irritation of the mammary tissue caused by the drug. IMM antibiotics distributed unevenly (Table 13.11) in an inflamed gland due to inflammation, swelling, and fibrosis that can block milk ducts, thereby preventing antibiotic diffusion throughout the gland (Owens and Nickerson, 1989; 1990). In addition, the intracellular location of some bacteria such as *S. aureus* means that estimates of *in-vivo* milk phase concentrations may not accurately reflect intracellular concentrations (Owens and Nickerson, 1989). Because antibiotics have variable penetration to the site of infection in mastitis (particularly in chronic infections), it is likely that MIC values determined *in-vitro* do not accurately reflect the *in-vivo* response to therapy (Constable and Morin, 2003).

Table 13.11: Distribution of antibiotics throughout the udder after intramammary administration (Ziv, 1980a).

Good	Moderate	Poor
Amoxycillin	Penicillin-G	Bacitracin
Ampicillin	Cloxacillin	Dihydrostreptomycin
Cephalexin	Cephalonium	Getamicin
Erythromycin	Cephapirin	Neomycin
Novobiocin	Cephacetrile	Polymyxins
Penethamate	Cefquinome	Framycetin
Quinolones	Tetracyclines	
Spiramycin	Other Sulphonamides	
Sulphanilamide		
Tylosin		
Trimethoprim		
Rifamycin		
Amoxycillin-clavulanic acid		
Lincomycin		
Pirlimycin		

Fibrin casts and micro-abscess formation interfere with distribution of infused drugs to the site of infection in the terminal alveoli. Furthermore, the typical 24 hours to 36 hours duration of therapy for intramammary infusions limits the time period of effective concentration in the gland necessary to eliminate more chronic or invasive IMI. It is for these reasons that systemic administration of anti-bacterials has received attention as an adjunct or alternative therapy to IMM therapy.

In addition, some *in-vitro* studies have shown that some antibiotics may disturb phagocytosis in the udder, when given intramammary (Nickerson *et al.*, 1986; Ziv *et al.*, 1983). Sodium Novobiocin had a more pronounced effect on neutrophil phagocytosis and killing than did benzathin cephapirin (Lintner and Eberhart, 1990). Commercial mastitis IMM tubes first became available in the 1960s and 1970s. Initial success suggested 75% cure rates in both lactating and dry preparations. Now numerous IMM products seem to have appeared on the market without supportive scientific data on their efficacy.

Intramammary preparations with combinations of two or even three antibiotics were introduced to mastitis therapy due to suggested synergistic action and to cover all pathogens, including Gram-negative organisms. The evidence of their efficacy against coliform mastitis is still lacking, and synergistic action was never proven in-vivo (Whittem and Hanlon, 1997).

Weakly basic and lipid soluble antibiotics tend to remain in the mammary gland following treatment. The degree of diffusion into glandular tissue is the same when either water or ointment is used as a vehicle for IMM infusion. Intramammary preparations are formulated either to provide quick release of the antimicrobial agent (for lactating cow therapy) or slow release (for dry cow therapy) of the antibiotic over an extended period.

Intramammary preparation for use in lactating cows should contain a readily available form, usually water soluble salt, of an antimicrobial agent with a low degree of binding to milk and mammary tissue proteins. The vehicle used and viscosity of the formulation should allow rapid release of the drug and ensure that effective concentrations are maintained throughout the recommended dosage interval. Quick release intramammary preparations have short withdrawal periods, typically slaughter times of 7 days and milk withholding times of 3 – 5 days or either may be less depending on the preparation (O'Rourke and Baggot, 2004). The intramammary preparations for lactating cow therapy should be with the following characteristic:-

1. Minimal irritation to the udder.
2. Quick release rate from ointment or vehicle base.
3. Low degree of binding to milk and udder proteins.
4. Low minimum inhibitory concentration (MIC).
5. Low degree of ionization in the udder.
6. Adequate exposure time for antibacterial action.
7. Short milk withholding time.

Dry cow formulation for the treatment of sub-clinical mastitis, are designed to produce extended duration of effective drug concentrations. This is achieved by using a higher concentration of active drug or the benzathine salt of the active drug in oil or repository vehicle. The intramammary preparations for dry cow therapy should be with the following characteristic:-

1. It should be completely non-irritant to udder tissue.
2. High degree of binding to udder secretions.
3. Slow release rate from the vehicle or base.

4. Drug should be bactericidal in action with long exposure time.
5. Large molecular weight.

Special attention should be paid on technique of infusion in the mammary gland. A proper intramammary administration technique should be followed, because faulty intramammary administration may increase the chance of more infection or worse condition (see dry cow therapy in prevention and control chapter for details). When teat ends are disinfected prior to intramammary infusion many bacteria are killed, but some lodge in the microscopic crevices around the orifice survive. When a treatment syringe cannula is fully inserted through the orifice, surviving bacteria may be carried into the teat cistern where a few resistant ones can multiply. However, teat end disinfection has no effect on bacteria that colonize teat canal keratin. Full insertion of the treatment syringe cannula may push bits of keratin with colonized bacteria into the teat cistern (Figure 13.2a), where again, a few resistant ones could multiply and infect milk-producing tissues. In addition, the syringe cannula may be up to eight times the diameter of the teat canal, causing temporary dilation of the sphincter muscle and providing an open passageway for bacteria. Studies have shown that partial insertion of the treatment syringe cannula only 3 mm (1/8 inch) into the teat canal avoids damage to teat end tissue and reduces new infections by 50 percent (Figure 13.2b).

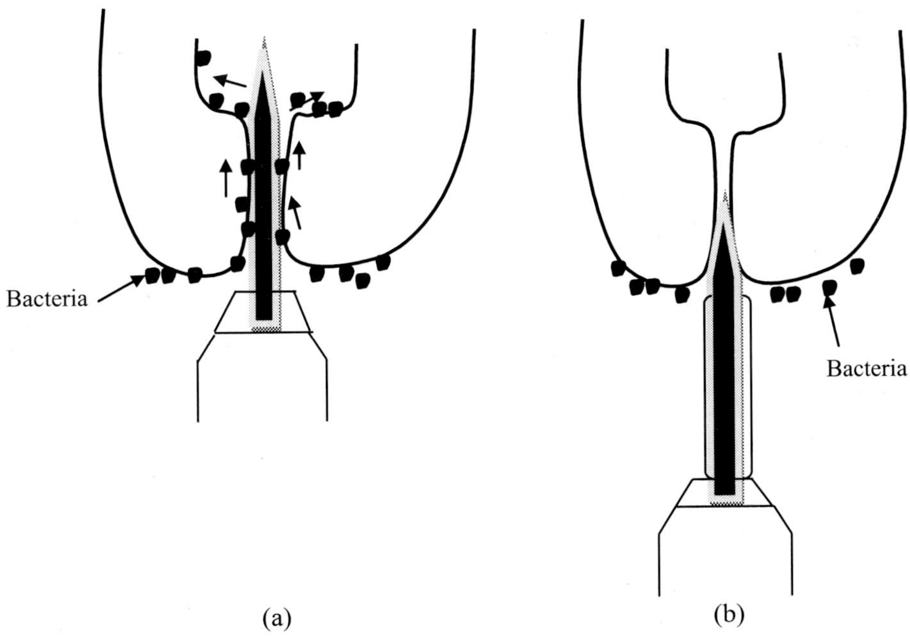

Figure 13.2: Insertion of intramammary tube: a) Complete insertion of tube cannula, b) Partial insertion of tube cannula

Strict hygiene and use of a short cannula (that just penetrate the external sphincter) is necessary during intramammary treatment to avoid the super-infections, caused by secondary invaders. These secondary invaders are mostly *P. aeruginosa, Candida* spp. and *Nocardia* spp. result in worse clinical implications than if no intramammary infusion was administered at all (Erskine *et al.*, 2003). Care must be taken to ensure that bulk containers of mastitis infusions are not contaminated by frequent withdrawals and that individual sterilized teat cannulas usually part of commercial, single dose ointment tubes, are used for each quarter.

Preparation should be infused after complete stripping milk and other products (e.g. cellular debris, pus) from the infected quarters. Complete emptying of the quarter before infusion, by parenteral injection of Oxytocin is advisable in cases of acute mastitis. Oxytocin, 5 - 10 units of diluted solution (10 units/ml), can be administered by slow intravenous injection to facilitate the completeness of stripping. The half life of Oxytocin is approximately 2 min.

After an intramammary infusion, emptying of gland, and thus losing the antibiotic or other drug, should be avoided for as long as possible by treating immediately after milking, preferably in the evening. The frequency of milking and the efficiency of milk out greatly influence the concentration of antimicrobial that could be attained in the udder. Since frequent stripping of the infected quarter(s) is recommended in cows with clinical mastitis, it follows that only quick release intramammary preparations are suitable for use in lactating cows.

In infections of the milk compartment such as Streptococcal mastitis, there is probably no advantage of the systemic administration. For example, concentration of Penicillin-G in milk remains after systemic administration 100 - 1000 fold lower than when given intramammary (Franklin *et al.*, 1986; Moretain and Boisseau, 1989).

Parenteral route

The parenteral route of administration was introduced in to mastitis therapy in the 1970s, mainly after Israel work (Ziv, 1980a). Twenty years earlier Swedish researchers had shown by radiographic studies that Penicellin G was distributed unevenly when administered by the intramammary route (Ullberg *et al.*, 1958). It was suggested that systemic treatment would penetrate throughout the udder better and be more efficient in therapy of mastitis. However, the superiority of parenteral treatment of mastitis over intramammary treatment has never been proven in comparative clinical trials (Pyorala, 2002). This route of administration is advisable in all cases of mastitis in which there is a marked systemic reaction to control or prevent the development of a septicemia or bacteremia and to assist in the treatment of the intramammary infection. Severe clinical mastitis is usually treated systemically, although intramammary therapy will often be used adjunctively. The antibiotics possessing following properties will be the drug of choice for the treatment of mastitis by parenteral routes.

1. High bioavailability (F) from extravenous injection site to systemic circulation.
2. Low minimum inhibitory concentration for majority of mastitis causing pathogens.
3. Low plasma protein binding.
4. Sufficiently lipid soluble.
5. Chemically weak base or otherwise predominately non-ionized in the blood circulation.
6. Longer elimination half-life in milk and udder tissue.
7. Retain activity in inflammatory secretions.
8. High value of volume of distribution [$Vd_{(area)}$] and tissue/plasma ratio.
9. No drug accumulation in any other body organs including blood.
10. Minimal adverse effects in animal.
11. Short withdrawal periods (milk withholding and slaughter).

It is finally concluded that for achieving therapeutic drug level in milk only drugs with good systemic bioavailability should be employed, those which are poorly or slowly absorbed from inject site should be given by intravenous route.

Pharmacokinetics of antimicrobials after parenteral administration into adult ruminants is problematic (Prescott *et al.*, 2000). Ruminants eliminate antibiotics very fast and half lives of many antibiotics are short. It is difficult to achieve and maintain therapeutic concentrations in milk or udder tissue via systemic administration (Ziv, 1980a). Intravenous administration would be in general produce higher concentrations in milk, but it is often unpractical in field conditions (Pyorala, 2002). The slowly absorbed antibiotic preparations for intramuscular use are the worst choice in mastitis, because they do not generally produce therapeutic concentrations in milk or tissues.

There are very few antibiotics, which from the pharmacokinetic point of view, would be ideal for systemic mastitis treatment. These antibiotics include Procain penicillin, Amoxycillin trihydrate-clavulanate potassium combinations, Trimethoprime-suphadiazine (or Sulphamethoxazole) combination and fluoroquinolones (Enrofloxacin). Although, only the fluoroquinolones have broad spectrum of activity against Gram-negative bacteria. In order to obtain effective concentrations in milk Oxytetracycline hydrochloride (conventional preparation or concentration of salt- 50mg/ml) should be administered by slow intravenous injection. Long-acting parenteral preparations of Oxytetracycline (Terramycin-LA, concentration of salt-200 mg/ml) are not indicated in treatment of mastitis (O'Rourke and Baggot, 2004). Macrolide antibiotics (Erythromycin) have good tissue penetration capacity and the ion-trapping effect favours the concentrations in milk. Macrolides, which are narrow spectrum drugs with activity against Gram positive bacteria only, would have ideal pharmacokinetic (Sanders *et al.*, 1992), but they have problems in pharmacodynamics. They are bacteriostatic and milk strongly interferes with their activity. These may reasons for the reported poor efficacy of macrolides in mastitis treatment (Pyorala and Pyorala, 1998; Owens *et al.*, 1999).

Cefquinome is a broad spectrum, fourth generation cephalosporin that has good tissue distribution and low minimum inhibitory concentration for Gram-negative bacteria (Shpigel *et al.*, 1994). It is resistant to â-lactamases produced by the majority of clinically important bacteria.

Drugs are transferred from the general circulation to the mammary gland by passive diffusion (Ziv, 1980a). Consequently, non-ionized lipid soluble agents that are not extremely bound to plasma proteins more readily reach the mammary gland (Table 13.12). Because milk is weakly acidic (pH 6.5-6.8), drugs that are weak bases (Trimethoprime, macrolides, lincosamides) are preferentially concentrated by ion-trapping (Baggot, 2000).

Table 13.12: Distribution of antibiotics throughout the udder after parenteral administration (Ziv, 1980a).

Good	Moderate	Poor
Fluoroquinolones	Penicillin-G	Dihydrostreptomycin
Erythromycin	Amoxycillin	Gentamicin
Trimethoprim	Ampicillin	Neomycin
Spiramycin	Cephalosporins	Polymyxins
Tylosin	Tetracyclines	
	Sulphonamides	

From clinical point of view, the successful intravenous or intramuscular anti-mastitic therapy depends on effective transport of the drug from blood into milk. Although concentration of an antibiotic in blood are commonly equated with therapeutic effect of drug in vacularized organs, but in avascular, fibrin rich infectious processes and in infections at sites separated from blood by physiological or anatomical membranes or barriers (i.e. udder, joints, brain and eye) the level of drug will not be reflected by that in blood.

Parenteral treatment is also advisable when the gland is badly swollen and intramammary antibiotic is unlikely to diffuse to all parts of the glandular tissue. Fortunately, the rate of diffusion is greater in damaged than in normal quarters. To produce therapeutic levels of antibiotic in the mammary gland by parenteral treatment it is necessary, for the various reasons, to use higher than normal dose rates and to give a course of 5 days rather than the conventional 3 days. Recently it has been pointed out that if parenteral administration of the drug achieves sufficient MIC at the site of infection for desirable period, intramammary infusion of the drug should be discouraged clinically. The recommended dose rate of commonly used antibiotics for the treatment of mastitis in bovines is given in table 13.13.

Table 13.13: Parenteral dosage of antibiotics used for the treatment of mastitis.

Antibiotic	Dose (mg/kg b.wt.)	Frequency	Route
Ampicillin	20	BID	IM
Amoxycillin/Clauvulanic acid	8.75	BID	IM
Penicillin-G	20000-25000 IU/kg b.wt.	OD, BID	IM
Polymixin	3-5	BID	IM
Gentamicin	5	BID	IM
Lincomycin HCl	10	OD	IM
Clindamycin	10	OD	IM
Erythromycin	125	BID	IM
Tylosin	20	BID	IM
Spiramycin	20	OD	IM
Tiamulin	20	OID	IM
Chloramphenicol	50	BID	IM
Doxycycline	10-20	BID	IV
Minocycline	10-20	BID	IV
Tetracycline HCl	10-20	BID	IV
Sulphonamide	50	BID	IV
Rifampin	10	-	IM/IV
Enrofloxacin	2-5	OD	IM

OD = Once in a day, BID= Bis in a day, IM= Intramuscular, IV= Intravenous

Through systemic administration of antibiotic and absorption of the drug into blood, it may be possible for greater contact with living in milk producing tissues. Thus, intramammary infused antibiotic could contact bacteria growing in the cisternal areas and large ducts, and systemic antibiotic could function synergistically with infused drugs by contacting bacteria residing deeper in the gland (e.g. *Staphylococcus aureus*). Hence, it appears that, through the process of combination therapy, that is intramuscular injections coupled with intramammary infusions over several days, greater amounts of drug may last for sufficient period of time, and be more effective than conventional intramammary therapy alone. In conclusion, the combination of multiple intramuscular injections together with intramammary infusions over a 3 day period resulted in the greatest tissue antibiotic concentrations and better results. The combination therapy increases the efficacy and reduces the duration of treatment than alone intramammary therapy (Table 13.14, 13.15).

Table 13.14: Percentage efficacy vis-a-vis route of administration (Sharma and Prasad, 2003).

Antibiotic	Anima-wise		Quarter-wise	
	IMM	IM + IMM	IMM	IM + IMM
Ampicillin + Cloxacillin[a]	78.57	84.21	70.83	76.92
Gentamicin[b]	63.63	80.00	68.42	83.33
Enrofloxacin[c]	54.54	80.00	50.00	71.42
Streptopenicllin[d]	44.44	55.55	45.50	63.63

a = IMM – 75mg + 200mg BID; IM – 8mg/kg OD
b = IMM – 100mg + 2.5ml distill water, BID; IM – 2.5mg/kg BID
c = IMM – 200mg + 6ml distill water; IM – 5mg/kg, OD
d = IMM - Pendistrin SH- 1 tube; IM – 2.5g, OD

Table 13.15: Comparative efficacy of various antibiotics in relation to duration (days) of drug therapy (Sharma and Prasad, 2003).

Drug	Duration of treatment (days)	
	IMM	IMM + IM
Ampicillin + Cloxacillin	4.80±1.02	3.50±0.78
Gentamicin	5.32±0.83	3.70±1.06
Enrofloxacin	7.80±1.30	4.80±1.20
Streptopenicllin	6.63±1.18	5.15±0.22

Dosage

The complete doses of antibiotics have a paramount importance in the treatment of clinical mastitis. Incomplete dosage may cause a severe problem of antimicrobial resistance. Early diagnosis and the prompt use of antibiotic in sufficient dose to treat mastitis will reduce the duration of infection, extent of tissue damage and will increase the rate of recovery and the return of milk production to or approaching the original level. Most antibiotics commonly used in bovine practice are believed to be most effective if concentrations at the site of infection are maintained above the MIC for a particular pathogen for the maximum amount of time between doses. This concept is termed "*time-dependent killing*". While gentamicin activity against pathogens (killing of pathogen) is depends on the magnitude of concentration of drug achieved above the MIC. This concept termed as "*concentration-dependent or peak-dependent killing*" (Erskine *et al.*, 2003). Doses are usually based on body weight and site of pathogen in the udder. Dosage calculations are also based on MIC which is assumed to be related to the concentration attained at the site of infection in the udder.

The recommended dose usually provides good blood and tissue levels that are effective against most susceptible pathogens, with minimal side effects. In most cases the recommended dose is the minimal dose (Andrews, 2004). Less susceptible organisms require higher levels to ensure success.

The constraints in calculating a dose of an antibiotics are :-

(1) The dose interval.

(2) Minimum inhibitory concentration of the drug.

(3) Route of administration.

(4) The pharmacological compartment of cow where the pathogen located or drug must act.

(5) The pharmacokinetic parameters of the selected drug.

(6) The withholding period of individual drug, and

(7) The possible toxicity of drug.

Pharmacokinetics of individual antibiotic in mastitis

[A] Penicillins

Kakavas (1944) was the first to report on the use of penicillin in bovine mastitis of both crude penicillin and the purified sodium salt of penicillin.

(1) Penicillin-G

Penicillin-G was reported to be highly effective because at that time most cases of mastitis were caused by *Streptococcus agalactiae* which was susceptible to low concentrations of penicillins. Penicillin-G sodium and aqueous suspension of penethemate hydroiodide are the only two agents recommended in acute clinical mastitis. Penethemate hydroiodide achieves a concentration in milk 5 – 7 times higher than that in plasma due to its hydrolysis in udder to benzyl penicillin which diffuses relatively poorly out of gland. Ulberg *et al.* (1958) found that intramammary infused penicillin was distributed unevenly and that certain areas contained no antibiotic 8 to 15 hours after administration.

Distribution of penicillin appears to be dependent on passage through the ductal system, because spread via diffusion through tissue is limited. Thus, duct patency is very important in intramammary therapy. Penicillin is not reached the site where fibrous tissue proliferation in the udder. In case of acute clinical mastitis, accompanied by visual abnormalities in milk, penicillin distribution is unsatisfactory, being limited to the larger milk ducts and a few lobules; therefore, intramammary administration would be of dubious value (Ulberg *et al.*, 1958). Penicillin-G shows that the drug is not detected in milk upto 2 hours after treatment and even during the first 14 hours the concentration of drug is lower in milk than in plasma. Only 0.0003 per cent of drug is detected in milk upto 36 hours (Face to Vet, 2007). Extended spectrum penicillins have activity against Gram positive and Gram negative aerobic and anaerobic bacteria (Dumka and Srivastava, 2003). Penicillin-G is today not a preferred choice of veterinarians because most of mastitis causing bacteria are resistant to penicillin (Singh *et al.*, 2005).

Intramuscular injection is the most common route of administration. Intramuscular administration of benzyl penicillin at the dose rate of 16000 IU/kg body weight maintained MIC in milk against streptococci for 15 hours (Rule *et al.*, 1991). Blood concentration of penicillin is consistently higher when penicillin is infused in infected quarters than when infused into normal quarters (Richard Adams, 2001). Procain penicillin-G is a buffered aqueous suspension available for intramuscular injection, having prolonged absorption. Recommended dosage, route, half life and time interval between consecutive injections of common penicillin antibiotics is given in table 13.16.

Table 13.16: Recommended doses for common penicillin antibiotics (Dumka and Srivastava, 2003).

Drug	Dose	Route of administration	Elimination half life ($t_{1/2}$)	Time interval (hours)
Procain penicillin-G	10,000-66,000 IU/kg	IM	0.5	12
Benzathine penicillin	10,000-66,000 IU/kg	IM, SC	-	48
Ampicillin	11 – 22 mg/kg	IM, SC	1.2	12
Amoxycillin	6 – 11 mg/kg	IM, SC	0.3	12 - 24

(2) Ampicillin

Ampicillin antibiotic is a valuable semi-synthetic penicillin that effective against both gram positive and Gram negative bacteria. Unfortunately, it is inactivated by beta-lactamase and is therefore ineffective against penicillin resistant Staphylococci. Its absorption at quarter level is faster the penicillin. Ziv (1980b) reported proportionately more ampicillin in serum of dairy cows than in tissue compartment and that distribution of the drug occurred rapidly as compared to elimination. Pharmacokinetic studies indicate that ampicillin has faster distribution as compared to elimination. Intramuscular administration of ampicillin at the dose rate of 20 mg/kg has been recommended to produce MIC against most of the causative bacteria of mastitis for 24 hours (Francis, 1989).

(3) Amoxycillin

Amoxycillin is a later derivative of penicillin than ampicillin. It has rapid absorption at the site of injection as well as higher tissue concentration in mastitic quarter(s) with better tissuephilic action especially in inflamed quarter(s) rather than normal quarter(s). Amoxycillin has synergistic property with clavulanic acid. Intramuscular injection of Amoxycillin and clavulanic acid in combination at the dose rate of 8.8 mg/kg body weight have better efficacy than alone Amoxycillin. Amoxycillin should be given by both parenteral and intramammary route at a time than intramammary infusion only. Owens and Nickerson (1989) found that concentration of Amoxycillin was 3 fold higher when using combination (parenteral and intramammary) therapy in comparison with intramammary infusion alone (0.25 vs. 0.09 μg/ml tissue).

(4) Cloxacillin

Cloxacillin came in existence for the treatment of mastitis when inactivation of Ampicillin and Amoxycillin by β-lactamse. Cloxacillin offers the great advantage of not being inactivated by β-lactamase produced by penicillin resistant staphylococci. Most of mastitis causing staphylococci are susceptible to cloxacillin, but not effective against coliforms. The combinations of Ampicillin/Cloxacillin and Amoxycillin/Cloxacillin are available in the market for the treatment of mastitis for last several years. These combinations have good efficacy against Gram positive and majority of Gram negative bacteria.

[B] Cephalosporins

Now a days cephalosporins are using by most of veterinarians in the treatment of mastitis due to its broad spectrum activity, but they also have some limitation. Cephalosporins have limited distribution in udder tissue resulting very high dose (10 – 15 mg/kg b. wt.) is required by parenteral route. All Cephalosporins are not recommended by parenteral route for the treatment of mastitis because of their high minimum effective concentration (MEC) against most of mastitis causing organisms. Among first general Cephalosporins, Cephapirin sodium and cephapirin benzathine are available for intramammary infusion in lactating and dry cows respectively. Similarly, the 3rd generation Cephalosporins e.g. Ceftiofur sodium and Cefoperazone in oil base are available for parenteral and intramammary use, respectively (Dumka and Srivastava, 2003).

Cephalosporins are rapidly absorbed following intramuscular or subcutaneous administration and their bioavailability varies with drug and species. The non-irritant properties of Cefoperazone along with the persistence of therapeutic concentrations of the drug in treated quarters for 3 - 4 milkings make this drug very useful for the treatment of bovine mastitis (Holmgren *et al.*, 1985). Single drug preparation of Cefacetrile or Cefoperazone and combination of intramuscular and intramammary routes have also been reported to give better clinical outcome in high yielding dairy cows affected by acute or chronic mastitis (Giersemehl, 1995). Owens *et al.* (1990b) carried out a kinetic study of Ceftiofur in dairy cows suffering from staphylococcal mastitis (*S. aureus*) showed that following intramammary injection (500 mg), the concentration of Ceftiofur was below detectable limits in udder and milk, and the causative agent was not eliminated from infected mammary glands by intramammary infusion (100 – 200mg). However, combination therapy by both routes reduced *S. aureus* count in milk and udder markedly. Ceftriaxone is one of the most widely recommended 3rd generation cephalosporin. It is highly stable in presence of betalactamases, both penicillinases and cephalosporinases of gram-negative and gram-positive bacteria. These two enzymes are majorly responsible for bacterial resistance. Ceftizoxime (an active metabolite of Ceftriaxone) being an amphoteric drug may cross blood milk barrier at a faster rate as the pH of the milk become alkaline during mastitis than Ceftriaxone (Sar *et al.*, 2010). Cefquinome is a fourth generation cephalosporin is most effective against Gram positive and negative bacteria than second and third generation cephalosporins.

[C] Aminoglycosides

Aminoglycosides have amino sugar linked to an aminocyclitol by the glycosidic bonds. The polarity of the molecules limits its poor solubility which in turn limits their use as parenteral antibacterials for the treatment of mastitis. Amongst aminoglycosides, Gentamicin, Streptomycin, Amikacin and Kanamycin are routinely used in veterinary practice while Neomycin and Paramycin are generally not used systematically on account of their well known, ototoxic and nephrotoxic effects. Aminoglycosides are still considered to be the drugs of choice for treating severe aerobic gram negative infections in veterinary medicine.

Ziv and Sulman (1974) have studied the pharmacokinetics and recovery of aminoglycosides in milk and serum of lactating cows. After single intravenous injection, the half-life values of antibiotics in serum ranged from 1.85 hours for Gentamicin to 4.65 hours for paromomycin. The drugs were calculated to occupy less than 20% of total body volume and only a very small fraction of dose was recovered in milk secreted from normal or inflamed mammary glands during the 12 hours after treatment. Penetration of Gentamicin into milk is poor (10 - 15%) and elimination from milk is slower than from plasma. It is suggested that the limited penetration of these drugs into milk is mainly due to their poor lipid solubility, which would curtail their potential usefulness in the parenteral treatment of mastitis (Srivastava, 2000). Altered pathophysiologic states may alter the distribution, clearance and half life of aminoglycosides by as much as 1000 fold (Zoske *et al.*, 1982). It has been observed in culture sensitivity test that more than 93% of isolates from mastitic cows are sensitive to Gentamicin (Sing *et al.*, 1994). The recommended intramuscular doses for the treatment of mastitis in lactating and dry cows are 3.5 mg/kg b. wt. (Hadded *et al.*, 1986) and 5 mg/kg b. wt. (Hadded *et al.*, 1987) respectively and repeat at every 8 hours intervals. Absorption of Gentamicin from intramuscular site is rapid and nearly complete. Peak bound levels are usually achieved within 30 - 90 minutes after intramuscular administration. In mastitic animals the recovery of aminoglycosides in milk of inflamed glands of cows was in general 40 to 80% higher than the recoveries from the normal glands after intramuscular administration (Ziv and Sulman, 1974). After intramammary administration of Gentamicin in inflamed quarters, antibiotic persisted in milk for 8 milkings after 250 mg and 9 milkings after 500 mg administration (Ziv and Sulman, 1974).

[D] Tetracycline

Tetracyclines are very commonly used, broad spectrum antibiotics in veterinary practice. They are effective against wide variety of organisms like bacteria, protozoa and many intracellular organisms. Amongst all Tetracyclines, Oxytetracycline injection is the most commonly used antibiotic in large animal practice, this is because of its broad spectrum activity and low cost of therapy. Normally, Oxytetracycline is not accepted in mastitis treatment because of their bacteriostatic action and therapeutic concentration in milk is observed only if the drug is administered at a high dose of 10 mg/kg b. wt.

[E] Fluoroquinolones

Fluoroquinolones are a relatively new class of potent synthetic antimicrobial agents, with long lasting bactericidal effect and broad spectrum antibacterial activity, including strains resistant to many other antimicrobial agents. Amongst fluoroquinolones, three drugs are commonly used in veterinary practice – Enrofloxacin, Ciprofloxacin and Norfloxacin. In general, fluoroquinolones are mostly effective against aerobic Gram negative organisms as well as Gram positive organisms, Mycobacteria, Chlamydia and *Mycoplasma pneumonia*. Most anaerobes are resistant to existing fluoroquinolones (Sharma *et al.*, 1994). The efficacy of quinolones towards Gram negative organisms is pH dependent. They are less effective at acidic pH. Quinolones readily penetrate intracellularly into phagocytic cells and Enrofloxacin reaches a concentration in neutrophils seven times higher than extracellular concentration, therefore allowing is to be effective in killing of intracellular bacteria. The MIC of Enrofloxacin for most Gram negative organisms is generally <0.25 mg/ml and rarely exceeds 1 mg/ml (Dawn, 1994).

Following intramuscular administration of Enrofloxacin at the dose rate of 3.5 mg/kg b. wt. (repeat at 24 hours interval), the buffalo suffering from acute mastitis was reported to be recovered within 5 days of daily treatment with supportive therapy (melonex and fluid therapy) (Sharma *et al.*, 2007). As per personal experience of first author of this book, the parenteral administration of Enrofloxacin and Gentamicin in combination is also sufficiently effective in the treatment of clinical mastitis and this combination is more useful where antibiotic sensitivity test is not available. The satisfactory and appropriate intramuscular dosage regimen of Enrofloxacin in buffaloes suffering from mastitis was calculated to be 5 mg/kg repeated at 24 hours interval (Srivastava, 2000).

[F] Macrolides

Macrolides are very promising anti-bacterials for systemic as well as for intramammary use, but have problems of poor intramuscular bioavailability when bases are organic solvents, although water soluble formulations achieve effective levels for longer periods. They are narrow spectrum drugs with activity against Gram positive bacteria only and are bacteriostatic in nature. Erythromycin, Spiramycin, Oleandomycin and Tylocin are among this group which are used clinically in veterinary practice and their plasma half life usually 1 - 3 hours (Srivastava *et al.*, 2002). Some imperative points regarding use of macrolides in the treatment of mastitis are as-

1. It is a drug of choice for mastitis caused by Gram positive organisms.
2. Following single administration, the MEC in milk is maintained for 18 to 24 hours.
3. Being organic bases with high lipid solubility, the concentration of drug in milk is very high.

4. Water soluble formulations achieve effective levels for longer periods as compared to preparations containing organic vehicle.

Spiramycin is one of the most promising drug for the treatment of mastitis caused by *Staphylococcal aureus*.

(I) Chloramphenicol

Chloramphenicol possesses a fairly wide spectrum of activity and MIC of Chloramphenicol is 5 – 10 μg/ml. it is suggested to be most important drug for the treatment of coliform mastitis. The recommended dose rate of Chloramphenicol for intramuscular route is 30 mg/kg b. wt., and for intramammary route is 250 mg/quarter and same dose repeat after 24 hours (Srivastava *et al.*, 2002). It has been reported that the drug concentration in mastitic quarter is higher than that in normal quarter(s). In case of acute mastitis, Chloramphenicol administration should be given by both intramammary and intramuscular route conjointly for better result.

(II) Polymixin-B

Polymixin-B is a membrane acting antibiotic and is considered to be one of the most toxic antibiotic for parenteral use. The pharmacokinetics of Polymixin-B, infused at the dose rate of 100 – 200 mg/quarter into the normal, chronically inflamed and acutely inflamed quarters of mammary gland of lactating cows was conducted (Ziv and Schultze, 1982). Polymixin-B was not found to be absorbed from normal and chronically inflamed quarters and more than 90% of the infused dose was recovered in milk within 24 hours after infusion. The concentration of drug in milk from acutely inflamed quarters was lower than in milk from normal quarters. These results indicated that Polymixin-B well absorbed from acutely inflamed quarters into the systemic circulation (Srivastava *et al.*, 2002).

[G] Sulfonamides

The sulfonamides were the first effective chemotherapeutic agents to be employed systemically for the prevention and cure of mastitis, but the emergence of resistance has limited their usefulness in clinical settings. Also the advent of newer agents has diminished the usefulness of sulfonamides. Allot (1937) was the first to report on the use of sulfonamides in the treatment of bovine mastitis. Now day's sulfonamide is not commonly used in the cases of clinical mastitis.

Finally based on the different studies, and author's experience, it is recommended that if parenteral administration of antibiotics achieves sufficient concentration at the site of infection that is in the udder tissue, for desirable duration, intramammary infusion should be discouraged.

Failure of Antibiotic Therapy

The mastitis is caused by numerous organisms, of which *Staphylococcus aureus* is the more dangerous organism. *Staphylococcus aureus* is difficult infection to clear, and the presence of cows with chronic mastitis poses a threat to other cows in the farm. Finally, mastitis results after bacteria penetrate streak canal keratin, overcome the defenses in udder/quarter(s), and multiply within the gland. A hallmark of acute inflammation is the formation of inflammatory exudates composed of necrotic tissue debris, leukocytes, bacteria, fibrin and other blood components that occlude milk ducts, draining area of secretory tissue. The frequent therapy failures during acute mastitis are due, in part, to poor or uneven distribution of the drug throughout the intensely swollen udder parenchyma in which the duct system is either compressed or blocked by inflammatory products.

The infecting organisms (bacteria) interact with udder defending cells (milk leukocytes), particularly neutrophils, these phagocytic cells greatly influences or prevent the establishment of intramammary infections. Neutrophils are the first line of defense and function by phagocytosing bacteria and killing the organisms intracellularly. However, phagocytosis is inefficient in the mastitis udder due to lack of an energy source, low opsonic activity, and interference caused by casein and butter fat. In addition, many bacteria (e.g. *S. aureus*) remains intracellularly and survive inside neutrophils once they have been phagocytosed, and most antibiotics can not penetrate inside the neutrophil to contact intracellular bacteria. Bacteria may later be released from the cell upon lysis, and multiply within the gland as the concentrations of antibiotic decrease. Unfortunately, successful antibiotic therapy occurs, at best, only about 50% of time. The success of mastitis therapy depends on factors like early and correct diagnosis, route of administration of drug, selection of drug, stage at which treatment is initiated, severity of udder pathology, supportive treatment, elimination of predisposing factors and some factors relating to the mastitis causing organisms themselves. Indiscriminate uses of antibiotics have to lead to the development of resistance and failure of antibiotic therapy. In the situation when lack of cultural and sensitivity facilities and presentation of mastitis case at late stage, many veterinarians try several antibiotics one after the other or in combination ending with success or many times failure. At field level use of right antibiotic in right concentration for right duration is rarely done, which results in poor rate of successful treatment and development of resistance.

Treatment failure may occur due to various factors like management and iatrogenic factors, mastitis causing organism factors, drug factors and, animal/ mammary gland factors. There are some factors which plays important role in the failure of antibiotic treatment-

[A] Drug/management factors

1. Antibiotics do not reach the site of infection in adequate concentrations due to:

a) Problems in maintenance of adequate levels of the antibiotic over a required period of time, too low a dose, too long dosing interval, too short a treatment period and,

b) Pharmacokinetic limitations
   - incomplete absorption, disposition, elimination
   - sequestration due to ionization
   - diffusion barriers during intramammary treatments (oedema, occluded milk ducts, abscess formation, fibrosis). Infections are frequently refractory to IMM therapy because of the inaccessibility to bacteria. This inaccessibility is in part due to deep tissue lesions, swelling and reduced patency of milk ducts.
   - problems in the delivery of antibiotics across the *blood-milk barrier* during parenteral treatment
   - binding of antibiotics to milk or serum protein
   - intracellular parasitism (*S. aureus*)

2. Delayed initial treatment.
3. Blind use of antibiotics may develop resistance.
4. Some antibiotics are detrimental to phagocytosis.
5. Inadequate supportive treatment.
6. Re-infections:
   - from remaining 'inoculum' when the host fails to clear the infection sup-pressed by the antibiotic;
   - from teat canal infections;
   - from external sources due to inadequate milking procedures etc.
7. Super-infections
8. Partial or full insertion of intramammary cannula.

[B] Mastitis causing organisms factors

1. Bacterial dormancy. Non-multiplying bacteria are not sensitive to most antibiotics.
2. L-forms of bacteria. Acapsular 'naked' forms are not sensitive to the ß-lactam group of antibiotics.

3. Escape from endogenous antibacterial factors :
   - Capsule or slime formation
   - Receptormediated adsorption of host proteins into bacteria
   - Intracellular parasitism (*S. aureus*)
   - Interference with phagocyte function, leukocidin production.
4. Avoidance of washout effects due to milkings :
   - Adherence to tissue linings
   - Flotation upwards with cream
   - Increase in replication rate.

[C] Endogenous/mammary gland factors

1. All endogenous antibacterial factors become very much diluted down in milk.
2. Problems in effective phagocytosis :
   - Too long milking intervals. Neutrophils are active only for a short period after entering the milkcompartment
   - The pH of milk is too low for optimal granulocyte function
   - Phagocytes waste their protective capacity in endocytosing fat and casein
   - The receptors for opsonins are covered by casein
   - Phagocytes are deprived of energy as the glucose content is low in milk
   - The oxygen tension is too low for phagocytes to operate effectively
   - Casein split products stimulate phagocytes (unspecific stimulation)
   - Opsonins are diluted in milk
   - Immunocomplexes in milk block the normal functions of phagocytes.
3. Lactoperoxidase does not have sufficient substrate (thiocyanate, hydrogen peroxide) for producing an effective antibacterial system in milk.
4. The lactoferrindependent ironbinding system does not effectively withhold iron from bacteria if the milk contains haemoglobin or other haem compounds as occurs in mastitic milk.
5. Components in milk mask or inactivate the effect of activated complement.

New treatment strategies are needed to improve cure rates for existing infection (mastitis) and reduce the incidence of new infections. The methods are needed to reduce the duration of established infections in order to maintain an overall low level of mastitis in the herd. There are four ways (Figure 13.3) to eliminate new intramammary infections caused by major udder pathogens. These are:-

a. Spontaneous recovery
b. Culling of chronically infected cows
c. Treatment during lactation, and
d. Treatment at drying off.

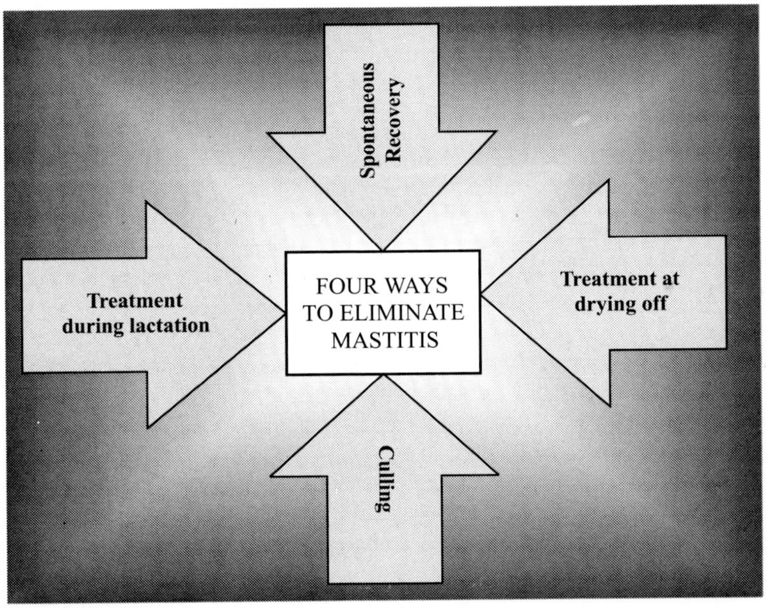

Figure 13.3: Four ways to eliminate intramammary infection.

Spontaneous recovery occurs when the infected cow cures herself of an intramammary infection, but this phenomenon takes place in at most 20% of established infections. Culling is often the only practical means to eliminate chronic infections from a herd. Obviously, both spontaneous recovery and culling have somber precincts in terms of usefulness for eliminating such infections from a herd. Thus, antibiotics continue to be relied upon in efforts to-

I. treat mastitic quarters during lactation, and
II. eliminate existing infections and prevent new infections during the dry period.

Before going to the treatment of clinical mastitis, a standard treatment protocol should be established at every dairy farm. In USA, most of dairy farms have established clinical mastitis treatment protocol (Figure 13.4), several things need to be considered.

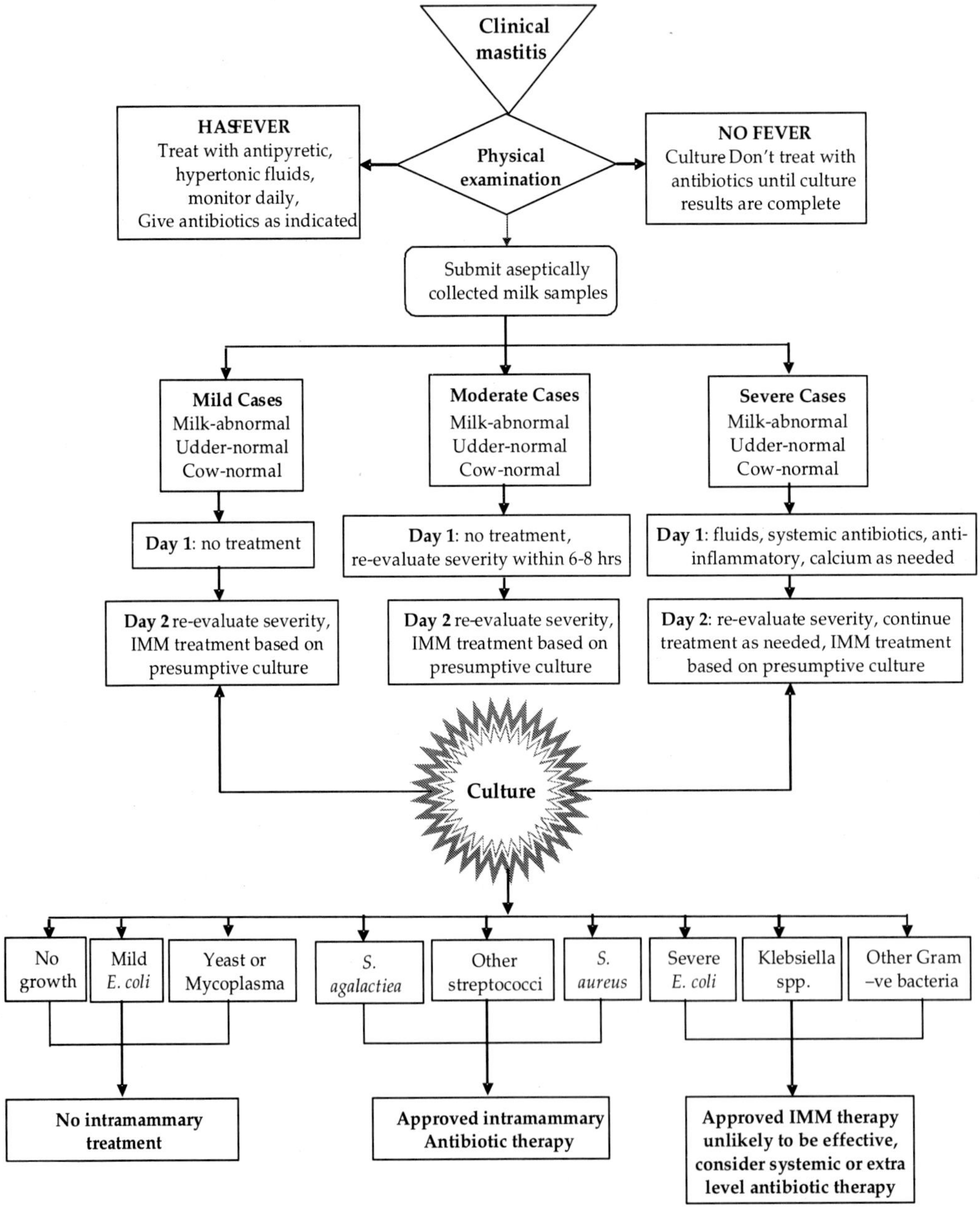

Figure 13.4 : Final decision making tree for clinical mastitis therapy (Modified from Roberson, 2003).

The first process in establishing a protocol is to identify cow or buffalo with clinical mastitis. When a cow with clinical mastitis is identified, some methods should be used to determine the severity of mastitis. The treatment selected should differ depending whether the infection is mild, moderate or severe (Roberson, 2003). Although, most agree to use the severity levels of mild, moderate and severe, the exact definition of each level is not completely clear (Smith and Hillerton, 1999). Mastitis severity can also be scored as 1 (abnormal milk), 2 (abnormal milk and gland) and 3 (abnormal milk and gland, and sick cow) (Figure 13.5). In general, mild cases (score 1) are those

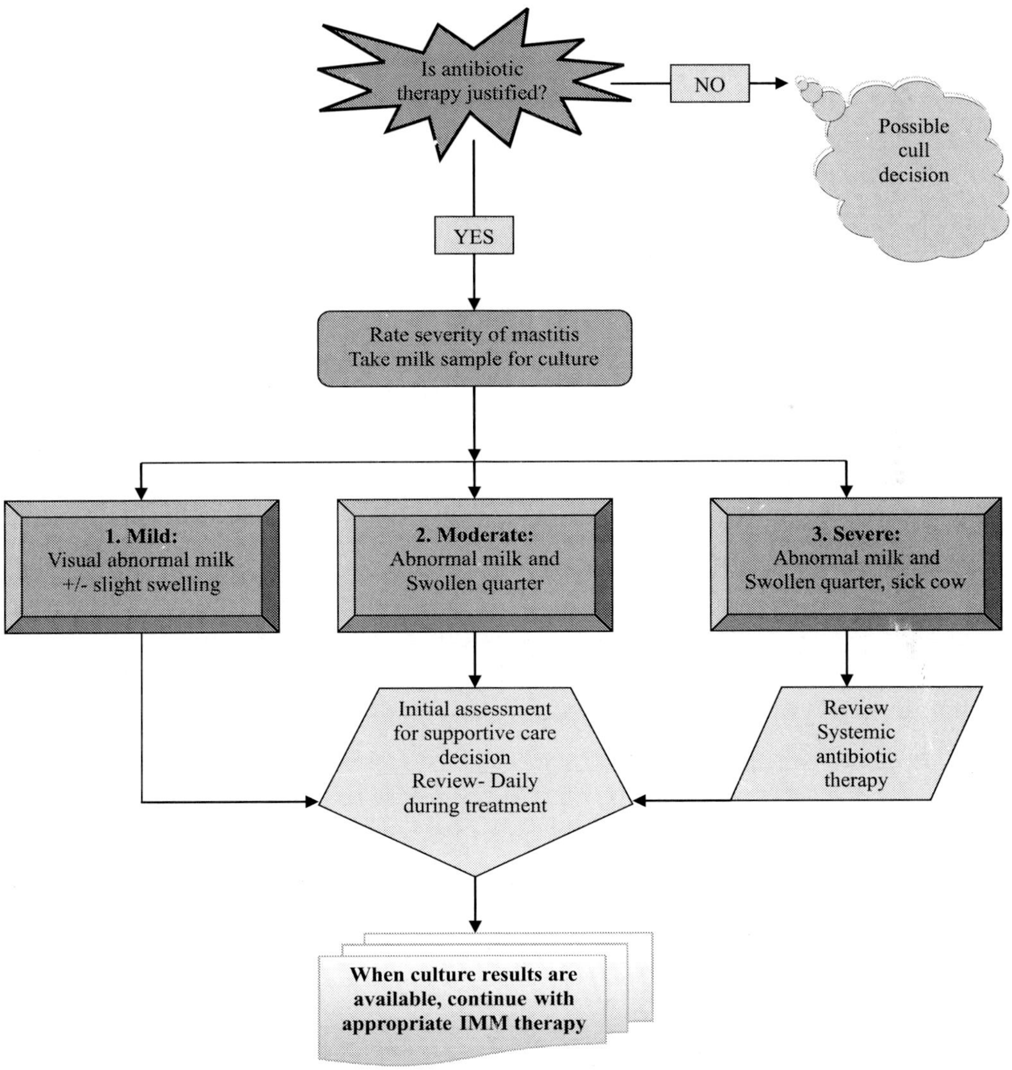

Figure 13.5: Severity score of mastitis on the basis of visual changes in milk and udder and systemic antibiotic decision.

that consist of abnormal milk. Moderate cases (score 2) may include external mammary gland signs such as redness, swelling, heat, and pain upon palpation and mild systemic signs of illness. Severe clinical mastitis (score 3) consists of abnormal milk, signs of systemic illness (such as elevated rectal temperature, heart rate, and respiratory rate, decreased or absent rumen strength or contractions, and dehydration, and possible external mammary signs (Roberson, 2003). A system developed by Roberson (1997), to determined severity of clinical mastitis consists of six parameters- rectal temperature, heart rate, respiratory rate, hydration status, rumen contraction strength and yellow serum like mammary secretion. Cases with no abnormal parameters are considered "*mild cases*", one abnormal parameter is considered a "*moderate case*", and when two or more parameters are abnormal, the case is "*sever*". Wenz *et al.* (2001b) also developed a grading protocol for acute coliform mastitis. They used four parameters- rectal temperature, hydration status, rumen contraction rate and altitude based on signs of depression (Figure 13.6).

When clinical mastitis cases are mild (a score of 1 or 2), treatment with oxytocin, with the quarter milked out, is generally sufficient until culture results are available (American Association of Bovine Practitioners protocol) . Only more severe cases (with a score of 2 or 3) need immediate attention if the cow exhibits pain and fever. These cows should be given an anti-inflammatory (e.g. Meloxicam) to reduce pain and fever, given fluids if necessary, and be rechecked in 12 hours. Further therapy decision can be made when the culture results are available the next day.

[A] Antimicrobial Therapy During Lactation

Historically, treatment during lactation involved regular "stripping out" of the infected quarters, application of various topical treatments and massage to encourage the "circulation". The advent of antimicrobials brought a "magic bullet" approach and drugs were developed with varying degrees of efficacy against the common mastitis causing pathogens (Biggs, 1998).

It appears that the "normal" three tubes used for a treatment course has become part of mastitis history but it is difficult to find any reference to the logic by which this three tube approach was chosen.

Treatment of severe clinical mastitis

As per the experience of field veterinarians most of mastitis cases presented at late stage and per-acute form of mastitis makes the treatment difficult, as sufficient damage would have been taken place and there would be no sufficient time for taking up culture and *in-vitro* sensitivity tests. The second problem in the field is that, the facilities for culture and *in-vitro* antibiotic sensitivity test are not usually available at near place and it is time consuming also.

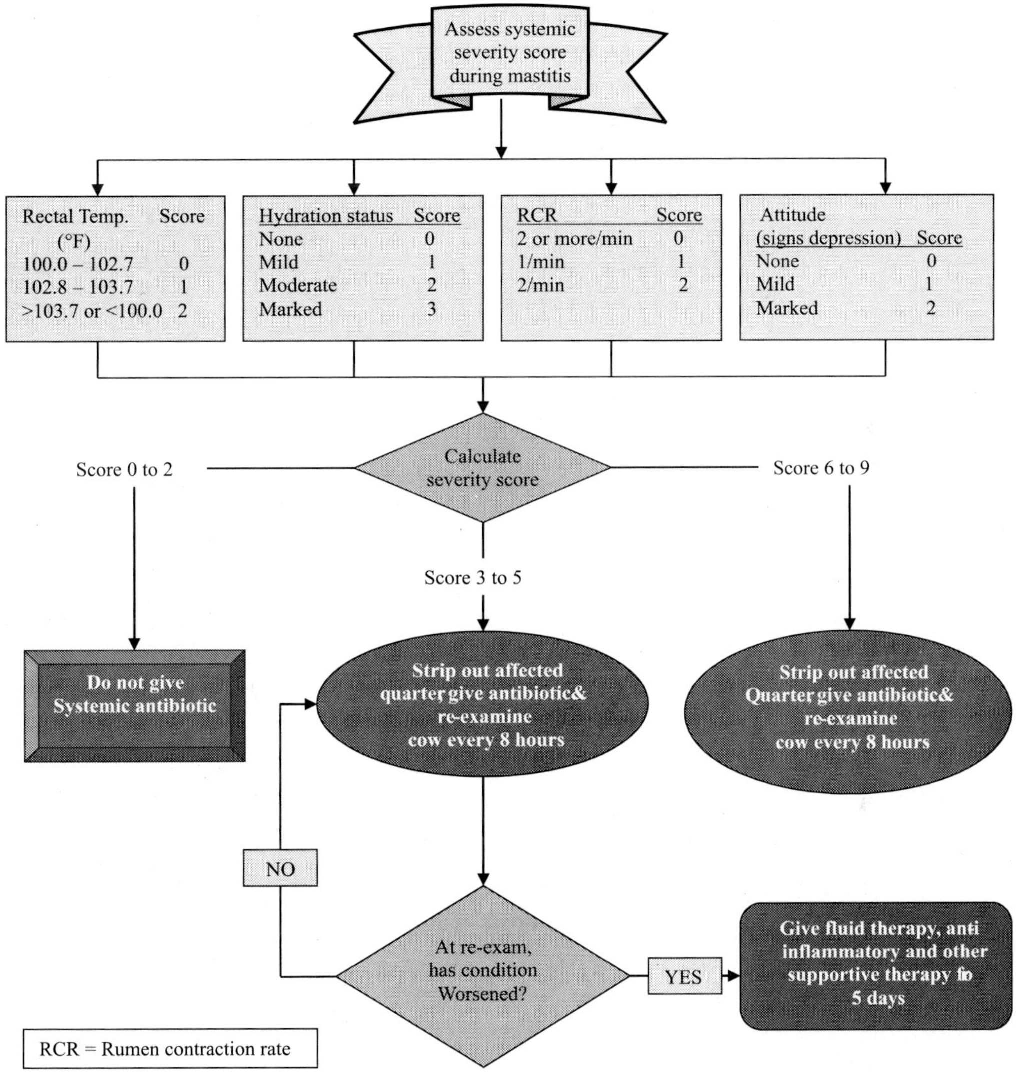

Figure 13.6: Systemic severity score of mastitis and systemic antibiotic decision.

Clinical mastitis cases that include systemic involvement are termed "*severe*". Coliform organisms (lactose-fermenting Gram negative rods of the family Enterobacteriaceae) are the most common cause of this form of mastitis in most dairy cows (Erskine *et al.*, 2003). However, numerous other pathogens including Gram positive cocci and mycotic organisms can all result in severe mastitis. Thus, primary therapy for severe clinical mastitis should be directed against coliform organisms, although secondary consideration must be given for causative agents other than coliform.

It is extremely important to have a treatment plan for clinical mastitis that is based upon the individual animal history and a likely diagnosis of the suspected pathogen. Clinical mastitis almost always demands treatment and there is no t time to identify the pathogen involved using a broad spectrum intramammary antibiotic is usually the line of approach for most veterinarians. There are very few veterinarians those culturing the clinical case milk samples, therefore most of treatments are based on clinical signs. The outcome is not always favourable but treatment is generally initiated and will reduce bacteria shedding even if a bacterial cure is not achieved. This is equally important in the treatment of sub-clinical mastitis (Biggs, 2002). Performing cultures prior to treatment and basing the treatment protocol on the diagnostic result is not generally done because it is difficult to receive results from diagnostic laboratory quickly enough to allow their use prior to treatment. A history of previous diagnosis and a careful physical examination should be used to guide treatment decisions from a cowside appraisal, treatment of severe clinical mastitis cases is a forced decision, i.e. treatment is indicated, if only to relieve the cow of systemic signs. Since mastitis results in the destruction and disturbances of the mammary gland and affects milk production and productivity, it needs serious and immediate action as soon as possible. Collectively, a therapeutic regimen for severe clinical mastitis should include – (i) administering supportive care, especially fluids for cows displaying shock, (ii) targeting antibacterial therapy to maintain effective concentrations in plasma; (iii) selecting a systemic antibacterial with a broad spectrum of activity, and (iv) administering appropriate intramammary antibacterial therapy.

Many of the inflammatory and systemic changes observed during the course of coliform mastitis with acute onset result from the release of lipopolysachharide endotoxin from *E. coli*. Lipopolysachharides released during the phagocytosis process. These endotoxin initiate the production of inflammatory mediators e.g. prostaglandins, leukotriens, thromboxanes etc. they cause the development of systemic signs and finally endotoxin induced shock. Signs of endotoxic shock may appear within a few hours of onset. All this time, the prognosis is guarded to poor. Recumbency, marked depression, progressive dehydration, diarrhea, and normal or below normal rectal temperature are associated with endotoxic shock. From a practical standpoint, the treatment of severe coliform mastitis can not begin until clinical signs appear. In addition, numerous other organisms including *Mycoplasma bovis*, Gram positive cocci, and mycotic organisms cause severe clinical mastitis that can be difficult to distinguish from cases caused by coliform at initial presentation. Thus the primary therapeutic concern is the treatment of endotoxin induced shock with fluids, anti-inflammatory drugs and other supportive care. In case of sever clinical mastitis fluid therapy should start as soon as possible. The administration of large amounts of balanced electrolyte solutions will counteract dehydration and cause forced dieresis to maintain renal function for the excretion of toxic metabolites. Frequent milking with oxytocin injection is also recommended for treatment of coliform mastitis.

Antibiotic therapy may be of secondary importance relative to immediate supportive treatment of endotoxic shock but it remains an integral part of a therapeutic regimen for severe clinical mastitis. The emphasis of clinical mastitis treatment has been on antimicrobial therapy and currently here are a number of conventional antibiotics with different degree of spectrums that are used for the treatment of mastitis in India. Generally, the efficacy of the antibiotic treatment in coliform mastitis has been questioned, as cure rates have been as high with or without antibiotics or with drugs inefficient *in-vitro* (Jones and Ward, 1990). Systemic and intramammary antibiotics are widely used in the treatment of coliform mastitis. Owens *et al.* (1990b), showed that a combination of parenteral and intramammary antibiotic therapy resulted in higher concentration of antibiotic in mammary biopsies and better bacteriological cure rates, when compared to intramammary treatment alone. Even though, mastitis has been treated with antimicrobials for more than decades, our knowledge about their efficacy is still very scarce. Selection of appropriate antibiotics for the treatment of coliform mastitis poses several problems for the clinicians. Selection of a potentially efficacious antibiotic for the therapy of severe clinical (coliform) mastitis is primarily dependent on the selection criteria discussed earlier in this chapter. Therefore, the primary goal should be to target the cow compartment with appropriate antibiotic to which implicated pathogens are generally susceptible and the duration of therapy should be sufficient as per type of infection. Caution should be employed in extending therapy for cows that have demonstrated marked clinical improvement, especially for cases of coliform mastitis, as recovering cows affected by these organisms have cleared the infection, and generally do not need antibiotics to complete recovery. Unnecessary extension of treatment in these instances results in increased discarded milk expense for the dairy producers and risk of antibiotics in marketed milk (Erskine, 1998).

The antibiotic spectrum of a therapeutic agent must be recognized when selecting a drug prior to knowing the invading pathogen. For example, drugs such as erythromycin and pirlimycin have no activity against coliform bacteria.

Author experience suggests that combination therapy of Enrofloxacin and Gentamicin parenterally along with intramammary administration of Enrofloxacin (200 mg Enrofloxacin plus 6 ml distilled water) gives good result in clinical mastitis. Yadav *et al.* (2002) and Sharma *et al.* (2007) found that Enrofloxacin along with supportive therapy have good effectiveness in the treatment of gangrenous/severe clinical mastitis in cows.

Broad spectrum antibiotics are recommended parenterally, preferably by the intravenous route initially, followed by intramuscular injections to maintain blood levels. For the treatment of severe coliform mastitis, Gentamicin, Amikacin and Cephalosporins are highly effective. Newer antibiotics such as beta-lactams amoxycillin-clavulanic acid combination, and the new quinolone norfloxacin have excellent activity. Ceftiofur sodium has been reported to have excellent activity against Gram negative pathogens, with a suggested MIC_{90} for *E. coli* of 0.50 μg/ml (Owens *et al.*, 1990b). Cefquinome is a broad spectrum 4th generation Cephalosporin with improved antibacterial activity against both Gram positive and Gram negative bacteria over the 2nd and 3rd generation Cephalosporin. Cefquinome is resistant to â-lactamases produced by the majority of clinically important bacteria (*S. aureus*). The *in-vitro* activity of Cefquinome against *E. coli* of bovine mastitis origin is comparable to, or better than 3rd generation Cephalosporins; the MIC_{90} and MIC_{50} values have been reported to be 0.13 mg/ml with a low resistance rate (Schmid *et al.*, 1994).

Roy *et al.* (2010) administer a combination of Ceftriaxone sodium (3000 mg) and Tazobactam sodium (375 mg) at the dose rate of 5 – 10 mg/kg b. wt. by intramuscular route for 5 days. They found marked clinical improvement and significant restoration of blood biochemical parameters (e.g. glucose, BUN, total protein, albumin, globulin, cholesterol) and SCC towards normal.

Sulphonamides and Trimethoprim combinations have been used for many years for the treatment of infectious conditions caused by susceptible organism. Although efficacy has never been established in clinical mastitis trials, this combination is still frequently used in the treatment of clinical mastitis in some countries (Ziv, 1992). The combination is problematic in the ruminant as pharmacokinetics of the components markedly differs from each other (Kaartinen *et al.*, 1999). It is evident that doses recommended by the manufactures are quite low for producing therapeutic concentrations in the milk. From the other hand, the range of concentrations of the combination, which offers synergistic activity, is rather large (Bushby, 1980).

Gentamicin has been used extensively for the treatment of acute and per-acute coliform mastitis because more than 90% of isolates from milk from affected cows are sensitive in-vitro (Radostits *et al.*, 2000).

Antibiotics might also exert possibly detrimental effects by causing massive bacterial endotoxin release induced by drugs (Shenep *et al.*, 1985) and by interfering with phagocytic activity in the udder (Linter and Eberhart, 1998; Hoeben *et al.*, 1998). Due to this controversy over the use of antibiotic in the treatment of coliform mastitis, emphasis should be given on immediate use anti-inflammatory drugs. A very important procedure in treatment of coliform mastitis infections involves frequent milking of the infected cow to remove leukocytes, bacteria and toxins from the mammary gland. Hourly milkings could be very helpful. An injection of oxytocin close to the milking will also aid in removal of residual milk that contains toxins.

As already discussed earlier, severe clinical mastitis is also caused by other organisms like Gram positive cocci and mycotic organisms. Hence, antibiotic should be given on the basis of sensitivity of individual organism or broad spectrum till receiving of laboratory results. Infections at all stages of lactation have 90% cure rates with Penicillin, Erythromycin, Cloxacillin, Amoxycillin and Cephalosporins. Procain penicillin-G is universally used as mammary infusion at a dose rate of 100,000 units. A mixture of Penicillin (1 lac units) and Neomycin sulfate (500 mg) as intramammary infusion, three infusions at interval of 24 hours to maintain adequate milk levels for 72 hours. Other antibiotics like Tetracycline (400 mg), Penicillin + Streptomycin combination (100,000 units + 250 mg), Novobiocin (250 mg), Penicillin-tylosin combination (100,000 units +240 mg), Erythromycin (300 – 600 mg) etc. as intramammary infusion for the treatment of severe clinical mastitis during lactation along with parenteral antibiotic. *S. aureus* mastitis is a difficult infection to clear and the presence of cow with chronic mastitis poses a threat to other cows in the herd. *S. aureus* intramammary infection often results in deep seated abscess. Therapy is difficult, especially because resistance to antibacterials (particularly â-lactams) is more common compared with streptococci, *S. aureus* may survive intracellularly following phagocytosis where antibacterial concentrations are reduced. In addition, *S. aureus* has numerous extracellular substances that impart an ability to survive in the presence of a hostile host immune system. Consequently, elimination of intramammary infection by antibacterial treatment is often not successful (Erskine *et al.*, 2003).

S. aureus causes the both clinical and sub-clinical mastitis. The cure rates for lactation therapy for *S. aureus* mastitis are considerably lower than for dry cow therapy (Sears and McCarthy, 2003). Because therapy during the dry period is successful in 40 to 70% of cases, the dry period is considered the best time to employ treatment (Nickerson, 1993). The combination of intramammary antibiotics along with systemic antibiotic therapy increased the clinical cure rate from 20 to 50% in lactating cows (Kirk, 1991). In another study in which cows were treated for 6 milkings with intramammary infusions of 62.5 mg Amoxycillin and 9 million units of intramuscular Procain penicillin G for 3 days, the combination treatment had a cure rate of 51% of the affected quarters compared with 25% of the quarters given intramammary infusion alone (Owens *et al.*, 1988). Because *S. aureus* is difficult to eliminate from infected glands, protocols have been developed to extend treatment over 6 to 8 days in order to maintain therapeutic levels of antibiotics. In a study, using

Pirlimycin, the bacteriologic cure rate for intramammary infections increased from 26% for two treatments to 51% for eight treatments when treatment was given at 24 hours interval (Costa *et al.*, 2000). The relative properties of the major types of antimicrobials for use in the lactating mammary gland is given in table 13.17.

Table 13.17: Comparison of common antibiotics to treat mastitis caused by streptococci (Hillerton and Berrry, 2003).

Antibiotic	Relative activity	Relative distribution
Penicillin G	+ + + +	Moderate
Penethemate	+ + + +	Good
Cloxacillin	+ + +	Moderate
Erythromycin	+ + +	Good
Cephalosporins	+ +/+ + +	Moderate

+ + = Moderate, + + + = Very good, + + + + = Excellent

Treatment of mild/chronic mastitis

The treatment of mild clinical mastitis (abnormal milk with or without local inflammation of the affected quarter, no systemic signs) is more or less similar to severe clinical mastitis except mild coliform mastitis (*E. coli*) because many mild cases of *E. coli* mastitis are resolved before treatment is necessary. Persistently elevated somatic cell count or repeated isolation of the same pathogen despite treatment will help differentiate these cows from transiently isolation of the same pathogen despite treatment will help differentiate chronically infected cows from transiently infected cows, which may either self cured or responded to treatment (Biggs, 1998). Chronic mastitis is more likely to be caused by *Staphylococcus aureus* or *Streptococcus uberis*. Other streptococci such as *Streptococcus agalactiae* or *Streptococcus dysgalactiae* can be relatively easily eliminated from individual infected quarters with antibiotic therapy. Commonly overlooked, coagulase negative staphylococci (CNS) are frequently isolated from milk samples and are a significant cause of mild inflammation and elevated SCC upto 2 to 3 fold greater than those found in uninfected quarters (Harmon *et al.*, 1986). However, chronic mastitis cows pose a significant infection risk to the rest of the herd and as culling is the only alternate they will often justify the increased expense of a specifically tailored treatment regime. These regimes are either a form of "*extended therapy*"- where treatment is prolonged in an attempt to improve success rates, or "*combination therapy*", where parenteral therapy is combined with intramammary tubes to improve the penetration of the udder tissue and improve success rates.

Common sense and individual herd history should determine the course of therapeutic planning for mild clinical mastitis cases. If standard therapy regimens are achieving less than desired results, then it would be better to extend therapy for a prolonged period rather than change to other antibiotic drug or increase the amount of each dose. Alternatively, treatment of mild cases should be given after getting culture and antibiotic sensitivity results.

Administration of intravenous Oxytetracycline and intramammary Cephapirin to cow with varying degrees of clinical mastitis severity resulted in a higher frequency of normal udder appearance by 10 days and bacteriological cure by 14 days for streptococcal intramammary infection compared with cows not administered antibacterials (Morin *et al.*, 1988). The goal is to eliminate the infection by causing fibrosis of the affected quarter, thus reducing the risk of further pathogenic change or systemic effects on the cow and the risk of infection for other cows. Infusion of 60 ml of 2% chlorhexidine-diacetate in the affected quarters twice at 24 hours intervals has been recommended (Erskine *et al.*, 2003). Other supportive treatments (e.g. fluid, anti-inflammatory, antipyretic etc) should also be given along with antibiotic therapy.

Early detection of reticulin fibre in the milk by silver impregnation technique thus, can serve as an excellent marker for detection of onset of fibrosis in the udder. Fibrinolytic agents such as hylase, streptokinase, streptodornase and hylurinidase should be used as an adjunct therapy in those cases of bovine mastitis where the milk samples were found to be reticulin positive.

Treatment of sub-clinical mastitis

In this form of mammary gland infection, cow does not show any physical changes in milk as well as in udder, hence its diagnosis is done by California mastitis test (CMT), SCC and cultural isolation of organisms. Sub-clinical mastitis does not require aggressive and urgent treatment because sub-clinical form is not so dangerous (acutely) to the potential loss of mammary gland or life to animal. However, many sub-clinical intramammary infections selected as potential therapy candidates are chronic and, particularly in the case of *Staphylococcus aureus*, prediction of therapeutic outcome by *in-vitro* testing is poor in chronically infected quarters compared with newly acquired intramammary infection (Owens *et al.*, 1993). Cultural isolation and antibiotic sensitivity test can be completed prior to initiation of the therapy.

Most often, the predominant pathogens causing sub-clinical mastitis are streptococci and staphylococcus. In particular, the contagious pathogens *Streptococcus agalactiae* and *Staphylococcus aureus* call for essentially opposite therapeutic strategies. With exception of *Streptococcus agalactiae* and

Staphylococcus aureus infections, treatment of cows affected with *sub-clinical* mastitis is usually discouraged because discarding saleable milk may result in considerable financial loss. Treatment of sub-clinical infections has generally occurred at dry off. Maintaining cows with sub-clinical mastitis infections within the dairy herd has some potential negative consequences. Cows with sub-clinical mastitis may have periodic clinical episodes that require milk withholding or antibiotic treatments. Untreated infections allow invasive pathogens the opportunity to establish chronic infections that are unlikely to respond to antibiotic therapy. The decision to treat sub-clinical mastitis is dependent upon the type of pathogens that are prevalent and diagnostic efforts (milk culturing) must be undertaken before developing a treatment protocol. When *Staphylococcus aureus* is prevalent, treatment of sub-clinical cases is only advised for animals that have a high probability of cure.

Prevalence of *Streptococcus agalactiae* intramammary infection can be rapidly reduced by "blitz" treatment (treating entire herd or more economically treating all four quarters of all infected cows) with intramammary â-lactam antibiotic, although use of Erythromycin has been successful, cure rates from 70 - 90% can be expected from blitz treatment (Erskine and Eberhart, 1990; Erskine *et al.*, 1996).

Effective treatment of sub-clinical mastitis caused by *Staphylococcus aureus* and/or environmental streptococci may require the use of intramammary therapy for upto 8 days (Deluyker *et al.*, 2001). Ruegg and Araujo (2002) treated cows suffering from sub-clinical infections (*Staphylococcus aureus* and environemental streps) for 5 days with intramammary therapy and found that 71% quarters were recover completely as compared to control quarters (46%) after 3 weeks of treatment.

Suresh *et al.* (2010) administer a single dose of long acting Enrofloxacin at the dose rate of 7.5 mg/kg b.wt. by intramuscular route and found 100% quarters cure rate in sub-clinical mastitic cows. While Akthar *et al.* (2004) reported 84.62% quarter cure rate in a clinical trial with Enrofloxacin.

Parenteral therapy in sub-clinical mastitis is not likely to offer any benefit over intramammary therapy and, in one study 90% cure rates were achieved with intramammary Penicillin/Novobiocin therapy as opposed to 9% with intramuscular Ceftiofur (Erskine *et al.*, 1996). Some cases of sub-clinical mastitis can be cured by regular teat dipping and proper hygienic conditions, while some cases self cured.

Chronic sub-clinical intramammary infection (mostly due to *Staphylococcus aureus*) should be treated by both intramammary and parenteral route for prolonged period to maintain MIC in the mammary gland for more effective time periods and resulted in better efficacy of antimicrobial. In experimental infections in lactating cows, the combined use of intramuscular Procain penicillin G and intramammary Amoxycillin alone (25%) (Owens *et al.*, 1988). Therefore, treatment of chronic sub-clinical mastitis may have the best probability of success by including parenteral therapy.

Sharma and Maiti (2005) have been reported that the effect of cefotaxime (@ 5 mg/kg b. wt.) treatment in SCM is greater in vitamin E (@ 500 I.U./ animal/day) and selenium (@ 6 mg/animal/day) supplemented animals than unsupplemented treated animals. The effectiveness was assessed on the basis of percentage reduction in somatic cell count (SCC). It was observed that in vitamin E and selenium supplemented animals the percentage reduction of SCC after cefotaxime treatment was higher (74.58%) than unsupplemented group (51.60%).

Sarode (2002) carried out a study on 60 cows affected with mastitis, administered the various antibiotics e.g. Chloramphenicol (100 mg/quarter), Penicillin G (1 lac IU/quarter), Ampicillin and Cloxacillin (200 mg/quarter), Pefloxacin (80 mg/quarter), Erythromycin (100 mg/quarter) and Gentamicin (80 mg/quarter) by intramammary route and found that Erythromycin cured 100% quarters followed by Pefloxacin (90%), Chloramphenicol (84.61%), Penicillin G (70.58%), Ampicillin-Cloxacillin (61.53%) and Gentamicin (50%). However, on *in-vitro* sensitivity test only 5.08% isolates of *Staphylococcus* spp. were sensitive to Erythromycin and remaining organisms (e.g. *Streptococcus* spp., Gram negative rods, *Bacillus* spp. and *Micrococcus* spp.) were resistant to Erythromycin. Only Chloramphenicol was showing maximum sensitivity to all isolates except *Micrococcus* spp. on in-vitro sensitivity.

Antimicrobial Therapy During Dry Period

Dry cow therapy is the use of long acting intramammary antibiotic therapy immediately after the last milking lactation. Now a day, most of farmers are also using the homeopathic drugs and immunomodulators (e.g. Vitamin E and selenium) in addition to antibiotics. Antibiotic therapy at drying off is more likely to be successful at eliminating intramammary infections than antibiotic therapy during lactation. The use of intramammary antibiotic to prevent intramammary infections in the dry period was originally developed as a control measure for summer mastitis (Pearson, 1950). The use of antibiotics to treat all quarters of all cows has been questioned in recent years because of concerns about the development of antibiotic resistant bacteria. There is no evidence that use of dry cow therapy contributes to the development of resistance to antibiotics and decreased resistance has been noted for some antibiotics (Erskine *et al.*, 2001; Makovec and Ruegg, 2003).

The dry period of the lactation cycle is a critical time for dairy animals. The dry periods are usually 45 to 60 days in length. During dry period mammary gland undergoes marked biochemical, cellular and immunologic changes. Involution (repair) of the mammary parenchyma begins 1 to 2 days after the end of lactation and continues for 10 to 14 days. The dry period is an ideal time to attain synergy between antibacterial therapy and immune function to eliminate pathogens from the gland, without incurring the extensive costs typical of lactating cow therapy (Erskine *et al.*, 2003). Both contagious and environmental mastitis pathogens have relevance to the dry period. Important contagious pathogens include *Staphylococcus aureus, Streptococcus agalactiea* and *Mycoplasma bovis*; significant environmental organisms are *Streptococcus uberis, Streptococcus dysgalactiea, E. coli, Klebsiella* and Enterobacter (NMC, 1999). Environmental organisms very frequently cause new intramammary infection in the dry period (Oliver, 1988; Smith and Hogan, 1995). Specifically, upto 95% of all intramammary infections caused by major pathogens in the dry period were shown to be caused by environmental pathogens (Oliver and Mitchell, 1983). By comparison, only 1% of quarters became infected with contagious organisms. This increased importance of environmental pathogens in the dry period may be attributable to continued exposure of cows to environmental organisms throughout the dry period, ineffective control measures against coliform bacteria, decreased spread of contagious organisms in the absence of milking, and reduced prevalence of contagious organisms in many herds (Eberhart, 1986; Bradley and Green, 2000).

Treating the dry cow with specially formulated, long acting antibiotics at drying-off, immediately following the last milking, is an effective practice in the battle against sub-clinical mastitis. Dry cow therapy eliminates existing infections and reduces the risk of new infections, thus, improving udder health. Dry cow therapy somewhat limited because most intramammary products available for dry cow therapy are effective against Gram positive cocci (*Staphylococcus aureus, Streptococcus agalactiea*) and environmental streps but inefficient against coliform bacteria.

It has been estimated that 70 to 98% of infections present at dry off can be eliminated with dry cow therapy (Neijenhuis *et al.*, 2000). Elimination of existing *Staphylococcus aureus* infections however, is considered to be lower and more variable (Sol *et al.*, 1994; Browning *et al.*, 1990). The cure rate of *Staphylococcus aureus* has been reported to be approximately 50% (Browning *et al.*, 1990; Osteras *et al.*, 1999). A plethora of reasons for a poor or reduced cure rate associated with *Staphylococcus aureus* have been examined and include resistance to antibiotics, poor distribution of antibiotic throughout the udder, induction of L-form variant strains, formation of micro-abscesses, decreased PMN cell phagocytosis, intracellular viability and expression of capsular polysaccharides affecting adherence (Leslie, 1994). The reduction of new intramammary infections during the dry period achieved by dry cow therapy has been reported to be approximately 50% (Eberhart, 1986; Berry and Hillerton, 2002).

Soback *et al.* (1990) administered Norfloxacin nicotinate subcutaneously at the start of dry period for *Staphylococcus aureus* compared with untreated cows and achieved a better cure rate and lower new infection rate over the dry period.

Only approved commercial antibiotic products formulated specifically for dry cow therapy in single dose containers for intramammary infusion should be used. These products contain high levels of one or more antibiotics in a slow release base which will maintain therapeutic levels in the dry udder for a significant length of time. An attempt to enhance immune function and clearance with immune modulators, either solely or synergistically with antibacterials, is also an area of potential future importance for mastitis therapy. A synergistic action of lactoferrin and antibiotic as has been reported for *E. coli* (Sanchez and Watts, 1999) and *Staphylococcus aureus* (Diarra *et al.*, 2002; 2003), with studies demonstrating that lactoferrin can restore the susceptibility of β-lactamase producing *Staphylococcus aureus* to penicillin by inhibiting β-lactamase activity. The more details on dry cow therapy is also discussed in the prevention and control chapter of this book.

Anti-inflammatory therapy

The goal of anti-inflammatory agents is to reduce pain (analgesic), inflammation (anti-inflammatory) and temperature (antipyretic) in animals that are suffering from clinical mastitis. Anti-inflammatory therapy seems logical since many of the physiological and pathological changes associated with clinical mastitis are a result of the inflammatory response to infection.

Mastitis is defined as the "inflammation of the mammary gland". The classical signs of acute inflammation (heat, redness, pain, swelling and loss of function) and the underline microcirculatory changes are produced by the release or synthesis of chemicals termed mediators and modulators. In mastitis, inflammatory changes in the udder are recognized increasingly to be crucial to the progress of the disease and increasing attention is now being directed towards the identification of which mediators and modulators are involved and the roles that they subserve.

Anti-inflammatory drugs are widely used to treat acute clinical mastitis. Most of the anti-inflammatory drugs currently in use inhibit the synthesis of eicosanoid group of inflammatory mediators including leukotriens, prostaglandins, and thromboxanes. Eicosanoids are formed from a 20-carbon unsaturated fatty acid, that is arachidonic acid (located in the cell membrane) is the principal precursor for eicosanoids. Bacterial endotoxins activate phospholipase A_2, which causes cell membranes to release arachidonic acid (AA) and make it available for the synthesis of eicosanoids. AA may serve as a substrate for two enzyme systems, cyclo-oxygenases and lipoxygenases. Cyclo-oxygenases catalyse the production of cyclic endoperoxides and further enzymatic action generates the prostanoids (PGE_2, PGD_2 and PGI_2) and thromboxanes (TXA_2). Lipoxygenases catalyse the synthesis of hydroxyeicosatetraenoic acids (HETEs) and leukotriens family of mediators. Eicosanoids contribute to localised and systemic inflammation, which may fulminate to multiple organ system failure. From a clinical point of view, it is important to realize that numerous other immune modulators, most notably leukocyte and endothelial derived cytokines, also contribute to the acute phase response and inflammation (Erskine *et al.*, 2003). In recent years evidence has accumulated to implicate nitric oxide (formerly known as endothelium derived relaxing factor) as an endogenous mediator of the vasodilator effects of a number of neurotransmitters and autacoids. It is synthesized from L-arginine in endothelial cells and, when released abluminally, activates guanylyl cyclase of adjacent smooth muscle cells. The resulting increase in cGMP levels causes vasodilation.

Eicosanoids, including prostaglandins, are undoubtedly implicated in mastitis. One difficulty in further defining the roles of eicosanoids is the limited information currently available on receptors. Thus, it is known that there are three PGE receptor sub-types (EP1, EP2 and EP3) and an IP receptor. Vasodilation is mediated by EP2 and IP receptors, whilst potentiation by PGE2 of bradykinin-induced edema is biphasic, the most potent phase being mediated by EP3 receptors and the less potent phase by EP2 receptors. Currently available ligands possess only limited selectivity and more selective drugs will no doubt facilitate elucidation of the roles of prostaglandins and other eicosanoids in inflammation. The importance of the arachidonic pathway in inflammation derives from the fact that the two most widely used groups of anti-inflammatory drugs, steroids and non-steroids (NSAIDs), may act at least in part by inhibiting enzymes in the arachidonic acid pathway. However, the inflammatory response has beneficial as well as harmful consequences for the cow and anti-inflammatory agents can produce detrimental side effects in some cases. The benefits and risks of anti-inflammatory therapy must be weighed. Some anti-inflammatory agents are quite expensive, making repeated doses potentially cost-prohibitive (Morin, 2004b).

Anti-inflammatory agents used to treat bovine mastitis include glucocorticoids and non-steroidal anti-inflammatory drugs (NSAIDs). These drugs reduce eicosanoid production by inhibiting arachidonic acid release (gluco-corticoids) or metabolism (NSAIDs), but a variety of other mechanisms contribute to their anti-inflammatory effects (Morin, 2004b).

Glucocorticoids

Glucocorticoids useful in the early stages of inflammation and of little value when dealing with established infections because arachidonic acid release, starts cascade early following endotoxin exposure. Glucocorticoid drugs inhibit the production of inflammatory molecules and the adhesion molecules that facilitate transport of inflammatory cells from the blood stream to the site of inflammation (Adams, 2001). Glucocorticoids also helps to maintain micro-circulation and cell membrane integrity, interfere with dissolution and disruption of connective tissue, decrease formation of histamine by injured cells, and antagonize toxins and kinins. These actions of glucocorticoid drugs could be expected to be of benefit to the mastitic cow, particularly one with mastitis caused by endo-toxin producing coliform bacteria (Erskine *et al.*, 2003). While glucocorticoid are less effective in chronic mastitis caused by Gram positive and may even be adversely affected.

Glucocorticoids prevent arachidonic acid release by stabilizing cell membranes and inducing lipocortin production. Liporcortin prevents phospholipase A2 from contacting cell membrane-associated arachidonic acid, effectively limiting availability of the precursor needed for eicosanoid production (Hirata, 1983).

Two glucocorticoids (Dexamethasone and Isoflupredone) are approved for the treatment of clinical mastitis in lactating cows. Both glucocorticoids are inexpensive and have no milk withholding requirement. However, dexamethasone may cause immunosuppression and abortion especially after 5 months of gestation. Isoflupredone is a less potent glucocorticoid than dexamethasone, does not cause abortion, and presumably less risk of immunosuppression. However, isoflupredone acetate has more mineralocorticoid activity, which can lead to hypokalemia and recumbency when repeated doses are used in sick cow (Sielman *et al.*, 1998; Sattler *et al.*, 1997). In India, dexamethasone is commonly used as anti-inflammatory agent in per-acute and acute mastitis cases, while isoflupredone does not use in India. Data on the activity of glucocorticoids for treatment of clinical mastitis are limited. In a study the administration of 30 mg dexamethasone as intramuscular to dairy cows immediately following the introduction of *E. coli* into the mammary gland had a number of beneficial effects like reduced local signs of inflammation (mammary gland swelling), impairment of rumen motility and milk production loss in treated cows (Lohuis *et al.*, 1988). Interestingly, treated cows had increased rectal temperature compared with untreated control, but their milk production losses were less than in untreated control (Lohuis *et al.*, 1988). In another study, a single intramuscular injection of 30 mg dexamethasone or 5 mg flumethasone at the time of endotoxin infusion in mammary gland reduced mammary gland swelling, rectal temperature and tachycardia compared with untreated controls (Lohuis *et al.*, 1989). Doses appears to be important in dictating the effects of dexamethasone administration to cows with endotoxic mastitis. In a study, cows were given the higher dose of 0.44 mg/kg b. wt. after 2 hours following the introduction of purified bacterial endotoxin into mammary gland. This higher dose also reduced inflammation of mammary gland. But in this higher dose study, it is observed that two effects of the higher dose of dexamethasone are opposite to those observed in the lower dose study; with high dose, increase in rectal temperature were reduced and milk production losses were increased (Anderson and Hunt, 1989). Isoflupredone acetate (20 mg intravenous) administered to endotoxin challenged cows after the onset of clinical mastitis had no beneficial effect on rectal temperature, heart rate, rumen contraction rate, mammary gland swelling, or milk production compared with untreated controls (Wagner and Apley, 2003). Because experimental mastitis is transient and resolves rapidly without treatment, the relevance of any of these studies to cows with naturally occurring clinical mastitis questionable. A particular concern about dexamethasone is that repeated dosing (0.04 - 0.8 mg/kg b. wt., intramuscular for 3 days) of cows with *sub-clinical* intramammary infections resulted in increased bacterial shedding in milk and development of clinical mastitis (Spier *et al.*, 1991; Burton and Kehrli, 1995).

The potential benefit of intramammary administration of glucocorticoids to reduce local inflammation without affecting the migration of neutrophils into the gland is an attractive therapeutic option. The absence of clear contraindications, the possible benefits to subsequent milk production, the possible relief of the effects of enterotoxemia, and the human relief provided by reduction of clinical signs suggest that a one time use of glucocorticoids drugs (Dexamethasone @ 30 mg, IM) is a rational consideration when treating clinical endotoxic mastitis (Erskine *et al.*, 2003).

Non-steroidal anti-inflammatory drugs (NSAIDs)

Non-steroidal anti-inflammatory drugs are substances other than steroids that inhibit some components of the inflammatory cascade. The NSAIDs are known for many years for their anti-inflammatory, antipyretic and analgesic activity. These activities are mediated by the inhibition of cyclooxygenase (COX) enzymes. COX has two isoforms, designated as COX-1 and COX-2. COX-1has been referred to as the "*housekeeping*" enzyme that is constitutively expressed in most tissues and responsible for maintenance of various physiological processes including maintaining gastrointestinal mucosal integrity, platelet aggregation, and renal blood flow (Smith, 2005). The COX-2 isoform is considered "*inducible*" and is upregulated in response to inflammatory stimuli that is pro-inflammatory enzyme. Nearly all currently used veterinary NSAIDs are non-selective COX-1 and COX-2 inhibitors. All

NSAIDs that are in common use in food animal medicine inhibit the formation of prostaglandin E2 in the brain, which effectively reduces fever (Anderson, 1989). Arachidonic acid metabolism is one of the key components of the inflammatory cascade, and the formation of eicosanoids such as thromboxanes is directly responsible for inflammatory process. The NSAIDs exert their actions by inhibiting the cyclooxygenase enzyme and thus suppress the formation of inflammatory mediators such as thromboxanes (Figure 13.7).

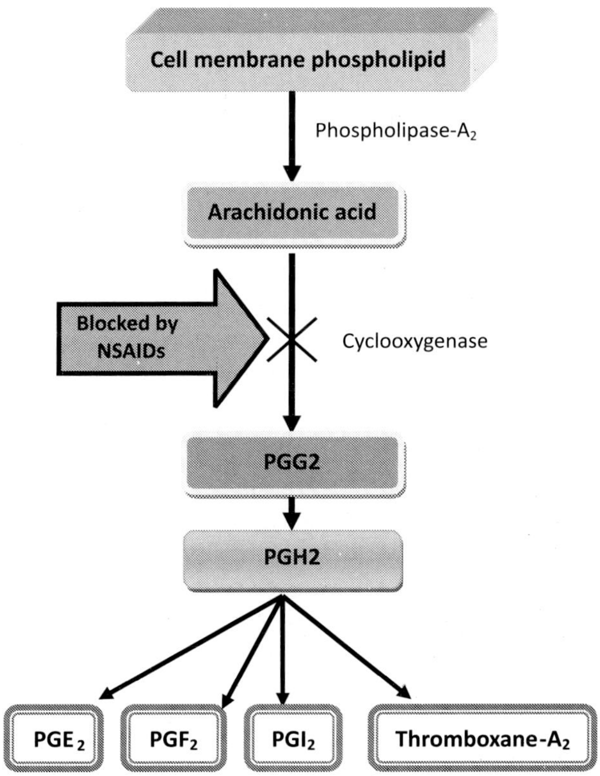

Figure 13.7: The arachidonic acid metabolism cascade and its inhibition by NSAIDs.

The NSAIDs have some other mechanisms, such as iron chelation, suppression of oxygen radical formation and lysosomal enzyme liberation, centrally mediated analgesic and anti-inflammatory effects and inhibition of bradykinin induced edema, may be attributed to other mechanisms than COX inhibition (Frey, 1992; Twomeny and Dale, 1992). The NSAIDs have been used for symptomatic relief of clinical signs of endotoxemic shock in acute mastitis. Flunixin meglumine, phenylbutazone, aspirin, dipyrone, nordihydroguaiaretic acid, flurbiprofen, carprofen, ibuprofen and ketoprofen have been studied as treatments of experimental coliform mastitis or endotoxin induced mastitis (DeGraves and Anderson, 1993; Rose *et al.*, 1991). But in

India, meloxicam (@ 0.2 – 0.3 mg/kg b. wt., intramuscular) is used as common anti-inflammatory agent in all inflammatory conditions including acute mastitis. Previously diclofenac was commonly used in veterinary practice in India but now it has completely been banned due to meal residual effects on vulture deaths. Hence, meloxicam is required a attention in India to detail study of its pharmacokinetic and pharmacodynamics in clinical cases of mastitis in field.

The various NSAIDs differ in their chemical structure, pharmacokinetics, anti-inflammatory, analgesic and antipyretic potency and toxicity (Frey, 1992; Higgins, 1985). Based on various experimental studies in animals, it has been found that flunixin meglumine, tolfenamic acid and ketoprofen can be classified as highly potent NSAIDs and phenylbutazone as a medium potency NSAID.

The NSAIDs do not have immunosuppressive effects but like glucocorticoids, do carry a risk of abomasal ulceration and renal damage (Morin, 2004b). Although these complications are not well documented in cattle and are probably of little concern, if hydration is maintained and administration is not prolonged. Flunixin meglumine is used at the dose rate of 1.1 to 2.2 mg/kg b. wt., once daily or divided twice daily for upto 3 days in the treatment of acute mastitis. Field trials using cows with naturally occurring clinical mastitis are more likely to indicate the true efficacy of NSAIDs for mastitis treatment. Flunixin meglumine can be expected to reduce the severity of clinical signs such as fever, depression, heart and respiratory rates, and udder pain (Erskine *et al.*, 2003). Ketoprofen has a shorter half life in cattle than does flunixin meglumine, and shorter milk residue duration. Also intramammary injection of ketoprofen is less irritating than intramuscular injection of flunixin meglumine (Pyorala *et al.*, 1999). In a field trial, a single dose of flunixin meglumine (1 g intravenous) or phenylbutazone (4 g intravenous) given to cows treated with gentamicin did not alter rectal temperature at 24 hours or milk yield over 10 weeks compared with saline treated controls (Dascanio *et al.*, 1995). Similarly, administration of 1g flunixin meglumine (2 doses at 24 hours interval) with or without intravenous fluids did not improve the outcome (survival rate, return to milk production) of toxic mastitis in 54 cows treated with antibiotics, oxytocin, stripping and calcium (Green *et al.*, 1997). Here it is questionable whether systemically administered NSAIDs are of benefit in cases of mastitis which are neither acute nor per-acute. However, another study found that cows treated with NSAIDs plus antibiotics (Trimethoprim-Sulfonamide) were 2.8 times more likely to recover than cows treated with antibiotic alone (Shpigel *et al.*, 1998). Cows treated with antibiotics plus ketoprofen (2g once daily) were 2.6 and 6.8 times more likely to recover (return to =75% milk production) than were cows treated with antibiotics alone or antibiotic plus a placebo, respectively (Shpigel *et al.*, 1994).

The appropriate NSAID have good potential as treatments for severe Gram negative mastitis (Erskine *et al.*, 2003).In conclusion, the administration of NSAIDs early in the course of infection is likely to be beneficial in the recovery of clinical signs in clinical mastitis cases.

Fluid therapy

Cows and buffaloes with clinical mastitis can develop fluid and electrolyte disturbances as a result of decreased feed and water intake, rumen stasis and diarrhea. Severely (per-acute) affected cows, particularly with coliform and gangrenous staphylococcal mastitis, may develop septic or endotoxic shock; in these cows death or organ damage can occur as result of decreased effective circulating volume (Morin, 2004b). Blood vessels dilate and as a result blood pressure starts to fall. Falling blood pressure leads to poor circulation and consequently poor tissue perfusion with blood. The animal appears dehydrated, as its body fluids are in the tissues and not in circulation. Dehydration may frequently reach 7 – 10% of body weight (Blowey and Edmondson, 2010). Most cows with clinical mastitis, even severe mastitis have normal acid-base balance or metabolic alkalosis; metabolic acidosis is uncommon and is associated with a poor prognosis (Morin, 2004b). Various studies suggest that there is no need for routine intravenous administration of alkalizing agents (e.g. bicarbonate or lactate), to cows with clinical mastitis (Cebra *et al.*, 1996; Katholm and Anderson, 1992). The oral products containing magnesium hydroxide should not be administered to mastitic cows, as these products can exacerbate metabolic alkalosis (Kasari *et al.*, 1990). Clinical mastitis is often accompanied by mild to moderate hypocalcemia. Therefore, calcium supplementation is logical.

The need for supportive therapy depends on the severity of the disease and usually is required only in the per-acute form. The administration of large amounts of balanced electrolyte solutions will counteract dehydration and cause forced diuresis to maintain renal function for the excretion of toxins or toxic metabolites. Administration of 5 – 10 liters in one hour may be sufficient; the cow may show marked improvement within 12 hours when shock is advanced, much larger volumes (60 – 110 mg/kg) of body weight may be needed with half the calculated dose given in the first 2 - 4 hours and the remainder in the next 6 hours (Radostits, 1970).

Intravenous administration

The common practice of balanced electrolyte or isotonic solutions administration is by intravenous route. Ringer's solution is the fluid of choice for rapid intravenous resuscitation of adult cows. Ringers solution is isotonic, mildly acidifying, and contains physiologic concentrations Na, Cl, K and Ca. However, administration of iso-osmotic crystalloid fluids or Ringers solution can be difficult due to the large volume of fluid required. The restraining of large animals is often difficult, hence administration of large volume of intravenous fluid is problematic. For these reasons, most veterinary practitioners do not administer complete dose of intravenous fluid, despite the fact that intravascular volume expansion is a fundamental goal in the clinical management of severe mastitis (endotoxic shock). Therefore, alternative to iso-osmotic intravenous fluid therapy is intravenous administration of hypertonic saline (7.5% NaCl solution). This is administered through a 16 gauze needle at a dose rate of 4 - 5 ml/kg b.wt. over 4 – 5 minutes period (approximately 2 liters for an average adult cow). Rapid administration is required in order to rapidly increase blood osmolality and creates an osmotic gradient to draw fluid from the intracellular spaces and rumen into the blood stream. The intravenous administration of hypertonic saline solution with administration of oral electrolyte solutions or water (without added electrolytes)can be extremely effective in rehydrating toxic or sick cow, and is much easier to administer than large volumes of isotonic fluids. The main force for water movement across the rumen wall is the gradient of osmolality between ruminal fluid (which is normally isotonic to plasma) and blood perfusing ruminal epithelium (Carter and Grovum, 1990). With the intravenous administration of hypertonic saline solution, plasma osmolality in adult ruminants is increased at the same time that rumen osmolality is decreased through oral administration of water or a hypotonic oral electrolyte solution. The increase in osmolar gradient across the rumen wall following this combined treatment is in part responsible for the movement of water from the rumen into the extracellular space, thereby expanding the plasma volume and correcting rehydration (Smith, 2005). Although hypertonic saline does not have a sustained effect and will not completely correct a large fluid deficit, it rapidly increases plasma volume and improves cardiac output and tissue perfusion. Administration of hypertonic saline solution alone without providing the cow fresh water is ineffective. Combined use of hypertonic saline solution with oral fluid should be considered to produce far superior resuscitation in the toxic cow than oral fluids alone (Smith, 2005).

Calcium borogluconate - 40% (Mifex)- 450 ml should be administer by slow intravenous route to restore calcium deficiency in clinical mastitis.

Oral fluid administration

The oral route is faster way of administering large volumes of fluid (10 - 20 liters). This route is least expensive and is often adequate for cows with mild to moderate dehydration, however, in cows that have severe dehydration or in those that are truly toxic, intravenous fluids are generally preferred. Until recently, the use of oral fluid therapy for cows has been limited by its practicability. A special device has been developed named as Agger's cattle pump (Figure 13.8) for the oral administration of fluid, which directly delivered the fluid into the rumen.

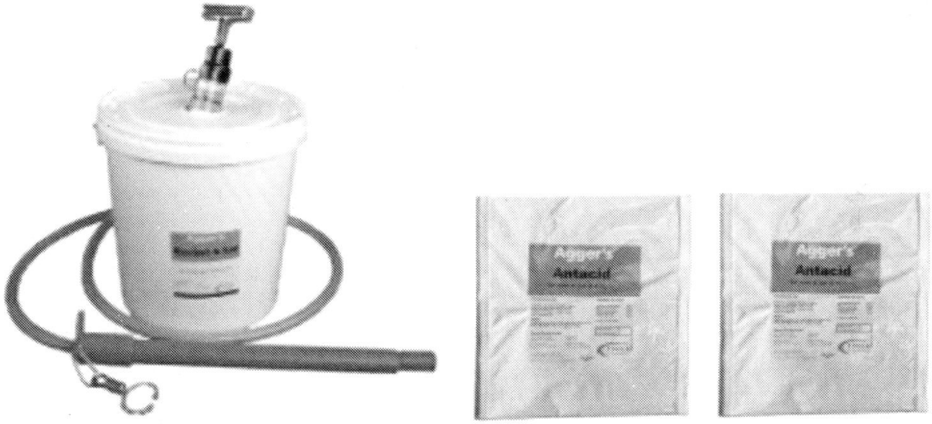

Figure 13.8: The Agger's cattle pump showing complete assembly.

The oral fluid should be hypotonic and contain sodium in order to create an osmotic gradient between ruminal fluid and blood, and enables sustained absorption of fluid and electrolytes (Morin, 2004b). Hypertonic oral fluids must be avoided because it will increase the tonicity of the rumen fluid. If this itself is made hypertonic, it will draw fluid from the circulation and so exacerbate the dehydration.

Most cases of dehydration in cows should not be treated with products designed for calves. Some of these products are hypertonic and most are alkalizing, because calves routinely have a metabolic acidosis. These properties of calf products makes them unsuitable for cows.

A man made oral rehydration formula for cows can be used in clinical dehydrated cattle.

Rehydration formula:

Sodium chloride	-	155g
Potassium chloride	-	50g
Calcium propionate	-	16g
Magnesium sulphate 7-hydrate	-	4g
Warm water	-	20 liters

Non-antibiotic treatment

Non-antibiotic approaches to the management of mastitis could occur through enhancement or manipulation of the natural defense factors in the mammary gland. As concern over the possible overuse of antimicrobials increases, attention has focused on reduction of their usage and trying to find some alternatives. Non-antibiotic approaches that would avoid residue problems have become the subject of common interest. A wide variety of other non-antibiotic measures are used to treat clinical mastitis cases. These include massage, application of liniments, homeopathy or herbal treatment, cytokine therapy, vitamin injections, clay therapy and other organic therapy.

Massage with different ointments is used to enhance blood circulation, but their effect is probably very limited.

[1] Homeopathy or herbal treatment

Homeopathy can defined as a specific stimulating therapy that activates the host defense mechanisms. Homeopathic medicine states that a substance that produces the symptoms of an illness can also be used in the treatment of any illness that causes similar symptoms. The precise method of action of homeopathic in bovine mastitis has not been determined, but they are prepared from a variety of plant, animal and mineral sources. The system relies on a series of dilutions being made, one part mother tincture to 99 parts of water and alcohol mixture. The mother tincture is an extract of natural substances e.g. of a culture of the bacteria that originally caused the symptoms (Blowey and Edmondson, 2010). Some homeopathic medicine which are frequently using in the treatment and control of mastitis are belladonna, bryonia, phytolacca, arnica etc.

Belladonna 1m - For acute post-partum mastitis. Udder very hot and red, painful to the touch. Animal is hot, and pulse is quick and strong. It results in swelling and tenderness of glandular system including mammary gland.

Dose: 1 dose every hour, 4 doses.

Belladonna 5CH - Hot red mammary gland that is painful to the touch, high fever. Prostrate animal.

Belladonna 5CH + Lachesis 5CH - Violet mammary gland, infiltration of underlying tissue with lateral preference. Prostrate animal.

Phytolacca 30c - It is useful in clinical and chronic cases. Clinical cases with sour, coagulated milk. Chronic cases with small clots at mid-lactation. It results in a state of restlessness and prostration together with glandular swelling.

Dose: Clinical- 3x/day for 3 days, followed by 1 dose a day for 4 days. Chronic- 1 dose every 3 hours, 4 doses.

Phytolacca alternating with Conium - Acute mastitis with hard gland, hot but pale. Strong pressure brings relief.

Bryonia alba 30c - Indicated for swollen and very hard udders. Pain is less intense when pressed. Animal is often lying down. Bryonia Alba is especially good for chronic mastitis cases with fibrosis.

Dose: Acute cases- 1 dose every 4 hours, 4 doses.

Chronic cases - 1 dose 2 times a week for one month.

Aconitum 6x - Routine treatment for all acute cases, particularly those that develop rapidly after exposure to cold dry wind. Relieves tension and anxiety.

Dose: 1 dose every half-hour, 6 doses.

Apis Mellifica 6c - Indicated for first calving, heifers with edema of and around the udder. Mammary vein is swollen.

Dose: 1 does every 3 hours, 4 doses.

Arnica Montana 30c - For mastitis resulting from udder injuries. There may then be blood in the secretions.

Dose: 3 doses per day for 3 days.

Belia Perennis 6c - As with Arnica, but for deeper injuries (e.g.: neglected milkers).

Dose: 3 doses per day for 4 days.

Urtica Ulens 6x - For clinical cases where edema forms plaques sometimes up to perineum.

Dose: 1 dose an hour, 4 doses.

S.S.C. 30c - Mixture of Sulphur, Silica and Carbo Vegetabilis that gives good results with clinical and *sub-clinical* cases. Lumps are usually big and yellowish, especially in first squirts of milk.

Dose: 3 doses a day for 3 days.

Ipeca 30c	- Useful for treating internal bleeding that produces pink or bloody milk. Dose: 3 doses a day for 3 days.
Silicea 200c	- Also useful for summer mastitis cases with purulent abscess and dry the pus. Dose: 2 doses a week for 4 weeks.
Hepar Sulphuris 6x	- Aids suppuration and cleaning of udder in summer mastitis cases (*Corynebacterium pyogenes*). Dose: 1 dose every 3 hours, 4 doses. 1 or 2 doses in greater dilution after udder is okay.
Lachesis 5 CH + Carbolicum acidum 5 CH	- Acute inflammation with edema, swollen veins, gangrenous tendency, extremely painful to the touch, quarter may feel cold. Weak heart, small quick pulse.
Vipera Reddi	- Marked glandular indurations. Chronic mastitis or end of mastitis. Little or no pain to the touch. Hypertrophy followed by atrophy.
Conium maculatum + Plumbum iodanum 5	- Hard quarter or nodes inside. Painful to the touch, retromammary ganglia. Cracking around teats.

Note: Legend- x, c and m refer to dilutions 10, 100 and 1,000

Phytolacca-200x, Aconite-200x, Bryonia-200x, Belladonna-200x, Camomilla-200x, Silasia-200x or Hypersulph-200x, at the dose rate of 4 to 10 drops every 6 hours for 6-7 days have been claimed to cure mastitis in animals (Varshney, 2000). Meaney (1993) stated that that the nosode had no effect in reducing the mastitis incidence or milk SCC. He evaluated the efficacy of a nosode formulated for *S. agalactiae, S.dysgalactiae, S. uberis, S. aureus, S. albus, S. epidermidis,Arcanobacterium pyogenes, E. coli and Mycobacterium bovis.* One group of 13 animals was treated with the nosode and a further group of 13 cows acted as an untreated control. The nosode was administered using a vulva spray technique and the experiment was conducted over an eight-month period.

The debate on the efficacy of homoeopathic medicines transcends both veterinary and human medicine. It is sometimes difficult to assess adequately conclusions drawn from some experiments due to poor experimental design and/or incomplete data. Day (1986) claimed to find some benefits from use of a nosode for unspecified periods in three herds while Sonnenwald (1986) found homoeopathic preparations were more successful than antibiotics in treating mastitis cases caused by Gram-negative bacteria but less effective than antibiotics in treating mastitis cases caused by Gram-positive bacteria. In a field study of 100 cases of acute clinical mastitis, it was found that homoeopathic treatments gave similar cure rates to antibiotics (Von Merck *et al.*, 1989). The authors also reported that homoeopathic treatments were more successful in mastitis cases caused by Gram-negative pathogens whereas antibiotic treatments were more effective in the treatment of mastitis caused by Gram-positive bacteria. Dorenkamp (1992), in a study of homoeopathic treatment on 580 *sub-clinical* cases of mastitis, achieved a cure rate of 97.9% after 4 days with only 28 (4.8%) showing relapses after 8 weeks. The same author reported that homoeopathic treatment of 218 clinical infections achieved 100% cure rate after 3 days with only 5 (2.5%) showing relapses after 8 weeks. The reports from Ireland indicate that there are no benefits from treating animals with some of the commercially produced homeopathic remedies in the market (Egan, 1998).

Chandel *et al.* (2009) used tetasule No 1 (composition: Apiswel 200, Pecacuanha 200, Bryonia 200, Plytolacca 200, Chamcmila 200, Urtica 200, Calc carb- Q.S.) and No.2 (composition: Belladona 200, Hepersulph 200, Calcflour 200, Silica 200, Conum 200, Calc Carb- Q.S.) in six divided doses of 5 ml in morning and evening respectively, in antibiotic treated clinical mastitic cows. Control group was treated with higher antibiotics only and tetasule was not used in control group. They found 95.56% recovery rate in tetasule treated animals, where as in control group except oedematous significantly lower than (50%) recovery rates were observed.

Coats *et al.* (1985) have been recommended 20 to 60 ml of aloes (in gel or juice form) intramammary administration at least once a day for the treatment of mastitis. Aloes is particularly indicated for treating udder injuries, which often leads to staphylococcal mastitis. Application of the aloes will quickly heal the tissue. Aloes helps to drain the infection, has anti-inflammatory properties and is a coagulant. It has a diuretic property also, which serves to soften the hardened udder. Once again, it is important to remember that the milk from cows treated this way cannot be put into the milk tank.

[2] Cytokine therapy

Soluble factors released by lymphocytes are termed "*lymphokines*" and those from monocytes and macrophages are termed "*monokines*", although they are now more commonly given the collective term cytokines. Cytokines are proteins that are produced naturally in the dairy cow, and function by regulating the activity of leukocytes involved in protecting the udder against mastitis causing bacteria. The term "*cytokine*" refers to a group of proteins produced by a spectrum of both immune or non-immune cells. Cytokines are water soluble regulatory peptides that provide relatively short range communication between cells of the immune system. The short range is important in limiting the effect of cytokines to the appropriate cells. The cytokines include interferons (IFN), interleukins (IL), growth and colony stimulating factors (CSF), tumor necrosis factor and a variety of other proteins with the capacity to modulate the activity of cells participating in immune and inflammatory processes. Cytokines have a tremendous potential to prevent and treat infectious diseases when normal host defense are compromised. One of the more exciting potential applications of cytokines is for the control of mastitis (VanMiert, 1990).

Cytokines may exert their effects in the udder by recruitment of effector cells (phagocytic cells), enhanced bacterial clearance by phagocytic cell populations and regulation of acute inflammation. There is increasing interest in the role of cytokines in enhancing immunity to mastitis.

(a) Interferon gamma (INFγ)

Interferon gamma is a cytokine, that modulates (enhanced) phagocytic activity of leukocytes, especially neutrophils and macrophages, as well as regulates the acute inflammatory response induced by bacterial toxins. Thus, it is believed that the use of INFγ shortly before or after calving could reduce the occurrence of coliform mastitis. *E. coli* infection is more prevalent during this time. Such infections occur because circulating leukocytes do not respond rapidly enough or in sufficient numbers to prevent establishment of these bacteria in the udder.

It is believed that prophylactic use of INFγ shortly before or after calving could reduce the incidence of coliform mastitis (Nickerson, 1994). Recombinant bovine INFã which is involved in upregulating Major Histocompatibility Complex (MHC) expression and the activation of macrophages, reversed suppressive effects.

(b) Colony stimulating factors (CSF)

Colony stimulating factors are a group of cytokines required for the proliferation and differential of bone marrow stem cells into functional mature leukocytes. Granulocyte-macrophage colony stimulating factor (GM-CSF) was first identified by its capacity to induce maturation of bone marrow cells into granulocytes (neutrophils0 and macrophages (Metcalf, 1985). Recombinant granulocyte macrophage colony stimulating factor, which stimulates growth and differentiation of cells of myelomonocytic lineage, enhanced the phagocytic capacity of neutrophils particularly in neutrophils isolated from mastitis cows (Reddy *et al.*, 1989) and induce leukocytosis into mammary gland which may have reduced new infections in cows treated with GM-CSG (Nickerson *et al.*, 1989). The administration of granulocyte colony stimulating factor (GCSF) to lactating dairy cows, markedly increase total leukocyte as well as neutrophil numbers in both blood and milk compared with placebo control. The GCSF treated cows challenged with *Staphylococcus aureus* exhibited a 47% reduction in new intramammary infection compared with control (Nickerson, 1994).

(c) Interleukins (IL)

'Interleukin is also an other group of cytokines. The term interleukin was originally introduced to describe cell free soluble factors that function as communicator between leukocytes. Now days IL-1 and IL-2 are the only bovine interleukins that have been cloned, sequenced and expressed. Interleukin-1 is synthesized by macrophages and activates lymphocytes involved in the immune responses. Interleukin-2 is produced by certain lymphoid cells and modulates lymphocyte activity by stimulating cell proliferation and maturation and as well as antibody production. The possibility of enhancing resistance level of the mammary gland with some cytokines as IL-2, has received considerable research attention. It has been reported that intramammary administration of some cytokines such as bovine IL-2 can enhance cellular and humoral immune responses against *Staphylococcus aureus* and coliforms. Prophylactic administration of IL-2 has been shown to protect the mammary gland from subsequent intramammary challenge with *Staphylococcus aureus* (Sordillo *et al.*, 1997).

The effect of recombinant bovine IL-2 on the treatment of *Staphylococcus aureus* mastitis in cattle showed that 3 intramammary infusions of the cytokine was 15 - 45% as effective as commercial antibiotic intramammary product (Hayes *et al.*, 1990). Similarly multiple infusions of recombinant bovine interleukin-1were 40 - 65% as efficacious as antibiotic in the treatment of *Staphylococcus aureus* infections (Dougherty *et al.*, 1990). Interleukin-1 enhanced therapeutic efficacy for antibiotic in established infections in cattle (Coyle *et al.*, 1992).

The use of these cytokines may improve therapeutic efficacy of lactating cow antibiotics, and the products are biologically inactive within 48 hours of treatment, thereby eliminating residues. The use of cytokines by intramammary administration routinely is not yet developed. However, research into the role of cytokines in bovine mastitis is in the beginning stages. Further developments in these areas are necessary before experimental findings can be transferred to field conditions.

[3] Bacteriocins therapy

Bacteriocins were first proposed for treatment of mastitis when the results of trials carried out by Taylor *et al.* (1949) indicated that a single intramammary infusion of nisin, a bacteriocin discovered in 1928 (Rogers and Whittier, 1928), was effective in treating both streptococcal and staphylococcal infections. Interest in the use of nisin as a therapeutic agent was renewed when Broadbent *et al.* (1989) showed that nisin was inhibitory to several Gram-positive, mastitis-causing pathogens.

Bacteriocins are non-toxic proteins, digested and inactivated by intestinal enzyme (protease) and thus potential less hazardous than antibiotic use in mastitis therapy. These proteins are larger molecules than antibiotics and are expected to persist in the udder longer. Bacteriocins kill targeted organisms rapidly by lysing the cell wall, and they do not require that the organism undergo cell division. Lysostaphin and nisin are the bacteriocins particularly active against staphylococci and streptococci; the major etiological agents of bovine mastitis. Both bacteriocins are rapidly bactericidal, equally active against dividing and non-dividing bacteria, and are active against antibiotic resistant isolates. They act as catalysts and are very specific to a single chemical reaction. For mastitis treatment, bacteriocins can be either infused as intramammary or used in solutions such as teat dips.

(a) Nicin

Nisin is a bacteriocin of commercial value used as a natural food preservative. Nicin is a natural product of *Lactococcus lactis* and it has broad spectrum antimicrobial activity. Nisin is easily deactivated by digestive enzyme like pancreatin and a-chymotrypsin and it is too small to induce antibody formation. Nicin has an activity against both Gram-positive (e.g. Staphylococci, Streptococci, Corynebacteria, Bacilli, Clostridia and *Listeria monocytogenes*) and Gram-negative bacteria such as *E. coli, Klebsiella pneumonia,* Salmonellae and *Pseudomonas aeruginosa* (Blackburn *et al.*, 1989). Because of its high antibacterial activity and nontoxicity for humans, nisin has already been employed as a food preservative for a long time, and licensed by 48 countries around the world (Deegan *et al.*, 2006). As an active ingredient, nisin has been formulated into some commercially available products for teat-dipping to prevent mastitis (Sears *et al.*, 1992). Although antibacterial activities of nisin have been reported.

Sears and Blackburn (1993) administered nicin in combination with lysostaphin by intramammary route and found promising results as 100%, 95% and 66% effective against *Streptococcus uberis, Strpetococcus agalactiea* and *Staphylococcus aureus*, respectively. Wu *et al.* (2007) treated cows with an intramammary infusion of nisin at a dose of 2,500,000 IU once daily for 3 days while the control cows received no treatment. Milk samples were collected from the affected mammary quarters before initiating, 1 and 2 weeks after treatments for analyses of bacteria, somatic cells and N-acetyl-β-D-glucosaminidase (NAGase). Results indicated that nisin therapy caused bacteriological cure rate of 90.1% for *Streptococcus agalactiae*, 50% for *Staphylococcus aureus*, 58.8% for coagulase negative staphylococci, and 65.2% for all cases. Meanwhile, only 15.9% spontaneously recovered in the no-treated cows. NAGase activiy in milk samples and the number of mammary quarters with milk SCC =500,000/ml were significantly decreased after nisin-treatment while no significant changes took place in the control group.

(b) Lacticin

Lacticin is a bacteriocin produced by *L. lactis* DPC3147 (Ryan *et al.*, 1998) that has a broad-spectrum of activity against all Gram-positive bacteria, including many mastitis-causing pathogens. The structure and mode of action of lacticin has been documented (McAuliffe *et al.*, 2000; Martin *et al.*, 2004). Ryan *et al.* (1998) examined the *in vitro* sensitivity of 24 mastitic streptococcal and staphylococcal isolates to lacticin 3147: all were inhibited.

(c) Lysostaphin

Lysostaphin is a potent peptidoglycan hydrolase and first time isolated from *Staphylococcus simulans*. It was first described in 1963. This antimicrobial protein has a potent anti-staphylococcal activity and its secretion into milk offers considerable resistance to infection caused by *Staphylococcus aureus*, on molar basis it 70 to 100 times more potent than penicillin. The gene for lysostaphin has been cloned and the recombinant product is produced as a secretory product by a non-pathogenic strain of *Bacillus sphaericus*. Now days lysostaphin gene is using for the development of mastitis resistant animals.

Lysostaphin is administered at the rate of 100 mg/60 ml phosphate buffer saline per quarter 24 hourly for 3 days.

[4] Oxytocin therapy

A very important procedure in treatment of coliform mastitis infections involves frequent milking of the infected cow to remove leukocytes, bacteria and toxins from the mammary gland. Frequent milking-out is a traditional and commonly used method to treat mastitis in many countries. When dairy industry has became more intensive and the units bigger, this practice has more or less disappeared. Scientific evidence on the effect of this treatment is not available, but probably frequent removing of the milk from the diseased quarter removes bacteria and toxins, and may relieve pain. Milking-out with oxytocin has often been recommended in the textbooks for treatment of coliform mastitis (Pyorala, 2003).

Oxytocin, a milk let-down hormone, released from the brain into the blood stream in response to the stimuli associated with milking. Oxytocin causes contraction of the milk producing alveoli within the mammary gland, resulting in the expulsion of milk. It is believed that administrating exogenous oxytocin further "squeezes out" or flushes residual bacteria laden fluid after milking, which may eliminate the infection. In addition, inflammatory byproducts, bacterial toxins, tissue debris and blood clots are removed. Similarly, evacuation of milk actually stimulates the production of more milk, enhances leukocyte movement into the quarter, and activates the other antimicrobial components of milk (Nickerson, 1994).

Oxytocin is frequently used to aid the stripping of affected quarter(s). Commonly, veterinarians recommend frequent stripping of affected quarter (6 times a day) following oxytocin administration at the rate of 40 to 50 IU, intramuscularly. Oxytocin is rapidly inactivated in the body and the potential for toxicity is low.

The optimal dosage of oxytocin and the optimal time of administration has not been established by research. Some clinicians have expressed the opinion that a small dose should be given at the end of milking to aid in the expulsion of residual milk and to reduce strippings. The label doses for aid in milk let-down is 10 to 20 IU, while that for obstetrical use in 100 IU (Guterbock, 1995). Nostrand *et al.* (1991) confirmed that 20 IU would elicit milk let-down in 1.5 to 2 minutes and would also aid in ejection of strippings milk. Guterbock *et al.* (1993) carried out a study to compared the efficacy of Cephapirin and Amoxycillin mastitis tubes to that of oxytocin alone in the treatment of mild clinical environmental mastitis. Oxytocin was administered at the rate of 100 IU intramuscularly just before milking. All the cows treated in the study had mild mastitis (abnormal milk with or without udder swelling, and no systemic signs). There were no significant differences in overall clinical cure (return of the affected quarter and milk to normal) rates by 9th milking after initial diagnosis and treatment or in bacterial cure (failure to isolate the primary pathogen present at the first milking) rate by day 21 (after initial treatment) between antibiotic and oxytocin treated quarters, although there was a significant effect of antibiotics on clinical cure in the category of other bacteria, which were pathogens other than coliforms and streptococci (Table 13.18).

Table 13.18: Bacterial and clinical cure (%) in oxytocin and antibiotic treated mastitis cows (Guterbock, 1995).

	Oxytocin	Amoxycillin	Cephapirin
Bacterial cure (%)			
Coliforms (n=63)	38.50	45.0	61.10
Streptococcus spp. (n=49)	60.00	60.0	54.50
Other bacteria (n= 26)	57.10	27.3	45.50
Clinical cure (%)			
Coliforms (n=94)	69.70	83.3	68.0
Streptococcus spp. (n=65)	52.80	48.0	64.0
Other bacteria (n= 34)	77.80	72.0	68.0

In some studies, high doses of oxytocin have been used but then there may be risk for adverse effects. In fact, inducing milk ejection does not need more than about 10 IU of oxytocin (Pyorala, 2003). In a field trial on mild clinical mastitis, Roberson (1997) suggested even harmful effects after frequent milking.

However, oxytocin therapy is also linked with some of the disadvantages-

- There is no economic advantage to oxytocin therapy due to longer time required to bring the animals to return to normal. In a study, oxytocin was administered intramuscularly at the rate of 100 IU every 12 hours for 2 or 3 milking, the clinical cure rate was 70%, but bacterial cure rate was 49% after 20 days of initial diagnosis and treatment (Nickerson, 19994).
- Higher rate (41%) in oxytocin treated cows. Administration of oxytocin (20 IU) for six consecutive milking eliminated 25% of infections, but 75% of the cows developed clinical mastitis due to relapse (Hillerton and Semmens, 1999).

Borsberry (2003) believed that oxytocin administration is contraindicated when-

- Teat canal is obstructed.
- In acutely inflamed quarters especially when the cow is toxic. Many of these cows have obstructed milk ducts. Administration of oxytocin can increase the pain experienced by increasing the pressure within the udder and cause a greater flow of toxins etc. from the alveoli through the damaged alveolar walls and hence into the blood circulation.

[5] Tri-sodium citrate

Normal udder (milk) pH (6.5-6.8) is unfavourable for bacterial growth but change in pH favours the bacterial growth. At normal milk pH (6.5) sodium citrate forms a strong soluble complex with Ca^{2+} which prevents it from clumping but variation in this complex result in shift of pH. Thus it forms an important buffer of Ca^{2+} and H^+ in milk. Citrate radical is concerned with synthesis of casein, lactose and fat in milk and its replenishment in animal system by tri-sodium citrate would make up the deficiency and initiate normal lactogenesis. The acidity of milk is due to free acidic groups of casein, citrate and phosphate as well as to the presence of dissolved CO_2. Extent of reduction in the level of citric acid may depend on the severity of inflammation. Citric acid deficiency causes retention of calcium in the milk secretary alveoli, adversely affecting the alveoli by causing necrosis of the secretary epithelium and thereby leading to cessation of milk. Administration of tri-sodium citrate orally replenished the citrate deficiency in animal system and restored the milk contents to normalcy. Tri-sodium citrate was found good in reducing the pH of milk (Dhillon *et al.*, 2000; Sindhu *et al.*, 2008). The milk pH is increased in case of mastitis due to inflammation. Citrate is essential for milk synthesis and it can be regarded as a harbinger for lactogenesis. Therefore, oral administration of tri-sodium citrate is effective in managing the cases of *sub-clinical* mastitis and it improved milk yield also (Sindhu *et al.*, 2008).

[6] Anti-oxidant therapy

Anti-oxidant therapy has utmost importance in the treatment and control of mastitis. Various anti-oxidants are using since last several decades e.g vitamin E, vitamin C, selenium, copper, zinc, manganese etc. Naturally body protects from any infecting organisms through various mechanisms including phagocytosis. During phagocytosis phagocytic granulocytes undergo respiratory burst to produce oxygen radicals to destroy intracellular pathogens. However, these oxidative products can in turn, damage healthy cells if they are not eliminated. Antioxidants serve to stabilize these highly reactive free radicals thereby maintaining the structural and functional integrity of cells. Therefore, antioxidants are very important to immune defense and health of animals. For detail of anti-oxidant therapy see chapter of prevention and control of this book.

[7] Ozone therapy

Ozone is polymerized oxygen (O_3) created by the passage of air or oxygen over high energy electrodes within an ozone generators or by ultraviolet light. The bactericidal and anti-fungal properties have been well established (Whistler and Sheldon, 1989a; Whistler and Sheldon, 1989b). Treatments utilizing ozone have been used in human medicine for over a century and a large number of hard-to-cure diseases have been safely remedied by ozone. Little attention has been paid to the clinical application of ozone in the veterinary practice. The application of ozone to bovine acute clinical mastitis, infusing of ozone into the inflamed quarter, appears to have great possibilities for sterilization of causative agents, and detoxicating of the inflamed quarter through oxidation with ozone. The ozone treatment involves the immersion of gas (50 - 100 ml) at different concentration directly in the affected quarters. Ozone treatment requires a minimum contact time, adequate volume and concentration of ozone to sterilize causative agents of mastitis, as the infused ozone needs direct contact with causative agents. The ozone therapy seems to have many advantages in treatment of bovine clinical mastitis-

- It can sterilized all the pathogenic organisms including bacteria, virus, mycetes, yeast etc. and their toxins also.

- Antibacterial effects are same or enhanced when mixed with milk.
- Local insufflations can reach the milk compartments of the glands.
- After ozone treatment, the relapse mastitis time is delayed.
- Milk of treated mastitis cases can be utilized immediately for industrial or nutritional purpose.
- No milk withdrawal time is required in ozone treated animals.
- It does not have any adverse interaction with other drugs.

Ogata and Nagahata (2000) states that ozone therapy is effective, safe, and cost effective and carries no risk of drug residues in milk and also reported that 65% of cows with acute clinical mastitis treated with ozone therapy, did not require any antibiotics for recovery. The potential therapeutic effect of ozone gas on bovine mastitis has been investigated HyunJoo *et al.* (2005) and it was concluded that ozone gas treatment (one ppm for 3 days) might be effective for the treatment of bovine mastitis. Pereira and Garcia (2006) administer ozone by intramammary route in sub-clinical mastitis cows and showed that ozone therapy is effective in reducing the intensity of infection.

However, the use of ozone has not come in the usual practice because- i) it is not easy to establish the right ozone concentration, ii) it has to be used in combination with antibiotics for desired efficacy and, iii) more clinical field trials are needed to develop good data base regarding its application and efficacy.

References

Adams, R.H. (2001). In: Vet. pharmacology and therapeutics, Ames (IA): Iowa State University Press; p. 229-267.

Akhtar, M.H., Roy, G.P., Singh, A.P., Sinha, B.K., Kumar, A. and Kumar, R. (2003). In: Proc. of 4th Round Table Conf. on Mastitis, Palampur, (India), 14-15 April, 2003. pp. 178-184.

Akthar, M.H., Roy, G.P., Singh, A.P., Sinha, B.K., Kumar, A. and Kumar, R. (2004). In: Proc. Round table Conf. on Mastitis, 14-15 April, Palampur, India. Pp. 178-184.

Allot, A.J. (1937). Am. Vet. Med. Assoc., 91: 588.

Altreuther, P. (1987). Vet. Med. Review., 2: 87-89.

Anderson, K.L. (1989). Therapy for acute coliform mastitis. Comp. Cont. Ed. Pract. Vet., 11: 1125-1133.

Anderson, K.L. and Hunt, E. (1989). Vet. Res. Commun., 13: 17-26.

Andrew, A.H. (2004). Antimicrobial agents. In: Bovine mastitis: Diseases and husbandry of cattle (2004), edited by Andrew, A.H., Blowey, R.W., Boyd, H. and Eddy, R.G., 2nd ed., Blackwel publishing Co., pp. 1035-1044.

Anonymous (1999). NCCLS document M31-A performance standards for antimicrobial disc and dilution susceptibility tests for bacteria isolated from animals; approved standard. Wyne (PA): National Committee for Clinical Laboratory Standards.

Anonymous (2000). Clin. Microbiol. Infect., 6: 503-508.

Baggot, J.D. (1977). Principles of drug disposition in domestic animals: the basis of veterinary clinical pharmacology. W.B. Saunders, Philadelphia.

Baggot, J.D. (2000). Priniciples of antimicrobial drug bioavailability and disposition. In: Antimicrobial Therapy in Veterinary Medicine (ed. by J.F. Prescott, J.D. Baggot & R.D. Walker), 3rd edn, pp. 50–87. Iowa State University Press, Ames, Iowa.

Baranski, W., Ras, M., Janowski, T., Zduñczyk, S., Dewulf, J., Kruif, A.D., Vliegher, S.D. and Opsomer, G. (2008). Medycyna Wet., 64(3): 301-305.

Bauer, A.W., Kieby, W.M.M., Shrenis, J.C. and Turck, M. (1966). Am. J. Clin. Pathol., 45: 453-496.

Berry, E.A. and Hillerton, J.E. (2000). In: Proc. 39th Ann. Mtg. Natl. Mastitis Council, Atlanta GA. Natl. Mastitis Counc., Inc., Madison, WI., Pp 213-214

Berry, E.A. and Hillerton, J.E. (2002). J. Dairy Sci., 85: 112–121.

Biggs, A. (1998). In: Proc. British Mastitis Conf., pp. 15-21.

Biggs, A. (2002). In: Proc. of the British Mastitis Conf., Brockworth, pp. 37-50.

Blackburn, P., Polak, J., Gusik, S. and Rubino, S. (1989). Nisin compositions for use as enhanced, broad range bacteriocides. In: International patent application number DCT/US89/06 2626; International publication number W089/12399. Applied Microbiology Inc. NY.

Blowey, R. and Edmondson, P. (2010). Mastitis control in dairy herds. 2nd edn., CABI International, UK.

Borseberry, S. (2003). In: Proc. Britich Mastitis Cong, Garstang. Pp. 63-71.

Bradley, A.J. and Green, M.J. (2000). J. Dairy Sci., 83: 1957–1965.

Broadbent, J.R., Chou, Y.C., Gillies, K. and Kondo, J.K. (1989). J. Dairy Sci., 72: 3342-3345.

Brown, M.B. and Scasserra, A.E. (1990). Am. J. Vet. Res., 51: 2015-2018.

Browning, J.W., Mein, G.A., Barton, M., *et al.* (1990). Aust. Vet. J., 67: 440-442.

Burton, J.L. and Kehrli, M.E. Jr. (1995). Am. J. Vet. Res., 56(8): 997-1006.

Bushby, S.R.M. (1980). J. Am. Vet. Med. Assoc., 176: 1949-1053.

Capuco, A.V. and Akers, R.M. (1999). J. Mammary Gland Biology and Neoplasia, 4(2): 137-144.

Carter, R.R. and Grovum, W.L. (1990). J. Anim. Sci., 68: 2811-2832.

Cebra, C.D., Garry, F.B. and Dinsmore, R.P. (1996). J. Vet. Int. Med., 10: 252-257.

Chandel, B.S., Dadawala, A.I., Chauhan, H.C., Parsani, H.R and kumar, P. (2009). Vet. World, 2(10): 383-384.

Coats, B.C., Holland, R.E. and Ahola, R. (1985). Creatures in our care: the veterinary uses of aloe vera. Published by the authors. Pp.299.

Constable, P.D. and Morin, D.E. (2003). Vet. Clin. Food Anim. Pract., 19: 139-155.

Costa, E.O., Benites, N.R., Guerra, J.L. and Melville, P.A. (2000). J. Vet. Med. B Infect. Dis. Vet. Public. Health. 47(2): 99-103.

Coyle, P. Furda, G.J., Tao, W., Daley, M. J. and Johnston, P. (1992). J. Dairy Sci., 75(1): 145.

Dascanio, J.J., Mechor, G.D., Grohn, T.Y. et al. (1995). Am. J. Vet. Res., 56: 1213-1218.

Dawn, M.B. (1994). Vet. Med., 89: 744-753.

Day, C.E.I. (1986). J. Vet. Homeopathy, 1: 15-19.

De Oliveira, A.P., Watts, J.L., Salmon S.A. and Aarestrup, F.M. (2000). J. Dairy Sci., 83: 855-862.

Deegan, L.H., Cotter, P.D., Hill, C. and Ross, P. (2006). Intl. Dairy J., 16:1058-1071.

DeGraves, F.J. and Anderson, K.L. (1993). Am. J. Vet. Res., 54:1128-1132.

Deluyker, H.A, Van Oye, S.N. and Boucher J.F. (2005). J Dairy Sci., 88: 604-614.

Deluyker, H.A., Michanek, P., Wuyts, N. *et al.*, (2001). In: Proc. 40th annual meeting of Natl. Mast. Coun., Reno NV, Natl Mast Coun. Madison, WI., pp. 170-174.

Dhillon, K.S., Singh, S., Varindra and Singh, T.J. (2000). Indian J. Dairy Sci., 53: 323-325.

Diarra, M.S., Petitclerc, D. and Lacasse, P. (2002). J. Dairy Sci, 85(5): 1141-1149.

Diarra, M.S., Petitclerc, D. *et al.* (2003). Vet. Immunol & Immunopathol, 95(1-2): 33-42.

Dorenkamp, B. (1992). Biologische Tiermedizin, 9: 76-86.

Dougherty, R., Williams, T. J., Coyle, P. A., Hayes, P., Walsh, J., Furda, G. J. and Daley, M. J. (1990). J. Dairy Sci., 73(Suppl. 1): 211.

Dumka, V.K. and Srivastava, A.K. (2003). In: Comp. Round Table Conf. on Mastitis, Palampur, India, 14-15th April, 2003. Pp. 97-111.

Eberhart, R.J. (1986). J. Dairy Sci, 69(6): 1721-1732.

Edmondson, P. (1989). Vet. Rec., 125: 591-593.

Egan, J. (1998). In: Proc. British Mastitis Conf., 1998, Axient/Institute for Animal Health, Milk Development Council/Novartis Animal Health, p22-28.

Erskine, R., Wagner, S. and DeGraves, F. (2003). Vet. Clin. North Am. Food Anim. Pract., 19: 109-138.

Erskine, R.J. (1998). In: Proc. British Mastitis Conf., Axient. Pp. 9-14.

Erskine, R.J. (2003). North Am. Vet. Conf., 2003. 13-16.

Erskine, R.J. and Eberhart, R.J. (1990). J. Am. Vet. Med. Assoc., 196: 1230-1235.

Erskine, R.J., Bartlett, P.C., Johnson, II G.L., *et al.* (1996). J. Am. Vet. Med. Assoc., 208: 258–260.

Erskine, R.J., Bartlett, P.C., VanLente, J.L. and Phipps, C.R. (2002). J. Dairy Sci., 85: 2571-2575.

Erskine, R.J., Kirk, J.H., Tyler, J.W. *et al.* (1989). Vet. Clin. North Am., 9: 499-519.

Erskine, R.J., Walder, R.D., Bolin, C.A., Bartlett, P.C. and White, D.G. (2001). J. Dairy Sci., 85: 1111-1118.

Face to Vet (2007). A clinical update (published by Intas Neovet pharmaceuticals Ltd., India). Volume 2, issue-3.

Foley, E.G., Lee, S.W. and Hartley, N.J. (1946). J. Food Technol., 8: 129-133.

Francis, P.G. (1989). Br. Vet. J., 45: 302-331.

Franklin, A. and Rantzien, M.H. (1983). Nord. Vet. Med., 35: 460-464.

Franklin, A., Horn a, R.M. Obel, N., Ostensson, K. and Astrom, G. (1986). J. Am. Vet. Res., 47: 804-807.

Frey, H.H. (1992). In: Proc. Intl. Symp. on the use of non-steroidal anti-inflammatory drugs in domesticated animals. 12, September, 1992, Nurnberg, Germany. pp. 11-20.

Garret, E.R. (1978). Scand. J. Infect. Dis., 14: 54-85.

Gentilini, E., Denamiel, G., Liorente, P., Godaly, S., Rebuelto, M. and DeGregorio (2000). J. Dairy Sci., 83: 1224-1227.

Giersemehl, K. (1995). Use of cephalosporins in therapy in bovine mastitis, Dissertation, pp. 138.

Green, M.J., Green, L.E. and Cripps, P.J. (1997). Vet. Rec., 140(6): 149-152.

Guterbock, W.M. (1995). In: Proc. 2nd Western large herd dairy management conf., Las Vegas, NV, 6 – 8 April, pp. 49-60.

Guterbock, W.M., Van Eenennaam, A.L., Anderson, R.I., Gardner, I.A., Cullor, J.S. and Holberg, C.A. (1993). J. Dairy Sci., 76: 3437.

Hadded, N.S., Ravis, W.R., Pedersoli, W.M. and Carson, R.L. (1986). Am. J. Vet. Res., 47: 808-813.

Hadded, N.S., Ravis, W.R., Pedersoli, W.M. and Carson, R.L. (1987). Am. J. Vet. Res., 48: 21-27.

Harmon, R.J., Crist, W.L., Hemken, R.W. and Langlois, B.E. (1986). J Dairy Sci., 69: 843-849.

Hayes, H.C., Dougherty, R., Williams, T.J., Coyle, P.A., Furda, G.J., Walsh, J. and Daley, M.J. (1990). J. Dairy Sci., 73 (Suppl.. 3): 211.

Higgins, A.J. (1985). J. Vet. Pharmacol. Therap., 8: 1.

Hillerton, J.E. (1998). Bulletin of the International Dairy federation No. 330, pp.4-5.

Hillerton, J.E. and Berry, E.A. (2003). Vet. Clin. Food Anim., 19: 157-169.

Hillerton, J.E. and Kliem, K.E. (2001). In: Proc. 2nd Intl. Symp. Mastitis and Milk Quality. Pp. 234-237.

Hillerton, J.E. and Kliem, K.E. (2002). J. Dairy Sci., 85: 1009-1014.

Hillerton, J.E. and Semmens, J.E. (1999). J. Dairy Sci., 82: 93–98.

Hirata, F. (1983). Lipomodulin: a possible mediator of the action of glucocorticoids. Adv. Prostaglandin Thromboxane Leukot Res., 11: 73-82.

Hoeben, D., Burvenich, C. and Heyneman, R. (1998). J. Dairy Sci., 81: 403-410.

Holmgren, N., Haggmar, B. and Tolling, S. (1985). Nord. Vet. Med., 37: 228-233.

HyunJoo, K., JianZhu, L., SungNam, J., KunHo, S., DuckHwan, K., MooHyung, J., SungWhan, C., MyungCheol, K. and HyoIn, Y. (2005). J. Vet. Clin., 22(4): 314-317.

Jones, A., Higgs, T.M., Neave, F.K. and Smith, A. (1967). J. Dairy Res., 34: 249-255.

Jones, G.F. and Ward, G.E. (1990). J. Am. Vet. Med. Assoc., 197: 731-735.

Kaartinen, L., Lohonen, K., Wiese, B., Franklin, A. and Pyorala, S. (1999). Acta. Vet. Scan., 40: 271.

Kakavas, J.C. (1944). North Am. Veterinarian, 25: 408.

Kasari, T.R., Woodbury, A.H. and Morcom-Kasari, E. (1990). J. Am. Vet. Med. Assoc., 196: 735-742.

Katholm, J. and Andersen, P.H. (1992). Vet. Rec., 131: 513-514.

Kehrli, M. and Harp, J. (2001). Vet. CLin. North Am. Food Anim. Pract., 17: 495-516.

Kirk, J.H. (1991). Agri-Practice 12: 5-8.

Knight, C.H., Fitzpatrick, J.L., Logue, D.N. and Platt, D.J. (2000). Vet. Rec., 146: 311-316.

Kung, K., Riond, J.L. and Wanner, M. (1993). J. vet. Pharmacol. Ther., 16: 462-468.

Lawrence, K. (2002). In: Proc. British Mastitis Conf., Brockworth. Pp. 30-36.

Leslie, K.E. (1994). Mastitis control in dairy herds. In: Radostits OM, Fetrow J, editors. Herd health: food animal production medicine. 2nd edition. Philadelphia: WB Saunders; pp. 229–276.

Lintner, T.J. and Eberhart, T.J. (1990). Am. J. vet. Res., 51: 533-542.

Lohuis, J.A., Van Leeuwen, W., Verheijden J.H.M., Van Miert, A.S.J.P.A.M. and Brand, A. (1988). J. Dairy Sci., 71: 2782-1789.

Lohuis, J.A.C.M., vac Leeuwen, W., Verheijden, J.H.M., Brand, A. and Van Miert, A.S.J.P.A.M. (1989). J. Dairy Sci., 72: 241-249.

Makovec, J.A. and Ruegg, P.L. (2003). J. Am. Vet. Med. Assoc., 222: 1582-1589.

Martin, N.L., Sprules, T., Carpenter, M.R., Cotter, P.D., Hill, C., Ross, R.P. and Vederas, J.C. (2004). Biochemistry 43: 3049-3056.

McAllister, T.A., Yanke, L.J., Inglis, G.D. and Olson, M.E. (2001). Advances in Dairy technology, 13: 229-247.

McAuliffe, O., Hill, C. and Ross, R.P. (2000). Microbiology 146: 129-138.

Meaney, W.J. (1993). In: Mastitis and Milk Quality: A Handbook for Veterinary Practitioners. (Editor W.J. Meaney). Teagasc Research Centre, Moorepark, Fermoy, Ireland, 59-71.

Metcalf, D. (1995). Science, 229: 16.

Milne, M.H., Barrett, D.C., Fitzpatrick, J.L. and Biggs, A.M. (2000). In: Proc. IDF Symp. Immunol. Rumin. Mamm. Gland. Stresa, Italy. pp 379-381.

Moretain, J.P. and Boisseau, J. (1989). Food Add Contamin., 6: 79-90.

Morin, D., Shanks, R.D., McCoy, G.C., *et al.* (1988). J. Am. Vet. Med. Assoc., 213: 676-681.

Morin, D.E. (2004a). Acute mastitis: Revisiting the goals of therapy. In: Proc. 23rd world Buiatrics Cong., Quebec city.

Morin, D.E. (2004b). In: Proc. National Mastitis Council, pp. 13-23.

Myllys, V., Louhi, M. and Ali-Vehmas, T. (1992). J. Vet. Med. B., 39: 723-731.

National Mastitis Council. (1999). Laboratory handbook on bovine mastitis. Revised edition. Madison (WI): National Mastitis Council.

Neijenhuis, F., Barkema, H.W., Hogeveen, H. and Noordhuizen, J.P.T.M. (2000). J Dairy Sci., 83: 2795–2804.

Nickerson, S.C. (1993). Vet. Med., 33: 368-373.

Nickerson, S.C. (1994). Alternatives to antibiotic therapy for treating mastitis. Dairy Research Report, Louisiana State University, Hill Farm Research Station, Homer, LA-71040. Pp. 123-140.

Nickerson, S.C., Owens, W.E. and Watts, J.L. (1989). J. Dairy Sci., 72(12): 3286-3294.

Nickerson, S.C., Paape, M.J., Harmon, R.J. and Ziv, G. (1986). J. Dairy Sci., 69: 1733-1742.

Nostrand, S.D., Gatton, D.M., Erb, H.N. and Baumari, D.E. (1991). J. Dairy Sci., 74: 2119.

O'Rourke, D.J. and Baggot, J.D. (2004). Antimicrobial therapy of mastitis. In: Bovine medicine: Diseases and Husbandry of cattle (Ed. Andrew, A.H., Blowey, R.W., Boyd, H. and Eddy, R.G.), 2nd edn. (2004), Blackwell Pub. Agency, Oxford, UK.

Ogata, A. and Nagahata, H. (2000). J. Vet. Med. Sci., 62(7): 681-686.

Oliver, S.P. (1988). Am. J. Vet. Res., 49:1789–1793.

Oliver, S.P. and Mitchell, B.A. (1983). J. Dairy Sci., 66: 1162–1166.

Osteras, O., Edge, V.L. and Martin, S.W. (1999). J. Dairy Sci., 82: 1221–1231.

Owens, W.E. and Nickerson, S.C. (1989). Agri-Practice, 10: 10-15.

Owens, W.E. and Nickerson, S.C. (1990). J. Dairy Sci., 73: 115-124.

Owens, W.E., Nickerson, S.C. and Ray, C.H. (1999). J. Dairy Sci., 82: 645-647.

Owens, W.E., Ray, C.H. and Washburn, P.J. (1993). J. Vet. Med. B., 40: 508-514.

Owens, W.E., Ray, C.H., Watts, J.L. and Yancey, R.J. (1997). J. Dairy Sci., 80: 313-317.

Owens, W.E., Watts, J.L., Boddie, R.L. and Nickerson, S.C. (1988). J. Dairy Sci., 71: 3143–3147.

Owens, W.E., Watts, J.L., Greene, B.B. and Ray, C.H. (1990a). J. Dairy Sci., 73: 1225-1231.

Owens, W.E., Xiang, Z.Y., Ray, C.H. and Nickerson, S.C. (1990b). J. Dairy Sci., 73: 3449–3456.

Payorala, S. (2002). In: Proc. British Mastitis Conf., Brockworth, pp. 20-29.

Pearson, J.K.L. (1950). Vet. Rec., 62: 166-168.

Pearson, J.K.L. (1964). Vet. Rec., 76: 409.

Pereira, M.T.C. and Garcia, C.A. (2006). Veterinária Notícias, 12(2): 109-115.

Prescott, J.F., Baggot, J.D. and Walker, R.D. (2000). Antimicrobial therapy in veterinary medicine. 3rd ed. Iowa State University Press, Ames, Iowa.

Pyorala, S. (2002). In: Proc. British Mastitis Conf., 2002, Brockworth. Pp. 20-29.

Pyorala, S. (2003). In: Proc. North Am. Vet. Conf., pp.76-77.

Pyorala, S. (2006). In: Proc. World Buiatrics Cong., 2006, Nice, France.

Pyörälä, S. and Pyörälä, E. (1998). J. Am. Vet. Med. Assoc., 212: 407-412.

Pyörälä, S. and Syväjärvi, J. (1988). J. Vet. Med. B, 34: 629-639.

Pyorala, S., Laurila, T., Lehtonen, S. et al. (1999). Acta Vet. Scand., 40: 145-150.

Pyorala, S., T. Laurila, S. Lehtonen, Leppa, S. and Kaartinen, L. (1999). Acta Vet. Scand., 40:145-150.

Radostits, O.M. (1970). In: Proc. IV International Conf. on cattle diseases, Philadelphia, p. 67.

Radostits, O.M., Gay, C.C., Blood, D.C. and Hinchkliff, K.W. (2000). Veterinary Medicine. 9th edn. ELBS & Baillier Tindall.

Rasmussen, F. (1966). Studies on the mammary excretion and absorption of drugs. Carl Fr Mortensen, Copenhagen.

Reddy, P.G., Blecha, F., Minocha, H.C., Anderson, G.A., Morrill, J.L., Fedorka-Cray, P.J. and Baker, P.E. (1989). Vet. Immunol. Immunopathol., 23(1-2): 61-74.

Richard Adams, H. (2001). In: Veterinary Pharmacology & Therapeutics. (Richards, Adam, M. ed.) 8th Edn., Iowa State Univ. Press, Ames. Pp. 783-946.

Roberson, J.R. (1997). In: Proc. of the 36th Annual Meeting of the National Mastitis Council, Albuquerque, NM. Arlington (VA): National Mastitis Council, pp. 152-157.

Roberson, J.R. (2003). Vet. Clin. Food Anim., 19: 223-234.

Rogers, L.A. and Whittier, E.O. (1928). J. Bacteriol., 16: 211-214.

Rose, D.M., Giri, S.N., Cullor, J.S. and Bushnell, R.B. (1991). Zentralbl Veterinarmed A., 38(2): 99-106.

Rossitto, P.V., Ruiz, L., Kikuchi, Y., Glenn, K., Luiz, K., Watts, J.L. and Cullor, J.S. (2002). J. Dairy Sci., 85: 132-138.

Roy, S., Vishwakarma, P. and Roy, M. (2010). Intas Polivet, 11(I): 34-36.

Ruegg, P.L and Araujo, T.P.B. (2002). In: Proc. 2nd Panamerican Congress on Milk Quality and Mastitis Control. Nov 25-27, 2002. Ribeirao Preto, Brazil.

Rule, R., Buschiazzo, P., Castillo, J.R., Porcelli, C. and Peretti, M.C. (1991). Medicine Veterinaria, 8: 211-215.

Ryan, M., Meaney, W.J., Ross, R.P. and Hill, C. (1998). Appl. Environ. Microbiol., 64: 2287-2290.

Salmon, S.A., Watts, J.L., Aarestrup, F.M., Pankey, J.W. and Yancey, R.J. (1998). J. Dairy Sci., 81: 570-578.

Sanchez, M.S. and Watts, J.L. (1999). J. Dairy Sci., 82(3): 494-499.

Sanders, P., Moulin, G., Guillot, P., Dagorn, M., Perjant, P., Delepine, B., Gaudiche, C. and Mourot, D. (1992). J. Vet. Pharm. Ther., 15: 53-61.

Sandholm, M., Kaartinen, L. and Pyorala, S. (1990). J. Vet. Pharm. Ther., 13: 248-260.

Sar, T.K., Mandal, T.K., Samanta, I., Rahaman, A. and Chakraborty, A.K. (2010). Indian J. Anim. Sci., 80(12): 1182-1184.

Sarode, D.B. (2002). In: Proc. Round Table Conf on Mastitis, Nagpur, India. 4-5th Feb, 2002. Pp. 40-42.

Sattler, N., Sweeney, R.W., Whitlock, R.H. et al. (1997). J. Am. Vet. Med. Assoc., 210: 240-243.

Schaeren, W. and Schaellibaum, M. (1987). Schweiz. Milchw. Forschung. 16: 69-70.

Schaeren, W. and Schaellibaum, M. (1993). Bestimmung der minimalen Hemmkonzentrationen bei Mastitiserregern. Report of the Federal Dairy Research Station, 18: 1-31.

Schifferli, D., Schaellibaum, M. and Nicolet, J. (1984). Arch. Tierheilk., 126: 23-34.

Schmid, P., Bottner, A. and Humke, R. (1994). In: Proc. 18th World Buiatric Congr., Bologna, Italy. 1: 539.

Sears, P.M. and Blackburn, P. (1993). Antibiotic alternatives: The role of antimicrobial proteins. In: Proc. Regional Meeting, National Mastitis Council, Inc. NY.

Sears, P.M. and McCarthy, K.K. (2003). Vet. Clin. Food Anim., 19: 171-185.

Sears, P.M., Smith, B.S., Stewart, W.K., Gonzalez, R.N., Rubino, S.D., Gusik, S.A., Kulisek, E.S., Progran, S.J. and Blackburn, P. (1992). J. Dairy Sci., 75: 3185-3190.

Sebastian, S.R. and Vijayakumar, K. (2002). In: Proc. of 3rd Round Table Conf. on Mastitis, Izatnagar, (India). Pp. 120-125.

Serieys, F., Raguet, Y., Goby, L., Schmidt, H. and Friton, G. (2005). J. Dairy Sci., 88: 93-99.

Sharma, A. and Kapur, M.P. (2000). In: Proceeding of 1st Round Table Conference on Mastitis, IVRI, Izatnagar, (India),18th -19th Feb., p.8-11.

Sharma, A.K., Khosla, R., Kela, A.K. and Mehta, V.L. (1994). Indian J. Pharmacol., 26: 249-261.

Sharma, Neelesh and Maiti, S.K. (2005). Indian J. Vet. Med., 25(2): 76-79.

Sharma, Neelesh, Gupta, S.K., Sharma, U. and Hussain, K. (2007). Buffalo Bull., 26(2): 56-58.

Sharma, Neelesh, Maiti, S. K. and Sharma, Kamal Kant (2007). Intl. J. Dairy Sci., 2(2): 145-151.

Shenep, J.L., Barton, R.P. and Mogan, K.A. (1985). J. Infect. Dis., 151: 1012.

Shpigel, N.Y., Chen, R., Winkler, M., Saran, A., Ziv, G. and Longo, F. (1994). Res. Vet. Sci., 56(1): 62-68.

Shpigel, N.Y., Winkler, M., Ziv, G., et al. (1998). Vet. Rec., 142: 135-137.

Sielman, E.S., Fecteau, G., Girard, C. et al. (1998). Vet. Rec., 143: 503-507.

Sindhu, O.K., Baby, P.G., Pillai, U.N., Kumar, S.A. and Alex, P.C. (2008). Indian J. Vet. Med., 28(2): 143-145.

Singh, P.J., Singh, K.B., Jand, S.K., Dhingra, P.N. and Nauriyal, D.C. (1994). Indian J. Dairy Sci., 47(9): 730-733.

Singh, R., Sharma, Neelesh, Soodan, J.S. and Sidhan, N.A. (2005). J. Res. SKUAST-J., 4(2): 223-224.

Smith, G.W. (2005). Vet. CLin. Food Anim., 21: 595-614.

Smith, K.L. and Hillerton, J.E. (1999). In: Proc. 38th Ann. Meeting Natl. Mastitis Conc., Arlington (VA): National Mastitis Council. Pp. 200-201.

Smith, K.L. and Hogan, J.S. (1995). The importance of coagulase-negative staphylococci. IDF Bulletin No. 20. Brussels, Belgium: IDF.

Soback, S., Adler, H., Van Damm, B., *et al.* (1990). In: Proceedings of the International Symposium on Bovine Mastitis, Indianapolis, IN. Madison (WI): National Mastitis Council, pp. 134-137.

Sol, J., Sampimon, O.C., Snoep, J.J. and Schukken, Y.H. (1994). J. Dairy Sci., 77: 75–79.

Sol, J., Sampimon, O.C., Snoep, J.J. and Schukken, Y.H. (1997). J. Dairy Sci., 80: 2803-2808.

Sonnenwald, B.M. (1986). Abstract 1438 Dairy Science Abstracts 50: 158.

Sordillo, L.M., Shafer-Weaver. K. and DeRossa, D. (1997). J. Dairy Sci., 80(8): 1851-1865.

Spier, S.J., Smith, B.P., Cullor, J.S. et al. (1991). J. Vet. Intern. Med., 5: 341-350.

Srivastava, A.K. (2000). In: Comp. Round Table Conf. on Mastitis, Bareilly, India, 18-19th Feb., 2000. Pp. 62-83.

Srivastava, A.K., Saini, S.P.S. and Gill, M.S. (2002).. In: Comp. Round Table Conf. on Mastitis, Nagpur, India, 4-5th Feb, 2002. Pp. 43-65.

Suresh, R.V., Srinivasan, S.R., Gowri, B. and Krishna, M.M. (2010). Intas Polivet, 11(I): 31-33.

Taylor, J.I., Hirsch, A. and Mattick, A.T.R. (1949). Vet. Rec., 61: 197-198.

Tijare, D.B., Chaturvedi, V.K., Srivastava, A.B., Dhaneskar, N.S. and Mehara, K.N. (2000). Indian Vet. J., 77: 969-971.

Twomey, B. and Dale, M. (1992). Biochemical Pharmacology, 43: 413-418.

Ullberg, S., Hansson, E. and Funke, H. (1958). Am. J. Vet. Res., 19: 84-92.

VanMiert, A.S.J.P.A.M. (1990). Cytokines: Modulation of host resistance against infection. In: Proc. Mastitis physiology and pathology, International Cong., Gent, Belgium.

Varshney, J.P. (2000). In: Comp. Round Table Conf. Mastitis, 18-19 Feb, 2000, Izatnagar, Bareilly, India. Pp. 1-7.

Vliestra, R.J. (2003). In: Proc. National Mastitis Council Regional Meeting, 2003. pp. 30-35.

Von Merck, C.C. , Sonnenwald, B. and Rollwage, H. (1989) Berliner und Münchener Tieräarztliche Wochenschrift 102: 272-274.

Wagner, S.A. and Apley, M.D. (2003). J. Dairy Sci., 86: 792-798.

Watts, J.L. and Salmon, S.A. (1997). J. Dairy Sci., 80: 788-791.

Wells, S.J., Ott, S.L. and Seitzinger, A.H. (1998). J. dairy Sci., 81: 3029-3035.

Wenz, J.R., Barrington, G.M., Garry, F.B. et al. (2001a). J. Am. Vet. Med. Assoc., 219: 976-981.

Wenz, J.R., Garry, F.B. and Barrington, G.M. (2001b). In: Proc. of the 2nd International Symposium on Mastitis and Milk Quality, Vancouver, BC. Madison (WI): National Mastitis Council and Rome (GA): Am. Assoc. Bovine Pract., pp. 111-115.

Whistler, P.E. and Sheldon, B.W. (1989a). Poult. Sci., 68: 1068-1073.

Whistler, P.E. and Sheldon, B.W. (1989b). Poult. Sci., 68: 1345-1350.

Whittem, T. and Hanlon, D. (1997). New Zealand Vet. J.. 45: 178-184.

Wilson, D.J., Gonzalez, R.N., Case, K.L., Garrison, L.L. and Grohn, Y.T. (1999). J. Dairy Sci., 82: 1664-1670.

Wu, J., Hu, S. and Cao, L. (2007). Antimicrobial Agents and Chemotherapy. 51(9): 3131-3135.

Yadav, G.U., Bhikane, A.U., Anantwar, L.G., Kale, S.B. and Bhokare, A.P. (2002). In: Proc. of Round Table Conf. on Mastitis, Nagpur, India, 4-5th Feb., 2002. Pp. 137-138.

Ziv, G. (1980a). J. Am. Vet. Med. Assoc., 176: 1109-1115.

Ziv, G. (1980b). Vet. Med. Small Anim. Clin., 75: 277-290.

Ziv, G. (1992). Vet. Clin. North Am. Food Anim. Pract., 8: 1.

Ziv, G. and Schultze, W.D. (1982). J. Vet. Pharma. & Therap., 5(2): 123-129.

Ziv, G. and Storper, M. (1985). J. Vet. Pharm. Therap., 8: 276-283.

Ziv, G. and Sulman, F.G.C. (1974). Res. Vet. Sci., 17: 68-74.

Ziv, G., Paape, M. J. and Dulin, M.T. (1983). Am. J. Vet. Res., 44: 385-388.

Zoske, D.E., Cipolle, R.J., Rotschafer, J.C., Solem, L.D., Mosier, N.R. and Strate, R.G. (1982). Antimicrob. Agents Chemother., 21: 407-411.

□□□

CHAPTER

14

Prevention and Control

Perhaps the single biggest advance in dairy health in the last 25 years has been the paradigm shift from treatment of clinical illness to disease prevention particularly in case of mastitis. A fundamental advancement has been recognition of the multifactorial nature of almost all diseases of importance in dairy cattle. Health management has been defined as "*the promotion of health, improvement of productivity, and prevention of disease in animals within the economic framework of the owner and industry, while recognizing animal welfare, food safety, public health, and environmental sustainability*".

With the proliferation of international trade, globalization, and global warming, the importance of the control of contagious and infectious diseases has increased dramatically. Implementation of mastitis control strategies has led to a change in the incidence and etiology of mastitis over the past 40 years. This change has resulted in a decrease in the prevalence of contagious mastitis pathogens and an increase in the relative, and arguably absolute, importance of the environmental pathogens such as *Streptococcus uberis* and *E. coli* on the vast majority of well-managed dairy units (Sharma, 2010). Accordingly, disease prevention, considered broadly, is no longer the sole domain of veterinarians. Conversely, to deliver health management and effective disease prevention veterinarians must integrate consideration of nutrition, housing, and whole farm management systems into recommendations of best practices (LeBlanc *et al.*, 2006).

The fundamental principle of mastitis control is that the disease is controlled by either decreasing the exposure of the teat ends to potential pathogens or by increasing resistance of dairy cows to infection. Controlling mastitis is not a matter of doing just one thing. Instead, it involves following a number of steps better referred to as a control programme. To be acceptable, such a programme must be economical, practical, effective under most management conditions, and reduce new infections. The programme should also shorten the duration of pre-existing infections, reduce the incidence of clinical mastitis, and be subject to easy modification as improved methods are developed through research. Fortunately, working toward the reduction of clinical mastitis is not in conflict with the long range objectives of a control program because most clinical cases are preceded by sub-clinical cases. Thus, a reduction in the more obvious clinical mastitis is evidence that the unnoticed sub-clinical infections are also being reduced.

A key factor in preventing mastitis is to reduce the number of bacteria present around the teat end. This is particularly important in the period from about two weeks before calving to two weeks after. The following points should be practiced to control the mastitis

1. Preparation of Animal

Clipping the hair on the udders, the flanks and inside the hindlegs. Before milking animal should be clean. Teats specially the orifice, should be cleaned and dried prior to milking. The milking of wet udders and teats may lead to increased mastitis and higher bacteria counts in herd milk. Correct washing and massaging of the teats and udders sends a signal to the pituitary gland at the base of the brain, which secretes the milk letdown hormone, oxytocin, into the blood stream. This hormone then travels to the udder and stimulates the myoepithelial cells surrounding the milk secreting tissues to contract and cause milk letdown.

2. Biosecurity

Introduction of new animals to the herd can be risky from the standpoint of biosecurity. No animals infected by a contagious pathogen (*S. aureus, S. agalactiae, Mycoplasma*) should be alowed to join the herd before the previous check in and quarantine (Dingwell, 2002.; Eberhart, 1986).

The safest way to keep the herd healthy is never introduce the new animal. Unfortunately on modern dairies that often grows very fast, raising their own quality heifers is not an option. On modern dairy farm every animal which is not pregnant heifer or lactation cow should not exist. Every calf (male or female) should leave the farm soon after the calving. There is a posssibility to send the female calves to the heifer raising farms, keep them there until get pregnant and buy them back as replacement heifers or new animals if herd will be expanded. If farmer have to buy a cows or heifers, investigation of their previous status is absolute necessity.

They should be free of all kind of contagious mastitis pathogens and also free of other contagious diseases such as bovine viral diarrhea (BVD), Johne's disease, leukosis etc.

Heifers that have not yet calved are less likely to be infected (especially with mastitis causing microorganisms) than milking cows. To decrease risk of introducing infected cows into the herd:

a) Know the herd that you buy from - Buy only from herd with documentation to prove the low prevalence or no cases of contagious mastitis such as individual somatic cell count (SCC), herd SCC, mastitis and other disease records (infectious disease, lameness, metabolic problems), routine individual milk sample cultures (Wilsson, 1980). Consider sampling the bulk tank a few days in a row for bacterial culturing.

b) Know the cow that you buy - From those herds buy only cows with a low SCC, a negative California mastitis test (CMT) and a negative bacterial milk culture.

New cows should be milked after the healthy cows but before the already infected cows until you are sure of their udder health status.

3. Milk Cows with Clean, Dry Teats and Teat Ends

Teats and teat ends should be washed with water and dried completely before the milk is taken by hand or machine. Preparation of the teats and udder for milking has a two fols purpose, namely, to stimulate milk letdown and reduce the number of contaminating micro-organisms on the skin. Proper teat and udder preparation will reduce microbial contamination of milk, decrease strippings, increase milk yield, decrease milking time, and reduce the spread of contagious pathogens, i.e. *Staphylococcus aureus* and *Streptococcus agalactiae*, as well as reduce incidence of new infections with the environemental micro-organisms (Nickerson, 1994). Udders should be clipped or signed as necessary to remove long hair and to reduce the amount of dirt, manure, and bedding that may contaminate milk.

Emphasis should be placed on the teat ends. An additional positive step may be predipping with a sanitizing solution similar to those used for post-milking teat dipping. Predipping with teat dip has become popular. A 30-second contact with sanitizer is needed to kill organisms. If contact time is not sufficient,then it's a very expensive premilking regime. Predipping may be beneficial in reducing mastitis, but the actual dipping, dip contact time, and wiping with a towel increase the total milking time. There are many effective teat dips, including iodine at 0.1%, 0.5%, and 1.0%. Also, although it is not labeled for teat dipping, hypochlorite at 4.0% with a sodium hydroxide content less than 0.05% was effective in field trials. There are many more teat dips on the market that are effective in preventing new infections. Effective coverage of the teats is more important than the type of dip being used. Teat diping in details is dicussed in the dry cow therapy section.

4. Prevent Transfer of Pathogens from Cow to Cow during Milking

This has been universally successful to control most contagious mastitis pathogens by preventing spread from one infected cow to non-infected cows during the milking process. Single use towels (paper, cloth, wipes) should be used in preparation of the udder and teats. Gloves for milkers are helpful and should permit constant washing with irritation to hands. Separate milking units for infected cows, established milking orders to protect the non-infected cows, hospital pens with separate milking equipment are all appropriate methods. Hospital cows should not be milked with the fresh cows. Post-milking teat dipping is very important. There is only one way to effectively stop the spread of mastitis in the dairy herd, and that is by applying teat dip to every quarter of every cow after every milking. Teat dips are used to remove milk residue left on the teat and kill organisms on the teat at the time of dipping. They also leave a residual film of sanitizer between milkings. Post-milking teat dipping is effective in eliminating environmental organisms *E. coli* and *S. uberis* on the teats after milking. Milk should never be stripped directly into the milker's hand because this procedure spreads micro-organisms from quarter to quarter and from cow to cow via contaminated hands.

5. Prevent Injury to the Teats and Udder during Milking

Any injuries to the teats or teat ends and udder will eventually end up with a new case of mastitis. Important steps are proper milking techniques (attachment, alignment and removal of machines), proper milking machine design/function, routine and timely changing of inflations, and continuous maintenance of the milking equipment (cleaning pulsators, etc.). Periodic assessment of teat end condition may be a useful indicator. Environmental sources of injuries should also be controlled (bedding, housing, free stall design and maintenance, frostbite).

6. Housing

Providing adequate space, ventilation, bedding, and lighting to ensure cleanliness and comfort at all times. Over crowding should be avoided. Bedding materials are a major source of teat end exposure to environemental microorganisms, and reducing the number of bacteria in bedding generally results in a decrease in mastitis caused by these organisms. Finely choped organic bedding materials such as sawdust, shavings, recycled manure, pelleted corncobs and chopped straw frequently contain very high numbers of coliforms and environmental streptococci. Low moisture containing inorganic materials such as washed sand, crushed limestone, and clay are preferable to finely chopped organic materials because they contain few nutrients for bacteria to utilize and are, therefore, associated with lower numbers of organisms (Nickerson, 1994).

7. Early Detection of New Infections and their Prompt Treatment

Prompt detection of mastitis will preclude severe mastitis outbreaks. Milking may begin with a check of all quarters for mastitis. Any cows that show clinical mastitis should be examined and appropriate action taken. If fore milking is not done, visual checking for inflamed quarters is done by milkers and herd health people. Early detection may be by prestripping prior to milking, observation of the udder and teats, California mastitis test, various forms of electronic somatic cell counting or electrical conductivity. Milkers should be trained to use these techniques and management feedback is important.

Just after confirmation of mastitis treatment with appropriate therapy should be started as early as possible.

8. Milking

Proper milking procedures are important for the prevention of mastitis and for insuring complete milk removal from the udder. Cows should be milk completely to prevent the occurrence of new cases. Standard milking techniques should be used. Follow proper milking procedures, milk clean, dry udders, apply milking units properly, and make adjustments to prevent the admittance of air into the teat cup liners and prevent liner slip.

Although the cow is usually exposed to the act of milking and associated events less than 15 minutes a day, this period is a prime time for increased susceptibility to new infections. Milking time should be consistent routine, and the cow should not be frightned or excited before milking because such stress results in epinepfrine release into the bloodstream, which interferes with normal milk letdown.

9. Fly Control

High number of flies may be found on cows and heifers teats. Flies can transmit pathogens such as *S. aureus* and *Arcanobacterium pyogenes* from one animal to the other by biting the thin skin on teats. Horn flies (*Hydrotea irritans*) also cause scores and scabs on teats – a reservoir of *S. aureus*.

Efficient fly control inside and outside the barn can improve udder health. Basic fly control involves prevention of breeding sites through routine removal of manure and decaying feeds. Flies breed in organic material such as manure and feed, so weekly removal of organic material in and around the barn is the most important way to reduce the fly population. Improving the barn ventilation, holding area in front of milking parlor and milking parlor also helps. Tunnel ventilation or big fans fixed above the cows can be used for ventilation.

Various mechanical, biological and chemical control measures can assist but never replace proper sanitation protocols. Insecticide ear tags and sprays may also helpful.

10. Selecting the Bulls

Selection of bulls for higher milk production and fast milking may unfortunately have increased susceptibility to mastitis. Bulls are now also rated according to SCC and mastitis susceptibility. That way dairy farm owners can choose semen from bulls whose daughters are more resistant to mastitis.

Heritability is quite low, only around 15%, meaning that 85% of variation is explained by other factors such as feeding, housing and management in general. Genetic influence is long term, sometimes have to wait few generation before visible succes, but it should not be ignored.

11. Dry Cow Therapy

The dry period is crucial to optimize the cow's health and milk production for the next lactation. It is a period of high risk for many diseases including the mastitis. New infections are frequent during this period causing clinical mastitis cases in early lactation. To optimize the subsequent lactation a 60 day dry period (40 – 70 days) has been recommended for years. If it is too short, the regeneration of milk producing cells may not be optimum. If it is too long, annual milk production will decrease. New information suggests the dry period may be shorter, even eliminated, with mature cows. Research is ongoing to find effects on mastitis, reproduction and culling rate. They already find negative influence on milk production if dry period is eliminated.

Treating or infusion of antibiotics in all four quarters of cows with specially formulated, long acting antibiotics at drying-off, immediately following the last milking, is an effective practice in the battle against sub-clinical mastitis, called dry cow therapy (DCT). The use of dry cow antibiotic therapy and the treatment of intramammary infection at drying-off has been a corner stone and mastitis management and control over the past six decades. The use of intramammary antibiotic to prevent intramammary infections in the dry period was originally developed as a control measure for summer mastitis (Pearson,

1950). The status or prevalence of mastitis at farm(s) is a result of two factors, the "new infection rate" and the "duration of infection". The intramammary infection rate is 2-12 times higher during at any other time during the dry period than at any other time during the lactation cycle of the cow (Vliestra, 2003). Dry cow antibiotic therapy fulfills both of the most important criteria for mastitis control namely "reduction of the duration of existing infections" and "reduction of the new infection rate". In other words, the dry cow therapy has two major objectives:

1. *Curing the existing infections* – dry cow antibiotic infusion has a more concentrated dose, for a longer period of time than a lactation therapy antibiotic infusion. So it is more efficient to cure subclinical infections. The cure rate is fairly high for most of the pathogens (70 - 90%). Cure rate is less for *S. aureus* infections, especially for old infections but still higher than lactation therapy
2. *Preventing new infections in the early dry period* – dry cow therapy reduces the incidence of new infections by 50 - 75% particularly by environmental streptococci during the risky period following drying off. Reducing new infections during the dry period reduces the number of clinical cases in following lactation. It has a limited effect on coliforms infections occuring immediately before and after calving.

Eliminating existing infections (reducing duration of infections) can be of importance with contagious infections such as Staphylococci and Streptococci. Many cows infected during lactation do not show signs immediately and in some instances many not have a clinical episode for the whole lactation. The infection remains sub-clinical (Biggs, 1998) and this may become clinical during dry period or just after parturition (Figure 14.1).

Prevalence of bacteria during dry period

The mammary glands are most vulnerable to new infections during the first weeks and last weeks of the dry period. The environmental pathogens e.g. *S. uberis* and may be contagious pathogens are more prevalent during the first weeks of lactation, while during last weeks of dry period environmental pathogens including coliform bacteria too, are more prevalent. The rates of new infection by the coliform bacteria are 4 to 5 folds greater during the dry period than during lactation (Smith *et al.*, 1985). The susceptibility of dry mammary gland to new intramammary infection with environmental organisms has been confirmed by various studies around the world (Williamson *et al.*, 1995; Berry and Hillerton, 2002; Bradley and Green, 2001). All recent studies, in conventionally managed herds, have confirmed that the environmental pathogens are the most significant cause of new intramammary infection during the dry period. A study demonstrated that new infection rates with environmental organisms as being upto 10 times higher than during lactation (Smith *et al.*, 1985). Coagulase negative staphylococcal infections showed a significant rise in prevalence during the dry period, but the vast majority of these resolved spontaneously post-calving (Bradley and Green, 2004). It is important to remember that infections acquired in the late dry and transition periods are more likely to have a major influence on clinical mastitis in the subsequent lactation (Green *et al.*, 2002).

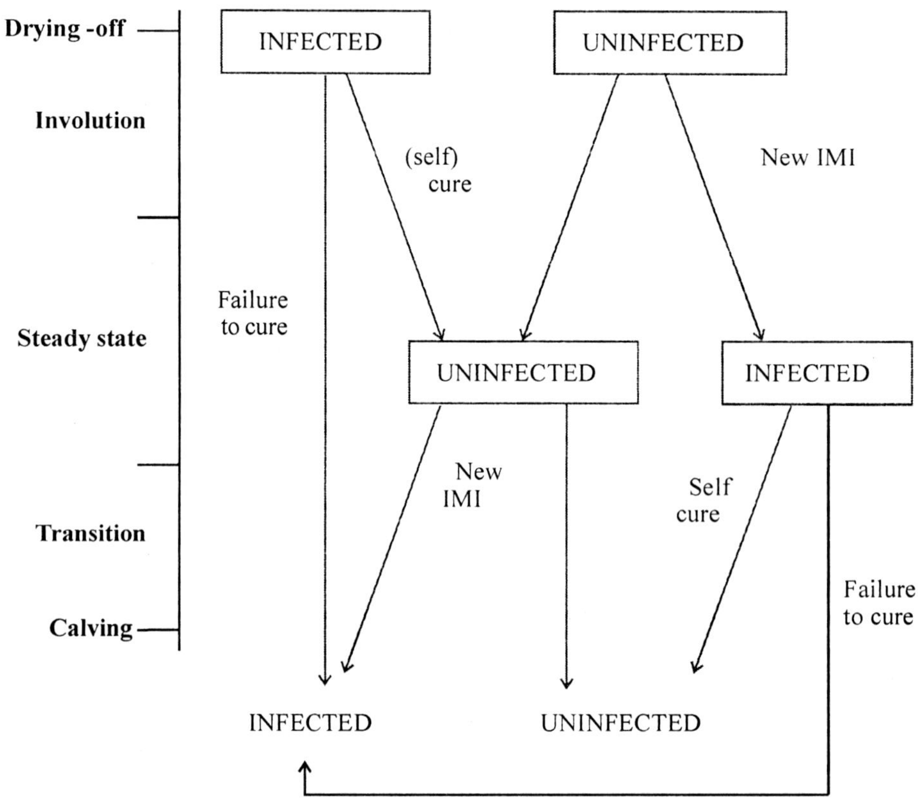

Figure 14.1: Possible outcomes for individual quarters during dry period.

The distribution pattern of mastitis pathogens causing new intramammary infections during the dry period vary between farms and in different parts of the world. However, mastitis causing pathogens also in different seasons and years on an individual dairy farm, hence it is important to take this into consideration when developing dry cow strategies on farm. However despite the progress made in contagious mastitis control, Gram positive infections, in particular *Staphylococcus aureus* and *Streptococcus uberis* are still the most significant cause of intramammary infection present at drying-off in the majority of dairy farms.

Infection dynamics and risk time for infection

Before going for the control strategies of infectious organisms in general and mastitis in particular, the basic knowledge of mode of entry of organisms is must. After knowing the dynamics of entry of organisms, controlling and elimination strategies can be made very effectively and cost effective.

New infections can be brought into the herd in four general ways:-

1. New infections during lactation
2. New infections during the dry period
3. Infected heifers entering the herds, and
4. Infected cows purchases.

Infections can be eliminated in four general ways:-

1. Spontaneous recovery, elimination by the animal's own defense mechanism, 20% effective.
2. Use of lactation therapy, usually 30-40% effective.
3. Dry period therapy, usually 80-90% effective, and
4. Lastly culling the animals, very effective (100%).

Infection rate from contagious and environmental Streptococci are high in the first two weeks of dry period for numerous reasons.

- Milking stops, which otherwise helps to flush out the microorganisms from the udder two or three times a day
- Pressure in the udder increases
- Teat canal dilates allowing microorganisms to enter more easily
- Teats are no longer disinfected pre- and post-milking which otherwise reduces the number of microorganisms (contagious) living on the teat skin

A few weeks after drying off the risk of infection drops because pressure in the udder decreases and the keratin accumulates, forming a plug in teat canal. There is also an increase in the concentration of immune factors such as leukocytes and antibodies. Some infections may even be eliminated during this period.

As calving approaches, the risk of infection by environmental pathogens (especially coliforms) increases once again. As the udder slowly fills with colostrum the concentration of defense mechanisms decreases and as the pressure in the udder increases the teat canal does not close as tightly. Bacterial population on teat skin at this time is very high, dry cow therapy is no longer effective and it is harder to maintain good hygiene during this period. Calving, start of milk production and start of milking increase stress.

Stress and the negative energy and protein balance around the calving reduce the efficiency of the various defense mechanisms. Many clinical cases in early lactation originate from infection that has started around the calving or in the early dry period. In herds where contagious mastitis has been controlled, aproximately 20% of all clinical mastitis cases in lactation occurred during the first week of lactation.

There are two major things to focus at calving to obtain as few infected quarters as possible:

- New infections mostly caused by environmental pathogens must be prevented.
- Infections present at the time of drying off mostly caused by contagious pathogens should be eliminated.

The response to treatment in the dry period is more complete or effective than lactating cow therapy in combating existing intramammary infections. This may be due to-

(I) Freedom to use higher doses of long acting antibiotics without risk of contamination of the bulk tank.

(II) Some physiological and immunological changes occurring during mammary gland involution-

- following the cessation of milking, leukocyte concentrations and the mammary environment becomes more conducive to leukocyte function (Sordillo and Nickerson, 1988) as fat and casein concentrations in the mammary secretion drop.
- immunoglobulin concentrations are also higher in the mammary gland of dry cows.
- increased concentration of the lysosomal enzymes in the dry mammary gland, and
- increased lactoperoxidase system in the dry mammary gland is likely to facilitate cure.

(III) Increased rate of cell renewal and apoptosis of senescent cells during a dry period (Capuko and Akers, 1999), this increased rate of apoptosis may lead to the release of intracellular organisms and the destruction of micro-abscesses in the alveolar ducts thereby increasing the exposure of pathogens to antibiotics (Bradley and Green, 2006).

(IV) The lactoferrin (iron binding) concentrations rapidly increased following the initiation of mammary involution. This increased concentration is associated with decreased in citrate level, which is well known to inhibit the growth of enterobacterial organisms (*E. coli*), mediated via the binding of iron (Sordillo *et al.*, 1997). Synergistic action of lactoferrin and antibiotic has been reported for *E. coli* (Sanchez and Watts, 1999) and *S. aureus* (Diarra *et al.*, 2003), with recent studies demonstrating that lactoferrin can restore the susceptibility of β-lactamse producing *S. aureus* to penicillin by inhibiting β-lactamse activity (Diarra *et al.*, 2002).

Advantages of dry cow therapy

The dry cow therapy has several advantages over lactation therapy-

1. A reduced incidence of new intramamary infections during the first 3 - 4 weeks of the dry period.
2. A reduced incidence of intramammary infection in the subsequent lactation.
3. A much higher cure rate than lactational therapy.
4. A much higher dose of antibiotic can be used safely.
5. Retention time of antibiotic in the udder is longer.
6. The risk of contaminating milk with drug residue is reduced.
7. An aid in the regeneration of damaged milk secretory tissues.
8. An avoidance of milk loss due to treatment of mastitis in lactation.
9. Translating into increased milk production.
10. Production of better quality milk and good market price of milk, because risk of contaminating milk with drug residue is reduced.

Disadvantages of dry cow therapy

1. Whilst considering those factors in the dry mammary gland, which increase the chance of cure, it is important not to overlook the fact that the dry mammary gland also passes through phases of increased susceptibility to new infection, exacerbated by factors such as delayed formation of the keratin plug (Dingwell *et al.*, 2001; Bradley and Green, 2006).
2. Discarded meat and milk, if the cow is slaughtered within the withdrawal time.

3. Large scale use of antibiotics increases selection pressure to spreading of antibiotic resistant bacterial strains.
4. A blind antibiotic therapy kills the normal bacterial flora of the teat end and teat canal allowing pathogenic and antibiotic resistant bacteria to colonize the area.
5. Unnecessary treatment of healthy quarters is expensive.

The effective dry cow therapy embraces mainly two options- Use of antibiotics and non-antibiotic approach. Non-antibiotic approach consist teat sealants, immunomodulator or anti-oxidant therapy (e.g. Vitamin E and Selenium) and other treatments. At present anti-oxidant therapy is also practicing commonly during dry period to reduce the incidence of intramammary infection.

Dry Cow Antibiotic Therapy

Dry cow antibiotic therapy is the most effective and widely used method for controlling mastitis in dry cows. It has been estimated that 70 to 98% of infections present at dry-off can be eliminated with dry cow antibiotic therapy (Neijenhuis *et al.*, 2000). The interesting report is that the use of intramammary antibiotic dry cow therapy increased the rate of development of a functional keratin plug. A study in UK demonstrated that only 20% of teats had formed a functional seal or keratin plug by late in the dry period in cows in organic herds, not receiving antibiotic dry cow therapy (Hayton, 2003). In one study it was found that quarters receiving dry cow therapy at drying-off had a significantly higher rate of closure of the teat canals in the first four weeks of the dry period than untreated quarters (Williamson *et al.*, 1995). This implies that dry cow treatment facilitates physical sealing of the canal. Although there is no obvious mechanism, the authors suggest the lining of the teat canal may be cleaner as- (1) the dry-cow antibiotic kills resident bacteria that colonise the teat canal and (2) there is minimal build-up of debris associated with the action of bacterial enzymes (Technote, 2000).

It is interesting and important to speculate about the reasons for failure of teat closure, because it may be a major risk factor for the acquisition of a new dry period intramammary infection (Bradley and Green, 2004).

Selection of antibiotic

The ideal antibiotic for dry cow therapy is to achieve high initial concentrations throughout the udder parenchyma in order to affect a kill of existing pathogens; this should then be followed by a prolonged period of release of antibiotic to prevent new infections (Bradley and Green, 2006). The details properties of intramammary antibiotics for dry cow have already been discussed in the treatment chapter. The rate of absorption and distribution of antibiotics from an intramammary formulation is governed by a number of factors. The dry cow preparations are formulated (vehicles, solvents, pH) to cause minimal tissue irritation, to avoid damaging the secretory tissue and to prevent fibrosis. It is advantageous if the antibiotic is bound to the tissues for an extended period and does not immediately diffuse from the udder into blood. The antibiotic should ne long-acting, as the purpose is to form a deposit in the milk ducts of the udder from which the antibiotic is slowly released. The duration of the effect of the antibiotic can be regulated by pharmaceutical manipulation of the intramammary drugs, e.g. precipitating the antibiotic, dissolving it in a slowly absorbing oil or micro-encapsulation (Janosi and Huszenicza, 2001).

Aluminium monosterate complexes penicillins and is used along with hydrophobic globules to facilitate prolonged release of antibiotic which would otherwise be rapidly distributed and absorbed into the systemic circulation (Bradley and Green, 2006). The spectrum of activity, of the antibiotics used in dry cow against the major pathogens is given in table 14.1.

Table 14.1: Typical spectrum of activity of antibiotics commonly found in dry cow therapy formulations (Source: Bradley and Green, 2006).

Antibiotic	Gram positives	Â-lactamse *S. aureus*	Gram negatives
Penicillin/Penethemate	+ + +	-	-
Ampicillin	+ +	-	+
Cloxacillin/Nafcillin	+ + +	+ + +	-
Cephalonium	+ +	+ +	+ +
Cefquinome	+ +	+ +	+ +
Dihydrostreptomycin	+	+ +	+ + +
Framycetin/Neomycin	+ +	+ +	+ + +

Because of change in the pattern of pathogens during different stages (early and late) of dry period, the dry cow treatment should be extended over the whole dry period. It is assumed that the involuted udder is naturally resistant to Gram-negative bacteria because of the high concentration of lactoferrin, and the low citrate/lactoferrin molar ratio in secretions inhibits their establishment, so their role in the dry period infections is minor in general. Dry cow antibiotic preparations, therefore, require good activity against *S. aureus* including β-lactamase producing strains, *S. uberis, S. dysgalactiae, S. agalactiae*.

The very limited antibiotics are available for dry cow therapy. High levels of benzathine penicillin, penicillin-novobiocin, penicillin-streptomycin, benzathine cephapirin, tilmicosin, cloxacillins, cephalonium and other products specifically for dry treatment are effective. Benzathine cloxacillin at the dose rate of 0.5 to 1.0g gives excellent results in dry cow therapy. Normally, procaine penicillin-G alone is not recommended but in combination with 500mg of either furatadone, neomycin, novobiocin or dihdrostreptomycin are widely used. Standard dose rate of procaine penicillin at 100,000 units plus streptomycin 0.5 to 1.0g, when increasing the amount of penicillin to 1 million units greatly enhances the activity of the product against staphylococci. These preparations are most commonly used because of their efficiency against Gram negative bacteria and cost effective, other products e.g. Cephalonium (250mg), Cephapirin benzathine (300mg) and Nitroquine (400mg) have excellent results against a wide range of bacteria especially bacteria (Radostits *et al.*, 2006). However, in India as per the knowledge of author the dry cow intramammary formulations are not available and lactation treatments are using as dry cow therapy for infected cows. In India the rate of dry cow therapy adoption is very less. Those farmers are adopting dry cow therapy, they simply using injectable formulations (i.e. lactating cow treatments) and inject directly in the mammary gland after last milking. While, some dairy farmers using parenteral antibiotics and antioxidant therapy (e.g. Vitamin E and selenium) either in combination or alone.

Route of antibiotic administration

The intramammary route is the route of choice for delivery of dry cow therapy and has the advantage of being well research, as well as allowing the delivery of high local concentrations of antibiotic and also allows the use of antibiotics that would not normally partition to the udder when administered systematically (Bradley and Green, 2006). There are two techniques of intramammary administration (Figure 14.2)-

1) Full insertion of infusion cannula into the teat cistern, and

2) Partial insertion of infusion cannula into the teat canal.

The cannula may force keratin against the interior teat wall, creating a larger than normal ductal lumen, thereby enhancing bacterial penetration. Full insertion of the cannula may also force bacteria colonizing teat duct keratin into the teat cistern. The partial insertion method of intramammary administration is recommended because it is more effective (85.7%) than full insertion method (57.9%) in the treatment of major pathogens during dry period (Boddie and Nickerson, 1986).

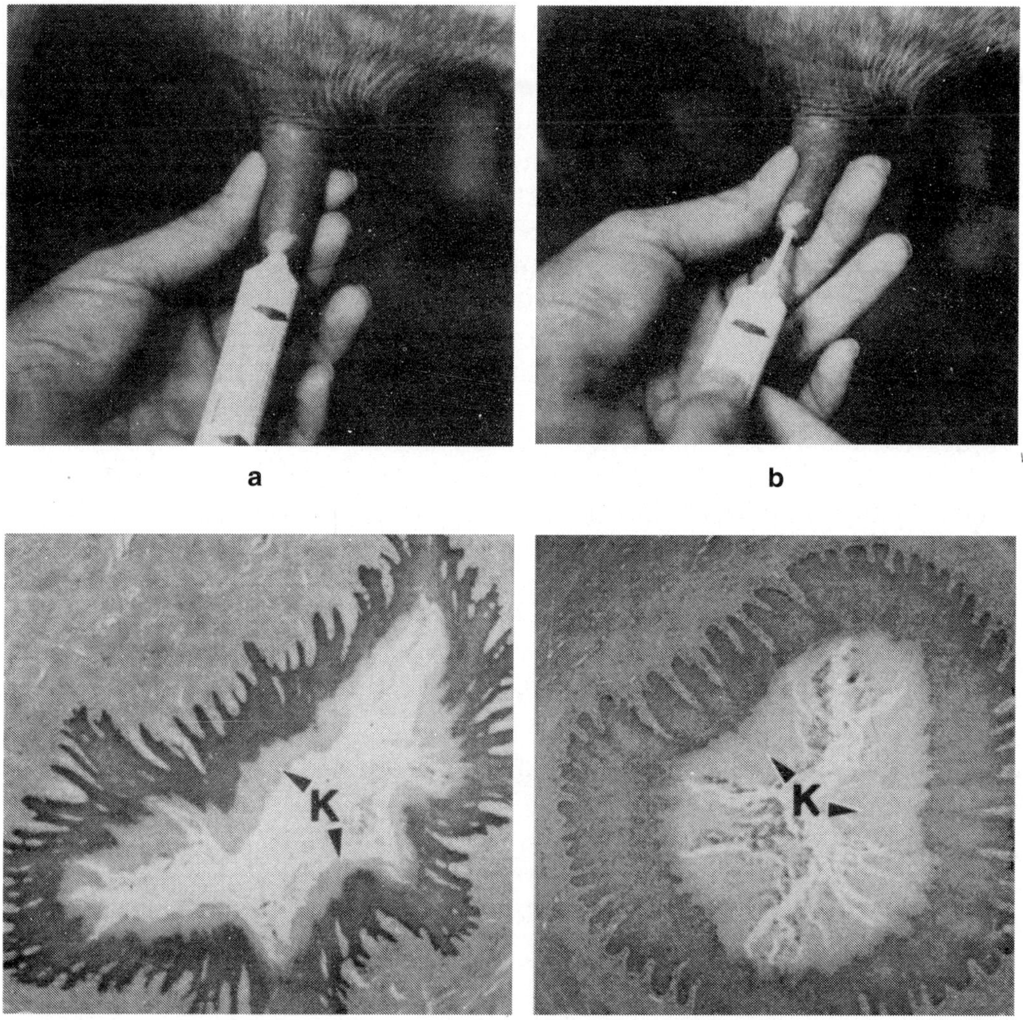

c d

Figure 14.2: Intramammary administration technique. (a) Full insertion of antibiotic syringe cannula into teat duct, (b) Partial insertion of antibiotic syringe cannula into teat duct, (c) Cross-section of mid teat duct from teat fully inserted with syringe cannula illustrating partial loss of keratin (K). Hematoxylin and eosin stain; × 300 and, (d) Cross-section of mid teat duct from teat partially inserted with syringe cannula, illustrating a thicker keratin layer in comparison with fully inserted teat (c) (Source: Boddie and Nickerson, 1986).

The intramammary route also has some disadvantages like intramammary penetration of intramammary tube cannulas may cause both physiological and anatomical damage (dilatation of the teat sphincter muscles) to the streak canal and inoculation of organisms at the time of infusion. Hence, the use of systemic antibiotic therapy is also recommended. Alternatively, systemic therapy at drying-off does not risk infection with organisms introduced via the teat duct during infusion. Antibiotic classes such as fluoroquinolone are well distributed in body fluids, have a long half life, and have broad spectrum activity. Soback *et al.* (1990) compared the subcutaneous injection of the fluoroquinolone Norfloxacin nicotinate (10mg/kg), the intramuscular injection of Oxytetracycline-HCl (20mg/kg), the infusion of 500mg Cephapirin benzathine, and an untreated control at drying-off. The numbers of existing *S. aureus* infections were reduced only in the Norfloxacin nicotinate group, and new infection rate was lower using systemic treatment. Overall, results indicated that use of the fluoroquinolone was more effective than the other treatments. Systemic use of macrolides is also being tested as a dry cow therapeutic because of the affinity of this class of antibiotic for mammary tissues (Nickerson, 1994). However, success rates for systemic treatments either alone or in combination with intramammary treatment have been no better than intramammary treatment alone. The use of systemic antibiotics at drying-off may pose an extra antibiotic residue risk, with antibiotics excreted in the urine and feces in possible sub-therapeutic concentrations (Berry, 2000).

Blanket dry cow therapy

Antibiotic dry cow therapy was developed in the 1950s, since then undoubtedly still plays an important role in the production of quality milk in modern dairy herds. Treatment of all quarters of all animals at the time of drying-off is called "*blanket dry cow therapy*". In this way, new infections arising shortly after drying-off are prevented and laboratory or screening procedures to decide which quarter to treat are eliminated. One of the difficult decisions about dry period treatment is whether or not all quarters should be treated (Figure 14.3).

In most developed dairy producing countries an antibiotic treatment is recommended for all quarters of all cows at drying off. Every cow needs protection during that critical period. Treating every quarter is only way to guarantee to treat every infected quarter, even those with low SCC. The opportunity to cure the infection will never be better.

These two reasons explain why dry - treated cows produce more milk in the following lactation, an economic justification to treat every cow.

The debate on "to treat or not to treat" uninfected cows at drying-off has been ongoing for many years and some researchers have recommended that dry cow antibiotic therapy should be reserved for infected cows and not applied as a routine prophylactic measure (Browning *et al.*, 1990).

On the other hand, it has been reported that the incidence of new intramammary infections increases when uninfected cows are left untreated, particularly in the early part of dry period. Woolford *et al.* (1998) showed that 16% of a sample of 528 untreated quarters, uninfected at drying-off, developed a new infection during the dry period. Berry (2000) also showed that between 30% and 50% of untreated cows at drying-off developed new infections during the dry period compared to a new infection rate of between 0% and 15% in cows treated with antibiotics.

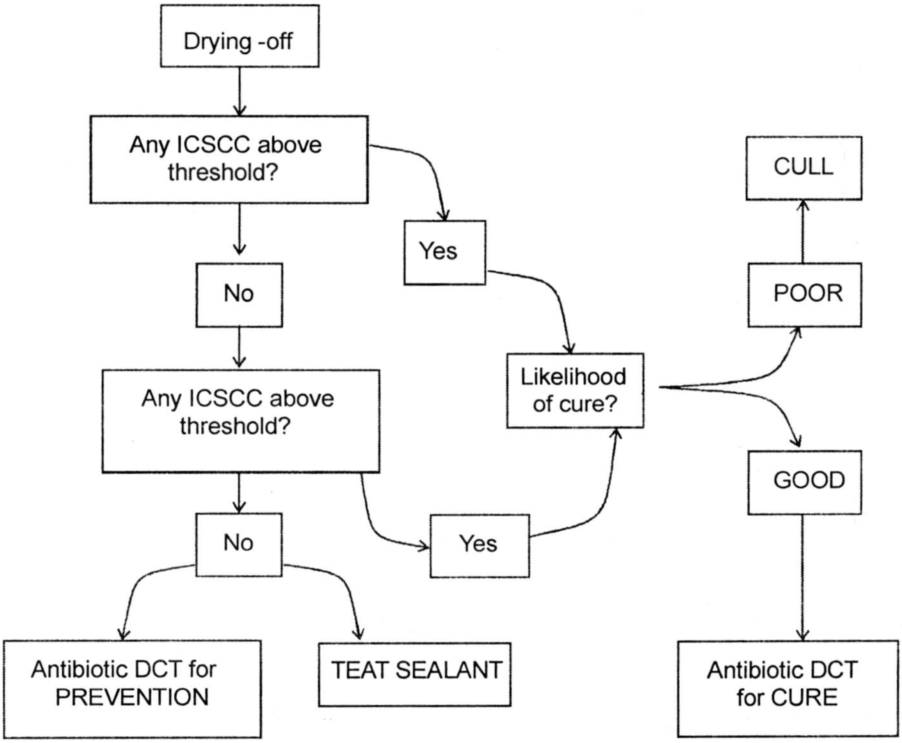

Figure 14.3: Illustration of a typical decision tree for the prescription of dry cow therapy. ICSCC = Individual cow somatic cell count

The general recommendation is that all quarters be treated. This is undoubtedly the correct procedure when the infection rate is 40-50% of quarters, but in herds with a low prevalence of infection and low average cell count no significant gain in production or profitability is achieved.

The advantages of blanket dry cow therapy over selective dry cow therapy are- 1) all infected quarters are treated at drying-off, 2) many new infections are prevented during the first week or two of the dry period, and 3) there are no testing costs or labor costs associated with efforts to determine hich quarters or cows should be chosen for selective dry cow therapy.

Selective dry cow therapy

Treatment of infected quarters at the time of drying-off is called "*selective dry cow therapy*". A continuing controversy concerning dry cow therapy resolves around the necessity to treat all quarters of all cows at the end of lactation. Reasons to avoid this prophylactic use of antibiotics include the cost, the lack of benefit associated with treating uninfected quarters and cows, avoiding elimination of protective minor pathogens, possible emergence of antibiotic resistant organisms and the risk of antibiotic residue in the food chain. One of the "keys' to a rational approach to dry cow therapy is the selection of which cows are appropriate to treat and which cows are appropriate to cull. A variety of criteria to help in this important decision have been put forward over the years (Figure 14.3). The advantages of selective dry cow therapy are the saving in cost, especially when only 8-10% of quarters are infected, and the avoidance of complete sterilization of all quarters, with a resulting possible increase in susceptibility to infection.

Selective dry cow therapy is hard to justify on the basis of cost. In a study comprising selective and blanket dry cow therapy on this merit alone, the benefits associated with blanket use of dry cow therapy included a low rate of clinical mastitis, a marked reduction in SCC and an increased milk production in the next lactation (Osteras and Sandvik, 1996).

Selective quarter treatment requires initial screening to identify an infection and general preventive benefits of total dry cow therapy are lost. One of the main reasons that selective dry cow therapy has not gained wide spread adoption in the increased cost that would be associated with defining the infection status of individual cows prior to dry-off.

Identifying the infected cow

There has been much debate worldwide about the most effective way to identify cows with an intramammary infection. The important key for successful dry cow udder health management is to establish a picture of the etiology and epidemiology of mastitis on a farm, thereby informing the veterinary practitioner's decision with respect to product selection. This is very challengeable and expensive job to identify each cow and at quarter level. The lack of a reliable test to detect infected quarters is a major obstacle for the successful implementation of these programs. Presently, there is no inexpensive and practical cow-side test with adequate sensitivity and specificity to determine the infection status of cows, relative to the expensive "*gold standard*" of microbiologic culture of quarter milk samples (Leslie, 1994). Attempts to utilize the California mastitis test, SCC thresholds, and clinical mastitis history as sufficient tests (either alone or in combination) have not been successful (Poutrel and Rainard, 1981; Kirk *et al.*, 1996), despite the fact that the California mastitis test may be a useful monitoring tool to identify infections in early lactation (Sargeant *et al.*, 2001).

The generally accepted method applied to identify infected cows at a dairy farm is the use of cow level somatic cell counts. The SCC threshold applied for identification of infected cows has been suggested by International Dairy Federation (IDF) i.e. 200,000 cells/ml. It is probably best to err on the side of caution, and if there is any doubt about a cow infection status she should be treated as infected- primarily because dry cow therapy provides the best opportunity to effect a cure in sub-clinically affected cows. Having differentiated likely "infected" from "uninfected" cows, the opportunity now arises to select dry cow therapy on the basis of optimal efficacy with respect to curing and preventing intramammary infections respectively (Bradley and Green, 2004). The selection of appropriate cows to not infuse at dry-off is essential. Until a practical test is developed or highly predictive risk profiles of individual cows are established, infusion of all quarters of all cows is probably the safest practice (Schukken *et al.*, 1993).

The cure of uninfected cows during the dry period also has paramount importance in the control of mastitis. Possibly the most exciting aspect of identifying uninfected cows and stratifying a dairy herd is that it provides the opportunity to use non-antibiotic approaches to preventing new intramammary infections during the dry period, as there is no need to use antibiotics to cure existing intramammary infections. The teat sealants now offer a real alternative to antibiotics for the prevention of new intramammary infections in cows uninfected at drying off (Bradley and Green, 2004).

Finally, the use of selective or blanket dry cow therapy depends on information available, herd situation and health situation. It could be hypothesized that the worse the health situation is the more effective – at least in the short run(?)- is the concept of blanket dry cow therapy, the better the health situation the better is the concept of selective dry cow therapy.

The advantages of selective dry cow therapy are- 1) reduced cost of antibiotics, 2) reduced impact on development of bacterial antibiotic resistance, 3) reduced probability of damaging streak canals during the infusion process, and 4) reduced likelihood of introducing pathogens into uninfected glands during the infusion process.

Which cow to treat or not to treat?

Here the recommendations are given as per the Janosi and Huszenicza (2001):

1. Cows with clinical mastitis are treated according to normal practice before drying-off.

2. Dry cow therapy is recommended for all cows that have had contagious mastitis during lactation (*Staphlococcus aureus, Streptococcus agalactiae* and *Streptococcus dysgalactiae*).
3. Cows which have had a high milk cell count are also treated.
4. Systemic dry cow therapy is recommended for herds with a high infection rate.
5. Dry cow therapy is also recommended in herds with low somatic cell counts and low prevalence of contagious mastitis pathogen.
6. Important point is that the cows that have had at least one case of clinical mastitis and high geometric mean of SCC in the last 5 to 6 months before drying-off should be considered for culling, because they retain a high risk of subsequently having a major pathogen (mainly *Staphlococcus aureus* and *Streptococcus agalactiae*).

Decision for choosing blanket or selective dry cow therapy

The selection of method of dry cow antibiotic therapy is really a challengeable job for veterinarian. During selection of method various factors/ data should be considered for better results, for this, a decision tree can be used (Figure 14.4). There are the following important points which should be consider before choosing between a blanket or selective dry cow therapy (Technote, 2000)-

- Prevalence of mastitis in the herd.
- Likely pathogens causing the mastitis in the herd.
- The economics of missing infected cows or treating uninfected cows.
- The risk of new infections in the dry period; and
- Management of antibiotic use to avoid residue violations in meat and milk.

Public concerns over the widespread prophylactic use of antibiotics have led to a search for alternatives to dry cow therapy for the prevention of intramammary infections. For this reason, it may be that, in the field, the best option for improving the "apparent" cure rate during the dry period may be the improvement of prophylaxis through the use of teat sealants.

Homeopathy

The current trends necesitates the use of aternative therapy (homeopathy) for the control of mastitis through enhancement of immune system of udder (Pachauri *et al.*, 2001). Homeopathy based dry-off concepts only provided satisfying results in the prevention against certail micro-organisms (Klocke *et al.*, 2006) or in combination with antibiotics (Klocke *et al.*, 2000). Preventive effects by using so called homeopathic nosodes produced by potentiatized microbial cultures or other pathologic secretions are very limited. Homeopathic nosodes (remedies) used to prevent mamastitis are administered in drinking water, by drenching and even sprying them into the vulva.

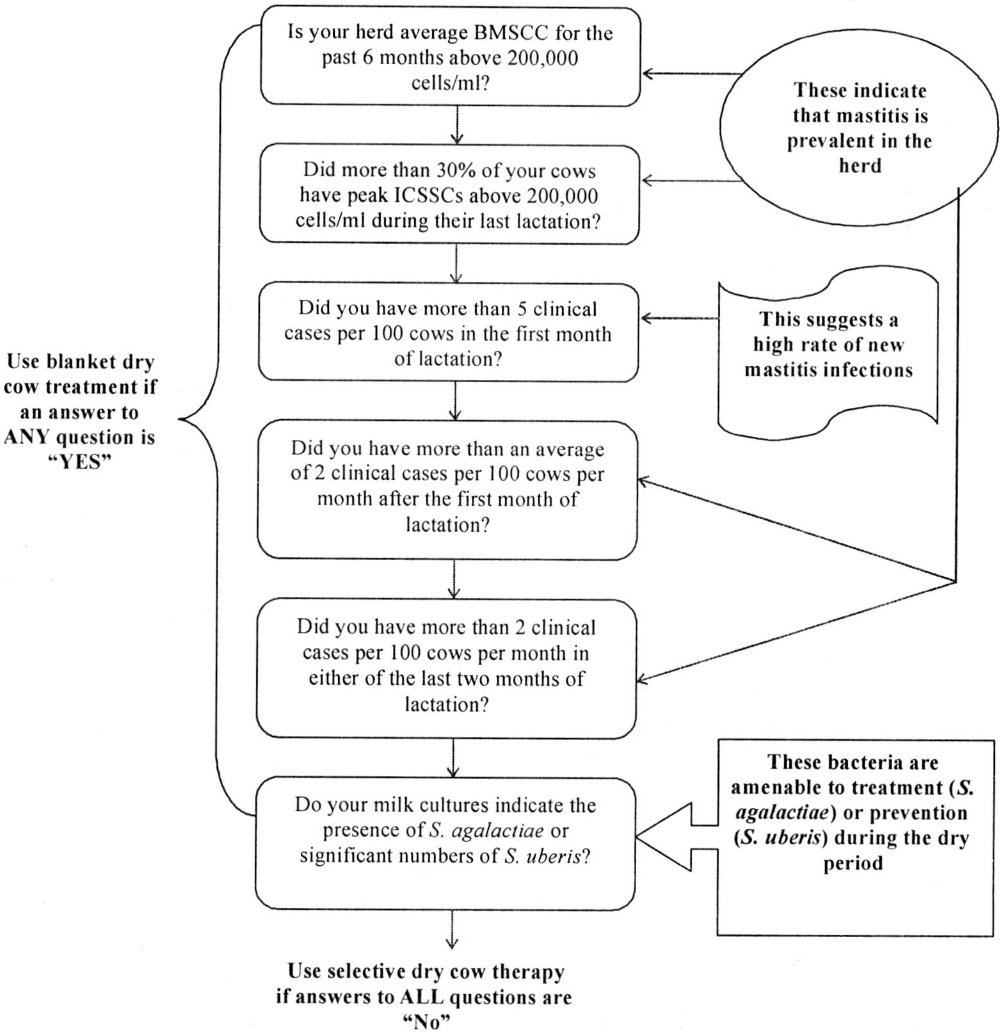

ICSCC = Individual cow somatic cell count, BMSCC = Bulk milk somatic cell count

Figure 14.4: A decision tree for the selection of dry cow therapy method.

Preventive homeopathic treatments are administered using nosodes on an entire herd rather than on individual animals. Nosodes are fragments of pathogenic cells that increase the immune response. Nosode preparation is established accordnig to the etiological agent prevalent at the herd.

Use of herbal preparations

Apart the dry cow antibiotic therapy, various herbal drugs are also used for the control of mastitis in dairy animals. In India, some topical herbal preparations as ointment are also available e.g mastilep, wisprec etc. However,there is much variation in the efficacy of these products from aothor to author. Nath and Dutta (2005) used ointment mastilep as topical application on the teats and found 88.3 – 88.8% efficacy. Each 100 g mastilep contains *Glycerrhiza glabra*- 5 g, *Curcuma longa*- 2 g, *Cedrus deodara*- 10 g, *Paederia foetida*- 5 g and Sulphur- 10 g in a gel base. Maiti *et al.* (2006) also reported that mastilep significantly controlled and prevented intramammary infection caused by *Escherichia coli, Staphylococcus, Streptococcus, Bacillus* and *Corynebacterium* spp. There was also a decrease in the number of animals positive for sub-clinical mastitis. No adverse effects on udder and suckling calves were observed.

Teat sealants

The main objection to dry cow antibiotic therapy comes from continued use of antibiotics in the dry period for either prophylactic or therapeutic purposes. The blanket and over use of antibiotics is associated with antibiotic resolve in milk or emergence of antibiotic resistant human pathogens (methicillin resistant *Staphylococcus aureus*) and animal welfare. Such concerns have prompted the World Health Organization to issue recommendations on global programmes to try to reduce the use of antibiotic therapies for both human and animal applications in the future.

Alternative strategies may be used other than blanket use of dry cow antibiotic therapy should be at the cow level and not the quarter level (Berry *et al.*, 2003). A traditional approach to protecting the dry cows, is use of teat sealants. It is believed that a teat canal keratin plug should form early during the dry period to establish a natural protective mechanism to prevent penetration of bacteria and reduce the incidence of new intramammary infection (Williamson *et al.*, 1995). This natural teat seal (keratin) may take a minimum of two weeks to form, and upto 23% of teats may never be closed naturally (Williamson *et al.*, 1995; Dingwell, 2002). While some studies claims that 50% of teats are still open after a week, 25% after 40 days and 5% remains open during the whole dry period. Most new infections occur in these "open" teat quarters so seal the teat canal may prevent new infections. Conventional teat dips are sometimes used after drying off and before calving. They don't really seal the teat canal but keep the bacteria population lower and this practice encourages mastitis detection (Woolford *et al.*, 1998; Timms *et al.*, 1997). Hence, internal and external teat sealants have been popularized to prevent entry of organisms through teat orifice or teat canal.

There are two types of teat sealant, internal and external.

Internal teat sealant

Studies on internal teat sealers began in 1972 (Meaney, 1976). The teat seal is a viscous non-antibiotic formulation and when it is infused into the teat canal and the teat sinus it forms an internal seal that provides a physical barrier to invasion by mastitis-causing pathogens. This type of sealant is infused into the teat cistern at drying off (Figure 14.5b). The gel fills the approximately half of the teat cistern, preventing the entrance of microorganisms into the udder for the entire duration of dry period. It reduces the risk of new infections up to calving date. Internal teat sealant might be used in combination with antibiotic dry cow therapy or as single preventive measure for healthy uninfected cows. It has been reported that use of teat sealer at the time of dry-off significantly reduced the level of new dry period infections.

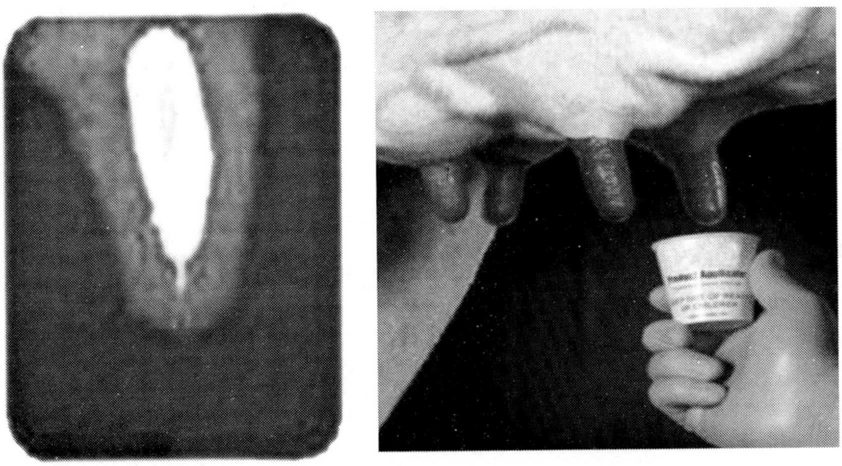

(a) (b)

Figure 14.5: (a) Internal teat sealant (white contrast in teat cistern on X-ray image), (b) External teat sealer.

The teat sealer consisted of a heavy inorganic salt (bismuth subnitrate) in a paraffin wax base, and it did not contain any antibiotic (Dingwell *et al.*, 2003). All aseptic precautions should be taken during administration of teat sealers. When the teat sealer alone was compared with dry cow antibiotic therapy alone, 3.5% of quarters with the sealer became infected versus 32% of quarters that received the dry cow antibiotic therapy (Meaney, 1977). Recent developments in non-antibiotic internal teat sealing technology have proved to be very effective in preventing new cases of mastitis during the dry period when infused into the teats of uninfected cows at drying-off. The teat seal formulation contains a heavy inorganic bismuth salt in a mineral oil base. Bismuth based teat seals are biologically inert and do not have an associated antimicrobial activity (Meaney *et al.*, 2001). This inert viscous paste infused into the quarter at the time of dry-off forming an immediate physical barrier in the distal portion of the teat cistern to prevent bacteria from ascending through the teat canal. The majority of internal teat seal product is stripped out at first milking after calving, with some residual product removed in the subsequent several milkings after calving (Godden *et al.*, 2003). It has been studied that the use of a teat seal containing 65% bismuth subnitrate in paraffin is significantly better than no therapy and equivalent to dry cow antibiotic therapy, in its ability to prevent new intramammary infections during the dry period and clinical mastitis in the following lactation (Woolford *et al.*, 1998).

Alternative non-antibiotic additives to enhance teat sealing formulations might include bacteriocins such as nisin or lacticin 3147. Bacteriocins are potent proteins produced by some bacteria that have the ability to kill other microorganisms. Bacteriocins were first proposed for treatment of mastitis when the results of trials carried out by Taylor *et al.* (1949) indicated that a single intramammary infusion of nisin, a bacteriocin discovered in 1928 (Rogers and Whittier, 1928), was effective in treating both streptococcal and staphylococcal infections. The incorporation of a bacteriocin into the seal may provide a method to prevent inadvertent contamination during infusion, improving the safety of the product in the hands of the untrained user (Crispie *et al.*, 2004).

A study on nisin has been reported by Sears *et al.* (1992) who showed that nisin in combination with lysostaphin cured 66% of *S. aureus*. 95% of *S. agalactiae* and 100% of *S. uberis* infections.

External teat sealant

A less invasive alternative to achieve teat end protection is the application of an external barrier product (external teat sealant) to teats during the dry period (Dingwell *et al.*, 2003). External teat sealants were originally developed for prevention of mastitis during lactation between milkings (Farnsworth *et al.*, 1980). An acrylic latex film is most commonly used as external teat sealant and it was found to have a statistically significant reduction in rates of infections with *S. aureus, S. epidermidis* and coliforms (Farnsworth *et al.*, 1980). Recently, external teat sealer with a better sealing capacity and extended effect has been developed to be used in combination with antibiotic dry cow therapy. It forms rubbery formation (second skin like) on a teat (Figure 14.5a)). If application is done under good conditions and upon the product recommendations it can be effective for up to a week. The adherence seems better if sealant is applied at refrigerator temperature. First application is immediately after dry cow therapy. Few applications might be useful in weeks before expected calving date. The OrbeSeal is the most commonly used external teat sealant in UK and has significant result in the control of intramammary infection.

Teat sealants are potentially beneficial to all cows, but particularly to those cows that have teat canals of wide diameter or less effective mechanisms for closure of the teat orifice, commonly called cows with *"open teat canals"*. Such cows are therefore vulnerable to infection (Berry and Hillerton, 2002), particularly in the early dry period before the keratin plugs have formed in the teat canals and around calving when they have been lost from many teats. However, it is important to stress that the use of antibiotics in high SCC cows at drying-off remains essential on the basis of the need to eliminate existing infections.

Conventional teat dips are sometimes used after drying off and before calving. They do not really seal the teat canal but keep the bacteria population lower and this practice encourages mastitis detection.

Technique of dry cow therapy

The following steps should be espoused during dry cow therapy.

1. Milk out the cow completely.

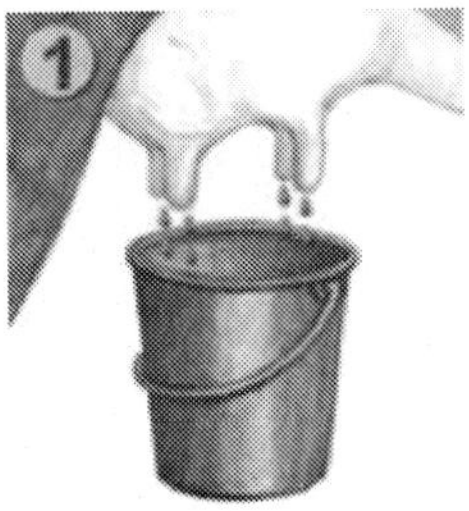

2. Clean the teats with a clean paper and wipe the water with sterilized towel.

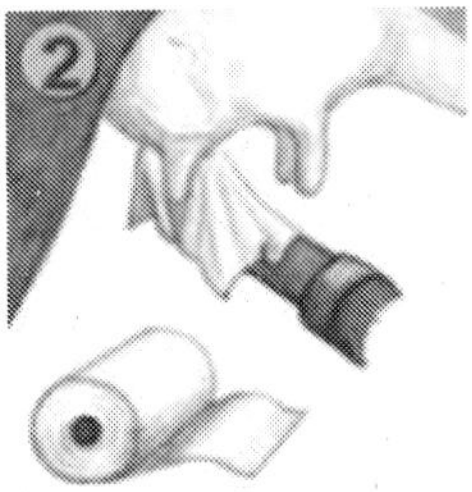

3. Pre-dip the teats in teat sealant for 5 to 10 minutes.

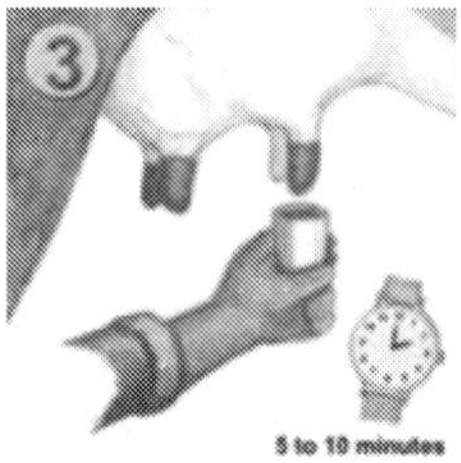

4. Pre-dip again

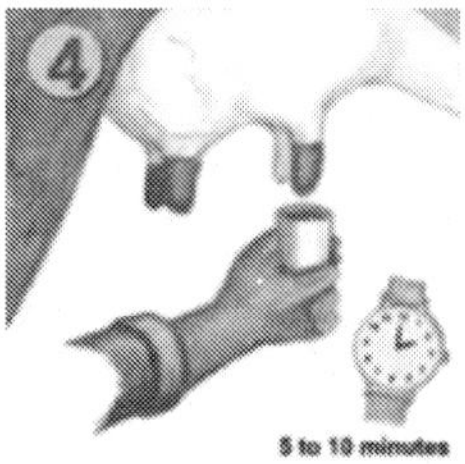

5. Give intramammary preparation as dry cow therapy.

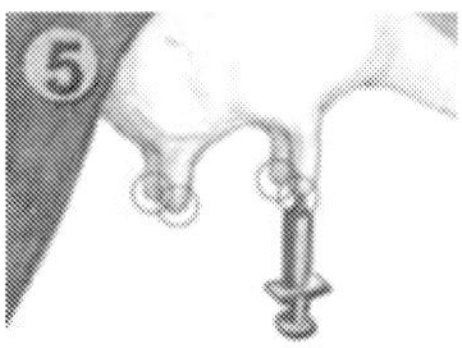

6. Ten days before calving, apply teat dip again to prevent the entry of organisms just before calving.

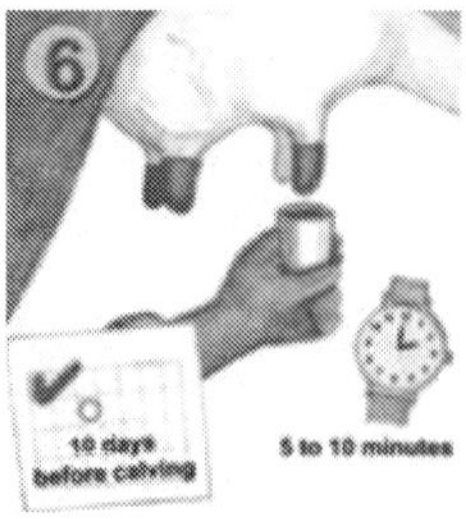

Dry cow observation

To minimize antibiotic and milk leakage do not let cows walk long distance few days following dry off. Quarters should be daily visually checked during the first week to detect a clinical mastitis (Figure 14.6). If clinical mastitis is detected the quarter should be stripped out and treated with lactating cow antibiotic. Quarters should be checked weekly through the whole dry period.

At the same time dry cow's environment should be checked too. One of the crucial points of mastitis prevention in dry period is checking the udders daily one week before the calving date to detect mastitis or/and udder edema.

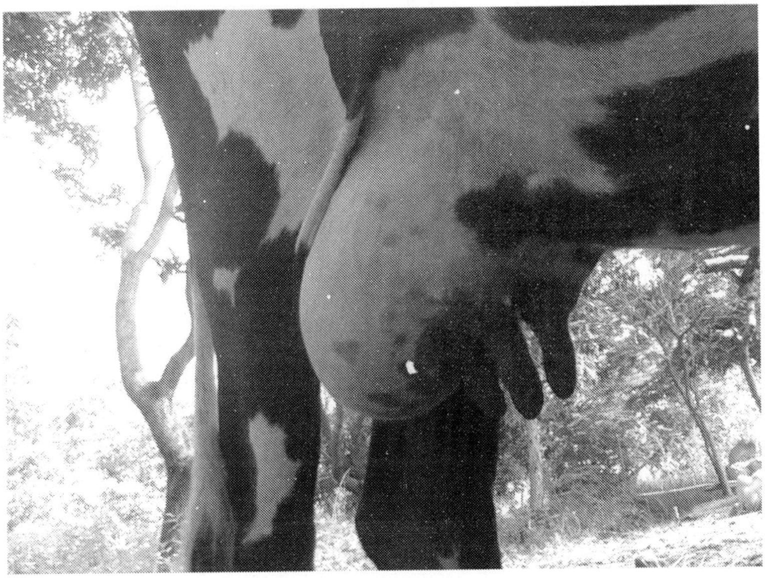

Figure 14.6: Dried off udder should be daily visually checked during the first week to detect a clinical mastitis.

Heifer mastitis

Most dairy farmers erroneusly consider their heifers free of intramammary infection (IMI) because clinical signs of mastitis do not appear before the first calving. But mastitis causing microorganisms can be found in mammary secretions from heifers as young as six months old. If we have that in mind, wherever imported heifers come from, they can introduce mastitis causing pathogens into the mastitis free milking herd or just add new pathogens to those already existing in the herd.

Udder infection during the first pregnancy decreases secretory tissue development and milk production in the following lactation. A study has shown that heifers having an SCC over 200.000 cells/ml at their first test produce 600 liters less per lactation than low SCC heifers (De Vliegher *et al.*, 2004).

Many different pathogens can infect heifer udder before the first calving. Infection pattern is similar to the older cows pattern. Environmental conditions at calving and later on affect environmental mastitis rate in *heifers*. Coagulase negative Staphylococci (CNS) infections are common but fortunately spontaneous cure rate is very high.

Heifers having spent more time with older cows, calving at older age, having udder edema[1] or leaking milk are more at risk for udder infection.

When *S. aureus* is common in the herd it is often transmitted from cows to heifers. Feeding fresh raw milk from *S. aureus* infected cows and calves suckling each other are considered the main risk factors. Feeding waste milk can also increase risk of transmitting Mycoplasma, Johne's disease and BVD. Alternatives are milk replacers or on - farm pasteurization of milk that uses for calves (Figure 14.7). During raising of heifer calves should be keep in dry and clean housing to avoid the infection. Woodan hutches should be preferred for the housing of heifer calves due to poor disinfection and cleaning (Figure 14.8).

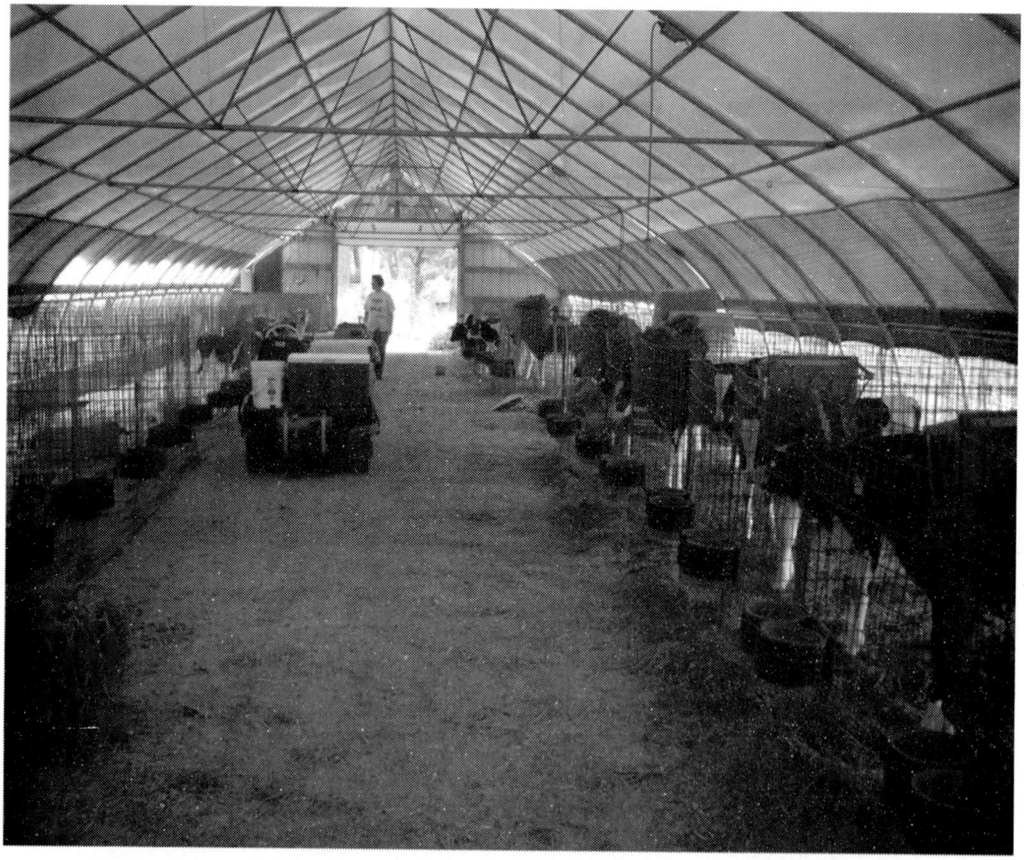

Figure 14.7. a) Keeping the calves in the same barn in separate boxes.

[1] Udder edema is not a disease but rather an excessive accumulation of fluid in the extravascular spaces of the udder and surrounding tissues in front or behind the udder. Edema is more likely in first calf heifers when they calve older.

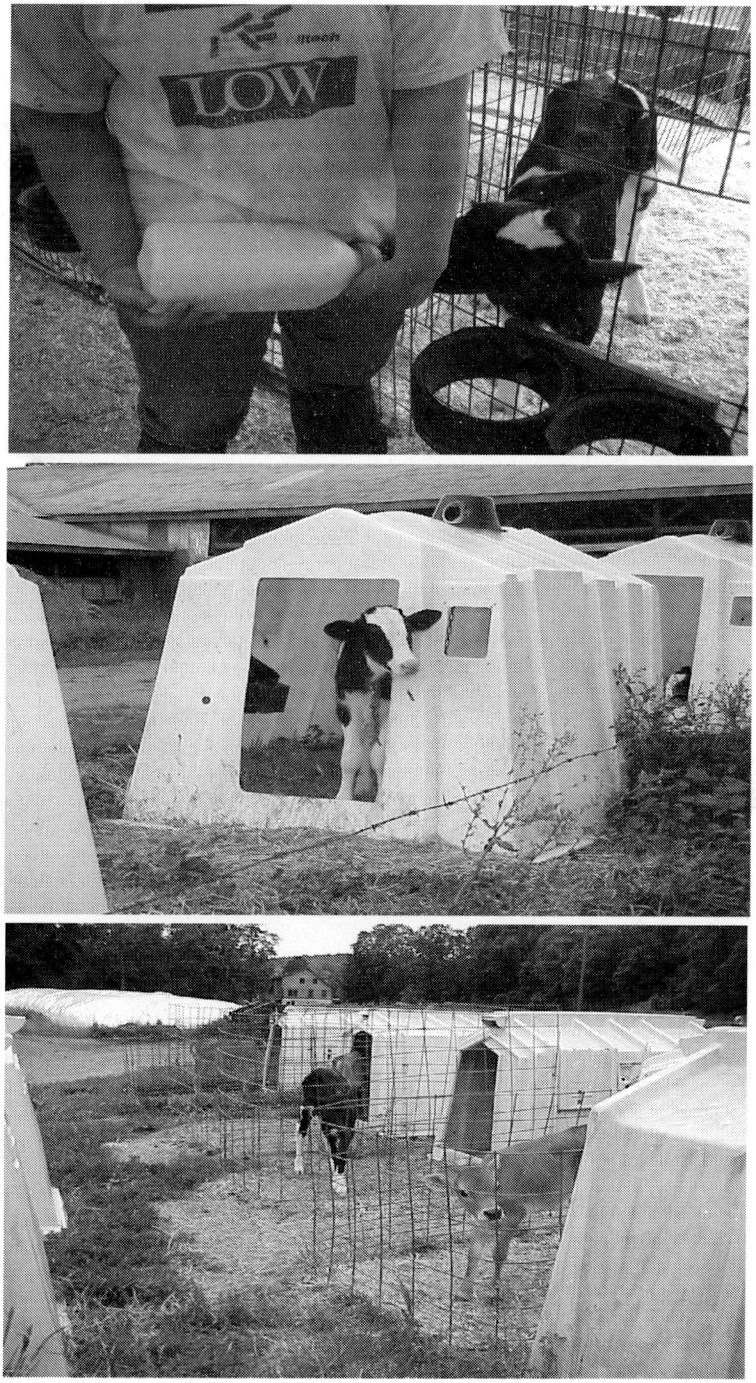

(b)

(c)

(d)

Figure 14.7 : b) Individual feeding with milk replacer, c) Individual calf housing in a plastic hutches, d) Individual calf housing in a plastic hutches with wire fence enclosure so the calf can move outside.

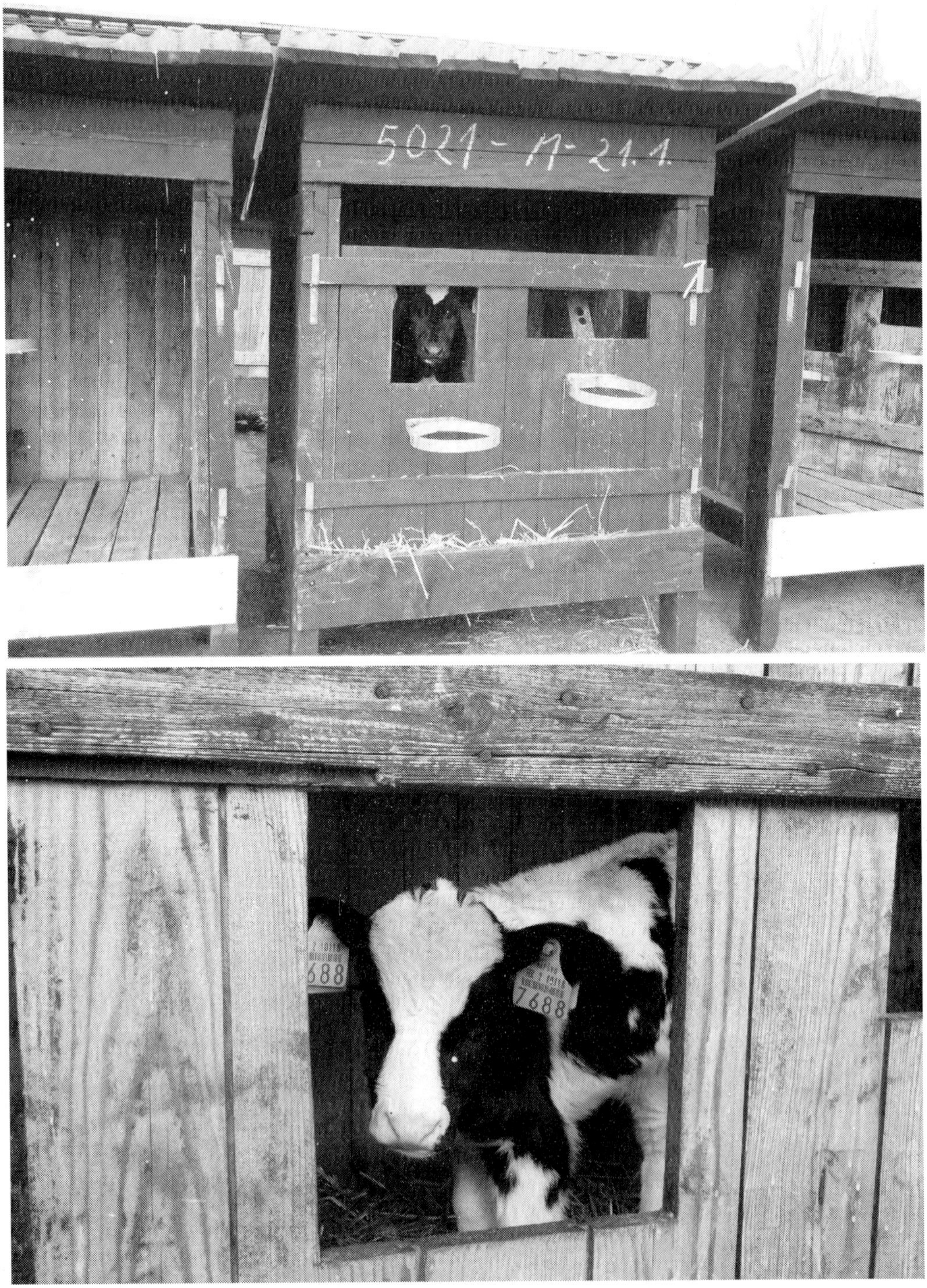

Figure 14.8. Keeping calves in wooden huches is not recommended due to poor disinfection and cleaning

Raising heifers individually until weaning is the best way to prevent suckling, keeping heifers in group restrained immediately after feeding may decrease it. Older heifers should be kept separatelly from adult cows as long as possible (Figure 14.9).

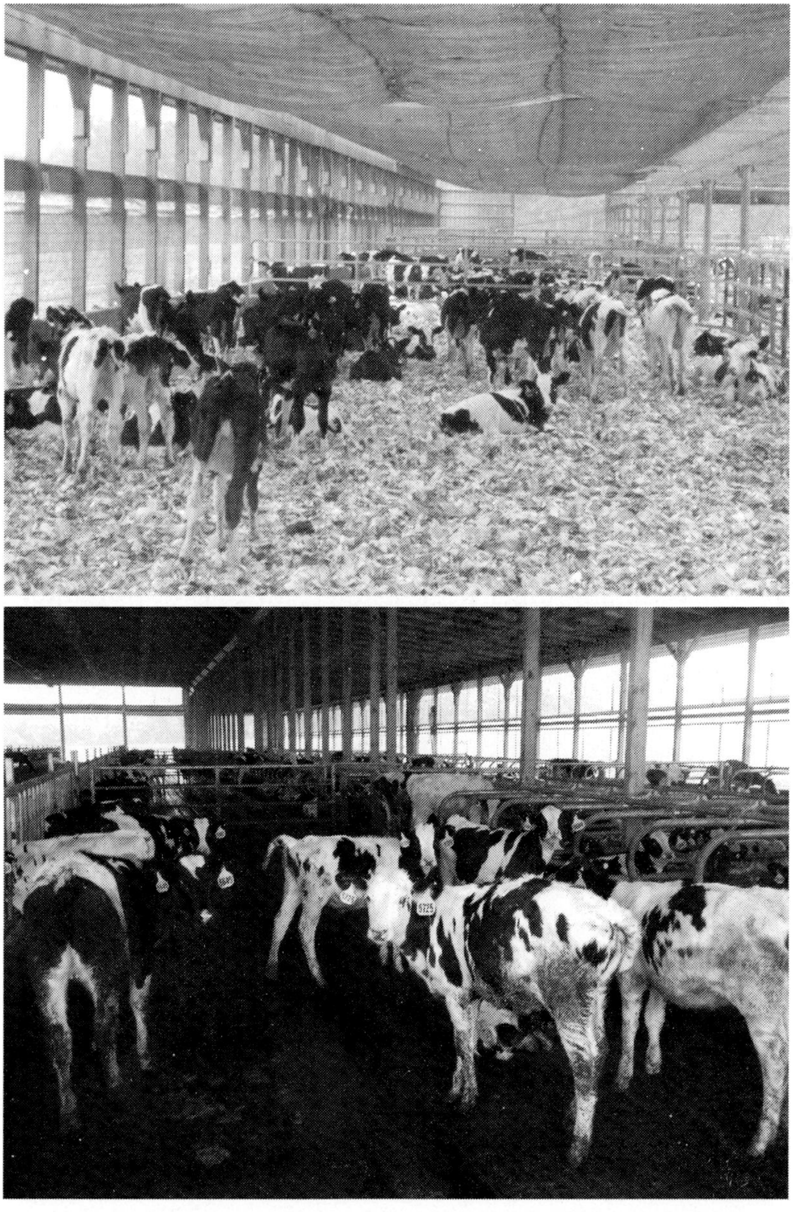

(a)

(b)

Figure 14.9. a) Group of young heifers in a separate barn on the recycled paper bedding, b) Group of older heifers in a barn that is look like barn for lactating cows – this will decrease postcalving stress and beginning of milking

- Flies can also transmit contagious pathogens from animal to animal.
- Extra teats on calves may make milking more difficult when grow older. Sometimes they open into the gland and may be another entrance for mastitis pathogens. Therefore they should be removed before the calf is one year old.
- Every modern milking management should consider training heifers to enter the milking area before they actually freshen and start milking.
- Taking the California Mastitis Test (CMT) or any other mastitis test after freshening and culturing the CMT positive quarters identifies the infected quarters and causing microorganisms (Schukken *et al.*, 1993).
- To preserve their udder health, it is suggested whenever is possible, to form a separate group of first lactation cows and to milk them first in the shift.

Milking order and segregation

Biosecurity within the herd should also be the part of general biosecurity program. The main point is that sick cows should not be housed together with fresh cows. Also waste raw milk from mastitic cows should not be fed to calves. Farms that needing to decrease the prevalence of contagious mastitis should segregating the infected cows and / or establishing milking order. Backflushing the milking units with disinfectant could be an alternative for some farms.

In addition to segregation or milking order, good management practices to decrease risk factors for contagious pathogens spread are (Bacic *et al.*, 2005):

- Wearing disposable latex gloves (Figure 14.10) for all milking procedures and cleaning and changing them regularly
- Minimizing contact beetwen the milker's hands and the cow's hair or the milk.
- Using single-use individual paper towels or previously laundered individual cloth towels for clining and drying the teats prior to milking.

How to milk cows infected by contagious bacteria in the barn?

In theory, the manual disinfection of the milking unit can also be used when milking in the barn. The important thing is; then the milking units should be rinsed, disinfected for at least 30 seconds, then rinsed again and dried. In practice, very few people will apply this procedures complete. In most tie-stall barn situations, the teatcups are quickly dipped in one or two pails and attached while they are still wet (Figure14.11). The only thing this procedure provides is a false sense of security.

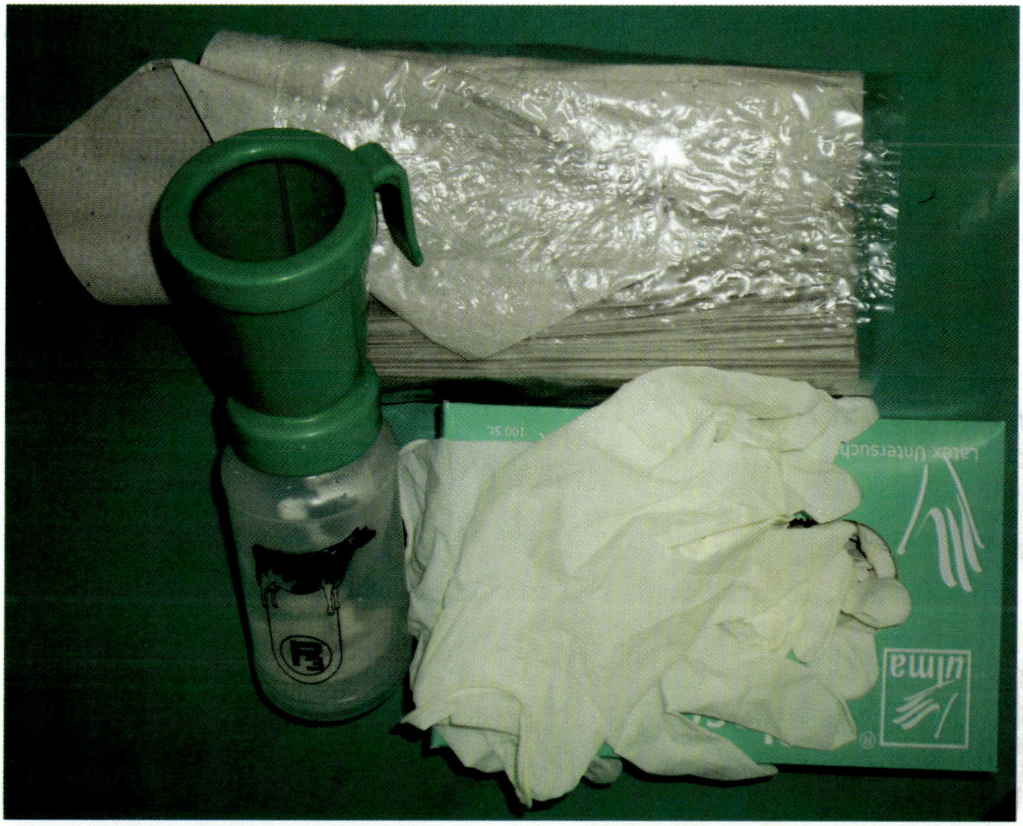

Figure 14.10: Single teat disinfectant cup, latex disposable gloves and single paper towels

There are three recommended ways to milk infected cows separately:

1. *Place infected cows at the end of the row* – all the cows that are confirmed positive infected by contagious pathogens are placed at the end of the milking order and milked last. This way all milkers will apply the milking order even if they don't know about it. Furthermore contamination of milkers hands and of the environment of healthy cows will be decreased and minimized.

2. *Skip infected cows and than come back to milk them after all healthy cows have been milked.* Using this method increases the risk of error, particularly if milkers are not aware of the reason for the milking order.

3. *Use separate milking unit only on infected cows.* All the infected cows are therefore milked with the same milking unit, which is then never used to milk healthy cows (Figure 14.12). Milkers hands, ideally wearing latex or rubber gloves, should be washed after milking these cows.

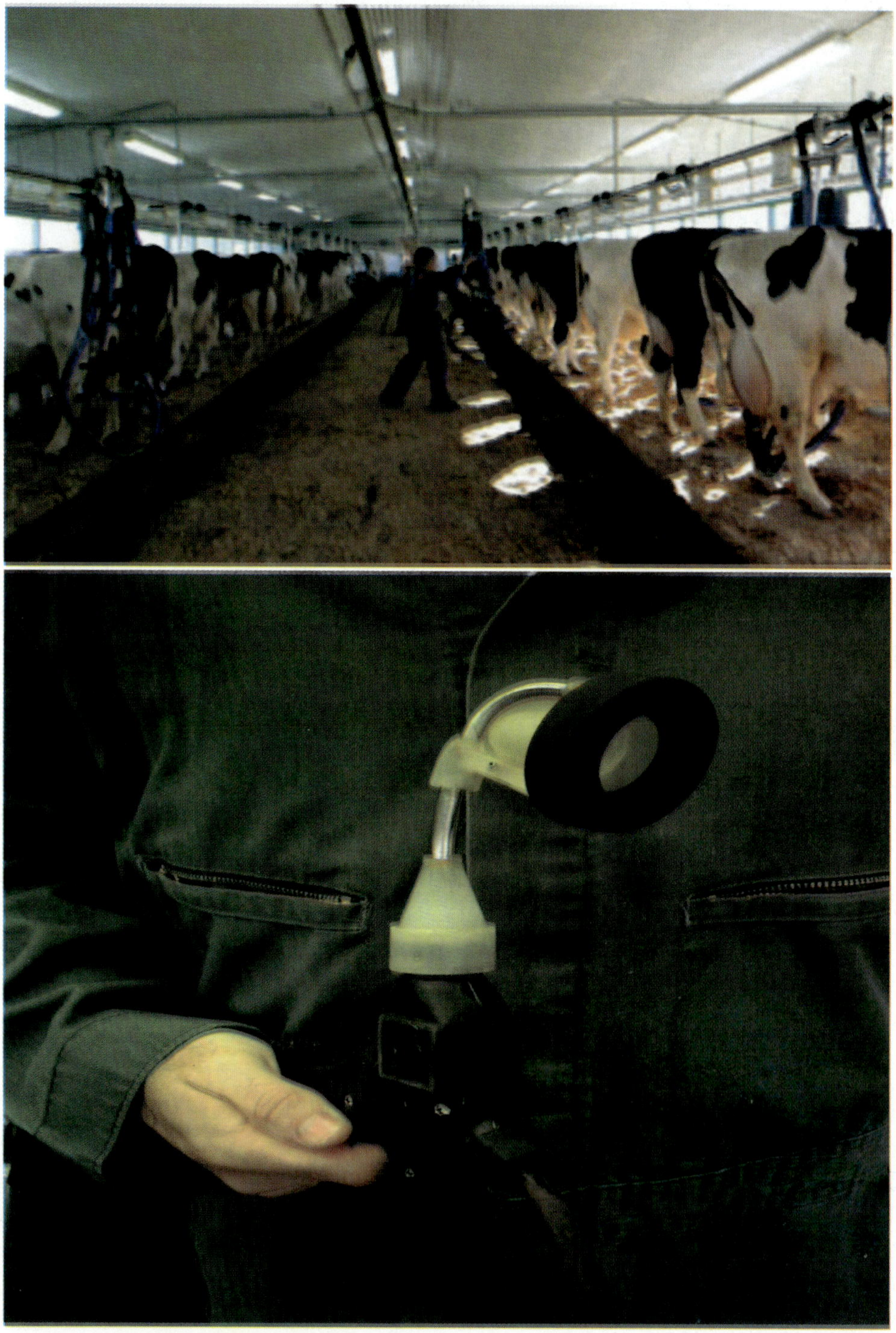

(a)

(b)

Figure14.11. a) Milking cows in tiestall barn with individual milking buckets, b) Vacuum gun for pre and after milking desinfection

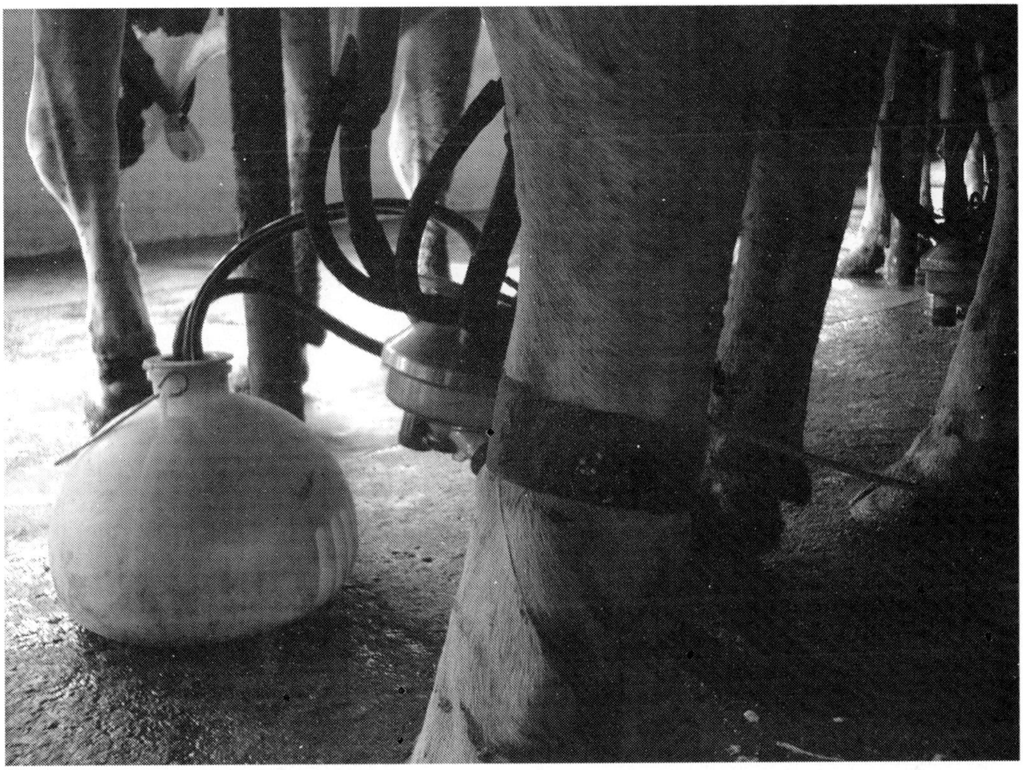

Figure 14.12. Special individual milking unit only for use on infected cows (note velcro bands around the legs – indicate infected cows, treated cows or healthy cows but milk still not suitable for use, different velcro colors for different cases).

How to milk cows infected by contagious pathogens in a milking parlor?

Again there are three ways to deal with this problem

1. *Form a group of infected cows.* This is the most efficient way. If the number of infected cows justifies it, group can be formed from all infected cows and this group will be milked last.
2. *Have a special unit for infected cows.* You can use a special milking unit for infected cows. Always make sure this unit is not used on treated cows and wash your hands after milking these cows.
3. *Disinfect the hands and milking units after milking an infected cow.*

Disinfection can be done in two ways but in practice results are not as good as with previous two methods.

- An automatic backflushing system can be installed in order to disinfect the milking units. This system will automatically rinse, disinfect, rinse again and dry the milking unit between the milking of each cow. Theortically efficient this method seldom justifies the additional investment.

- After having milked an infected cow milking unit can also be disinfected manually. First rinse both exterior and interior of the milking unit. Than dip the unit in the sanitizing solution containing 25 - 50 ppm of iodine (pH 3 - 4). Be sure the solution will stay in contact with the interior of the teatcups and whole milking claw for at least 30 seconds, then rinse the milking unit and let id dry.

Treating heifers before calving

In herds where infections are frequent among the heifers, the veterinarian should be consulted in order to set up a preventive antibiotic treatment program (Ziv *et al.*, 1981). This technique has proven to be effective and profitable in certain cases (Borm *et al.*, 2006; Compton *et al.* 2007; Janosi and Huszenicza, 2001).

It should only be used if several bacteriological cultures taken after the heifers have freshened show the presence of pathogenic microorganisms despite the fact that all the methods of management have been improved.

The preventive treatment involves infusing antibiotics designed for the dry cow therapy eight to twelve weeks before the calving date. In high risk herds every heifer may also be treated.

It could also be possible to palpate quarters and to check secretions two months prior to the expected calving date. Normal precalving secretions are thick and like honey. If secretion is like whey, thin, watery and/or shows flakes or cloths, it's recomended to take a sample for bacteriological culture and treat infected cows.

Another alternative is suggested when facilities to treat heifers are not available two months prior to calving. You can examine udders two to four weeks before calving to detect infected quarters or treat every quarter with an approved mastitis antibiotic for lactating cows 14 days before expected calving date (Oliver *et al.*, 2004; Oliver *et al.*, 2003).

Although the increased milk production usually more than makes up for the cost, antibiotic treatment in heifers may not be needed or cannot be managed on every milking farm. This is so called extra-label antibiotic use and veterinarian must be consulted in advance.

As there is a risk of inserting pathogens at the same time, as with intramammary infusion, the partial insertion technique is recommended.

Precautionary measures should also be taken in order to avoid the risk of milk residues, especially with early calvings.

Heifers are not used to having their teats manipulated so a proper milking facility is necessary to do it safely. Treating the heifers in the milking parlor will associate the milking parlor and procedure with a painful experience and will interfere with milk letdown when they enter the parlor for normal milking.

An alternative to prepartum treatment would be to take a mastitis test on days 2 - 4 post calving and/or sample for bacteriological culturing and to treat infected quarters. If quarter is infected with *S. aureus,* this is by far the best opportunity to cure the infection.

Days before and after calving

Familiarizing heifers with the milking environment, milking machines, milking parlor before calving may decrease their post calving stress. In the US and some countries of EU it is a common practice to clip or flame hair from the udder and tail before calving. Few days before due date cows should be placed into clean and dry maternity pens. A deep layer of dry and clean bedding can provide them comfort footing and hygiene. Maternity or calving pen should be clean and disinfect thoroughly when the cow is moved to fresh cow barn. Fresh cows are highly susceptible for all kind of diseases so keeping sick cows close to maternity pen or together with fresh and lactating cows will increase the risk of transmitting diseases.

Fresh cows should be milked out completely as soon as possible after calving (maximum 12 hours). It is use to be *"old school practice"* to leave the milk in the udder to prevent milk fever but that's increases the risk of mastitis. Hypocalcemia or milk fever should be controlled by proper feeding management before and at calving and with calcium treatment if necessary (Costello, 1998).

Before selling that milk check if the cow has passed withdrawal period following dry cow therapy especially if the cow has aborted or has calved sooner than expected. Fresh cows during the first week after calving are more at risk so udders and foremilk should be checked even more carefully for clinical mastitis.

Pre-partum milking

When udder edema is serious or when milk is leaking it is common practice to start milking one week before expected calving. It is important to freeze colostrum for the calf and to respect the withdrawal period following dry cow therapy. Udder edema is not a disease but rather an excessive fluid

accumulation in the extravascular spaces of the udder and surrounding tissues (Figure 14.13). It generally appears between two weeks before calving and after calving. During that period blood flow through the udder increases three fold, udder is warmer than usual, swollen and red. It affects all four quarters. Udder edema is more likely in heifers, especially when they calve older (Melendez *et al.*, 2006.). Long dry period and genetics may be other predisposing factors. Udder edema can cause problems such as discomfort, incomplete milking, due to increase of weight udder ligaments tears. All earlier mentioned factors increase risk of mastitis. Transition nutrition is very important in udder edema prevention so usual recommendations for minimizing the problem include avoidance of excessive potassium, sodium, energy and proteins before calving. It is helpful to allow dry cow to exercise and walk around pen or pasture. Adding antioxidants such as vitamin E, selenium, beta-carotene and zinc in food might improve prevention.

If udder edema occurs make the cow more comfortable and encourage better circulation – moderate exercise in a dry, clean backyard, frequent milking, massage with udder balm. Bathing the udder with cold water or cold compresses (2 times daily / 10 - 20 minutes) also might help. In most cases edema will disappear within a day or two.

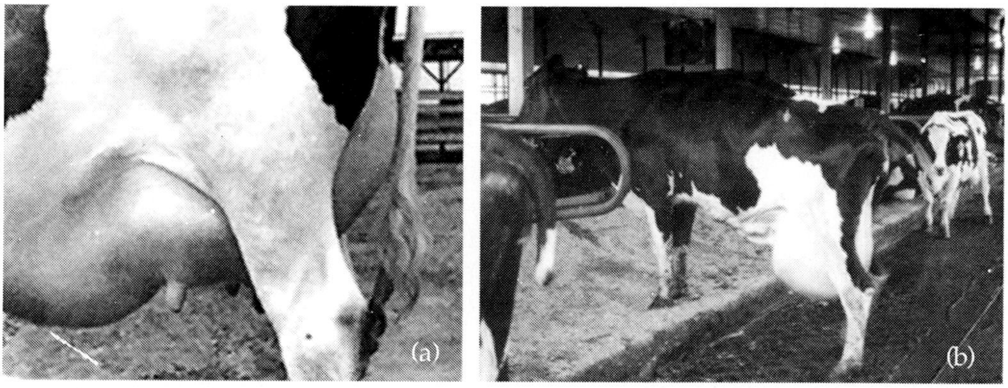

Figure 14.13: (a) Udder edema in heifer, (b) Udder edema in third lactation cow

In serious cases of udder edema when milk is leaking it may be recommended to start milking few days earlier than expected calving date (do not forgot to freeze colostrum). To reduce the risk of suspensory ligaments tearing avoid exercise and have the cow wear an udder support.

A treatment plan involving the use of corticosteroids, diuretics and non steroid anti-inflammatory drugs (NSAID) should be discussed with veterinarian. Sharma *et al.* (2005) reported that in severe cases furosemide (500mg, i/m) and dexamethasone (20 mg, i/m) along with massage is

sufficient to recover the animal within 3-4 days. In severe cases, physical support to udder may be essential as it prevents the udder tissue from damage and helps in early recovery. Salt in diet should be restricted.

12. Provide adequate nutrition to preclude increased susceptibility to mastitis

The occurrence of mastitis is an outcome of interplay between the infectious agents and management practices stressing the defense of udder (Sharma *et al.*, 2003). Traditionally, the mastitis control programmes are focused at use of chemical disinfectants, antiseptic or herbal teat dips (Maiti *et al.*, 2004) and antibiotic therapy. It is well established that the changes in incidence and severity of mastitis are related directly to changes in the composition, magnitude, and efficiency of the udder's immune system. In order to address the future needs of the dairy industry, researchers are investigating ways to enhance the natural defense mechanisms of the udder to prevent and effectively eliminate mastitis. Any control procedure employed that tries to improve the dairy animal ability to fight off environmental pathogens is reactionary and implies that the cow needs to respond to an infection. It is much more logical to place the majority of our control efforts by enhancing the immune status of animal. Since past 20 years researchers are emphasizing on the control of mastitis by enhancing immunity through nutrition. Mastitis exhibits the characteristic of an inflammatory disease rather than an infectious disease; hence the mechanism of the host defense has to be focused. Balanced nutrition is essential in ensuring the maintenance of health and productivity of dairy cows and gross abnormalities in diet are likely to lead to increased clinical mastitis. Nutrition indirectly affects teat end exposure via changes in the amount of manure produced and by altering characteristics of manure (e.g., moisture concentration, pH), but effects on mastitis would probably be small. Conversely, nutrition can have significant effects on the immune system thereby affecting infection rate and severity of mastitis. It has been clearly shown that the dietary intake of the vitamins (e.g. vitamin E, vitamin A and ß-carotene) and the trace minerals (e.g. selenium, copper and zinc) affect the immunological systems of the cow and deficiencies are clearly related to increased rates of new infection during both the dry period and during lactation. The major role of micronutrients is either as cell membrane anti-oxidants, vitamin E and β-carotene, or as essential elements of cytosolic antioxidants, selenium dependent glutathione-peroxidase (GSHPx); copper and zinc-dependent superoxide dismutases (SOD). Antioxidants protect the cell against the free oxygen radicals produced in the phagolysosome of phagocytes following ingestion of pathogens and are thus implicated in efficient mammary gland phagocyte function. The monitoring of herd anti-oxidant status should be considered as part of a mastitis control programme.

The highest rates of mastitis generally occur at or shortly after parturition. Early lactation is also the time when most cows experience short-term malnutrition, i.e., intake of nutrients does not meet nutrient requirements. The mastitic cows have lower Vitamin E and Selenium concentration (Nauriyal and Pachauri, 1997). Inadequate dietary concentrations lead to reduced phagocytic cell function and recruitment of phagocytic cells to sites of infection including the mammary gland. The micronutrients being important for proper immune cell function and protection, deficiencies of these micronutrients can have serious consequences on mammary gland health and thus supplementation could provide great benefit to the control of bovine mastitis (Sharma, 2008).

The immune system, as any physiological system, does not function optimally during periods of malnutrition. In addition, the immune system has high requirements for specific nutrients and when these nutrients are not provided in adequate amounts, immune function may suffer. The majority of published evidence is for vitamin E and selenium and both vitamin E and selenium are important components of the antioxidant defenses of tissues and cells (Smith *et al.*, 1997). The risk of low blood and tissue concentrations of vitamin E and selenium appears to be greatest around calving, a period of known high susceptibility to the environmental pathogens. Diets of dry cows are often low in vitamin E as poor quality forages are frequently fed to dry cows. In addition, forages in many parts of the world are deficient in selenium. Inadequate concentrations of vitamin E and selenium during the dry period have been associated with increased prevalence of infected quarters at calving, higher somatic cell counts during lactation and increased cases of clinical mastitis with greater severity.

Suggested levels of supplementation (amount/cow/day):

Selenium	6 mg (Lactating cows) 3 mg (Dry cows)
Copper	200-250 mg
Zinc	900-1200 mg
Vitamin A	100,000 – 150,000 IU
Vitamin E	500 IU (Lactating cows) 1000 IU (Dry cows)

Why mastitis researchers are emphasing on use of Vitamin E and Selenium in mastitis?

Mastitis is a multietiological complex disease; there is no simple solution to control it. Well over 250 different microorganisms can cause mastitis. Even

also no single vaccine is successful to control mastitis due to its multietiolgical nature of disease. However, antibiotics were introduced in mastitis therapy from 50 year back for the control of mastitis. But the problem in dairy animals remain as same as it was prior to antibiotic era. The antibiotic treatment may help in minimizing the losses but may lead drug resistance (Sharma, 2008). The efficacy of antibiotics in treatment of clinical coliform mastitis is questionable, and antibiotic treatment for *S. aureus* induced mastitis is not economically sound because of low bacterial cure rate (Kirk *et al.*, 1994). Further factors such as pharmacokinetic problems, and phagocytosis depressing effect of certain antibiotics (Hoeben *et al.*, 1998; Hoeben *et al.*, 2000) and residue in milk limit the success of antibiotic therapy in mastitis. Therefore, attention is being paid to find alternative approaches to control mastitis (Sharma, 2003). These approaches are directed to enhance udder defense and antibacterial system in milk by using immunoregulatory micronutrients (vitamins and minerals), vaccines and cytokines.

Vitamin E

Vitamin E was recognized more than 60 years ago as factor required for normal gestation in rats. Evans *et al.* (1936) isolated the vitamin from wheat germ oil. Vitamin E is an essential fat-soluble vitamin. Recently, the National Academy of Sciences defined vitamin E as the 2*R* stereoisomers of alpha-tocopherol. The most active source of vitamin E is alpha tocopherol. Gamma tocopherol and alpha tocotrienol each have approximately 30 percent the vitamin E activity of alpha tocopherol in terms of preventing or resolving symptoms of vitamin E deficiency.

Vitamin E has long been recognized as a natural biological antioxidant. Vitamin E appears to be the first line of defense against peroxidation (Sharma *et al.*, 2005).

To identify the kind of vitamin E in a supplement, it is necessary to read the chemical names in the content description. Natural vitamin E begins with d and synthetic vitamin E with dl. Fresh, green forage is an excellent source of Vitamin E. Vegetable oils are also good source of vitamin E e.g. wheat germ oil contains alpha-tocophero- 133 mg/100 gm oil, soyabean oils alpha-tocopherol- 8 mg and delta-tocopherol- 80 mg/100 gm oil.

Selenium

Selenium is an essential trace element in human and animal nutrition. It is involved in the defense against the toxicity of reactive oxygen species, in the regulation of thyroid hormone metabolism and the regulation of the redox state of cells. Interest in selenium (Se) in animal nutrition initially was focused on its toxic effects. The toxic factor was identified as selenium in 1934. Selenium was discovered in 1817 by Berzelius who named it after Selene, the Greek goddess of the moon. Selenium has been known to be an essential dietary element for animals since the 1950s. Selenium is found in human and animal tissues as L-selenomethionine or L-selenocysteine. The selenoproteins are comprised of four selenium-dependent glutathione peroxidases (GSHPx-1, GSHPx-2, GSHPx-3 and GSHPx-4), three selenium-dependent iodothyronine deiodinases, three thioredoxin reductases, selenoprotein P, selenoprotein W and selenophosphate synthetase. The glutathione peroxidases, and possibly selenoprotein P and selenoprotein W, are antioxidant proteins. The selenium-dependent iodothyronine deiodinases convert thyroxine to triiodothyronine, thus regulating thyroid hormone metabolism. The biochemical function of selenium in higher animals was defined by Rotruck *et al.* (1973) to be as a component of the enzyme glutathione peroxidase. The glutathione peroxidase enzyme has antioxidant activity in cytosol. The specific function of glutathione peroxidase is the coversion of hydrogen peroxide to water and lipid peroxides to the corresponding alcohol.

Synergistic effect of Vitamin E and Selenium in mastitis

In recent years, Vitamin E and Selenium have been frequently discussed together because of their close relationship. Both Vitamin E and Selenium protect cells from the detrimental effect of oxidation but they do so in different ways. Compounds having vitamin E activity are known chemically as tocopherols but biologically most active form is a-tocopherol. Vitamin E is a fat soluble antioxidant which is found in cell membrane prevents the formation of harmful free radicals. Because of this localization within cell membrane, vitamin E can not protect the cytosol from free radicals. Selenium has biological function related to Vitamin E in that selenium is an essential component of glutathione peroxidase (GSHPx), an enzyme involved in detoxification of hydrogen peroxide and lipid hydroperoxides (Rotruck *et al.*, 1973). Selenium is found in cytosol and its functions throughout the cell to destroy peroxides and other harmful compounds. This localization also explains the relationship between selenium and vitamin E. Vitamin E and selenium appear to enhance host defenses against infections by improving phagocytic cell function. Selenium spares vitamin E or reduces the requirements for vitamin E by preserves the integrity of pancreas which allows normal fat digestion and thus normal vitamin E absorption, reduces the amount of vitamin E required to maintain integrity of membranes via GSHPx and aids in some unknown ways in the retention of vitamin E in blood plasma (Uppal *et al.*, 2005). Likewise, vitamin E appears to reduce the requirements for selenium by maintains body selenium in active form and prevent its loss from the body and, prevents the destruction of membrane lipids within the membrane thereby inhibiting the production of hydroperoxides and reducing the amount of selenium dependent enzyme (GSHPx) needed to destroy peroxides formed in the cells.

Oxidants (free radicals), oxidative strees, oxidative damage and anti-oxidants

Normal cell processes, environmental insults (certain mycotoxins, nitrates etc.), and inflammatory responses produce compounds called reactive oxygen speies (ROS) or free radicals. Oxidation is a (normal part of metabolism like "combustion" in animals "internal combustion engine") chemical process whereby an element or compound acquires a positive electrical charge, usually by reaction with an oxygen containing molecule. Free radicals are chemicals possessing an unpaired electron, which are usually very reactive. Free radicals can attack enzymes, fat and proteins disrupting normal cell activities or cell membranes, leading to a destructive chain reaction (Sharma *et al.*, 2006). The major free radicals found in biological systems are superoxide ($O.-_2$), hydrogen peroxide ($H_2O._2$), hydroxyl radical (OH..) and fatty acid radical. Hydrogen peroxide found primarily in the cytosol of the cells and fatty acid radicals are found in cell membranes. Superoxide and hydroxyl radicals can be found in both cell components. Oxidative stress occurs when the production of reactive oxygen metabolites (ROM) exceeds the capacity of the antioxidant system of the cell, tissue, or body. Free radicals can be extremely damaging to biological systems.

Free radicals cause severe oxidative damage and due to tissue injury mastitis may develop. Damages at cellular level are produced by free radicals in various organs in which they are produced. They causes damages due to following reasons-

- formation of lipid peroxides
- breakdown of cellular substances.
- accumulation of inert substances such as lipofuschin.
- alteration of membrane characteristics like fibrosis of vessel walls and destruction of microbes.

The damage occurs from free radicals are due to the fact that whenever an atom is split, energy is released. A severe oxidative stress, however, induces cascade of biochemical reactions leading to injury at cellular site including DNA strand breakage, increase in intracellular free calcium, and damage to membrane proteins and ionic transport, and peroxidation of lipids (Figure 14.14). Hydrogen peroxide radicals can degrade heme proteins such as hemoglobin and myoglobin. Tissue injuries due to free radicals contribute to the development of disease conditions, mastitis being one of them.

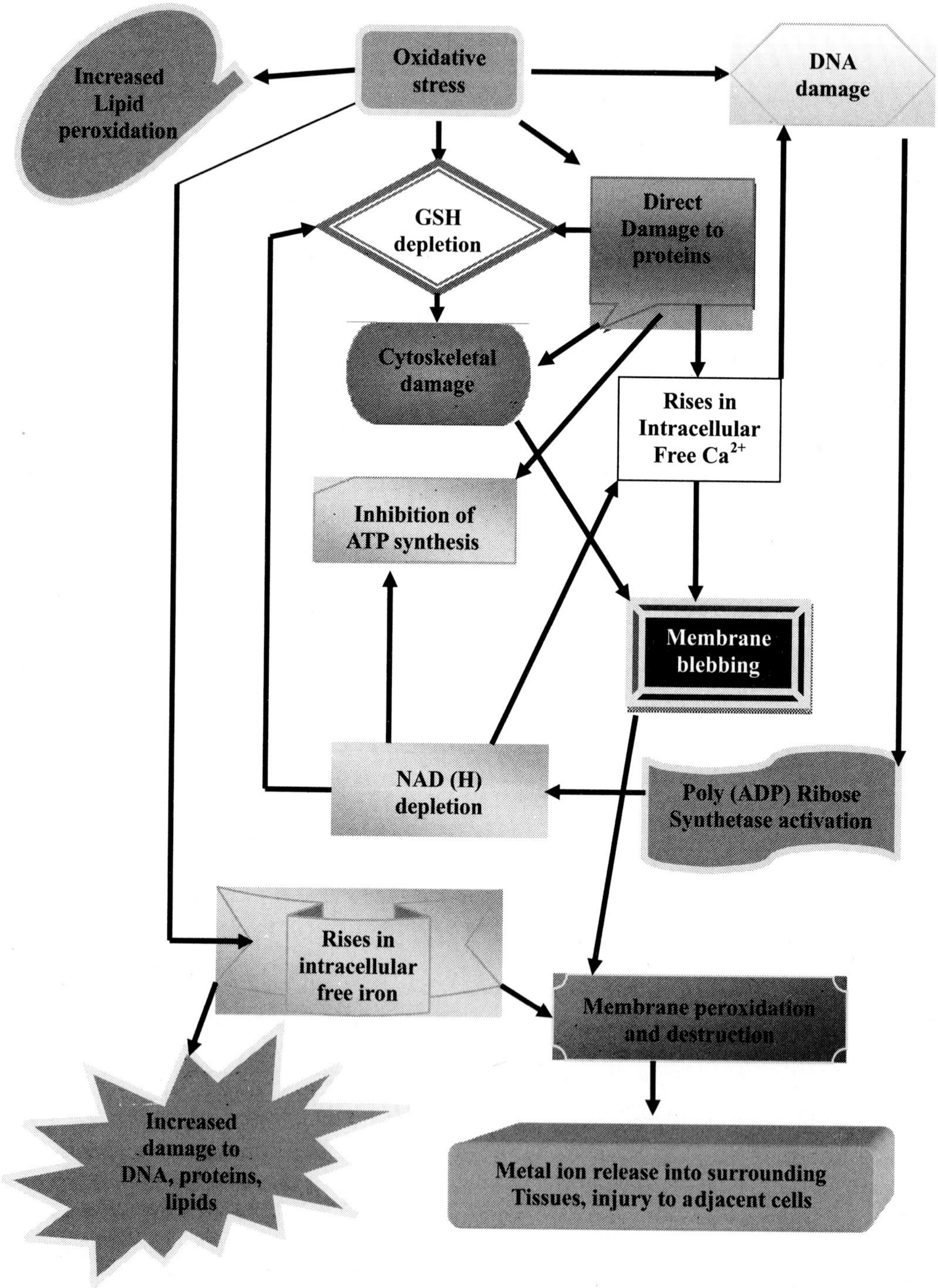

Figure 14.14: Diagram to illustrate the complex multifactorial nature of oxidative damage to cells. Adopted from: Halliwell (1991).

Antioxidants are molecules which can easily and harmlessly give up an electron. An *antioxidant* is a substance that when present in low concentrations compared to those of an oxidizable substrate significantly delays or prevents oxidation of that substrate.

The term "*oxidizable substrate*" includes almost everything found in living cells. Including proteins, lipids, carbohydrates and DNA (Halliwell, 1991) Chemically antioxidants work by one of the following mechanisms:

- removing O_2
- scavenging free radicals
- inhibiting free radical formation
- binding metal ions needed for catalysis of free radical production
- up regulation of indigenous antioxidant defenses.

Selenium comes in to picture as a part of GSHPx in second line of defense. Generation of free radicals under normal condition is a continuous process and these are neutralized by antioxidants. Hydrogen peroxide (produced from superoxides by superoxide dismutase) is converted in to waters by the selenium contains enzyme GSHPx and fatty acid radicals (free radicals) generated by superoxide and hydroxyl radical, attacks other fatty acids, producing free radicals which are ultimately neutralized by antioxidant systems vitamin E and selenium (Sharma *et al.*, 2003).

Natural body defense mechanism against Free Radicals

Cows and buffaloes experience oxidative stress around calving. Vitamin E is able to decrease oxidative stress by scavenging free radicals. Normally, the formed vitamin E radicals will be regenerated by an antioxidant network. This network is called the *'vitamin E regeneration system'* (VERS). In case of supplementation, VERS should be sufficient to regenerate these vitamin E radicals. If not, oxidative stress might increase instead of decrease.

Even under healthy conditions, potentially toxic free radicals are produced in the body. But antioxidant defenses in the body effectively neutralize them. Normally the body is protected against oxidative stress and free radical injury by a host of defense system (Sharma *et al.*, 2005). But when free radicals/ROS are produced faster than scavenging capability of antioxidant defenses in the body, the condition of oxidative stress arises. So, why are antioxidants important?

Because free radicals are extremely toxic to cells, the body has developed a sophisticated antioxidant system (Table 14.2). Superoxide dimutase (an enzyme that contain Cu and Zn) converts superoxide to hydrogen peroxide.

Hydrogen peroxide is converted to water by the enzyme GSHPx (contain selenium) (Figure 14.15). These two enzymes effectively control most free radicals within the cytosol. Superoxide and hydroxyl radicals can migrate into cell membrane where they attack fatty acids (especially polyunsaturated fatty acids) and produce fatty acid radicals (a process called initiation). Fatty acid radicals then react with other fatty acids producing a chain reaction. Vitamin E reacts with fatty acid radicals and stops the chain reaction. It explains importance of vitamin E as antioxidant. There are also some macromolecules such as transferrin, ceruloplasmin and albumin involved in the body defense mechanism. Vitamin E and selenium are important for optimal immune functions associated with T and B lymphocytes (Bendich, 1990).

Table 14.2: Antioxidant system of mammalian cell.

Component and location in cell	Nutrients involved	Function
Ceruloplasmin (Water phase)	Cu	An oxidant protein, may prevent Cu and Fe from partipating in oxidation reactions
Superoxide dimutase (Cytosol)	Cu and Zn	An enzyme that converts superoxide to hydrogen peroxide.
Superoxide dimutase (Mitochondria)	Mn and Zn	An enzyme that converts superoxide to hydrogen peroxide.
Glutathione peroxidase (Cytosol)	Se	An enzyme that converts hydrogen peroxide to water.
Catalase (Cytosol)	Fe	An enzyme (primarily found in liver) that converts hydrogen peroxide to water.
α-tocopherol (Membrane)	Vitamin E	Breaks fatty acid peroxidation chain reactions.
β-carotene (Membrane)	Carotene	Prevents initiation of fatty acid peroxidation chain reaction.
Ascprbic acid (Cytosol)	Vitamin C	React with several types of free radicals.

How vitamin E and selenium helps in Mastitis Control ?

Effective management of mastitis is a major challenge to dairy farmers and modern veterinarians. One of the most important approaches to control mastitis and to enhance therapeutic efficacy of antimicrobial treatment is to enhance udder defense against pathogens. Antioxidants such as vitamin E and selenium have been tried with encouraging results in this direction. Vitamin E is the most important free radical scavenger within cell membrane (Rice and Kennedy, 1986). Tocopherols, apart from being radical scavengers,

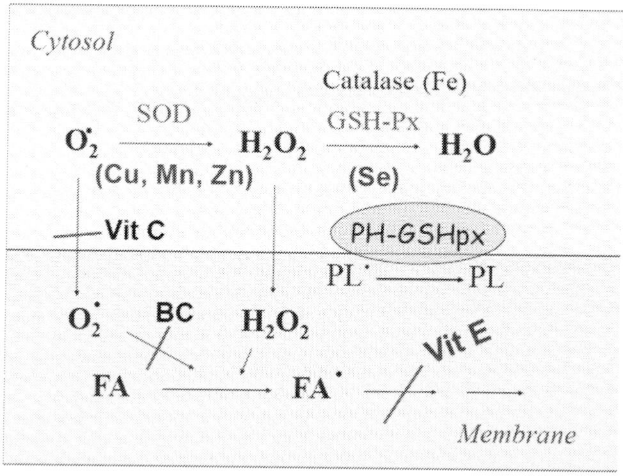

Figure 14.15: Simplified illustration of antioxidant system showing relationship with antioxidant nutrients. (Source: Weiss, W.P. http://nmconline.org/articles/nutrition.pdf, downloaded on 31/10/2009)
[SOD – superoxide dismutase, GSHPx – glutathione peroxidase, PH-GSHPx – phospholipid hydroperoxide glutathione peroxidase, BC – α-carotene, FA – fatty acid, PL- phospholipids]

react with singlet molecular oxygen (Kaiser *et al.*, 1990; Diplock *et al.*, 1989). Polyunsaturated fatty acids (PUFA) of membranes are particularly vulnerable to attack by free radicals, and the free radicals can initiate a chain reaction of lipid destruction that destroys the cell membrane. An important PUFA in cellular membranes is arachidonic acid (AA). AA protects DNA of the cells from the free radicals damage, prevents infections by strengthening cell membranes, and helps protecting phagocytic cells from oxidative damage. Arachidonic acid can be metabolized to leukotriens, prostaglandins etc. by the cyclooxygenase enzyme complex (Kuehl and Egan, 1980). Leukotriens act as chemotactic agent for PMN, eosinophils and monocytes. The main function of vitamin E in udder defense is linked to maximize polymorphonuclear (PMN) cells activity as it protects polyunsaturated fatty acids in the PMN membrane from destruction by free oxygen radicals that are produced during phagocytosis (Boxer, 1986). The prostaglandins are known to influence the function of smooth muscel tissue (Monicada and Vane, 1979). Smooth muscle, which surrounds the streak canal of the bovine teat, helps to keep the canal tightly closed. So, altered, prostaglandin synthesis results failure of complete tight closure and consequently the pathogens may enter into the gland more easily (Sharma *et al.*, 2003). This explains as to how vitamin E deficient dairy cows become prone to mastitis. Vitamin E inhibits peroxidation of arachidonic acid by scavenging peroxyl radicals thus slowing the chain reaction (Figure 14.16). This free radical scavenging vitamin is an important component of udder defense and has been proved effective in augmenting therapeutic efficacy of antimicrobial treatment in mastitis. Primary source of α-tocopherol (Vitamin E) in the normal milk is the fat globule membrane. But during inflammation, neutrophils are rich source of vitamin E and contain about 17.6 mg α-tocopherol/million cells. It is reported that neutrophil can account for 10% of milk α-tocopherol in non-infected and nearly 25% in milk from mastitic udder. Therefore, the increase in somatic cell count (SCC) is associated with increase in -tocopherol content in milk (Barret *et al.*, 1997).

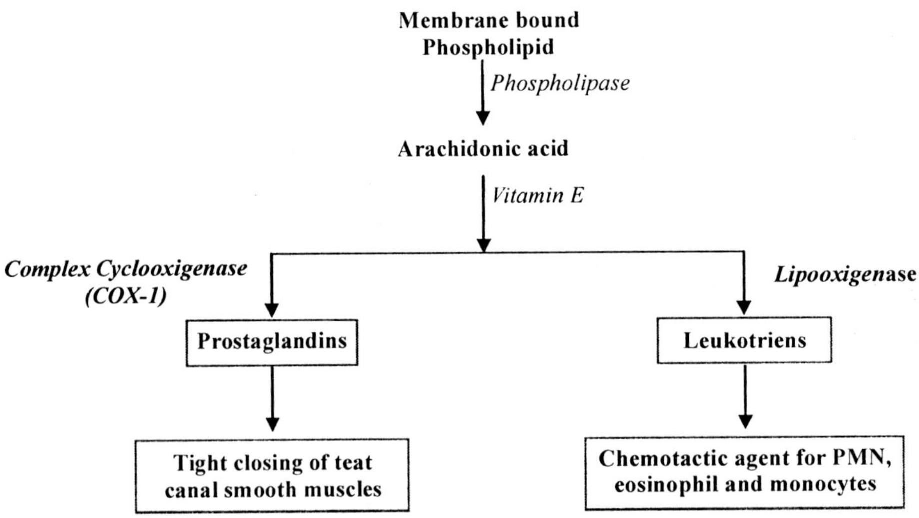

Figure 14.16: Diagram to illustrate the role of vitamin E in the control of mastitis by alteration of arachdonic acid metabolism.

Selenium is an essential component of an enzyme glutathione peroxidase (GSHPx). GSHPx is a major intracellular antioxidant that catalyzes the reduction of hydrogen peroxide and organic hydroperoxides to nontoxic compounds. If an animal is selenium deficient, GSHPx will not be present in adequate amounts, which allows free radicals to interact with cell membranes. When selenium is deficient, additional vitamin E is needed to protect cell membranes. If a cow is deficient in vitamin E, more free radicals are produced in the cell membranes, some of which interact with compounds in the cytosol, which increase the need for selenium.

In mastitis neutrophils are the predominant cell type found in mammary tissues and in mammary secretions during early inflammation and can constitute >90% of total mammary gland leukoytes (Sordillo *et al.*, 1987). When a pathogen invades the mammary gland of a cow, a cascade of events occurs. First, neutrophils move from the blood to mammary gland in response to variety of inflammatory mediators (Person *et al.*, 1993). When the mastitogens enter the mammary gland, they are engulfed and killed by these neutrophils, through the process of respiratory burst (Figure 14.17). This process produces a high concentration of free radicals help to kill the bacteria i.e. without sufficient free radicals, neutrophils can not function properly. However, the level of free radicals must be controlled, otherwise they will damage or kill the neutrophils before the neutrophils can kill the bacteria. Neutrophils contain large concentrations of a-tocopherol to protect it from free radicals. This is where vitamin E important. It appears, vitamin E in cellular and sub cellular membranes is the first line of defence against peroxidation of phospholipids, but even with adequate vitamin E, some peroxides are formed.

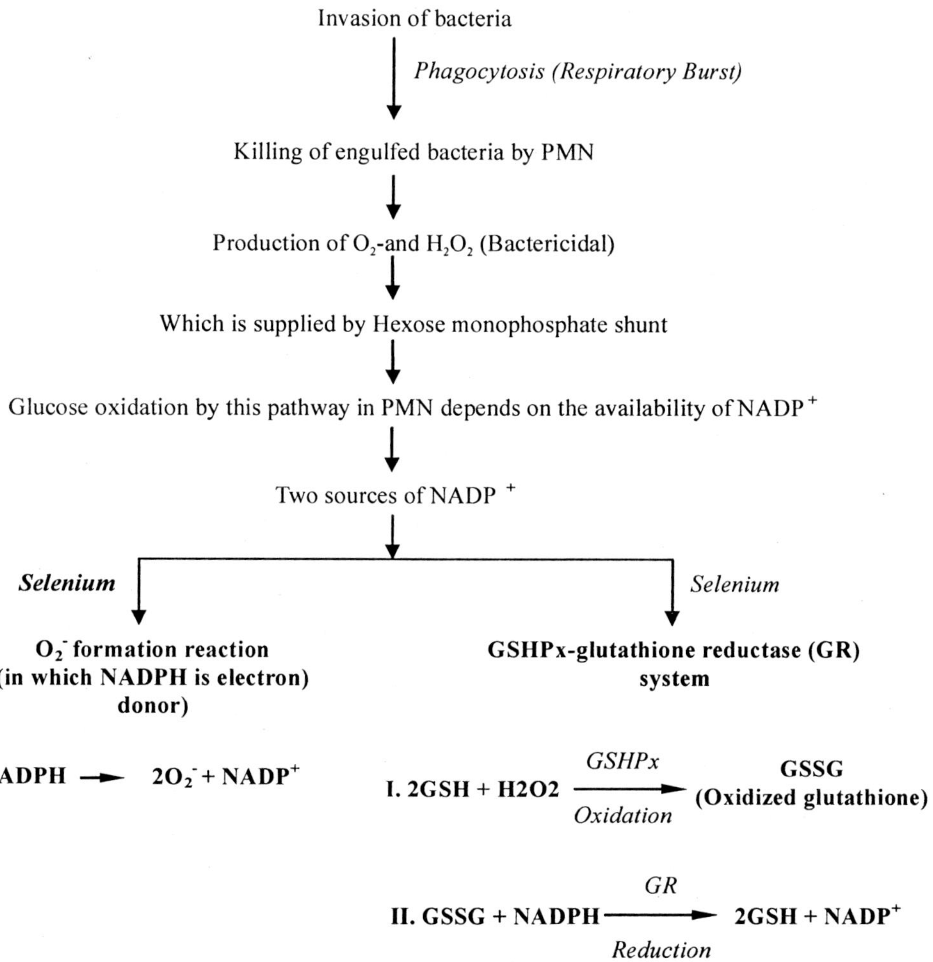

Figure 14.17: Diagram to illustrate the action of selenium in the control of free radical production and killing of bacteria. *[Source: Sharma (2007)].*

Selenium as part of GSHPx is a second line of defence that destroys these peroxides before they have an opportunity to cause damage to membranes. Therefore, selenium, vitamin E and sulphur containing amino acids, through different biochemical mechanisms (Figure 14.18) such as prevention of hydroperoxide formation by vitamin E, role of sulphur containing amino acids as a precursor of glutathione peroxidase (GSHPx) and selenium as an integral component of GSHPx. Antioxidants can however scavenges and minimize the formation of these free radicals/ROS, but not 100% effective. When ROS are not effectively and safely removed, oxidative stress may impair health in dairy animals both directly (peroxidative damage to important lipids and macromolecules) and indirectly (changes induced in cellular membranes and components).

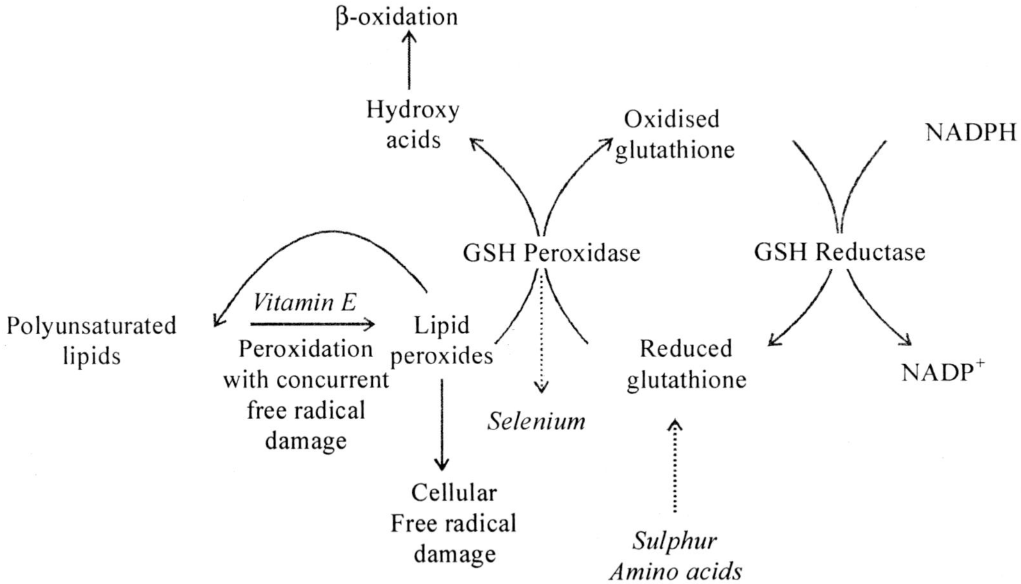

Figure 14.18: Diagram to illustrate interaction among selenium, vitamin E and sulphur amino acids.

Supplementation of Vitamin E and Selenium

The antioxidants viz. vitamin E and selenium have extensively used in bovine mastitis therapy. Deficiencies of either vitamin E or selenium have been associated with increased incidence and severity of intramammary infection (IMI), increased clinical mastitis cases and higher somatic cell count in milk. The important thing is that the blind (without estimation of blood vitamin E and selenium level) treatment with vitamin E and selenium for long duartion should be avoided, otherwise it may cause toxicity.

Plasma vitamin E concentrations in dairy cows are normally lowest when rates of intramammary infection are highest and when neutrophil functions are depressed during the periparturient period. Low plasma concentration of a-tocopherol at parturition is considered as a significant risk factor for intrammamary infection during first week of lactation (Samanta *et al.*, 2005). The plasma a-tocopherol decreases during the periparturient period is may be due to a combination of reduced dry matter intake in dry cows, decrease transport capacity for the vitamin in plasma and loss of vitamin E into milk of lactating cows. Cows are immunosuppresed during the time when plasma concentrations of vitamin E are low (especially from 7days prepartum to 1 or 2 weeks postpartum). The effect of vitamin E supplementation particularly on neutrophil function (Table 14.3).

Table 14.3: Effect of Vitamin E supplementation on neutrophil function in dairy cows.

Type of cows	Supplementation	Response	Reference
Lactating cows, 30 days in lactation	1000 IU/day of dietary vitamin E during the dry period and 500 IU/day during the first 30 days of lactation	• Phagocytosis not affected • Ability to kill *S. aureus* and *E. coli* was improved	Hogan *et al.*, 1990
Fresh Cows (<3 days in lactation)	3000 IU of vitamin E injected at 10 and 5 days before anticipated calving	• Phagocytosis not affected • Ability to kill *E. coli* was improved	Hogan *et al.*, 1992
Dairy cows from 4 wk to 5wk postpartum	3000 IU/day of dietary vitamin E from 4 wk pre to 8 wk post partum + 3000 IU of vitamin E injected 1 wk prepartum	• Neutrophil chemotaxis was improved	Politis *et al.*, 1996
Fresh cows (<7 days in milk)	3000 IU/day of dietary vitamin E from 4 wk pre to 8 wk post partum + 3000 IU of vitamin E injected 1 wk prepartum	• Overall neutrophil function was improved	Politis *et al.*, 1995

Dietary supplementation of cows with vitamin E and selenium results in a more rapid PMN influx into milk following intramammary bacterial challenge and increased intracellular kill of ingested bacteria by PMN. The killing ability of blood neutrophils has been correlated with the concentration of a-tocopherol in neutrophils (Weiss *et al.*, 1994). NRC (1989) recommendation for total not supplemental, vitamin E for dry and lactating cows is 15 IU/kg of dry mater (DM) based on typical dry mater intake (DMI), that amount is equivalent to about 300 and 150 IU/day for dry and lactating cows, respectively.

The first clinical study on the effect of vitamin E and selenium on mastitis was conducted by Smith *et al.* (1984). In that study, dry cows were fed high forage diets based on hay and silage that provided 0 or 740 IU/day of supplemental vitamin E and were fed no supplemental selenium or injected with 0.1 mg of selenium/kg of body weight 21 days before anticipated calving. Diets fed to lactating cows were not supplemented with vitamin E and selenium. Supplemental vitamin E with or without a selenium injection reduced the incidence of clinical mastitis during the subsequent lactation by 37% compared with cows not fed supplemental vitamin E or injected with selenium. Selenium without supplemental vitamin E reduced the incidence of clinical mastitis by 12% compared with unsupplemented cows, vitamin E without selenium injections reduced the duration of clinical mastitis by 44% and by 62% when selenium was injected.

Smith *et al.* (1985) also concluded that diets of heifers were either unsupplemented or supplemented with selenium (0.3 ppm) and vitamin E (1000 IU/day total intake) from 60 days prepartum and continuing throughout lactation. Supplemented heifers had significantly fewer quarters infected at calving, reduced prevalence of infection throughout lactation, fewer cases of clinical mastitis, infections of shorter duration and lower milk SCC compare with unsupplemented heifers.

Bendich (1990) stated that vitamin E and Selenium are important for immune function associated with T and B lymphocyte. Effective management of mastitis is a great challenge to dairy industry, strengthening the defense mechanism against pathogen may prove an important tool. Reports are available showing encouraging results of vitamin E and selenium in improving defense mechanism. Vitamin E maximize polymorphonuclear (PMN) cell activity by preventing polyunsaturated fatty acids (PUFA) in PMN membrane from destruction by free oxygen radicals which are produced during phagocytosis (Boxer 1986).

Politis *et al.* (1995, 1996) fed cows either 0 or 3,000 IU/day suplemental vitamin E during the last 28 day prepartum and the first 56 day postpartum (base ration supplied 300 IU/day vitamin E). Cows in the supplemental group also received a single injection of 5,000 IU vitamin E ~1 week before calving. Selenium status of cows was more than adequate at 88 ng/ml plasma. Somatic cell count (log 10) was significantly lower in the vitamin E supplemented cows (2.1 vs 2.5), and several measures of leukocyte function were improved by supplementing vitamin E at these levels. It is concluded that "vitamin E prevented suppression of leukocyte function during the early postpartum period".

Weiss *et al.* (1997) conducted a trial to examine effect of feeding of various amounts of vitamin E during the dry period on the prevalence of clinical mastitis during the first week of lactation when all cows were fed 0.1 mg/kg of diet DM of selenium. In that study cows at dry-off (approximately 60 days before calving) were fed diets with 0.1 mg/kg of selenium and 100 or 1000 IU/day of supplemental vitamin E (all-*rac*- a-tocopherol acetate). At 14 days before anticipated calving, cows that were fed 1000 IU/day of supplemental vitamin E either continued to receive 1000 IU/day or were fed 4000 IU/day of supplemental vitamin E. Total intramammary infections during the first week of lactation were not different among cows fed 100 or 1000 IU/day throughout the dry period (30 and 28% of lactating quarters, respectively) but cows fed 4000 IU/day of supplemental vitamin E during the 14 days prepartum period had fewer intramammary gland infections (13% of lactating quarters). The incidence of clinical mastitis was 24, 17 and 3% for cows fed 100, 1000 and 4000 IU/day of supplemental vitamin E, respectively.

Baldi *et al.* (2000) also reported that significantly lower somatic cell count (log 10) in cows fed 2,000 IU/day supplemental vitamin E vs 1,000 IU/day from 14 day prepartum through 7 day postpartum in rations with 0.3 ppm added selenium. Plasma and milk vitamin E were increased in cows fed 2000 vs 1000 IU/day. Taken together, these studies sub stantiate the cooperative roles of vitamin E and selenium in maintaining mammary immune function and suggest that 2,000 and 4,000 IU vitamin E/day during the prepartum period can be beneficial to dairy cows in terms of udder health and milk quality.

Sharma *et al.* (2004) also reported that antibiotic (Cefotaxime @ 5mg/kg/b. wt. for 4 days i/m) in vitamin E (@ 500 IU/animal/day) and selenium (@ 6 mg/animal/day during early lactation for 60 days) supplemented cows is more effective in the control of sub-clinical mastitis as compared to unsupplemented animals.

Sharma and Maiti (2005) dietary supplemented vitamin E (@ 500 IU/animal/day) and selenium (@ 6 mg/animal/day) in sub-clinical mastitic cows during early lactation (for 60 days) caused 40% reduction in the infection rate. Both somatic cell count and total bacterial count were gradually reduced in supplemented groups. Supplementation of vitamin E (@ 1000 IU/animal/day) and selenium (@ 3 mg/animal/day) during dry period (last 60 days) caused 50% and 71.42% reduction in incidence of sub-clinical mastitis in subsequent lactation (after calving) on animal and quarter wise basis, respectively.

Adverse effects of oral vitamin E supplementation

It is cleared that not every dairy cow needs to be supplemented with high vitamin E amounts during the dry period to reduce mastitis incidence post partum, because higher doses of oral vitamin E may cause adverse effect on animal production. The level of oxidative stress and the vitamin E status might be important conditions to evaluate prior to supplementation. Boustra *et al.* (2010a) conducted a study on 5 farms, 296 cows were randomly divided into two groups. Both groups received a mineral mix between dry-off and calving that contained 3,000 IU vitamin E or 135 IU, respectively. Cows were sampled at dry-off and 2 weeks before expected calving day. In two non sufficient VERS subgroups, the supplemented group had higher levels of free radicals at two weeks ante-partum compared to the control group. Relative risk calculation was used to study the effect of oxidative stress at two weeks ante-partum on incidence of mastitis in the first 100 days of lactation. Higher levels of oxidative stress at two weeks ante-partum was related to higher risk of clinical mastitis. Finally they concluded that not every dairy dry responded well to high vitamin E supplementation.

A study demonstrated an adverse effect of vitamin E supplementation during the dry period on mastitis incidence in early lactation (Boustra *et al.*, 2010b). On 5 dairy farms dry cows were randomly divided into two experimental groups, a high and a low group. Both groups received a dry cow mineral mix between dry-off and calving containing 3,000 IU vitamin E or 135 IU, respectively. The results showed that vitamin E supplements increased both absolute vitamin E and the ratio of vitamin E to cholesterol in blood. In the high group significantly more sub-clinical and clinical cases occurred showing the same trend on all farms. In this study, an initial vitamin E level at dry-off above 14.5 μ mol/L was a risk factor for clinical mastitis, suggesting that the vitamin E status at the start of the dry period is important. It is recommended to work out exactly at which threshold vitamin E is harmful for udder health before new trials with high dosages of vitamin E are started. Therefore, further research is required to investigate the mechanism by which vitamin E affects udder health.

Some studies have been done on the effects of other antioxidant micronutrients on the incidence and severity of mastitis including vitamins A, vitamin C, β-carotene, copper and zinc (Goff, 2006; Scaletti *et al.*, 2003; Spears, 2000; Wilde, 2006).

Vitamin A and β-carotene

The effects of vitamin A and β-carotene on mastitis measures have been inconsistent. Limited research is carried out on the potential effects of vitamin A and its precursor β-carotene in controlling mastitis in dairy cattle documented a reduction of plasma retinol in peri-parturient animals and speculated on an association with an increased risk of mastitis (Chew, 1987; Goff *et al.*, 2002). Michal *et al.*, (1994) found positive effects on neutrophil and lymphocyte function when cows are supplemented with approximately 70,000

IU/day of vitamin A or 300 to 600 mg of β-carotene, but in clinical study similar treatments had no effect on mammary gland health (Oldham *et al.*, 1991). Low concentrations of plasma vitamin A (<80 μg/100 ml) and α-carotene (<200 μg/100 ml) are associated with severity of mastitis (based on California Mastitis Test scores) (Chew *et al.* 1982).

However, some previous studies presented conflicting data on vitamin A and a possible relationship on udder health. Both vitamin A and β-carotene have been shown to have stimulatory effects on immune cell populations and have been correlated with a generally increased resistance to mastitis (Sordillo *et al.*, 1997).

Antioxidant properties of carotenoids include scavenging singlet oxygen and peroxyl radicals, sulfur, thiyl, sulfonyl and NO_2 radicals and provide protection of lipids from superoxide and hydroxyl radical attack. Carotenoids can actively quench singlet oxygen (O^-_2) and prevent lipid peroxidation caused by O_2 and they can intercept the propagation step of lipid peroxidation. One molecule of beta-carotene is able to quench 1000 molecules of O^-_2 before it reacts chemically. Although the principal antioxidant carotenoid is beta-carotene, other carotenoids (*e.g.* lutein, lycopene and zeaxanthin) have strong antioxidant activities.

Cows with mastitis had lower levels of plasma vitamin A and cows supplemented with β-carotene prior to involution had lower rates of new intramammary infections during the dry period when compared to un-supplemented animals (Chew, 1995). However, some studies found that vitamin A and β-carotene have no impact on mastitis resistance in dairy cattle (Oldham *et al.*, 1991). The potential impact of vitamin A or β-carotene on mastitis susceptibility remains uncertain. Vitamin A deficiency has been linked to increased glucocorticoid response to stress, which has an immuno-suppressive effect. Beta-carotene can act independently as an oxygen radical scavenger and is incorporated into cell membranes as such. Jukola *et al.* (1996) suggested that plasma concentrations of β-carotene in dairy cows should be >3 mg/L to optimize udder health. Supplemental β-carotene may have some benefit if cows are in low β-carotene status.

Vitamin C

Despite the fact that vitamin C is not a required nutrient in healthy dairy cattle due to hepatic synthesis, recent data also suggest that it may play a role in development of mastitis (Chaiyotwittayakun *et al.*, 2002; Weiss and Hogan, 2007). An increased incidence of mastitis and the severity of clinical symptoms have been correlated with decreased concentrations of plasmatic vitamin C (Weiss and Hogan, 2007; Weiss *et al.*, 2004).

Vitamin C is the most important antioxidant in extracellular fluids and can protect biomembranes against lipid peroxidation damage by eliminating peroxyl radicals in the aqueous phase before the latter can initiate peroxidation. Vitamin C is located in the aqueous phase of cells, where it contributes to radical scavenging. Vitamin C is a potent antioxidant, easily giving up electrons to stabilize reactive oxygen species (ROS).

Most forms of vitamin C are extensively degraded in the rumen, therefore the cow must rely on tissue synthesis of vitamin C. The concentration of ascorbic acid is high in neutrophils (important immune cells with respect to mastitis) and increases as much as 30-fold when the neutrophil is stimulated. Various supplement forms are available like calcium ascorbate - buffered form of vitamin C and ester C which is very expensive but can be tolerated better by those who experience gastrointestinal side effects from other forms of vitamin C. The health benefits of taking Sodium Ascorbate are remarkable and have far reaching implications for many health conditions. In addition sodium ascorbate has a leading role to play in the elimination of chronic and acute infections. Ascorbate is essential for the hydroxylation of the amino acid Proline which forms hydroxyproline - a major component of collagen. Collagen is an essential structural protein in the body accounting for around a quarter of all the protein in our bodies and is critical to the structural integrity of our bodies.

Udder infections reduce the amount of ascorbic acid in the milk, the reduction being correlated in general with the severity of the infection. In early stages of mastitis the ascorbic acid of the milk is reduced about by 10% and in advanced cases it may reduced by as much as 30 to 50%. There is a trend toward an inverse relationship between ascorbic acid and chlorides in mastitic milk and also in the milk produced following perfusion of the mammary duct system with a hypertonic solution.

Kleczkowski *et al.* (2005) reported that markedly low level of ascorbic acid concentration in the serum of cows affected with mastitis (29.4 μ mol/dml) as compared with the control group (64.9 μ mol/dml) was observed.

Copper (Cu)

Copper is an essential element in the antioxidant Cu-dependent enzyme superoxide dismutase (SOD) and in the serum protein ceruloplasmin, which is recognised as an acute phase protein in cattle. These two proteins are important to immune function, partially because of their protection of cells from oxidative products released by phagocytosis and killing by leukocytes (Sordillo *et al.* 1997). Cu deficiency results in a decline in ceruloplasmin and SOD levels in blood, and could potentially compromise host defense. Ceruloplasmin may function as anti-oxidant, scavenging oxygen free radicals,

and could serve as an endogenous modulators of the inflammatory response. It modulates the tissue injury associated with production of free radicals by phagocytes during inflammation.

Superoxide dismutase neutralize the free radicals by converting into water.

$$O^{2-} + O^{2-} + 2H^{+} \xrightarrow{\text{SOD}} H_2O_2 + O_2$$

This reaction is essential in protecting host tissues from membrane oxidation by oxygen derived free radicals from neutrophils and macrophages during the inflammatory response. The importance of copper in immunity has been documented in numerous species, but evidence for its potential role in bovine mastitis is lacking (Spears, 2000).

Inadequate Cu status may be related to an increased incidence of infections at calving, increased severity of infections, and a higher SCC than that seen in Cu adequate level. Current recommendations are to maintain Cu between 10 - 15 ppm of the diet. If excessive interfering minerals such as Mo, S, Fe and Zn are present, dietary levels may be increased slight. Gakhar *et al.* (2010) given injection copper glycinate (75 mg/ml) at the dose rate of 2 ml per animal subcutaneously in brisket region before drying off, followed by second injection at the same dose rate after parturition. They found that a reduction in occurrence of postpartum mastitis in supplemented cows (50%) as compared to un-supplemented control group (70%). A study, however, concluded that dietary copper supplementation in dairy cows enhanced resistance to experimentally challenged *E. coli* mastitis as measured by a reduction in bacterial and somatic cell counts, lower clinical mammary scores and lower peak rectal temperatures (Scaletti *et al.*, 2003). Due to the large copper demand of the fetus, copper status of cows tends to be lowest at calving. Supplementation of copper reduced the severity of clinical signs but unaffected the duration of mastitis.

Zinc (Zn)

Zinc deficiency in cattle and buffaloes results in weakening of skin and other stratified epithelia (e.g. keratinocytes), that is Zn is important for keratin production. Keratin lines the inside of streak canal and helps to keep out microorganisms that cause mastitis. Streak canal keratin act as physical barrier and have bactericidal properties. Cows receiving supplemental Zn methionine had significantly more teat canal keratin. Moderate to severe blood hypozincemia during mastitis particularly acute coliform mastitis, has been documented. Zinc is an integral part of immune system. It is a structural component of cell membranes. Zn stabilizes membrane structure by binding to the sulphur and nitrogen groups in proteins and to phospholipids via their phosphate groups. Zn is also known to be associated with enzymes involved in the phagocytic oxidative burst, in cellular maturation, and functioning of B- and T-lymphocytes and macrophages. As such Zn boosts immune functioning.

The relationship of zinc and mastitis in dairy cattle has received little attention despite experiments that have documented a decrease in Zn plasma concentrations following intramammary challenge with *E. coli* and *Staphylococcus aureus* (Erskine and Bartlett, 1993; Middleton *et al.*, 2004). The ability of Zn to decrease the percentage of infected quarters at calving and a reduction in SCC in Zn supplemented cows has been reported (Harmon and Torre, 1994). Singh and Pachauri (2001) supplemented Zn at the dose rate of 260 mg per day, during last three weeks of pregnancy and 390 mg per day for first 100 days after calving as zinc sulphate. They found 33.33% recovery in sub-clinically infected cows. Now several studies have examined the effect of supplemental zinc methionine on SCC and in most cases supplementation statistically or numerically reduced SCC (O'Rourke, 2009). Organic forms of Zn appear to be better absorbed and retained by the animal. NRC recommendation for pregnant cows is 22.8 ppm zinc in the diet or approximately 300 mg per day.

13. Vaccination

Vaccination is an important aspect in disease prevention but in mastitis vaccination is not much successful due to its multifactorial complex etiology. However, vaccine against major mastitis pathogens like *Staphylococcus aureus, Streptococcus uberis, E. coli* have been developed, but they are costly. There are some additional treatments that could act preventively on mastitis such as vaccination and application of teat sealant. The role of vaccines is to stimulate antibodies to fight certain pathogens. Unfortunately there are no vaccines that could be used against all microoranisms that cause mastitis. There are various vaccines specifically for coliforms that can be used at drying off and after calving in some countries (UK and USA). Implementing proper milking procedures and providing a clean environment for dairy cattle can help prevent mastitis, but it can also be important to use an effective mastitis vaccine. Two vaccines are dominant on the market; MERIAL J-VAC® and UPJOHN J-5 BACTERIN®. MERIAL J-VAC® is the proven and probably the most effective *E. coli* mastitis vaccine with the exclusive convenience of only two doses - all competitive vaccines require three doses. MERIAL J-VAC® also protects against endotoxemia caused by *E. coli* and *Salmonella typhimurium*. You can administer MERIAL J-VAC® at dry-off and then boost two to four weeks later, or give J-VAC to your whole herd at any stage of lactation and boost two to four weeks later. Whichever administration program one will choose, the two-dose regimen is less labor intensive than conventional three-dose protocols.

MERIAL J-VAC® can be administered intramuscularly or subcutaneously, and there's no milk withholding.

UPJOHN J-5 BACTERIN® is made up of special *E. coli* 0111:B4(J-5) mutant bacterial strain. Here's how it works:

- The bacterial strain possesses exposed core antigens, which are identical among many gram-negative bacteria, including *Klebsiella, Salmonella, E. coli, Pasteurella,* and *Serratia.*
- In UPJOHN J-5 BACTERIN® the core antigens are exposed, prompting the cow to produce antibodies that will attack subsequent challenge infections early.
- This reduction in bacterial load subsequently reduces the level of endotoxins released in the cow's system.

This is why cows vaccinated with UPJOHN J-5 BACTERIN® will experience fewer and milder cases of coliform mastitis. Generally vaccination is useful measure of prevention especially in developed dairy countries and it always pay offs. But in some countries success might be diminished by higher costs of vaccine and on farm management.

References

Bacic, G. (2005). In: Comp. 6th Middle European Buiatrics Congress, Cracow, Poland, 2005. Pp. 446-448.

Baldi, A., Savoini, G., Pinotti, L., Monfardini, E., Cheli, F. and Dellorto. V. (2000). J. Vet. Med. Assoc., 47: 599.

Barret, J.J., Hogan, J.S., Weiss, W.P., Smith, K.L. and Sordillo, L.M. (1997). J. Dairy Sci., 80: 2826-2832.

Bendich, A. (1990). Ann. New York Acad. Sci., 587: 168.

Berry, E. and Hillerton, J.E. (2002). J. Dairy, Sci., 85: 112-121.

Berry, E.A. (2000). In: Proc. British Mastitis Conf., Shepton Mallet. Pp. 37-43.

Berry, E.A., Johnson, W.T. and Hillerton, J.E. (2003). J. Dairy Sci., 86: 3912-3919.

Biggs, A. (1998). In: Proc. British Mastitis Conference, pp. 15-21.

Boddie, R.L. and Nickerson, S.C. (1986). J. Dairy Sci., 69: 253-257.

Borm, A.A., Fox, L.K., Leslie, K.E., Hogan, J.S., Andrew, S.M., Moyes, K.M., Oliver, S.P., Schukken, Y.H., Hancock, D.D., Gaskins, C.T., Owens, W.E. and Norman, C. (2006). J. Dairy Sci., 89(6): 2090 - 2098.

Boustra, R.J., Nielen, M. and Werven, T.V. (2010a). Not every dairy cow needs to be supplemented with high vitamin e amounts during the dry period to reduce mastitis incidence post partum. In: Proc. XXVI World Buiatrics Cong. Nov. 14-18, 2010 Santiago de Chile, Chile.

Boustra, R.J., Nielen, M., Werven, T.V. and Jorritsma, R. (2010b). Adverse effect of oral vitamin E supplementation during the dry period on incidence of mastitis post partum in dairy cattle. In: Proc. XXVI World Buiatrics Cong. Nov. 14-18, 2010 Santiago de Chile, Chile.

Boxer, L.A. (1986). In: Proc. Nutri. Soc., 45: 333-338.

Bradley, A.J. and Green, M.J. (2001). In: Proc. 40th Annual Meeting of the National Mastitis Council, Reno, Nevada; 2001.

Bradley, A.J. and Green, M.J. (2004). Vet. Clin. Food Anim., 20: 547-568.

Bradley, A.J. and Green, M.J. (2006). The use of antibiotics in the treatment of intramammary infection at drying-off. In: Proc. World Buiatrics Cong., Nice, France, 2006.

Browning, J.W., Main, G.A., Barton, M., Nicholls, T.J. and Brightling, P. (1990). Aust. Vet. J., 67: 440-442.

Capuco, A.V. and Akers, R.M. (1999). J. Mammary Gland Biology & Neoplasia, 4(2): 137-144.

Chaiyotwittayakun, A., Erskine, R.J., Bartlett, P.C., Herd, T.H., Sears, P.M. and Harmont, R.J., (2002). J. Dairy Sci., 85: 60-67.

Chew, B.P. (1987). J. Dairy Sci., 70: 2732–2743.

Chew, B.P. (1995). J. Nutr., 125: 1804S–1808S.

Chew, B.P., Hollen, L.L., Hillers, J.K. and Herlugson, M.L. (1982). J. Dairy Sci., 65: 2111-2118.

Compton, C.W.R., Heuer, C., Parker, K. and McDougall, S. (2007). J. Dairy Sci., 90(9): 4171-4180.

Costello, S. (1998). http://www.moormans.com/dairy/DairyFF/dairysept98/mastitis.htm

Crispie, F.,Flynn, J., Ross, R.P., Hill, C. and Meaney, W.J. (2004). Irish Vet. J., 57(11): 652-656.

De Vliegher, S., Laevens, H., Barkema, H.W., Dohoo, I.R., Stryhn, H., Opsomer, G. and de Kruif, A. (2004). J. Dairy Sci., 87(4): 937-947.

Diarra, M.S., Petitclerc, D. and Lacasse, P. (2002). J. Dairy Sci., 85(5):1141-1149.

Diarra, M.S., Petitclerc, D., Deschênes, E., Lessard, N., Grondin, G., Talbot, B.G. and Lacasse, P. (2003). Vet. Immunol & Immunopathol, 95(1-2): 33-42.

Dingwell, R.T. (2002). Management strategies for the prevention and elimination of intramammary infections in non-lactating dairy cows. DVSc thesis, Guelph, Ontario: University of Guelph.

Dingwell, R.T., Conklin, J., Schlothauer, D., Martin, A., Sargeant, J. and Timms, L. (2001). In: Proc. 40th Annual Meeting National Mastitis council, 2001.

Dingwell, R.T., Kelton, D.F. and Leslie, K.E. (2003). Vet. Clin. Food Anim., 19: 235-265.

Diplock, A.T., Machlin, L.J., Packer, L. and Pryor, W.A. (1989). Ann. NY. Acad. Sci., p. 570.

Eberhart, R.L. (1986). J. Dairy Sci., 69: 1721-1732.

Erskine, R.J. and Bartlett, P.C. (1993). J. Dairy Sci., 76: 408-413.

Evans, H.M., Emerson, O.H. and Emerson, G.A. (1936). J. Biol. Chem. 113: 319.

Farnsworth, R.J., Wyman, L. and Hawkinson, R. (1980). J. Am. Vet. Med. Assoc., 177: 441-444.

Gakhar, G., Ranshawa, S.S., Ranshawa, C.S., Bansal, B.K. and Singh, R.S. (2010). Indian J. Anim. Sci., 80(8): 727-728.

Godden, S., Rapnicki, P., Stewart, S., Fetrow, J., Johnson, A., Bey, R. and Farnsworth, R. (2003). J. Dairy Sci., 86: 3899-3911.

Goff, J.P. (2006). J. Dairy Sci., 89: 1292-1301.

Goff, J.P., Kimura, K. and Horst, R.L. (2002). J. Dairy Sci., 85: 1427-1436.

Green, M.J., Green, L.E., Medley, G.F., Schukken, Y.H. and Bradley, A.J. (2002). J. Dairy Sci., 85(10): 2589-2599.

Halliwell, B. (1991). Am. J. Med., 91: 14-22.

Harmon, R.J. and Torre, P.M. (1994). In: Proc. National Mastitis Council Annual Meeting, Madoson, WI. pp. 54.

Hayton, A.J. (2003). An investigation into the efficacy of an external teat sealant and of factors affecting new intramammary infection rate during the dry period on organic farms. RCVS Diploma, RCVS, 2003.

Hoeben, D., Burnevich, C. and Heyneman, R. (1997). J. Dairy Sci., 81: 403-410.

Hoeben, D., Burnewitch, C. and Hamann, J. (2000). J. Dairy Res., 67: 485-502.

Hogan, J.S., Smith, K.L., Wiess, W.P., Todhunter, D.A. and Shockey, W.L. (1990). J. Dairy Sci., 73: 2372-2378.

Hogan, J.S.; Wiess, W.P., Todhunter, D.A., Smith, K.L. and Schoenberger. P.S. (1992). J. Dairy Sci., 75: 399-405.

Janosi, Sz. And Huszenicza, G. (2001). Vet. Med.-Czech, 46(2): 55-60.

Jukola, E., Hakkarainen, J., Saloniemi, H. And Sankari, S. (19996). J. Dairy Sci., 79: 838-845.

Kaiser, S., Di Mascio, P., Murphy, M.E. and Sies, H. (1990). Arch. Biochem. Biophys., 227: 101-108.

Kirk, J.H., Berry, S.L., Reynolds, J.P., *et al.* (1996). J. Am. Vet. Med. Assoc., 288: 1054-1057.

Kirk, J.H., Degraves, F and Tyler, J. (1994). J. Am. Vet. Med. Assoc., 204: 1152-1158.

Kleczkowski, M., Klucinski, W., Shaktur, A. and Sikora, J. (2005). Bull. Vet. Inst. Pulawy., 49: 203-207.

Klocke, P., Garbe, S., Spranger, J. and Merck, C.C. (2000). Homeopathic supported udder health control regarding cow associated factors in Brandenburg (D). In: Proc. 13th International IFOAM Scientific Conference, Basel, pp 343

Klocke, P., Ivemeyer, S., Walkenhorst, M., Maeschli, A. and Heil, F. (2006). Handling the dry-off problem in organic dairy herds by teat sealing or homeopathy compared to therapy omission. In: Proc. organic joint congress, Odense (DK), May 30th to 31st, 2006.

Kuehl, A.K. Jr. and R.W. Egan (1980). Science (Wash DC).. 210: 978-984.

LeBlanc, S.J., Lissemore, K.D., Kelton, D.F., Duffield, T.F. and Leslie, K.E. (2006). J. Dairy Sci., 89: 1267-1279.

Leslie, K.E. (1994). In: Radostits, O.M., Fetrow, J., editors. Herd health: food animal production medicine. 2nd edition. Philadelphia: WB Saunders, pp. 229–276.

Maiti, S.K., Sharma, Neelesh and Koley, K.M. (2004). Vet. Practitioner. 5(2):105-106.

Maiti, S.K., Sharma, Neelesh and Mukherjee, K. (2006). Indian J. field Vet. 2(1): 36-39.

Meaney, W.J. (1976). Vet. Rec., 99: 30.

Meaney, W.J. (1977). Ir. J. Agric. Res., 16: 293-299.

Meaney, W.J., Twomey, D.P., Flynn, J., Hill, C. and Ross, R.P. (2001). In: Proc. British Mastitis Conf., Garstang, pp. 24-32.

Melendez, P., Hofer, C.C. and Donovan, G.A. (2006). Prev. Vet. Med., 76(3-4): 211-221.

Michal, J.J., Heirman, L.R., Wong, T.S., Chew, B.P., Frigg, M. And Volker, L. (1994). J. Dairy Sci., 77: 1408-1421.

Middleton, J.R., Luby, C.D., Viera, L., Tyler, J.W. and Casteel, S. (2004). J. Dairy Sci., 87: 976-979.

Monicada, S. and Vane, J.R. (1979). In: The Prostaglandin System: Endoperoxides, prostacyclin, and Thromboxanes. Eds. F. Berti, G.F. velo. Plenum Press, New york. pp. 203-221.

Nath, K. and Dutta, J.B. (2005). Intl. J. Cow Sci., 1(1): 63-65.

National Research Council (1989). Nutrient requirement of dairy cattle. 6th rev. ed. Natl. Acad. Sci., Washington, DC.

Nauriyal, D.S. and Pachauri, S.P. (1997). In Proc. Of Natl. Symp. Of Indian Soc. For Vet. Med., held at Bangalore, Feb.20-22.

Neijenhuis, F., Barkema, H.W., Hogeveen, H. and Noordhuizen, J.P.T.M. (2000). J. Dairy Sci., 83: 2795-2804.

Nickerson, S.C. (1994). In: Comp. dairy research report, Hill Farm Research Station, Lousiana State University, pp. 1-11.

O'Rourke, D. (2009). J. Irish Vet. 62:15-20.

Oldham, E.R., Eberhart, R.J. and Muller, L.D. (1991). J. Dairy Sci., 74: 3775-3781.

Oliver, S.P., Gillespie, B.E., Ivey, S.J., Lewis, M.J., Johnson, D.L., Lamar, K.C., Moorehead, H., Dowlen, H.H., Chester, S.T. and Hallberg, J.W. (2004). J. Dairy Sci., 87(6): 1727 - 1731.

Oliver, S.P., Lewis, M.J., Gillespie, B.E., Dowlen, H.H., Jaenicke, E.C. and Roberts, R.K. (2003). J. Dairy Sci., 86(4): 1187-1193.

Osteras, O. and Sandvik, L. (1996). J. Vet. Med. B, 45: 555-575.

Pachauri, S.P., Singh, S.V. and Nauriyal, D.S. (2001). Indian Vet. Med. J., 25: 317-321.

Pearson, J.K.L. (1950). Vet. Rec., 62: 166-168.

Person, K., Larsson, I. and Hallen, S.C. (1993). Vet. Immunol. Immunopath.. 37: 99.

Politis, L., Hidiroglou, M., Batra, T.R., Gorewit, R.C. and Scherf, H. (1995). Am. J. Vet. Res. 56: 179-184.

Politis, L., Hidiroglou, M., White, J., Gilmore, J.A., Williams, S., Scherf, H. and Frigg, M. (1996). Am. J. Vet. Res., 57: 468-471.

Poutrel, B. and Rainard, P. (1981). J. Dairy Sci., 64: 241-248.

Radostits, O.M., Gay, C.C., Blood, D.C. and Hinchkliff, K.W. (2006). Veterinary Medicine. 10th edn. ELBS & Baillier Tindall.

Rice, D. and Kennedy, S. (1986). In: Proc. Roche Symposium, London, England. Pp.1-23.

Rogers, L.A. and Whittier, E.O. (1928). J. Bacteriol., 16: 211-214.

Rotruck, J.T., Pope, A.L., Ganther, H.E., Swanson, A.B., Hafeman, D.G. and Hoekstra, W.G. (1973). Science, 179:585.

Samanta, A.K., Sharma, R.K., Ramachndran, M., Mandal, G.P. and Rastogi, A. (2005). In: Proc. of XXI Annl. Conv. and Natnl. Symp. Of ISSAR Nov. 23rd – 25th Nov., F.V.Sc. & A.H., R.S. Pura, Jammu. P. 214.

Sanchez, M.S. and Watts, J.L. (1999). J. Dairy Sci., 82(3): 494-499.

Sargeant, .JM., Leslie, K.E., Shirley, J.E., Pulkrabek, B. and Lim, G.H. (2001). J. Dairy Sci., 84: 2018-2024.

Scaletti, R.W., Trammell, D.S., Smith, B.A. and Harmon, R.J. (2003). J. Dairy Sci., 86: 1240–1249.

Schukken, Y.H., Vanvliet, J., Vandegeer, D. and Grommers, F.J. (1993). J. Dairy Sci., 76: 2925-2930.

Sears, P.M., Wilson, D.J. and Gonzalez, R.N. (1992). In: Proc. XVII World Buiatrics Cong. (Williams, E.I. ed), Am. Assoc. Bovine Pract., Stillwater, Ok, USA, pp. 138-142.

Sharma, Neelesh (2003). Epidemiological study on sub-clinical mastitis in dairy animals: Role of vit E and Selenium supplementation on its control in cattle. M.V.Sc. thesis, IG.KVV., Raipur (C.G.) India.

Sharma, Neelesh (2007). Asian J. Anim. Vet. Adv., 2(2): 50-62.

Sharma, Neelesh (2008). Vetcare Bulletin, pp. 1-11.

Sharma, Neelesh (2010). SMVS Dairy Year Book-2010. Published by Sarva Manav Vikash Samiti, Gurgoan, India. pp. 47-65.

Sharma, Neelesh and Maiti, S.K. (2004). In: Proc. of IV Ann. Conf. Indian Soc. Vet. Pharmacol. and Toxicol., 22-24 Dec., Anjora, Durg (C.G.), p. 101.

Sharma, Neelesh and Maiti, S.K. (2005). Indian J. Vet. Med., 25(2): 76-79.

Sharma, Neelesh, Gautam, A., Upadhyay, S.R., Hussain K., Soodan, J.S. and Gupta, S.K.(2006). Indian J. Field Vet., 2(1): 73-76.

Sharma, Neelesh, Gupta, S.K., Soodan, J.S. and Upadhyay, S.R. (2005). In: Mineral Imbalances in Livestock and their Impact on Animal Health and Production, (ed. Singh, R. and Srivastava, A.K.). pp.139-148.

Sharma, Neelesh, Maiti, S.K. and Roy, S. (2003). Vet. Practitioner. 4(2): 140-143.

Sharma, Neelesh, Maiti, S.K., Mukherjee, K., Ghosh, S.C. and Roy, S. (2005). Indian Vet. J., 82: 675-676.

Smith, K.L., Conrad, H.R., Amiet, B.A. and Todhunter, D.A. (1985). Forschungsber., 37: 482.

Smith, K.L., Harrison, Hancock, D.D., Todhunter, D.A. and Conrad, H.R. (1984). J. Dairy Sci., 67: 1293.

Smith, K.L., Hogan, J.S. and Weiss, W.P. (1997). J. Anim. Sci. 75:1659-1665.

Smith, K.L., Todhunte,r D.A. and Schoenberger, P.S. (1985). J. Dairy Sci., 68(2): 402-417.

Soback, S., Ziv, G., Winkler, M. and Saran, A. (1990). J. Dairy Sci., 73: 661.

Sordillo, L.M. and Nickerson, S.C. (1988). Am. J. Vet. Res., 49: 1112.

Sordillo, L.M., Nickerson, S.C., Akers, R.M. and Oliver, S.P. (1987). J. Dairy Sci., 72: 228.

Sordillo, L.M., Shafer-Weaver, K. and DeRosa, D. (1997). J. Dairy Sci., 80(8):1851-1865.

Spears, J.W. (2000). In: Proc. Nutr. Soc., 59: 587-594.

Taylor, J.I., Hirsch, A. and Mattick, A.T.R. (1949). Vet. Rec., 61: 197-198.

Technote, 14 (2000). Decide dry cow mastitis strategy - drying off dates and dry cow treatment. Jan, 2000. Pp. 1-6. www.dairyautralia.com.au

Timms, L.L., Steffens, A., Piggot, S. and Allen, L. (1997). In: Proc. National Mastitis Council, pp. 201-203.

Uppal, S.K., Dua, K. and Randhawa, C.S. (2005). In: Mineral Imbalances in Livestock and their Impact on Animal Health and Production, (ed. Singh, R. and Srivastava, A.K.). pp98-108.

Vliestra, R.J. (2003). In: Proc. National Mastitis Council Regional Meeting, pp. 30-35.

Weiss, W.P. and Hogan, J.S. (2007). J. Dairy Sci., 90: 731-739.

Weiss, W.P., Hogan, J.S. and Smith, K.L. (1994). Agri. Practice., 15(7): 5.

Weiss, W.P., Hogan, J.S. and Smith, K.L. (2004). J. Dairy Sci., 87: 32-37.

Weiss, W.P., Hogan, J.S., Todhunter, D.A. and Smith, K.L (1997). J.Dairy Sci., 80: 1728.

Wilde, D. (2006). Anim. Reprod. Sci., 96: 240-249.

Williamson, J.H., Woolford, M.W. and Day, A,M. (1995). New Zealand Vet. J., 43(6): 228-234.

Woolford, M.W., Williamson, J.H., Day, A.M. and Copeman, P.J.A. (1998). New Zealand Vet. J., 46: 12-19.

Ziv, G., Storper, M. and Saran, A. (1981). Vet. Quart., 3: 74-79.

□□□

About the Authors

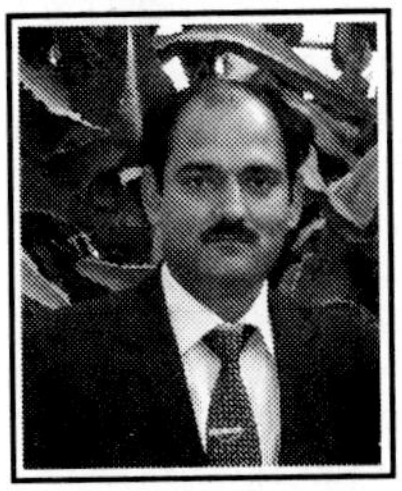

Dr. Neelesh Sharma is graduated in Veterinary Science & Animal Husbandry in 2001 from the College of Veterinary Science, Mhow (J.N.K.V.V., Jabalpur), Madhya Pradesh, India and post-graduated in Veterinary Medicine from College of Veterinary Science, Anjora, Durg (I.G.K.V.V., Raipur), Chhattisgarh, India. He has more than 8 years of experience in teaching research and extension. Dr. Sharma started his professional career as Research Fellow at Faculty of Veterinary Science and Animal Husbandry, Jammu and later he joined as Assistant Professor in September, 2005, in the same faculty. Dr. Sharma is an "*ICAR-International Fellow*". He is recipient of The Bronze Standard International Award by HRH The Duke of Edinburgh. Dr. Sharma has conferred for "IAAVR Merit Award-2011" by Indian Association for the Advancement of Veterinary Research, Bareilly, India. He has also received the best paper award by Indian Association for the Advancement of Veterinary Science (IAAVR), India and appreciation award from RIAM, Delhi. Dr. Sharma has worked as collaborating scientist in two National and one International (Angila Ruskin University, Cambridge, England) research projects. He has published more than 75 publications in journals of National and International repute. He has authored a practical manual of Veterinary Clinical Medicine-II and three books in veterinary science, and contributed 09 chapters in books. His recent book is on "*Production Diseases of Dairy Animals*" by Satish Serial Publishing House, Delhi. He is a member of various scientific societies. He had reviewer and technical editor of International Journal of Dairy Science, Research Journal of Veterinary Sciences, Asian Journal of Animal Sciences, Asian Journal of Animal and Veterinary Advances, Vet Scan and regional editor of Pakistan Journal of Life & Social Sciences. He is also a chief editor of a Scientific Journal. "The Journal of Animal Research". Dr. Sharma presently focusing on stem cell therapy in Mastitis at Jeju National University, South Korea. At present he is working as Assistant Professor, Division of Veterinary Clinical Medicine & Jurisprudence, Faculty of Veterinary Sciences & Animal Husbandry, SKUAST-J, R.S. Pura, Jammu, India.

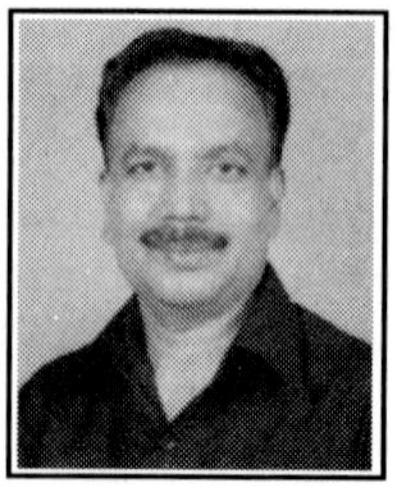

Dr. Anil Kumar Srivastava, Director & Vice-Chancellor of National Dairy Research Institute (Deemed University), Karnal, India has obtained B.V.Sc. & A. H. and M. V. Sc. degrees from Veterinary College, Mathura and Doctoral degree from PAU, Ludhiana. He is recipient the coveted German Academic Exchange Fellowship to work as DAAD Fellow at Munich (Germany).

Dr. Srivastava started his professional career as Assistant Professor at Panjab Agricultural University Ludhiana, where he served for 20 years in different capacities including Professor & Head, Department of Pharmacology and Toxicology and Controller of Examinations. Before assuming the office of the Director & Vice-Chancellor of NDRI Deemed University, he was Director, Resident Instructions and Dean Postgraduate Studies and Dean, Faculty of Veterinary Sciences and Animal Husbandry at Sher-e-Kashmir University of Agricultural Sciences & Technology, Jammu (J&K). To his credit he has authored 09 books and manuals, edited 18 books/ proceedings/ monographs and bulletins and published more than 220 research papers in journals of National and International repute. He has guided 14 M.V.Sc. and 10 Ph.D scholars.

He has been decorated with numerous prestigious awards including ICAR Jawaharlal Nehru Award; International NOCL Award on "Pesticides: Toxicity, Safety and Risk Assessment; National Alarsin Award by Indian Veterinary Association and Best Paper Awards by Indian Science Congress Association and other societies.

Dr. Srivastava has been conferred with fellowships by a number of professional bodies and associations which include: National Academy of Agricultural Sciences, National Academy of Veterinary Sciences, Indian Association for Advancement of Veterinary Research, Society of Toxicology, Society of Environmental Sciences, Society of Sciences, International Society for Ecological Communications and Member of National Academy of Sciences. Dr. Srivastava has organized 15 International and National Conferences/ Symposia/ Seminar and ICAR & CSIR training. He had held important positions in many professional societies *i.e.* Founder chief Editor, Indian Journal of Veterinary Pharmacology & Toxicology, Member advisory Board, Indian Journal of Toxicology, Editor, Polivet Journal, Technical Advisor, Vets Bulletin, Member Editorial Board, Journal of Current Sciences and Journal of Research, SKUAST-J, Member Advisory Board, Vetspex, Member, Editorial Board, Councilor, Punjab Academy of Sciences and Member, J&K Council of Science and Technology. Presently he is also the Secretary of National Academy of Agricultural Sciences.

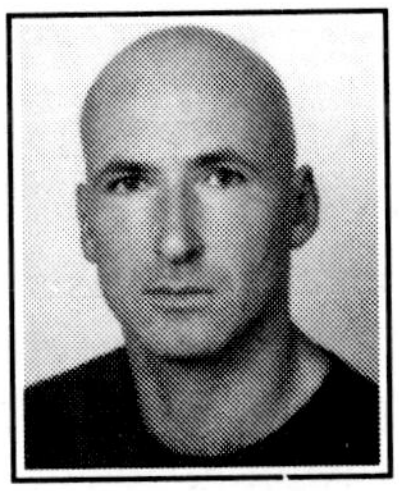

Dr. Goran Bacic received his Bachelor of Veterinary Sciences in 1990 at Veterinary College, Zagreb Univeristy, Croatia. He accomplished his postgraduation study in 1994 and PhD in 1999. Dr. Bacic spent year 2001 at Veterinary College, Cornell University, Ithaca, NY, USA for specialization in Herd Health and Production Management. Dr Bacic participated in numerous visiting veterinarian programs at Large Animal Hospital Veterinary College Cornell University, Ithaca, NY, USA.

Dr. Bacic has experience of various research and teaching posts since 1994. Together with Assistant Professor Tugomir Karadjole and Teaching Assistant Nino Macesic. Dr Bacic was a founder of Laparoscopic Team for Small Animal Gynecology Surgery at the Clinic For Reproduction and Theriogenology. He became Professor at the Clinic For Reproduction and Theriogenology and Ambulatory Service with Herd Health Management, Veterinary College University of Zagreb in 2007 and then became a Head of the Ambulatory and Herd Health Department at 2009.

Dr Bacic has published more than 80 international and domestic papers, wrote one University text book "Diagnostic and treatment of mastitis in cows", participated in some chapters and in numerous domestic and foreign Conferences. He is a member of AABP, ESDAR and Croatian Veterinary Society and reviewer in Journal Croatian Veterinary Archive. Dr Bacic was successful mentor in numerous student graduate thesis and in a few MSc and PhD thesis. Dr Bacic participated as invited lecturer in USAID - CROATIA training program "Best Milking Farm Practices" together with international expert Dr. Arun Phatak from UC Davis, California.

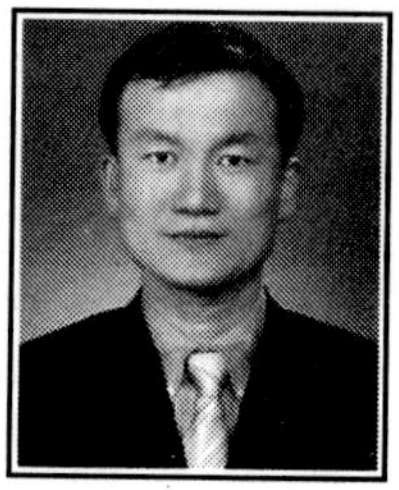

Dr. Dong Kee Jeong received Bachelor degree of agricultural education in 1992 at College of Education, Sunchon National University, South Korea. He finished Master degree and defended MSc thesis "The study on the chromosome karyotype of Korea wild pig" in 1994. He studied during Ph.D. period on focused production of transgenic animal using stem cells and defended Ph.D. thesis "Studies on the efficient separation of primordial germ cells and introduction of foreign DNA in the chicken" in 1999. After finished his Ph.D. in Animal Science and Biotechnology from the Seoul National University, South Korea. He has worked Korean NIH. His research project in the Korea NIH is transgenic mouse production as an animal disease model, embryonic stem cell establishment and genetic diagnosis of human genetic disease during 2 years. He moved to USA and had worked at Washington State University and Johns Hopkins University as a researcher. He worked as a Post-doc fellow about spermatogonial stem cell research field and gene regulation in the genome. Also, he worked hematopoietic stem cells in the human clinical trial and gene signal pathway in the stem cell field. He has authored and coauthored about 60 papers on Biotechnology, stem cells and transgenic animal including long-term culture and transplantation of murine spermatogonial stem cells. J. of Andrology(2004), improved germline transmission in chicken chimeras produced by transplantation of gonadal primordial germ cells into recipient embryo(2003), Gene transfer into long-term cultured murine spermatogonial stem cell (2005). In 2005 he accepted the position of Assistant professor at Jeju National University for the Animal Biotechnology and stem cell biology. At year 2009 he became Associate Professor and Head of Department during 2 years. He is now working for the cancer stem cell and stem cell therapy for the livestock at Universityof Calgary, Canada as a visiting professor from 2010-2011.

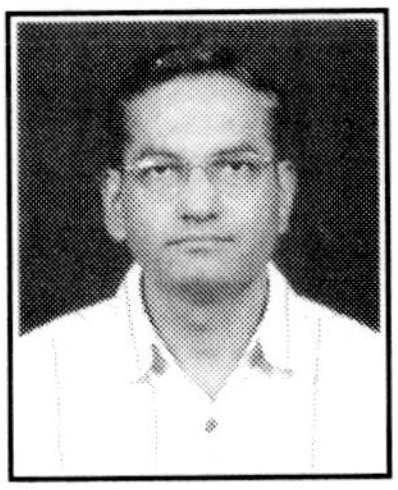

Dr. Rajesh Kumar Sharma received his Bachelor degree of Veterinary Sciences and Animal Husbandry in 1987 at College of Veterinary Science and Animal Husbandry, Jawaharlal Nehru Krishi Vishwa Vidyalaya, Jabalpur (M.P.), India. He accomplished his postgraduation in Veterinary Pharmacology and Toxicology in 1989 and received Shri Ramlal Agrawal Memorial National Award (1990) on his Research Work. Thereafter, he joined as Veterinary Assistant Surgeon, Madhya Pradesh State Government Services and continued till 1994. In 1994 he joined as Assistant Professor and I/C, Department of Pharmacology and Toxicology, College of Veterinary Science and Animal Husbandry, Mhow (M.P.), He did his PhD in 2003.

Dr. Sharma has experience of various research and teaching posts since 1994, he has Guided Postgraduate students for their research work in Veterinary Pharmacology, Veterinary Medicine, Veterinary Surgery, Veterinary Microbiology, Veterinary Obstetrics and Gynaecology, Veterinary Physiology and Veterinary Biochemistry and has been Major advisor for six M.V.Sc. Student and Minor Advisor for 20 students. He is a life member of a number of academic associations and is Life Member of Indian Society of Veterinary Pharmacology and Toxicology and Indian Association for Advancement of Veterinary Research.

Dr Sharma has published more than 50 National and International papers and has delivered a number of lectures; he is an active participant in extension work. He has also written a monograph on Anti-Inflammatory drugs published by Indian Journal of Indigenous Medicine. At present he is the Principal investigator in two projects. At present he is Associate Professor, Department of Veterinary Pharmacology & Toxicology, College of Veterinary Science and A. H., Jabalpur (M.P.), India.